Jonathan E. Rhoads

EIGHTIETH BIRTHDAY SYMPOSIUM

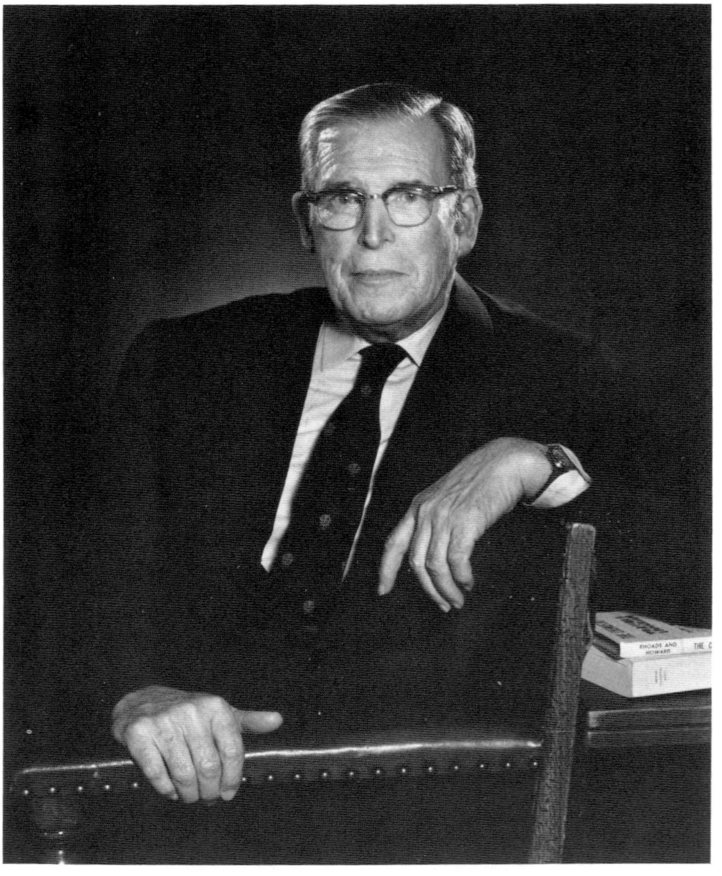
RHOADS AND HOWARD
THE

Jonathan E. Rhoads

EIGHTIETH BIRTHDAY SYMPOSIUM

EDITED BY

Clyde F. Barker, M.D.

John M. Daly, M.D.

May 9, 1987

The authors and publisher have exerted every effort to ensure that drug selection and dosage set forth in this text are in accord with current recommendations and practice at the time of publication. However, in view of ongoing research, changes in government regulations, and the constant flow of information relating to drug therapy and drug reactions, the reader is urged to check the package insert for each drug for any change in indications and dosage and for added warnings and precautions. This is particularly important when the recommended agent is a new or infrequently employed drug.

For information write J. B. Lippincott Company, East Washington Square, Philadelphia, Pennsylvania 19105.

1 3 5 6 4 2

Library of Congress Cataloging in Publication Data
Main entry under title:

Jonathan E. Rhoads: Eightieth Birthday Symposium

Bibliography: p.
1. Surgery—Congresses. 2. Rhoads, Jonathan E.
I. Rhoads, Jonathan E. II. Barker, Clyde F.
III. Daly, John M.
RD9.2.J66 1989 617 89-2428

ISBN 0-397-51006-3
Printed in the United States of America

Table of Contents

Symposium Contributions (presented at the scientific meeting on May 9, 1987)

Commemorative Articles

These written communications were contributed in honor of Dr. Rhoads by his trainees, but were not presented at the scientific meeting on May 9, 1987.

Foreword

FOR THOSE who were in Philadelphia for Dr. Rhoads' Eightieth Birthday Symposium, this volume may recall some of the special moments in which his trainees (now leaders in American Surgery) reminisced about their residency days and exchanged expressions of affection and esteem with their chief. The warmth and intimacy of this reunion, a scientific program worthy of any national meeting, and the attendance of many of the country's senior surgeons combined to make the weekend of May 9, 1987 a remarkable one.

The last section of this volume would in itself justify the publication since it contains the remarkable curriculum vitae and bibliography of Jonathan E. Rhoads. Dr. Rhoads is a Philadelphian, born in Germantown on May 9, 1907 to Margaret and Edward Rhoads who were also Philadelphians. In 1885, his father, Edward Rhoads, served his internship under D. Hayes Agnew and William Osler at the Hospital of the University of Pennsylvania, the nation's first University Hospital that had opened only 11 years before. Jonathan Rhoads was educated at Haverford College where he was Phi Beta Kappa and an outstanding varsity athlete, and then at Johns Hopkins where he was AOA, as was his classmate and wife to be Terry Folin, the daughter of Otto Folin, Chairman of Biochemistry at Harvard. Returning to Philadelphia in 1932 as an intern at the Hospital of the University of Pennsylvania, Dr. Rhoads completed his surgical residency training there under I. S. Ravdin in 1939. Less than a year later, Dr. Ravdin endorsed his young lieutenant by selecting Rhoads as his personal surgeon when he required an operation for acute cholecystitis. Dr. Rhoads later served the University of Pennsylvania as J. William White Professor of Surgical Research, Provost (1956 to 1959), and succeeded Dr. Ravdin in 1959 as John Rhea Barton Professor and Chairman of the Department of Surgery and Director of the Harrison Department of Surgical Research.

As noted in the introductions of the symposium speakers, Dr. Rhoads' list of 343 publications contains many that are pertinent to the modern state of almost every subject discussed during the Symposium. Furthermore, from the earliest days the bibliography contained entries that would prove to be of seminal importance in fields as varied as nutrition, cancer, renal failure, immunology, and gastrointestinal hormones and physiology. As an editor, Dr. Rhoads has served the *Journal of Surgical Research*, the *Journal of Clinical Surgery*, the *Annals of Surgery* (as chairman from 1971 to 1973), and *Cancer* (which he still edits). In his book "A Century of Surgery," Mark Ravitch credits Rhoads and his co-editors Alan, Harkins, and Moyer with initiating the first of the great multiauthored surgery texts.

Surgical colleges of other nations that have honored Dr. Rhoads with honorary fellowships include those of England, Edinburgh, Canada, Poland, South Africa, Holland, Germany, and India. He has been president of many of his 65 professional societies, including the Society of Surgical Chairmen, the Society of Clinical Surgery, the Philadelphia County Medical Society, the International Surgical Group, the International Federation of Surgical Colleges, the College of Physicians of Philadelphia, the Association of American Medical Colleges, the American Surgical Association, the Society for Surgery of the Alimentary Tract, the American College of Surgeons, the American Cancer Society, the Philadelphia Academy of Surgery, the Surgical Infection Society, and the American Philosophical Society. His special awards and honors include the following: the Distinguished Service Awards of the American Surgical Association, the American Trauma Society, and the American Cancer Society; the Strettmater Award of the Philadelphia County Medical Society; the Sheen Award of the American Medical Association for Scientific Accomplishment; and the Philadelphia Award as the city's first citizen, which he won in the bicentennial year of 1976. It is virtually impossible to summarize his record in government services, National Institutes of Health study sections, or civic, educational, and professional boards, such as the trustee boards of Bryn Mawr and Haverford colleges, the latter of which he has chaired. Almost as numerous are his honorary degrees from universities such as the University of Pennsylvania, Haverford, Swarthmore, the Medical College of Pennsylvania, Jefferson, Hahnemann, Georgetown, the Medical College of Ohio at Toledo, and Duke.

The tribute to Dr. Rhoads given at the Symposium banquet by Dr. Francis Moore, another giant of twentieth century surgery, was particularly effective in assigning historical prospective to his scientific contributions. Dr. Moore praised Dr. Rhoads for the "bull dog tenacity" with which for 20 years he pursued an obsession to perfect parenteral nutrition, a pursuit culminating in one of the great classic experiments in all of medicine that was concisely recorded in an abstract appearing in *Federation Proceedings* in March 1986 entitled "Total Intravenous Feeding and Growth in Puppies" by S. J. Dudrick, H. M. Vars, H. M. Rawnsley, and J. E. Rhoads. It read as follows:

> To date 12 week old male beagle pups have received their total nutritive requirements by a near-continuous intravenous infusion for 175, 72, 30 and 30 days. The daily per kilo intake of water, calories, glucose, amino acids (Aminosol), Ca and P has been 150–180 ml, 120–140, 25 gm, 4 gm, 2 meq was infused separately. All vitamins and other minerals known to be required for the dog were supplied also by vein. Only tapwater was available for oral consumption. . . . Body size and metabolic responses were comparable to those observed in their littermate controls which received orally a standard ration at the same caloric level. The animal which was infused the longest period increased in weight from 3.4 to 11.2 kg.

That puppies fed only by vein grew normally was an entirely new phenomenon that needed no statistical analysis. This was work that Dr. Moore ranks with only a few other landmarks to which the entire world of biology and medicine owes a debt to surgery, instead of the more usual other way round. The other examples he cited were extracorporeal oxygenation, the allotransplantation of organs, microvascular anastomosis, the endocrine treatment of cancer, and the functional localization of areas in the cerebral cortex. Drs. Longmire and Bell, the other after dinner speakers, praised Dr. Rhoads for his statesman-like contributions to surgery and his place in the broad scientific community as President of the American Philosophical Society.

However, many of us feel that his greatest contribution has been as a teacher, the leader of a great school of surgery at the University of Pennsylvania that in his 13 years as chairman turned out 62 surgeons who have served as faculty members in 34 different medical schools, 28 as full professors and 10 as chairmen. It was his impact as a teacher that inspired the Birthday Symposium and shaped its format. The idea came to me first (as many things in my life have) from my brother, Dr. Harold G. Barker, Hospital of the University of Pennsylvania Chief Resident from 1951 to 1952, Professor of Surgery at Columbia, and a medical historian. He showed me volumes commemorating the birthdays of greats of other generations, such as Harvey Cushing, William Welsh, and Lord Lister, whose trainees after themselves achieving prominence met to honor their chiefs with symposia of their scientific accomplishments. Our plan was to invite a group of Dr. Rhoads' former residents to present papers, to entertain them and some of his close friends in surgery with a party, and perhaps to publish a small commemorative volume. However, his residents responded with such enthusiasm that it was soon evident that our most difficult task would be limiting the occasion to controllable (and affordable) dimensions. The following former Hospital of the University of Pennsylvania residents of international fame were selected as speakers: Ted Copeland, Bill Curreri, Gordon Danielson, Stan Dudrick, Cleon Goodwin, Jim Hardy, John Howard, Scott Jones, Ed Kaplan, Carter Nance, Marshall Orloff, Frank Rosato, Harvey Sugerman, Jim Thompson, John Waldhausen, and Doug Wilmore. This list included only a few of the ex-residents who would have been logical choices for speakers. It was also unfortunate that in a one day program there would be no time available to hear from current Penn faculty members, whose research I therefore undertook to summarize.

The decision to invite some of Dr. Rhoads' closest friends from other institutions converted the Symposium from a small reunion of his former residents to a major national meeting. Accepting invitations to attend the meeting were senior surgeons from all parts of the country, such as Charles Huggins, the Nobel laureate, Harry Muller, Claude Welch, Stan Levenson, David Skinner, Harry Shoemaker, Lloyd Nyhus, Isidore Cohn, Frank Spencer, William Beck, George Stephenson, Dick Myers, Bill Glenn, Ward Griffen, Basil Pruitt, Mark Ravitch, Clarence Dennis, Frazer Gurd, Lasalle Leffal, and others. Bill Longmire, Francis Moore, and Whitfield Bell agreed to give after dinner talks. The growing size of the acceptance list soon presented a particular problem with regard to the banquet that was to be held at Philosophical Hall. This historic facility on Independence Square, so appropriate because Dr. Rhoads presided there from 1977 to 1984 as President of the American Philosophical Society, was large enough to accommodate only Dr. Rhoads' chief residents, family, surgical faculty colleagues, and out of town guests. Therefore, his former junior residents, friends, and colleagues from other disciplines presented their respects the evening before at a reception attended by over 400 people at another historic site, Lincoln Hall of the Union League of Philadelphia.

The organizing committee included Jack Mackie and Gordon Buzby, in addition to John Daly (the J. E. Rhoads Professor) and myself. Also contributing to the planning (and doing most of the work) were my wife Dode and my secretary Fran Ramirez. Dr. Rhoads' editorial assistant Donna Muldoon, Dr. Rhoads' classmate and life-long amateur photography expert Ted Hetzel, and Dr. Rhoads' family and neighbors were invaluable in unearthing old documents and photographs that were background material for presentation. Drs. John Howard, Doug Wilmore, Bob Welty, and Mr. Dave Douglas also took photographs of the Birthday Symposium, some of which are included in the section entitled "Symposium Highlights." Dr. Daly's secretary Carla Tolino-Panaccio provided valuable editorial assistance.

Both the scientific and social aspects of the weekend were successful. Many regarded the quality of the scientific program as equal to that of major national surgical societies. Dr. Rhoads and his family seemed to enjoy the whole affair immensely. All six of his children and eleven of his grandchildren were in attendance, some having come from as far away as Australia. Terry Rhoads appeared to be particularly vivacious and pleased. Her participation in the planning included the contribution of some important personal family material for presentation at the banquet. I was seated next to her and will not soon forget her exclamation that the after dinner speeches were "marvelous."

Only three days later, Terry Rhoads died suddenly while attending a luncheon with Mrs. William Altemier and other friends. For many of us the shock of this put a pall on the Birthday Symposium for months and was an unnerving reminder that the volume commemorating Harvey Cushing's seventieth birthday appeared after his death. However, as time went by and the manuscripts that had been asked for appeared and began to pile up, it became clear that this volume must be prepared and that Dr. Rhoads was looking forward to it.

Since time constraints allowed so few of the many logical choices as speakers to be invited to participate in the Symposium, invitations were sent to all former Hospital of the University of Pennsylvania residents to contribute to the published volume. Papers that were received are included as Commemorative Articles. Because of an aversion of pressing people for papers (or being pressed for them) this invitation was not repeated. The number of commemorative articles could have undoubtedly been increased had our objective been a comprehensive collection, but this section was included only to provide an opportunity for those anxious to be represented. Nevertheless, the 39 Commemorative Articles provide an interesting sample that in addition to a number of fine scientific papers (some original, some reprinted) includes the presidential address of John Daly (the Jonathan E. Rhoads Professor) at the American Society of Parenteral and Enteral Nutrition, a paper on AIDS by Surgeon General Koop, a personal recollection of the Hospital of the University of Pennsylvania's surgical service at the time of Dr. Rhoads' internship by Charles McLaughlin, and even a poem to Dr. Rhoads by James Long.

All of the papers delivered at the Symposium are included under Symposium Contributions. As noted, several of these papers had also been delivered or published elsewhere. Perhaps of even more interest than the scientific content of these papers were the anecdotes included by the speakers regarding their residency experiences and Dr. Rhoads' influence on their careers. Fortunately, since this symposium was recorded it was possible through the considerable efforts and skills of my secretary Fran Ramirez to include many of these priceless stories.

Although Dr. Rhoads had informed me several years before of his intent to stop operating when he reached 80, it hardly seemed possible to those of us trained by him and to his current faculty colleagues that 7 weeks after the Symposium Dr. Rhoads would actually do this, especially since there was a Whipple procedure on his schedule only a few days before. However, in every other way he remains as busy and productive as ever. He continues to write, see patients, edit the journal *Cancer*, and is in many ways the most productive member of the faculty. He continues to be the most consistent participant in departmental conferences and meetings, when his incredibly busy travel schedule and commitments to trustee boards and the like allow it. If it were not for these activities he would probably be kept busy simply by collecting the honors that he continues to accumulate. Since the Birthday Symposium he has had named in his honor the annual Oration of the Philadelphia Academy of Surgery (first delivered in 1881 by Samuel D. Gross) and has been awarded the Benjamin Franklin Medal of the American Philosophical Society (its highest honor), the Medal of the Surgeon General of the United States, the Swanberg Award of the American Medical Writers Association, membership in the Institute of Medicine of the National Academy of Science, and the Distinguished Service Award of the College of Physicians of Philadelphia. The presentation of the later award was reminiscent of Dr. Moore's after dinner speech at the Birthday Symposium in placing Dr. Rhoads' contribution in prospective with others of his and earlier eras. Only four awards were given by the College at this special meeting that marked its 200th anniversary. One award went posthumously to John Gibbon for extracorporeal circulation, another to Britton Chance and Mildred Cohn for magnetic resonance imaging, one to Robert Gallo for work on monoclonal antibodies. and one to Dr. Rhoads for his work in nutrition.

Many have commented before and after the eightieth birthday on the special place in American surgery occupied by Jonathan Rhoads. David Sabiston often refers to him as the Dean of American Surgery, a title that Dr. Rhoads says he is not particularly fond of. However, I think he may have enjoyed another particularly fitting tribute that came during last year's annual D. Hayes Agnew Lecture at the University of Pennsylvania from John Cameron, the current Chief of Surgery at his alma mater. Dr. Cameron recalled that in 1889 William Osler had been recruited from the Penn faculty to head the Department of Medicine at Johns Hopkins' new school. Dr. Cameron said, "When Jonathan Rhoads left Baltimore in 1932 to become an intern at the University of Pennsylvania, Hopkins finally returned the favor in kind."

While reviewing the material that has been collected for this publication, I was struck by the possibility that the volume may eventually prove interesting not only to Dr. Rhoads' residents, family, and friends, but also to those who will write the history of medicine in the last two thirds of the twentieth century, a period spanned by Dr. Rhoads' career. Videotapes of the symposium and banquet speeches will reside in the Archives of the American College of Surgeons under Dr. George Stephenson's care. It is also hoped that this collection will be of some value to the eventual biographers of Jonathan Rhoads by recording a few of the highlights of his first 80 years. In any case, it has been a privilege to be involved with the collection, just as it has always been a privilege to be associated with Dr. Rhoads as his trainee and colleague.

Clyde F. Barker, M.D.
November 15, 1988

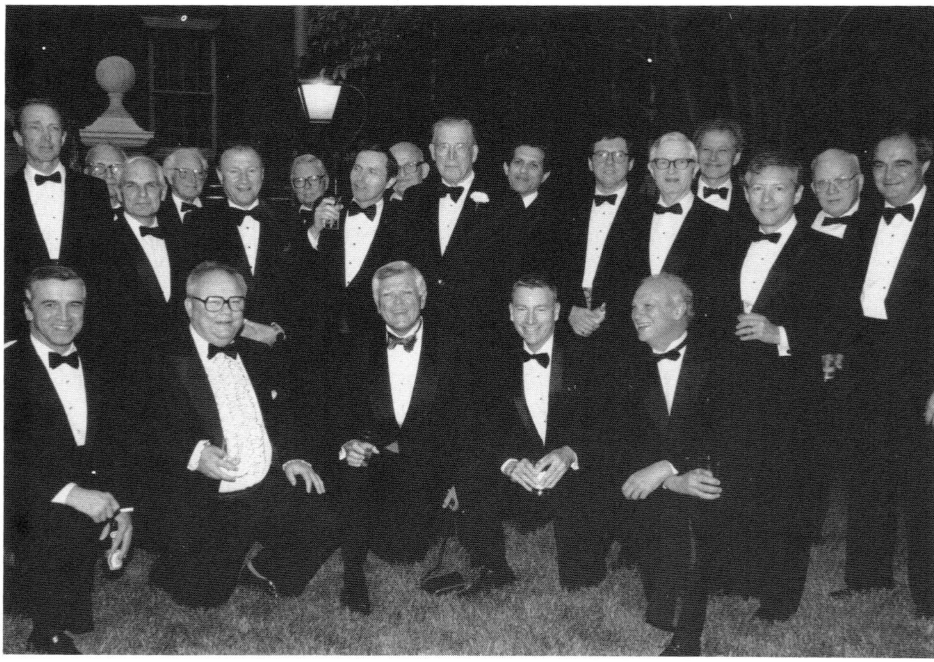

The speakers at the Jonathan E. Rhoads Birthday Symposium. Front row (left to right)*: Stanley J. Dudrick, C. Francis Nance, James C. Thompson, Clyde F. Barker, and Francis E. Rosato. Back row* (left to right)*: Gordon Danielson, Mark Ravitch, John A. Waldhausen, Francis D. Moore, Marshal J. Orloff, William Longmire, R. Scott Jones, John M. Howard, Jonathan E. Rhoads, Edwin L. Kaplan, Cleon W. Goodwin, James D. Hardy, Douglas W. Wilmore, Harvey J. Sugerman, Whitfield J. Bell, and P. William Curreri.*

Symposium Speakers

Clyde F. Barker, M.D.
Professor and Chairman
Department of Surgery
University of Pennsylvania

Edward M. Copeland, III, M.D.
Professor and Chairman
Department of Surgery
University of Florida

P. William Curreri, M.D.
Professor and Chairman
Department of Surgery
University of South Alabama
College of Medicine

Gordon Danielson, M.D.
Professor of Surgery
Mayo Clinic

Stanley J. Dudrick, M.D.
Professor and former Chairman of Surgery
University of Texas at Houston

Cleon W. Goodwin, M.D.
Associate Professor of Surgery
Cornell University Medical College

James D. Hardy, M.D.
Professor and Chairman
Department of Surgery
University of Mississippi

John M. Howard, M.D.
Professor of Surgery
Medical College of Ohio
Former Chairman of Surgery
Hahnemann and Emory Universities

R. Scott Jones, M.D.
Professor and Chairman
Department of Surgery
University of Virginia

Edwin L. Kaplan, M.D.
Professor of Surgery
University of Chicago

C. Francis Nance, M.D.
Professor and Chairman
Department of Surgery
St. Barnabus Medical Center

Marshal J. Orloff, M.D.
Professor and former Chairman of Surgery
University of California at
San Diego

Francis E. Rosato, M.D.
Professor and Chairman
Department of Surgery
Thomas Jefferson University

Harvey J. Sugerman, M.D.
Professor of Surgery
Medical College of Virginia

James C. Thompson, M.D.
Professor and Chairman
Department of Surgery
University of Texas
Medical Branch

John A. Waldhausen, M.D.
Professor and Chairman
Department of Surgery
Pennsylvania State University
College of Medicine

Douglas W. Wilmore, M.D.
Professor of Surgery
Harvard Medical School
The Brigham and Women's
Hospital

Current Status of the Department of Surgery and Projects of the Harrison Department of Surgical Research

CLYDE F. BARKER, M.D.

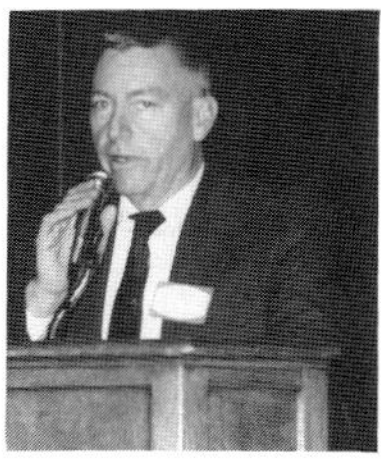

GOOD MORNING and welcome to the University of Pennsylvania and the Jonathan E. Rhoads 80th Birthday Symposium. Since there will be no time for presentations by the current University of Pennsylvania faculty, I will try to summarize recent activities in the Department of Surgery, especially the Harrison Department of Surgical Research. Those of you who have not visited recently will note major changes in the Hospital since the 1950s and 60s when most of our guest speakers were residents. In this photograph of the current Medical Center we can see the I. S. Ravdin Institute (completed in 1963), the Silverstein Building that was completed in 1978 and which is the locus of our surgical offices and most of the surgical inpatient service, and the brand-new 100 million dollar Founders Pavilion that will, in another few months, house our operating rooms and intensive care units.

Listed here is the current HUP surgical faculty with the following divisions: Cardiothoracic, Plastic, Pediatric Surgery, Neurosurgery, Urology, Transplantation, Vascular, Oncology, and Trauma and Critical Care, the later five being components of General Surgery.

General Surgery

Clyde F. Barker	Leonard J. Perloff
Henry D. Berkowitz	Jonathan E. Rhoads
Gordon P. Buzby	Brooke Roberts
John M. Daly	John L. Rombeau
Clifford W. Deveney	Ernest F. Rosato
Karen E. Deveney	Cletus W. Schwegman
Ira J. Fox	Larry W. Stephenson
Julius A. Mackie	John W. Thomas
Leonard D. Miller	Michael T. Torosian
James L. Mullen	Moritz M. Ziegler
Ali Naji	

Cardiothoracic Surgery

L. Henry Edmunds	W. Clark Hargrove
V. Paul Addonizio	Larry W. Stephenson

Neurosurgery

Frederick Murtagh	Thomas W. Langfitt
Steven J. Barrer	Luis Schut
Richard A. Davis	Frederick Simeone
Thomas A. Gennarelli	Leslie N. Sutton

From the Department of Surgery, Hospital of the University of Pennsylvania, Philadelphia, Pennsylvania.

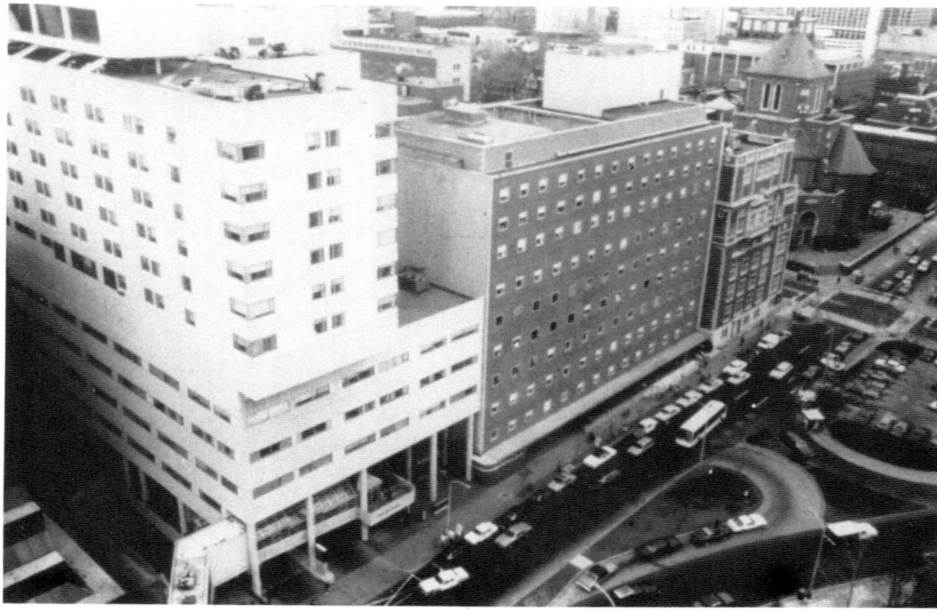

Current Silverstein, Ravdin, and White Buildings.

Plastic Surgery

Scott P. Bartlett	Don LaRossa
Howard S. Caplan	R. Barrett Noone
Ralph W. Hamilton	Peter Randall
Hazel I. Holst	Linton A. Whitaker
Paul W. Jackson	

Surgical Oncology

John M. Daly
Michael H. Torosian

Trauma

C. William Schwab

Urology

Harry M. Burros	John J. Murphy
Victor L. Carpiniello	Howard McC. Synder, III
John W. Duckett	Keith N. VanArsdalen
Philip M. Hanno	Alan J. Wein
Terrence R. Malloy	

Vascular and Transplantation

Clyde F. Barker	James A. O'Neill, Jr.
Henry D. Berkowitz	Leonard J. Perloff
Ira J. Fox	Brooke Roberts
Ali Naji	Moritz M. Ziegler

Significant changes in faculty composition have occurred recently or are about to occur. Since I became chairman 4 years ago, a number of new faculty members have joined us. John Daly, the first Jonathan E. Rhoads Professor of Surgical Sciences, came from Memorial Sloan–Kettering to head a new division of Surgical Oncology. Bill Schwab is forming a new division of Trauma and Critical Care, after heading similar divisions at East Carolina Univer-

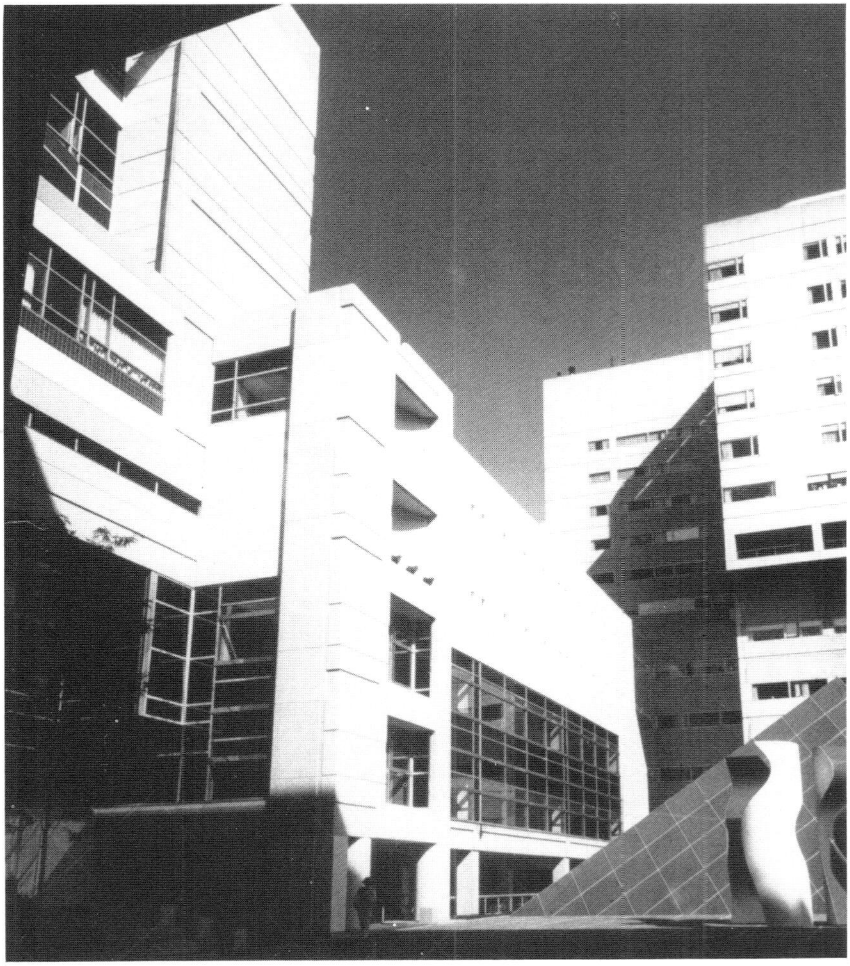

Present Founders and Silverstein Buildings.

sity and the Robert Wood Johnson School of Medicine in New Jersey.* Other new appointees include: Clark Hargrove and Paul Addonizio in the Cardiothoracic Division, both from our own program; Ira Fox, a liver transplant expert from Pittsburgh; Cliff Deveney, Chief of Surgery at the Veterans Administration (VA), and his wife Karen (both gastrointestinal surgeons from the University of California at San Francisco); Michael Torosian from Memorial in Oncology; and Don Dafoe in Transplantation and Dan Dempsey, both former Hospital of the University of Pennsylvania (HUP) residents who will be moving here in July from their current faculty positions at Michigan and Temple, respectively. Linton Whitaker will soon assume the role of Chief of Plastic Surgery, succeeding Peter Randall who is completing a distinguished career in this role. Linton is building a major new interdisciplinary program, the Center for Human Appearance.

On the other end of the spectrum, we very much miss Bill Inouye and Julian Johnson who both died recently. Alden Harken moved to Colorado in 1984 as Chairman of Surgery and Dick Edie recently moved to Jefferson as Chief of Cardiothoracic Surgery Dutch Dyson gave up surgery in 1985, although he still practices psychiatry at HUP. Brooke Roberts and Clete Schwegeman have both stopped operating, but remain active in the Department (among other things, they jointly manage the Surgical Clinic). Tom Langfitt has recently made a decision to conclude his distinguished career in Neurosurgery and tenure as Charles Harri-

* In 1988, a sixth division of GI surgery was added to the inclusive "Division" of General Surgery with Ernest F. Rosato as its chief.

son Frazier Professor to assume the leadership of the Glenmede and Pew Memorial Trusts, which have assets of about six billion dollars and are among the largest charitable trusts in the country.

In research, the Department remains active. The Harrison Department is comprised of 27,087 square feet, 19,645 belonging to General, Cardiothoracic, and Plastic Surgery, 4,820 to Neurosurgery, and 2,545 to Urology. Of this space, 17,458 square feet are in the Medical School and 9,525 are in the Hospital. Since 1982, the Department's annual research grant support has increased from $1,775,858 to $3,045,112, not including grants to the Division of Pediatric Surgery and Plastic Surgery that are administered by Children's Hospital and estimated at an additional one million dollars. Contributing substantially to these funds are six National Institutes of Health (NIH) R01 grants currently held by members of the full-time faculty in General and Cardiothoracic Surgery, which Bill Longmire tells me are as many as held by any other Department of Surgery. Substantial additional NIH funding exists in Neurosurgery, Urology, and Pediatric Surgery. The publication record of the Department appears to be solid, with 180 papers coming out in 1987.

In the remaining few minutes, I will show a few borrowed slides and describe briefly some of the many research projects going on in the Harrison Department.

Cardiothoracic Surgery

L. Henry Edmunds has built a Division of Cardiothoracic Surgery with a research record that I believe is second to none. The Division is currently funded by four NIH R01 grants, two belonging to Dr. Edmunds who has served two tours of duty on Surgery Study Section, one as chairman. The first of Dr. Edmunds' grants is entitled, "Extracorporeal Perfusion for Acute Myocardial Infarction," and seeks to determine the best extracorporeal perfusion system for patients in whom cardiogenic shock develops after an acute myocardial infarction. Because extracorporeal membrane oxygenation (ECMO) can be rapidly implemented without thorocotomy and because it supports both right and left ventricles, it has great potential for treatment of patients in cardiogenic shock. Arterial and venous cannulae are inserted through peripheral cutdowns; the apparatus is portable, reliable, and simple to operate. A study of venous cannulae indicates that necessary flow rates can be achieved if the catheter tip is in the right atrium as opposed to a peripheral vein or the inferior vena cava.

In sheep, the changes that occur in left ventricular wall stress during ECMO have been studied in normal and postischemic poorly contracting hearts using sonomicrometry. Small changes in left ventricular dimensions throughout the cardiac cycle can be measured using sonomicrometry and from these measurements changes in left ventricular volume and wall stress can be calculated using computer software developed in Dr. Edmunds' laboratory by Dr. Mark Ratcliffe. With Joe Bavaria, Dr. Edmunds has noted that increasing flows of ECMO cause a progressive *decrease* in left ventricular wall stress in the normal ejecting heart but, somewhat surprisingly, a progressive *increase* in wall stress in the postischemia dilated heart. (Figs. 3A and 3B) These data indicate that ECMO should be combined with an intra-aortic balloon pump that reduces afterload and therefore wall stress. Current studies will quantitate the changes in left ventricular wall stress using the combination of ECMO and a two-stage intra-aortic balloon wherein the second balloon remains constantly inflated.

After the best method to reduce left ventricular wall stress during mechanical circulatory assistance is worked out, studies of acute myocardial infarction will be done. When a coronary artery is acutely blocked, part of the myocardium infarcts while a surrounding zone of well-perfused myocardium ("stunned myocardium") also stops contracting. In 2 weeks, stunned myocardium recovers contractibility. By reducing left ventricular wall stress, it seems likely that recovery of stunned myocardium can be accelerated.

The Edmunds' second NIH-funded program is entitled, "Physiology of Blood Elements During Extracorporeal Bypass." Although heparin prevents clotting when blood contacts any nonendothelial cell surface, this contact activates platelets, leukocytes, and the intrinsic coagulation proteins. Although actual clotting does not occur, platelets stick to synthetic surfaces and are consumed and partially destroyed. Previous studies by Dr. Edmunds' group have led to a clinical trial by his colleague Dr. Addonizio of Iloprost, a prostaglandin analog that temporarily inhibits and therefore protects platelets during cardiopulmonary bypass. The group has also shown that platelets adhere to synthetic surfaces by a fibrinogen receptor

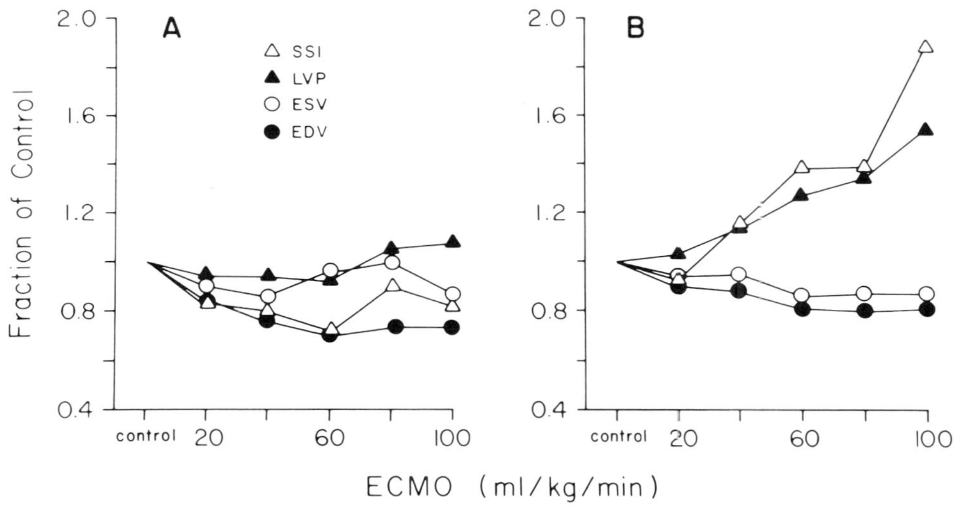

FIGS. 3A AND 3B. (A) Effect of extracorporeal membrane oxygenation (ECMO) on the normal heart. The fraction of control (measurement during ECMO divided by mean control measurement) is shown for the integral of left ventricular (LV) systolic wall stress (SSI), LV pressure (LVP), LV end-systolic volume (ESV), and LV end-diastolic volume (EDV). Data were obtained from all sheep except for ECMO flow = 100 ml/kg/min where N = 4. (B) Effect of ECMO in the postischemic heart. For ECMO flow = 0 to 100 ml/kg/min, N = 11 sheep. Note that while the reductions in LV volumes are similar to those seen in the normal heart, both LVP and SSI are markedly increased. (Reprinted [with permission from The Society of Thoracic Surgeons] from Babavaria JE, Ratcliffe MD, Gupta KB, Wenger RK, Bogen DK, Edmunds LH Jr. Changes in left ventricular systolic wall stress during biventricular circulatory assistance. Ann Thorac Surg 1988;45:530.)

and cannot react if this receptor is absent (as in the case of thrombosthenic platelets). Albumin pre-coating of extracorporeal synthetic devices prevents platelet attachment *in vitro*, but this does not work *in vivo*. Currently, Tregranun, a specific inhibitor of the platelet fibrinogen receptor, is being studied to determine if the reaction of platelets to synthetic surfaces can be inhibited without preventing platelet function in wounds.

Recent studies have shown that cardiopulmonary bypass causes neutrophils to secrete elastase, a powerful proteose. During bypass, serum elastase increases significantly and may be responsible for some of the morbidity associated with cardiopulmonary bypass. Measurement of C1 inhibitor complexes using specific immunosorbent enzymatic assays (ELISA) indicates that the contact coagulation pathway is activated by blood surface contact and that complement is activated by the classical pathway. This is the mechanism causing release of neutrophil elastase. *In vitro* elastase release can be inhibited by prostaglandin E1 and arginine 15-apoprotinin. These studies indicate that it may be possible to selectively inhibit release of elastase and thereby reduce the morbidity associated with long-term bypass for respiratory and circulatory support.

Some of the most interesting work ever done in the Harrison Department is that of Larry Stephenson, Associate Professor of Surgery, who has been exploring the use of skeletal muscle to assist or replace the failing myocardium. The technical feasibility of this approach was first demonstrated by grafting vascularized, innervated diaphragm into the right ventricle of dogs. Stimulation of the phrenic nerve caused the muscle graft to develop active tension and thicken substantially. With indirect or low-level direct stimulation, the graft could be induced to contract during any phase of the cardiac cycle. With direct stimulation at higher current levels, the heart could be "captured" by electronic spread and paced synchronously so that electrical stimulation would always be required and the graft could not be excited by the endogenous activity of the surrounding myocardium.

The impact of chronic electrical stimulation on morphology and collateral circulation of diaphragm grafts was conducted. In addition to thickening of the muscle, degeneration and fiber atrophy were seen histologically, although damage was less in stimulated than non-stimulated muscle. Perfusion studies with technetium-labeled microspheres and silicone demonstrated collateral circulation in the host ventricle as early as 28 days. Although the blood flow to grafts was only 32% of that in the normal ventricle, this represented a fivefold increase above flow to normal diaphragm muscle *in situ.*

The mechanical and histochemical properties of chronically stimulated muscles were studied and the possibility of conditioning the diaphragm muscle before making the graft was investigated. Conversion of skeletal muscle to fiber types of the fatigue-resistant form characteristic of cardiac muscle was demonstrated, indicating for the first time that such muscle transformation could occur at a stimulation frequency as low as the dog's own heart rate. If stimulation was delivered directly to the muscle, slow-twitch fibers were seen only within a 2-cm to 3-cm radius of the electrode. However, if stimulation of the muscle was accomplished by its motor nerve, far more extensive conversion was achieved. For complete transformation to fatigue-resistant type of muscle, 6 to 8 weeks were needed.

The histochemical and fatigue characteristics of the latissimus dorsi were evaluated after a 6-week period of electrical stimulation of the thoracodorsal nerve at either 2 Hz or 10 Hz. Conditioned muscles were compared with their unconditioned contralateral counterparts on the basis of histochemical fiber type composition, myosin isoforms, contraction characteristics, and rates of fatigue. Stimulated muscles had a much greater proportion of Type I (fatigue-resistant) fibers than controls. Electrophoresis of nondissociating gels revealed an increase in the slow myosin isozymes and a decrease in the fast myosin isoforms in stimulated muscles.

Dogs were studied in which diaphragm muscle was stimulated at the normal canine heart rate (2 Hz) or somewhat above (4 Hz) continuously by their motor nerve for 1 year. The stimulated muscle appeared normal by gross and microscopic inspection and was still contracting vigorously. By histochemical and immunohistochemical criteria, it had acquired a uniformly Type I character, in contrast to the mixed fiber composition of the unstimulated hemidiaphragms. This transformation was also reflected in myosin isozymes and enzyme activity.

It was noted that muscles are somewhat ischemic immediately after mobilization, perhaps because of ligation of collateral blood vessels. When stimulated, these muscles turned purple and, if stimulation was continued, they became necrotic. Blood flow studies with microspheres indicated that stimulation led to a tenfold increase in blood flow, but produced no increase in blood flow if collateral blood vessels were divided. However, if the collateral blood supply was divided and the muscle rested for 3 weeks before stimulation, there was a substantial recovery of exercise-induced increase in electrically conditioned muscles.

To quantify the amount of work done by a muscle graft, a hydraulic pouch model of the left ventricle has been developed. Such a device allows assessment of fatigue resistance, and could eventually be used as an auxiliary ventricle. The latissimus dorsi, which unlike pectoralis and rectus muscles has only one motor nerve, was particularly well suited for construction of skeletal muscle ventricles. The length of time that the electrically stimulated "ventricle" could generate flow in a hydraulic test system was measured. Artificial ventricles that had both chronic electrical conditioning and a vascular delay were found to be able to generate substantial flow for 4 hours. Skeletal muscle ventricles were then connected to the animal's own circulation and could generate significant pressures and pump significant amounts of blood against the systemic arterial resistance for 8 to 48 hours.

Since it was crucial to determine whether the skeletal muscle ventricles could perform useful work for extended periods, a totally implanted mock circulation device was developed that allowed the animal to move freely with no wires or tubes crossing the skin barrier. Pouches of lattisimus dorsi muscle were constructed that had previously had their collaterals cut, had been rested for 3 weeks, and had then been connected to an implanted mock circulation device. These devices have been shown to generate significant pressures and flows for as long as 10 weeks (Fig. 4).

The bioenergetic components of conditioned latissimus dorsi muscle are being studied using phosphorous-nuclear magnetic resonance (NMR) spectroscopy in collaboration with Dr. Britton Chance's group. Phosphorous-NMR spectroscopy was performed on conditioned and unconditioned muscle during successive periods of increasing stimulation. The ratio of inorganic phosphorous to phosphocreatinine, which reflects the muscle's ability to maintain energy balance, was measured. In unconditioned muscle, the inorganic phosphorous to phosphocreatinine ratio was increased and fatigue occurred. The ratio changed very

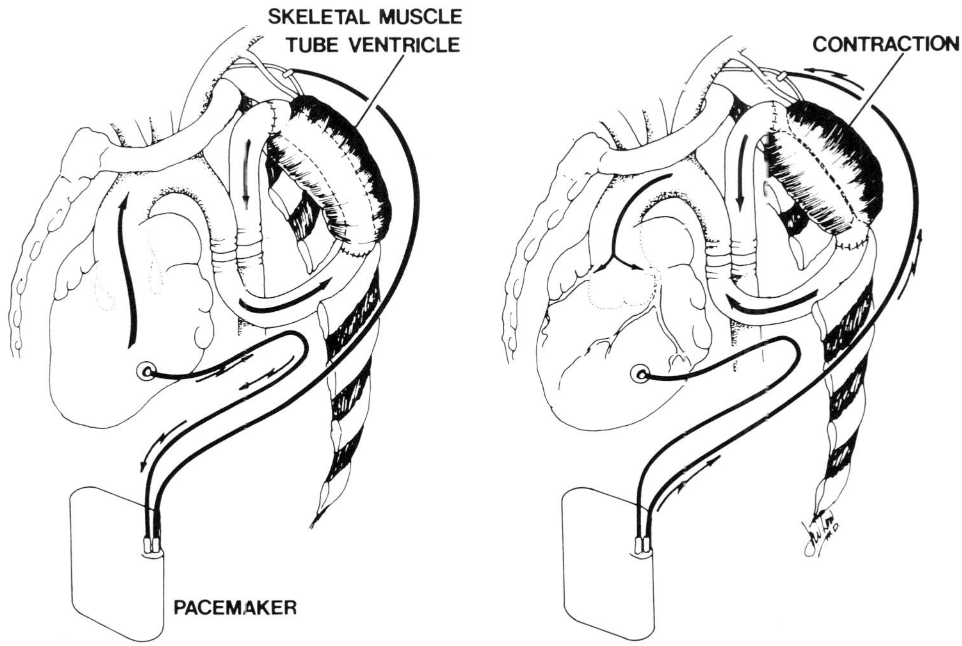

FIG. 4. This skeletal muscle ventricle, when implanted in dogs, has been able to contract and function as a circulatory assist device for many weeks.

little in electrically conditioned muscle and there was no fatigue as the intensity of the stimulation was increased. Thus, the increased fatigue resistance in electrically conditioned muscle is related to increased aerobic capacity of the transformed muscle that has assumed the work capability of cardiac muscle.

Dr. Stephenson's work, which has been published in a variety of journals (*i.e., Science, American Journal of Physiology,* and *The New York Times*), has been thorough and innovative. It has special appeal since the basic concept is simple, but it may lead to a major clinical breakthrough.

Clark W. Hargrove, III, who was appointed Assistant Professor of Surgery in 1984, has been studying intraoperative mapping techniques with multiple bipoplar electrode pairs and investigating local electrical activity in the area of the ventricular tachycardia circuit in collaboration with Dr. Mark Josephson, continuing work began in the Harrison Department by Alden Harken. This has led to improved care of patients with tachycardia arising from prior inferior wall infarction. These patients have been commonly found to have tachycardia maps compatible with macrorereentry and the isthmus of ventricular muscle between the ventriculotomy and the mitral valve annulus to be critical in the initiation and/or maintenance of the ventricular tachycardia. Destruction of this area surgically or with cryoablation has resulted in control of ventricular tachycardia in more than 90% of this subgroup of patients as compared with 50% with previous techniques. In addition, in patients with ventricular tachycardia and those with coronary artery disease, Dr. Hargrove has studied tissue anisotropy (*i.e.,* local conduction and wave-front propagating properties) that appears to be important in the genesis and maintenance of these arrhythmias.

With Larry Markowitz, a research fellow in the Harrison Department, and Dr. Edmunds, Dr. Hargrove has developed a large animal model for left ventricular aneurysm. The technique involves ligation of the left anterior ascending coronary artery plus one or more diagonal branches. The sheep is ideal for this experiment because due to the lack of a collateral coronary circulation in this species, a transmural infarct and subsequently an aneurysm is reproducibly created. Echocardiography and angiography are being carried out and regional myocardial wall motion in the non-infarcted myocardium is being evaluated by sonomicrometry. The latter technique uses computer software programs developed by Dr.

Mark Ratcliffe, and should help determine the optimal method of reconstruction of the ventricle after left ventricular aneurysmectomy. It has also been possible to induce ventricular arrhythmias in sheep with such aneurysms.

Dr. Paul Addonizio interrupted his clinical training in surgery for a postdoctoral fellowship at Penn with Dr. Robert Colman who is now head of the Thrombosis Center at Temple University. During this time, he did basic investigation in the field of hemostasis and thrombosis and was awarded a Young Investigatorship from the NIH. After completion of his general surgery and postgraduate training in cardiothoracic surgery at HUP, he was appointed Assistant Professor in the CT division in 1984.

Dr. Addonizio's basic research interests are hemostasis and thrombosis. He has applied his knowledge of basic physiology in this area to three courses of study. His interest in the role of platelets and leukocytes as mediators of acute coronary thrombosis led him to establish a model that uses a Langendorff heart preparation and NADH fluorescent photography to quantitate zones of ischemic muscle, allowing determination of the ability of various hemostatic elements, selectively added to the perfusate, to modify ischemia. Using this model, he is attempting to characterize the evolution of acute coronary thrombosis and establish the relative importance of formed blood elements *versus* clotting proteins in the thrombotic event. He is also attempting to manipulate the thrombotic process pharmacologically.

Another related area of Dr. Addonizio's research is acute lung injury. An animal model has been established for studying the role of formed blood elements as mediators of endothelial damage and acute noncardiac pulmonary edema. Because hemorrhage features so prominently in the clinical course of acute lung injury, attempts are being made to characterize the ability of the injured lung to alter a patient's hemostatic profile.

Finally, Dr. Addonizio is interested in blood synthetic surface interactions. His most recent work in this area involves the evaluation of a new prostacyclin analogue to prevent adverse platelet changes during acute cardiopulmonary bypass in humans, work that might eventually allow successful implementation of an *in situ* artificial lung and implantation of very small artificial blood vessels (less than 2 mm in diameter) or avoidance of coagulation abnormalities in patients with ventricular assist devices. These devices, particularly the one developed by Bill Pierce (another of Dr. Rhoads' trainees), are another area of Paul's interests that he plans to bring into clinical use at HUP shortly.

Since hemostasis and thrombosis are such fundamental areas, it is not surprising that Dr. Addonizio's work has attracted the interest of a wide range of collaborators from different disciplines. With members of the cardiology section of the Department of Medicine, he is exploring the kinetics of platelet activation in the atherosclerotic coronary systems after stress-induced angina, cigarette smoking, and coronary angioplasty. He is also collaborating with members of the Department of Obstetrics and Gynecology in characterization of procoagulants in amniotic fluid that may contribute to preeclampsia and disseminated intravascular coagulation, which can accompany abruptio placentae.

Dr. Addonizio has unusual promise as an investigator, a view endorsed by the Hartford Foundation that recently awarded him a career development fellowship and by the NIH that funds his R01 grant.

Transplantation

In 1965, Dr. Rhoads arranged for me to work as a fellow in the laboratory of Dr. Rupert Billingham, one of the originators of the field of transplantation biology and then the Chairman of Medical Genetics at the University of Pennsylvania. I was blessed not only with this unique mentor whom I worked closely with for 8 years, but subsequently with an unusually talented group of research fellows, mostly HUP residents, who are responsible for most of the work of recent years. This group included Leonard Perloff, Howard Silberman, Craig Reckard, Moritz Ziegler, Leo Frangiopane, Ali Naji, Richard Spence, Donald Dafoe, Stephen Bartlett, John Francfort, Manfred Woehrle, Kenneth Brayman, James Markmann, Jill Jacobson, and Michael Choti. Willys Silvers has also provided much help and support.

For the last 5 years, the responsibility for directing the surgical transplantation laboratory has been shared by myself and Dr. Ali Naji who after completing his residency and transplant fellowship returned to the lab to get a PhD in immunology. The recent work has

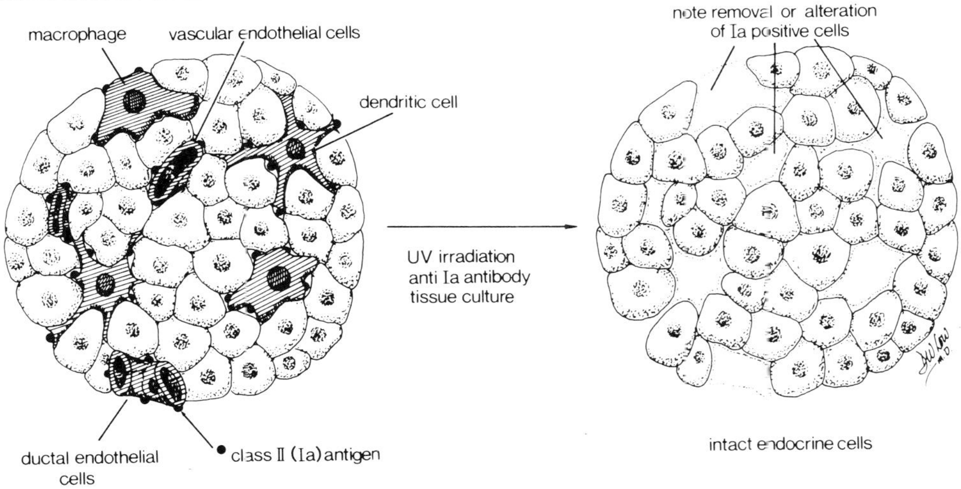

FIG. 5. Several treatments (tissue culture, ultraviolet irradiation, and specific antibodies) as capable of removing or inactivating immunogenic components of islet allografts. The endocrine cells alone are unlikely to provoke rejection, although they can serve as targets for either rejection or autoimmune attack.

focused on the following two areas: (1) transplantation of isolated pancreatic islets for treatment of diabetes and (2) the immunologic basis of Type I (insulin-dependent) diabetes mellitus.

Experimental Islet Transplantation

Studies done in this laboratory in the early 1970s were the first to demonstrate that transplantation of syngeneic isolated islets could totally reverse the hyperglycemic state in chemically induced diabetes in rodents (Ballinger and Lacy had previously demonstrated partial amelioration of diabetes) and that virtually all abnormal metabolic indices of diabetes could be corrected by islet transplantation. Moreover, our laboratory was the first to demonstrate successful reversal of diabetes by allogeneic islets and the fact that such islet allografts were vulnerable to rejection but that this could be overcome with immunosuppression.

Techniques of altering the immune response to transplanted islets have now been developed to permit successful transplantation without the need for immunosuppression. *In vitro* maintenance of islets in tissue culture is one method we have employed to decrease immunogenicity. The commonly held explanation of this finding is that *in vitro* culture deletes the intra-islet Class II major histocompatibility complex (MHC) antigen-bearing "passenger" leukocytes (macrophages and dendritic cells) that are the immunogenic components of the allografts (Fig. 5). Immunohistochemical staining with monoclonal antibodies has revealed only occasional Class II antigen-bearing cells (APC) after *in vitro* culture of islets.

Efforts have been made to dissect the cellular basis of islet allograft rejection. In particular, immunologic phenomena favoring unresponsiveness to allografts in nonimmunosuppressed hosts have been considered. We found that APC free islet allografts enjoy prolonged survival in recipients *incompatible* with the donor at the major histocompatibility complex locus. However, depleting APC from endocrine allografts has no beneficial effect in MHC *compatible* donor/host combinations. To explain these unexpected results, we invoked the involvement of MHC restriction in allograft immunity. It implies that transplantation antigens are only recognized in association with the MHC of APC, and that if the MHC of these cells is different from that of the MHC of the graft. The graft will not be recognized as foreign. We have also obtained evidence of the validity of this concept for other endocrine allografts such as parathyroid and thyroid. If MHC restriction does indeed apply to allograft immunity, the elimination of APC from allografts, in conjunction with MHC mismatching, may obviate the need for immunosuppression.

Immunologic Basis of Type I (Insulin-Dependent) Diabetes Mellitus

Studies in this laboratory were among the earliest to provide convincing experimental evidence that autoimmunity plays a pivotal role in the pathogenesis of Type I diabetes. We were possibly the first to conduct an extensive analysis of the immune pathogenesis of diabetes in spontaneously diabetic (BB) rats. While several investigators (including ourselves) noted that immunosuppression prevents or reverses diabetes in these animals, our demonstration that BB rats inoculated neonatally with bone marrow from normal rat donors are protected against the disease was even more interesting. To understand the reason(s) for alteration in susceptibility, we conducted a functional and phenotypic analysis of the immune system and noted that BB rats were immunodeficient. Animals protected from diabetes after bone marrow transplantation were found to have restoration of various parameters of T-cell immunodeficiency, especially with regard to the suppressor T-cell mechanisms, suggesting that these abnormalities might be related to its pathogenesis.

Islet transplantation studies in BB rats were important not only as a therapeutic modality, but also as a probe for defining the cause of diabetes. Islet transplantation can only succeed if transplanted islets are exempt from the aberrant autoimmune response that destroyed the native islets. We made the observation that unless immunosuppression is used, hyperglycemia recurs in BB rats after islet transplantation. Interpretation of this funding was complicated since syngeneic transplants were not possible in the outbred BB rat and failure of islet allografts could be attributed to either rejection or autoimmunity. To exclude rejection as a cause of islet allograft failure, donor-specific immunologic tolerance was induced by neonatal inoculation of prospective BB recipients with bone marrow cells. Although these rats permanently accepted donor skin allografts, their spontaneous diabetes was only transiently cured by transplantation of the donor islets (Fig. 6).

The finding that MHC compatible islet allografts are subject to autoimmune destruction by the original disease process raises several important questions, including the role of MHC restriction in the autoimmune reaction against islets. To assess the role of MHC restriction in islet autoimmunity, we have used *in vitro* culturing of isolated islets from MHC compatible or incompatible donors before their transplantation to BB recipients. In contrast to early failure of MHC compatible islet allografts, MHC incompatible islets survived permanently indicating that pretransplant tissue culture prevents damage from both rejection and autoimmunity.

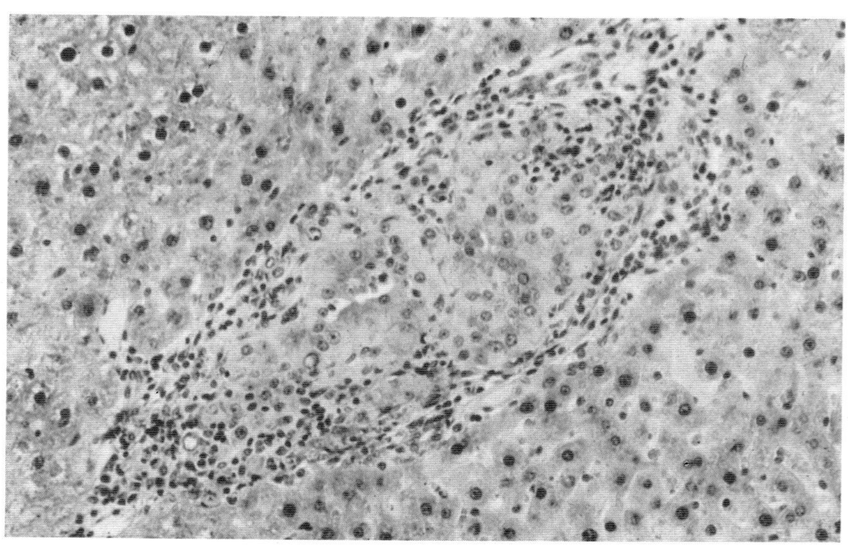

FIG. 6. This islet, transplanted to the liver of an immunologically tolerant diabetic BB rat recipient, is being destroyed by infiltrating mononuclear cells as a result of the autoimmune disease to which BB rats (and islets transplanted from normal non-diabetes–prone donors) are vulnerable.

Other studies done in this area and funded by the NIH have analyzed the following: genetic factors and interferon in viral models of diabetes, comparisons of the outcome of vascularized pancreas and islet allografts, the role of weak transplantation antigens in rejection of endocrine allografts, prevention of cytomegalovirus disease by vaccination, the role of activated T-cells and the thymus in diabetes.

In addition to this, Dr. Naji has his own NIH R01 grant that has funded the study entitled, "Role of Major Histocompatibility Complex (MHC) Antigens in the Allograft Response." Dr. Naji has focused his attention on the nature of cells within allografts that are important in provoking a host response. Immune responses are initiated by the presentation and processing of antigen by antigen presenting cells (APC) to antigen reactive T-lymphocytes. It has recently become clear that dendritic cells are the most efficient APC. It has also been demonstrated that small grafts such as pancreatic islet and thyroid allografts, if depleted of APC, may be exempt from rejection. However, the task of removing APC from complex vascularized organ allografts is formidable and cannot be accomplished by tissue culture as in the case of endocrine grafts. Thus, other maneuvers may be required to remove passenger leukocytes from complex organs. One such maneuver is temporary "parking" of grafts by transplantation to intermediate hosts. After a period of residence in the interim host, it is anticipated that donor APC will disappear and that the graft will become repopulated with APC of the interim host. In rats, cardiac allografts parked in interim hosts for 100 days and retransplanted to hosts syngeneic with the interim host were rejected, despite the fact that an identical protocol of parking was effective in protecting islet allografts. The most plausible explanation for this discrepancy is the considerably larger population of APC in cardiac grafts, possibly necessitating a longer period of parking to completely deplete APC from complex organ grafts as compared with small pancreatic islet grafts. In support of this interpretation, immunohistochemical studies of heterotopic cardiac allografts parked in interim hosts for 100 days have demonstrated persistence of donor antigen presenting cells; this was not true of islets.

In recent years, it has been noted that the expression of MHC antigens on cell surface is not a constant phenomena but may be induced or amplified. Increased cell surface expression of MHC antigens has been noted to result from the action of various lymphokines, particularly gamma interferon released by activated T-lymphocytes. Therefore, during allograft rejection modulation of donor MHC antigen, expression on either the nonparenchymal components (passenger leukocytes) or indigenous cellular elements of the graft may profoundly influence susceptibility of the graft to allospecific cytotoxicity.

It has been found that pancreatic endocrine cells do not normally express Class II MHC antigens, but do so after *in vitro* exposure to recombinant gamma interferon. We are currently using Class II positive islets in *in vitro* assays to assess their capacity as APC. Moreover, the fate of Class II positive pancreatic islets is being evaluated *in vivo* by islet transplantation experiments.

Dr. Leonard Perloff has focused on two areas of transplantation biology: (1) semibiologic vascular prostheses and (2) pancreatic allografts.

Glutaraldehyde-tanned, mandrel-grown, Dacron mesh supported vascular prostheses were created in ovine donors and transplanted to canine, rat, and human recipients. Based on earlier findings in his laboratory that venous allografts (whether fresh, frozen, or tanned with dialdehyde starch) maintained their antigenicity but were still able to function well as vascular conduits, the semibiologic ovine xenograft was developed in collaboration with Dr. Bruce Christie, a visiting research fellow from Australia. The grafts were tested in Philadelphia and Melbourne and were found to be quite satisfactory as small (0.5 to 1 mm) and medium (3 to 6 mm) conduits. Although retaining their antigenic nature, as evidenced by the development of anti-sheep hemagglutinating antibodies in the rat and canine hosts, the grafts demonstrated patency rates comparable with the best synthetic prostheses. They were pliable, smooth, and essentially nonreactive. Follow-up studies of the xenograft in clinical settings such as arterial and venous replacements are underway in several surgical centers internationally.

Immediately vascularized whole pancreatic allografts in diabetic rats were compared with allografts of isolated islets of Langerhans. The grafts were evaluated in terms of the influence of histocompatibility matching and adjunctive immunosuppression, vulnerability to humoral antibodies, and function in tolerant hosts. Immediately vascularized cardiac and renal grafts served as functional and histologic controls. Additional studies included the determination of the efficacy of donor-specific transfusion with untreated and Class II antigen-depleted whole blood in an effort to develop a model of donor-specific unresponsiveness. In virtually all respects the vascularized graft proved superior to the isolated islets.

Dr. Ira Fox, an Assistant Professor recruited from Pittsburgh 2 years ago to establish the liver transplant program, is studying cellular and molecular mechanisms of immunologic tolerance. Using lethal irradiation and syngeneic bone marrow reconstitution as a model of adult nonchimeric tolerance in rats, he is able to prevent rejection of pancreatic islet and cardiac allografts. Having established this model of immunologic unresponsiveness *in vivo*, he is now studying *in vitro* correlates of immunologic reactivity with assays quantitating cytotoxic T-lymphocytes, mixed (helper) lymphocyte reactivity, and interleukin-2 (IL-2) production.

Since the immature lymphocytes from bone marrow are presumably responsible for immunologic unresponsiveness in this model, he is growing bone marrow cells in culture to standardize the population of cells used for reconstitution of the irradiated hosts. These cells are phenotyped for analysis of subpopulation growth characteristics that are caused by the addition of hematopoietic growth factors to the tissue culture media. By using these bone marrow cells in the tolerance model, he intends to analyze the functional development of hematopoietic precursors and their role in immunologic self recognition. In addition, he is interested in looking at organ-specific antigens and immunologic techniques for identifying cytotoxic T-lymphocytes that identify and lyse pancreatic islets.

Nutrition and Metabolism

Dr. James L. Mullen is now the leader of the famous nutrition program begun in the Harrison Department by Dr. Rhoads. His research activities fall into the following three categories: (1) a clinical nutritional research core resource; (2) clinical nutrition research training; and (3) individual research projects.

Clinical Nutrition Research Core

This core includes a data management center and a bedside metabolic testing laboratory for performing indirect calorimetry, and a whole body counter that can measure total body potassium in humans. The nutrition reference library has hardcopy files of more than 13,000 scientific publications and is indexed on a computerized data management system that allows on-line searching of mainframe data bases such as *MedLine* through *BRS Colleague.*

Clinical Nutrition Research Training

Dr. Mullen is the PI of a National Cancer Institute (NCI)-funded Nutrition and Cancer Research Training Grant, the co-principal investor (PI) of an NIH Clinical Nutrition Research Training Grant of which David Kritchevsky is the PI, and for the past 10 years has also been the PI of an American Cancer Society (ACS) Institutional Research Fellowship.

Individual Research Projects

Dr. Mullen has been the PI of NCI-funded projects evaluating body composition in cancer patients and the use of electrical impedance as an indirect measure for total body water. He has also studied body compartments in patients with anorexia nervosa using serial determinations of energy expenditure and physical performance in these starved persons.

Dr. Mullen's group has also been investigating the caloric requirements of critically ill patients. The recent conclusion from this work, which employed indirect calorimetry, was that some patients have been grossly overfed. A more quantitative approach may result in better nutritional repletion, while reducing the possibility of complications such as hepatic dysfunction, respiratory failure, and overhydration. In animals, Dr. Mullen has explored protein and amino acid metabolism in tumor-bearing and septic rats. Another project involves the body composition and energy metabolism aspects of triathalon athletes. Working with the obesity research group, he has evaluated the relationships between body composi-

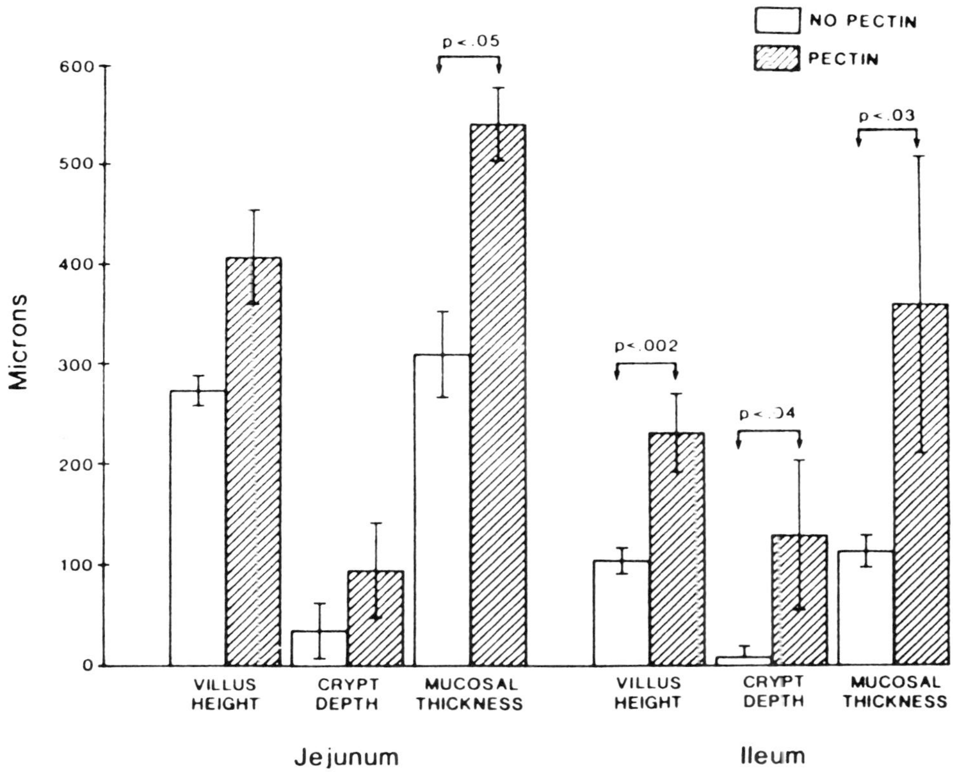

FIG. 7. Effect of a pectin-supplemented elemental diet on intestinal adaptation to massive small bowel resection. Changes in the histologic parameters for each intestinal segment for resected animals fed the no pectin and pectin diets. (Reprinted with permission from Koruda MJ, Rolandelli RH, Settle RG *et al.* The effect of a pectin-supplemented elemental diet on intestinal adaptation to massive small bowel resection. Winner 1986 Harry M. Vars Research Award. J Parenteral and Enternal Nutrition 1986;10:343–350).

tion changes and energy metabolism in the obese population. Several patient groups have been studied including the morbidly obese undergoing surgical treatment and the moderately obese undergoing dietary and pharmacologic therapy. Another focus has been the interaction between host energy metabolism and tumors. Since only 25% of cancer patients are hypermetabolic, this cannot be the mechanism of cancer cachexia in most patients. The determinants of energy expenditure in cancer patients seem to be related to their dietary intake, body composition, and tumor type. No effect of tumor burden on energy expenditure has been detected. In animal models, the interrelationships between body composition and tumor responsiveness to chemotherapy have been explored using cell-cycle kinetics and complex substrate supply timing regimens. Substrate supply and withdrawal can be manipulated to enhance tumor response to chemotherapy. The energy metabolism of head trauma patients and the capability of pharmacologic agents such as barbituates to reduce the hypermetabolic states have been studied. Dr. Mullen has also been the PI for the Philadelphia component of the nationwide multi-institutional VA Cooperative Study evaluating the effectiveness of preoperative total parenteral nutrition on patients undergoing major surgery.

Dr. John L. Rombeau, Associate Professor of Surgery, is another leader in the nutrition field. In fact, he is the President of the Association of Parenteral and Enteral Nutrition. John's recent research, which has been funded by VA merit review grants, has been focused on the following two areas: (1) the use of NMR as a test of nutritional function and (2) the effects of the noncellulosic fiber pectin as a supplement to enteral nutrition (Fig. 7).

Studies With Nuclear Magnetic Resonance (NMR)

With Danny Jacobs, a research fellow, Dr. Rombeau correlated liver dysfunction caused by carbon tetrachloride-induced fatty liver infiltration with changes in NMR. They also used phosphorus 31 magnetic resonance spectroscopy to study striated muscle during starvation, finding significant changes in the ratio of phosphocreatinine to inorganic phosphate.

Jacobs and Rombeau also investigated the diagnostic potential of NMR in experimentally induced appendicitis, finding that the associated tissue edema could be readily identified. Identification of edematous changes in the colon were similarly noted in a model of experimentally induced colitis in rats in studies carried out with Roland Rolandelli, another research fellow.

Dr. Rombeau also found NMR to be useful in differentiating second and third degree burns in studies with another fellow, Mark Koruda.

With Albina, Dr. Rombeau found that elemental diets consisting of short peptides rather than free amino acids allowed improved nitrogen utilization in monkeys.

In other particularly interesting experiments the effect of dietary pectin has been studied. With Rolandelli, Dr. Rombeau found that pectin-supplemented feedings promoted healing of colonic anastomosis in the rat as evidenced by higher bursting pressures. The by-products of pectin degradation (short chain fatty acids) appear to be responsible for these changes, and a similar beneficial effect on healing of colonic anastomosis has been obtained with intraluminal short chain fatty acids. With Koruda, Dr. Rombeau noted that pectin also had a beneficial effect on adaptation to massive small bowel resection in the rat, with regard to both morphologic and functional indices of the remaining intestine.

In the last few years, Dr. Rombeau has published three books on nutrition and has developed a new gastrostomy-jejunal feeding tube that is now in worldwide use for patients at increased risk for aspiration. One of his research fellows, Danny Jacobs, received the National Resident Research Award from the Association of Academic Surgery for his work on the detection of experimentally induced appendicitis with NMR, while another one of his research fellows, Mark Koruda, received the Harry M. Vars Research Award of American Society of Parenteral and Enteral Nutrition (ASPEN) for his work on the effect of pectin on intestinal adaptation in massive small bowel resection.

Dr. Gordon Buzby, Assistant Professor of Surgery, has used total parenteral nutrition (TPN) in the rat to characterize metabolic alterations in a variety of disorders and to explore methods of ameliorating undesired sequelae of TPN. The effects of cancer on nutritional status and substrate utilization have been investigated. The impact of a rat mammary adenocarcinoma on energy expenditure was characterized, and alternative fuel substrates were investigated for their impact on nutritional repletion and tumor growth. Dr. Buzby was intrigued by the observation that the rate of tumor growth is influenced by exogenous nutrient supply. Using flow cytofluorometric techniques, he determined that cell-cycle kinetics were exquisitely sensitive to the quantity and quality of exogenous caloric substrate provided to the host. It was possible to synchronize S-phase activity within the tumor, suggesting that tumor sensitization of S-phase specific chemotherapy may be feasible. It was also shown that tumor sensitivity to Adriamycin (doxorubicin, Adria Laboratories, Columbus, OH) and methotrexate could be increased by appropriate manipulation of caloric substrates provided.

The effect of stress and sepsis on host metabolism and exogenous nutrient efficacy was also studied in the rat. Cecal ligation/perforation was used as a standard of stress and sepsis, and the impact determined on energy expenditure and substrate metabolism as evaluated by an indirect calorimetry system for small animals. The degree of hypermetabolism and the severity of altered substrate utilization can be altered by pharmacologic agents such as prostaglandin inhibitors and beta-blocking agents. Attempts to provide more effective nutritional support through altering the exogenous caloric substrate supply have been less successful. Carnitine-dependent fatty acid transport could not be improved by administration of exogenous carnitine. Use of alternative substrates including medium chain triglycerides was similarly unsuccessful, but xylitol appears to be more promising.

The effect of ischemia on cellular metabolism in rats was investigated by NMR spectroscopy. Objectives were to evaluate NMR as a potential clinical tool for early detection of

ischemia (*e.g.*, with mesenteric ischemia) and to characterize the alterations in cellular metabolism associated with an ischemic event. Ischemia was evident after 20 minutes of arterial occlusion through alterations in phosphate metabolite concentrations and pH. For study of cellular changes associated with ischemia, a rat hind limb model was used. Alterations occurred in phosphate metabolites and intracellular and extracellular sodium and potassium. Cell death could be predicted reliably from membrane potentials calculated by the Nernst equation.

Studies of various methods for nutritional support have been evaluated in surgical patients. Objective means to identify malnourished patients were developed that are now widely used. A major national multicenter study of preoperative parenteral feeding in malnourished surgical patients was performed between 1980 and 1986, with Dr. Buzby serving as Study Chairman for a ten-hospital, 500-patient study funded through the VA Medical Research Service. The study is now in the final phase of data analysis.

Dr. Buzby was a recipient of an NCI Junior Faculty Clinical Fellowship from 1982 to 1985 while also serving as preceptor for two postdoctoral fellows funded by the NCI for training in nutrition and cancer. He has authored 52 original papers during the last 6 years.

Surgical Oncology

In the 16 months since John Daly, the Jonathan E. Rhoads Professor, has been part of our faculty, he has gathered around him a research team that includes Milad Bitar, John Reynolds, Arleen Thom, and Zhu Zhang, a surgeon from the Peoples Republic of China. They have been studying the efficiency of various antitumor drugs and the importance of tissue drug levels. A cell culture system has been developed that allows *in vitro* growth of VX-2 carcinoma cells for the first time. The sensitivity of these cells to various chemotherapeutic drugs and calcium channel blockers has been determined.

They have also studied colon cancer cell lines obtained from the Wistar Institute. Rabbits with tumor implants in the liver or hind limbs have been used to investigate methods of improving drug intake by tumors. NMR spectroscopy has been used in these animal to evaluate the distribution of fluorine in the tumors after drug infusions. In other studies, the effects of arginine supplementation on wound healing and on the immune system have been studied in mice implanted with immunogeneic and nonimmunogenic tumors. Interesting early results indicate that arginine significantly augments immune function.

Dr. Daly has also initiated four clinical oncology trials. The first is a continuation of a study he began at Memorial Sloan–Kettering comparing intravenous and intraarterial chemotherapy in patients with colorectal hepatic metastases. The second trial investigates the use of degradable starch microspheres to enhance drug uptake in hepatic tumors. The third evaluates the effects of arginine supplementation as an immunomodulator. Finally, clinical and biologic studies of the infusion of monoclonal antibodies in the extremities of patients with malignant melanoma are being carried out in collaboration with Drs. Koprowski and Herlyn of the Wistar Institute.

Michael H. Torosian, M.D., Assistant Professor of Surgery in the Division of Surgical Oncology, has been conducting animal studies that have demonstrated that exogenous nutrient administration can significantly stimulate tumor growth, a potential clinical concern in cancer patients receiving nutritional support. An approach to this potential problem is utilization of this phase of nutrient-induced tumor stimulation to therapeutic advantage.

Initial studies using a rat-tumor model in Lewis–Wistar rats have demonstrated an enhanced tumor response to chemotherapy during the administration of short-term (48 hours) TPN. This phenomenon occurred independent of changes in host nutritional status and without increased toxicity. Subsequent studies revealed that the effect was primarily due to the amino acid moiety in TPN and occurred only with cycle-specific chemotherapeutic agents (*i.e.*, methotrexate and Adriamycin [Adria Laboratories, Columbus, OH]).

To elucidate the biologic mechanism responsible for this potentiated tumor response to emotherapy, tumor growth kinetics were investigated. Significant alterations in tumor rowth occur within hours of initiating TPN. Biochemical changes included r protein synthesis and an increase in tumor DNA synthesis after

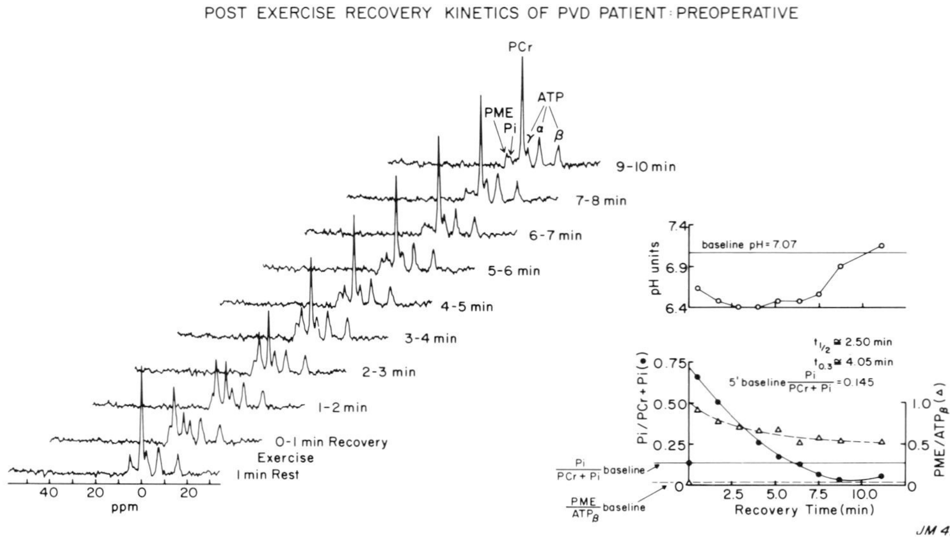

FIG. 8. Serial measurements of P^{31} NMR spectra in Limb with PVD at rest and at 1-minute intervals after excersize. The NMR index $\left(\frac{Pi}{Pcr + Pi}\right)$ reflects the ratio of inorganic phosphate (Pi) to phosphocreatinine (Pcr). Normally, this ratio is low (baseline index, .15) but after excersize Pcr falls and Pi becomes high (Index, .6) at 1 minute postexcersize and then returns to normal values. The time to recover $t_{1/2}$ or $t_{0.3}$ is prolonged with recovery time proportional to degree of ischemia. Note intracellular pH also falls and recovers by 10 minutes.

initiation of TPN. A significant change in tumor cytokinetics was also observed with an increase in the percentage of tumor cell synthesizing DNA (S-phase cells). These biochemical and cytokinetic alterations in tumor metabolism may explain the potentiated tumor response to chemotherapy that has been noted in this animal model. Underway are further investigations of the interaction between host and tumor, the biology of tumor metastasis, and the immunologic changes associated with malignant disease.

Vascular Surgery

Dr. Henry D. Berkowitz, Associate Professor of Surgery, is using 31-NMR spectroscopy as a means of studying patients with peripheral vascular disease. Patients have been studied in a 1.5 Tesla NMR spectroscope, in collaboration with Britton Chance, to determine whether NMR may be more sensitive than standard noninvasive vascular studies in characterizing peripheral vascular disease. These studies (thought to comprise the largest such series) have shown that the resting limbs of patients with severe peripheral vascular disease have elevated levels of inorganic phosphate. Although this indicates a failure in oxidative metabolism, depletion of ATP has not been seen unless actual muscle death has occurred. Since resting studies delineate only severe ischemia, patients have been made to exercise in an attempt to distinguish normal patients from those with mild and severe disease. Exercise produces a significant increase in inorganic phosphate (Pi) and depletion in phosphocreatinine (Pcr). The ratio of Pi to Pcr increases significantly and Pi equals or exceeds Pcr in the most severely ischemic limbs. Significant changes in muscle pH are detected by the shift in the distance of the Pi and Pcr peaks. Although significant abnormalities in Pi and Pcr are measured, no change in ATP is seen unless actual muscle death has occurred. Interestingly, after arterial revascularization of severely ischemic limbs, the return of these parameters to normal occurs only slowly, over a period of 6 months, suggesting a significant abnormality in mitochondrial metabolism that is not entirely dependent on blood flow (Fig. 8).

Noninvasive Diagnosis of Carotid Artery

During the past several years, Dr. Berkowitz has also been interes
morphology of carotid artery plaques removed from patients. Thes

graphed and catalogued for the presence of ulceration, and hemorrhage within the lumen or beneath the plaque. Plaque morphology appears to be an important predictor of disease progression and thus may allow identification of those asymptomatic plaques that should be operated on. With Dr. Goldberg from Radiology, plaques are being categorized by NMR imaging in patients who have been studied preoperatively in a whole-body NMR imager. After surgical removal, the plaque itself has been examined by NMR proton, imaging, and computed tomography (CT) scanning, intraoperative B-mode imaging, and histology. These studies showed that NMR imaging is far more sensitive than CT scans in identifying fresh and old hemorrhage within the plaque, while CT scans primarily detect calcification but not hemorrhage.

Noninvasive Diagnosis of Femoral-Popliteal and Femoral-Tibial Bypass Grafts

In the last 5 years, noninvasive studies of 500 patients with femoral-popliteal and femoral-tibial bypass grafts have been reviewed. Serial measurement of segmental pressures and pulse volumes and Doppler imaging and flow velocity were found to be more sensitive than clinical evaluation in early identification of vein graft stenosis. There was a 23% incidence of graft stenosis and treatment of such (often asymptomatic) lesions has led to an improvement in long-term graft patency. The 70% 5-year patency of femoral-tibial vein grafts in this series exceeds that reported by most others.

Gastrointestinal Surgery

The research studies of Clifford and Karen Deveney are focused on peptide hormones and membrane binding sites of cholecystokinin. They are examining the satiety effect of cholecystokinin in dogs by looking at the effect of cholecystokinin on the pyloric sphincter. They are experienced in the performance of radioimmunoassays of peptide hormones such as cholecystokinin and gastrin and have found that cholecystokinin causes pyloric sphincter contraction, delays gastric emptying, and may produce its effect by this mechanism.

With Dr. Arlene Thom, one of John Daly's fellows, Cliff Deveney is also studying the effect of various manipulations in blood flow on the uptake of chemotherapeutic agents in a transplantable rabbit sarcoma. They are studying the effect of intraarterially administered starch particles that embolize to tumors and slow blood flow through them. Chemotherapeutic agents are then inoculated to determine whether increased uptake of these agents occurs on the basis of the flow changes as measured by radioactive xenon clearance.

Plastic Surgery

Linton A. Whitaker, who in July will succeed Peter Randall as Chief of the Division of Plastic Surgery, is internationally respected for the major contributions he has made to the spectacular new discipline of craniofacial reconstruction. He also directs an active program in basic research.

Craniofacial Growth

To understand facial growth and the impact of changes in the calvarium on the face, Dr. Whitaker has studied facial growth in rabbits with cephalometrics after removal of different amounts of calvarium. With Scott Bartlett, Dr. Whitaker has also compared the healing of devascularized segments of bone with that of vascularized bone segments or free bone grafts, consistantly noting a more predictable outcome for arterialized bone flaps than for free bone grafts.

Bone Replacement

Experiments by Dr. Whitaker's fellows Jim Zins, Joe Kusiak, Scott Bartlett, and Craig VanderKolk demonstrated the superiority of membranous bone grafts from the calvarium over endochondial bone grafts and probed the biologic basis of the finding. These experiments and Dr. Whitaker's clinical results have led to general acceptance of the superiority of calvarial bone grafts for facial reconstruction. As the result of laboratory studies of several substitutes for facial bone, proplast and hydrozyapatite are now being used successfully in patients.

Electrical Stimulation of Cranial Bones

With Stalnecker, Dr. Whitaker attempted to stimulate extra bulk and cranial bone growth in instances of hypoplasia by using indwelling electrodes to accelerate the healing of cranial bone grafts and maintain volume during the healing state. Success was so limited that the technique currently appears to have little applicability for cranial bone.

Peter Randall's recent research has been focused on cleft lip and palate. He pioneered the use of muscle reconstruction in cleft lip, noting the abnormal orientation of the orbicularis oris muscle in children with clefts and using several techniques to reorient and reconstruct the muscle. In clefts of the palate the most important muscle for speech is the levator palatai, which is incorrectly oriented in the longitudinal direction instead of being in the transverse position. Studies have been directed toward reconstructing and reorienting the levator muscle and, more importantly, studying means to measure the results. This has been done by speech evaluations and video fluoroscopy, as well as direct nasendoscopic evaluations.

Dr. Randall's group has the world's largest series of children whose cleft palates have been repaired with the novel Furlow technique. These patients are under evaluation of the nasal airway, after posterior pharyngeal flap operations for velopharyngeal incompetence. Dr. Randall reports that during the last three meetings of the International Congress of Cleft Palate (held every 4 years) the Children's Hospital has presented more papers on the program than any other clinic in the world.

Don La Rossa, Associate Professor of Surgery, has been interested in microsurgery, assessment of blood flow in ischemic tissues, melanoma, and cleft lip and palate. Dr. La Rossa has investigated blood flow in skin flaps measuring the distribution of intravascularly injected fluorescein dye with a fluorometer designed and built by David Silverman of the Department of Anesthesia, finding the rate of uptake and washout of fluorescein dye to be good determinants of tissue viability. Dr. La Rossa's research fellow John Gatti demonstrated that hemodilation improved flow kinetics and skin flap survival. Determination of the minimum amount of blood flow needed for tissue survival has particular importance in reconstructive plastic surgery where flaps used for reconstruction are eventually severed from their blood supply. They were able to demonstrate neovascularization of skin flaps in animals after 4 to 5 days by both fluorometric methods and injection of the vessels with Microfil. They also demonstrated clinical applicability of the method and successfully divided flaps at 10 to 12 days instead of the usual 21 days. Perfusion fluorometry also proved useful in burn patients in whom survival of tissue was predicted accurately by using the technique. Additionally, the technique was used at Children's Hospital in the division of Siamese twins.

Dr. La Rossa directs the Division's microsurgery laboratory in which studies have been carried out on the patency of micro-arterial grafts with hemodilution and magnetic resonance imaging (MRI) has proved useful in assessing viability in limb replants done in cats.

As the director of the cleft palate program at Children's Hospital, Dr. La Rossa has evaluated a new double-reversing Z-plasty procedure for cleft palate, a triangular flap in cleft lip, bone grafting in alveolar clefts, and the use of premaxillary orthopaedics in the management of the bilateral cleft.

Basic Scientists

Space will permit only a brief mention of the activities of the basic scientists who have worked in the Harrison Department. We greatly miss the contributions and companionship of the deceased members, including Harry Vars (who figured prominently in the development of parenteral nutrition as noted elsewhere), Otto Rosenthal, and K. C. Tsou. Most of the basic scientists who remain active will be remembered by Dr. Rhoads' residents who have returned today. These scientists include David Cooper, Henry Sloviter, Heinz Schleyer, Shakunthala Narasimhulu, Sidney Levin, Elizabeth Miller, and David Kritchevsky whose laboratory is at the Wistar Institute.

David Cooper's classic paper in *SCIENCE* on the discovery of the P-450 enzyme system was recently reprinted as a "citation classic." He has collaborated in recent years with Heinz Schleyer, Sidney Levin, and others on continued study of this heme protein that is now the subject of more investigations than hemoglobin. To obtain information about the *in vivo* metabolic role of P-450, long-term bile fistulae have been studied. Investigations of the hepatic metabolism of representative chemicals have been carried out ranging from endogenous substances such as testosterone to drugs such as phenobarbital and toxic and carcinogenic compounds such as aftatoxins.

Dr. Narasimhulu's research has been focused mainly on the biochemistry of adrenal steroid 21 hydroxylase.

Henry Sloviter is exploring the possible uses of a new emulsion of perfluorochemical that he has developed in which the emulsified particles are coated with phospholipid. After intravenous infusion of this promising blood substitute, retention of the perfluorochemical in the circulation can be prolonged by injections of lecithin.

Elizabeth Miller's research is concerned with the biochemistry and immunology of cancer, working with long-established tumor lines in rats and mice.

David Kritchevsky, who collaborates with Dr. Mullen, is working with fascinating systems of experimental arteriosclerosis in rabbits and primates, the influence of dietary fat and fiber, and experimental carcinogenesis.

Neurosurgery

Since Tom Langfitt's appointment as Charles Harrison Frazier Professor and Director of the Division in 1968, the central hypothesis that has driven Neurosurgery's highly successful research is that brain ischemia is the final common denominator of irreversible brain damage and neuronal death in patients with head injuries.

Since 1969, the Division has been the recipient of a major NIH-funded grant as a Head Injury Clinical Research Center. A major focus of the program has been the measurement of regional cerebral blood flow initially by using the 133 Xenon intracarotid injection method and later by using a noninvasive technique developed by Walter Obrist for administering the 133 Xenon (either intravenously or by inhalation), which was demonstrated to be as accurate as the intracarotid method.

A second direction in the 1970s was the development of biochemical methodologies by Frank Welch for studying the regional and microregional alterations produced in the brain in response to global ischemia and hypoxia, demonstrating that even with the most uniform insult the response of the brain was heterogenous. Some regions with total energy failure demonstrated complete bioenergetic recovery, whereas others went on to tissue necrosis. Welch measured microregional blood flow and a variety of other parameters in an attempt to find the cause of the heterogeneity, observations that were important contributions to the understanding of experimental ischemia.

A third arm of the research program was Thomas Gennarelli's development of a primate model closing mimiking closed head injury in humans. Since 1975, the research efforts of the Division have been coordinated by Wayne Alves who replaced Obrist as Director of Research.

Clinical Research Programs

The central piece of Neurosurgery's clinical research efforts in the last few years has been the application of the noninvasive 133 Xenon technique to the study of acute head injuries. More than 150 patients were studied, with the major observation being that patients with acute head injuries are divided about equally into a group with increased cerebral blood flow and a group with reduced flow. In the former group, the major management problems are brain swelling and increased intracranial pressure. In the latter group, there is suggestive evidence that hyperventilation, which is standard therapy in patients with head injuries, can produce iatrogenic ischemia.

Drs. Gennarelli and Langfitt developed a new classification of head injury based on the length of coma and computed tomography (CT) diagnosis, entering more than 1,000 patients with severe head injuries into the classification. With this large data base they were able to define the morbidity and mortality within each category of the classification. Subdural hematoma was the big killer. The nature of the injury (hematoma, contusion, or diffuse injury) proved to be as important in predicting outcome as the Glasgow Coma Score.

Experimental Head Injury Program

In recent years, the efforts of the experimental head injury laboratory have been directed toward developing several reproducible models of clinically relevant head injury in primates and studying the biomechanics, physiology, and neuropathology of the injuries. Since 1983, the scope of research has been broadened to include studies of axonal damage in the giant axon of the squid and in the optic nerve of the guinea pig. These *in vivo* studies were paralleled by nonbiologic models, mathematical stimulations, and computer reconstructions of various segments of the head injury problem.

The principal achievement of the studies has been the demonstration that diffuse axonal injury, a term coined by Dr. Gennarelli, is the major cause of prolonged coma in patients with head injuries. The primate data demonstrated that a particular set of acceleration conditions produced a constellation of clinical and pathologic features that was unique to those conditions. In the case of diffuse anxonal injury, the direction in which the head was accelerated was a critical factor. It occurred only if the head was accelerated side to side, not in a sagittal plane. The close correlation between diffuse axonal injury and prolonged coma was demonstrated by the fact that the depth and duration of coma as well as the neurologic outcome were proportional to the amount of axonal damage demonstrated at postmortem examination in the primates.

The nature of the axonal injury was studied with light and electron microscopy and by axonal transport studies with horseradish peroxidase. Axonal damage was not maximal at the time of injury. Instead, transected or axotomized axons increased in number for the first 24 hours, suggesting a secondary injury phenomenon. The site of damage almost always occurred at the nodes of Ranvier. The most exciting and potentially important observation from the electron microscopy studies was the presence of large numbers of damaged axons with degeneration of the axoplasm but intact axon sheaths, suggesting the possibility that axons damaged in continuity could regenerate.

Experimental Ischemia

During the past 6 years, Frank Welsh has characterized, in great detail, the biochemical changes that accompany ischemic brain damage with the elusive goal of identifying the sequence of events that leads to irreversible neuronal damage. In the past 2 years, he has turned his attention to the putative role of excess neurotransmitters in producing delayed ischemic damage, especially in the hippocampus and basal ganglia. According to one hypothesis, the release of excess glutamate causes prolonged post-synaptic nuronal excition that, in the absence of sufficient O2, causes selective ischemic death of those neurons. He is testing this hypothesis by measuring high-energy phosphates, lactate, glutamate, glutamine, and aspartate in picogram samples of the layers of the hippocampus.

Brain Imaging and In Vivo *Biochemistry*

Beginning in 1980, Dr. Langfitt along with Britton Chance, Stanley Baum (Chairman of the Department of Radiology), and Martin Reivich (Director of the PET Center) initiated a plan for the development of morphologic and functional brain imaging. Chance and his colleagues had conducted some of the earliest studies with *in vivo* NMR spectroscopy. Baum had a long-standing relationship with the General Electric Company in the development of CT imaging. The first PET center funded by the NIH was established at the University of Pennsylvania in the late 1970s under the leadership of Reivich and Abass Alavi.

As an outcome of the collaboration, the first MRI unit built by the General Electric Company (a .12 Tesla system) was used to examine several hundred patients. NMR spectroscopy was added to the General Electric system this year as well as an imaging system for animals, which have been used to study models of experimental brain ischemia and elevated intracranial pressure in the cat.

In the summer of 1986, a 2.0 Tesla 1-m bore spectrometer was installed that under the direction of John Leigh and his colleagues in the Johnson Foundation is producing superb spectra of the human brain and will be used to develop clinical multicenter spectroscopy and metabolic imaging, particularly of lactate. The opportunities at the University of Pennsylvania for studying brain disorders with morphologic and functional imaging are second to no other institution in the world.

Urology

Alan Wein, who succeeded John Murphy as Chief of Urology in 1983, has built a research program that we believe is as productive in basic research as any in the country. In the last few years, Urology's research efforts have been concentrated in the following two fields: (1) neurophysiology and neuropharmacology of the lower urinary tract and (2) urinary tract infection and intrinsic defense mechanisms of the lower urinary tract. In the field of neurourology, these efforts have been concerned primarily with the neuromorphology, neurophysiology, and neuropharmacology of the lower urinary tract and alterations in these parameters under specific conditions. Considerable progress has been made in correlating the functional and metabolic characteristics of detrusor smooth muscle and in developing experimental models with clinical problems in voiding. Peer review funding has been consistently obtained (NIH and VA Merit Review) for these projects that Drs. Levin and Wein direct and in which Drs. Ruggeri, Hanno, and VanArdalen also participate.

In addition, an excellent laboratory model for the study of erectile function has been developed. A transrectal stimulator has been developed that may have clinical applicability in the diagnosis and treatment of erectile dysfunction. Research in infertility has primarily concentrated on clinical parameters related to semen analyses, and on the effects of various pharmacologic environments on sperm motility.

Pediatric Surgery

Dr. James O'Neill is Surgeon-In-Chief of the Children's Hospital of Pennsylvania (CHOP) and Chief of the Division of Pediatric Surgery, having succeeded Chick Koop who left to become Surgeon General of the United States in 1981. Jim is an internationally respected academic surgeon of the first order who is known particularly for his work in burns, vascular surgery, and trauma.

He has built a research program at CHOP that is funded by a variety of sources including the NIH–NCI, the McCabe Fund, the Glenmede Foundation, and the Surgical Associates Research and Education Foundation. Usually two fellows participate in the research activities of the Division. Last year they published 26 papers, 21 chapters, and 1 book. World class research programs exist in the Divisions of Urology and Neurosurgery, which I have neither the time nor expertise to describe here. A few of the research projects in General Surgery include:

1. Development of a reproducible model of hepatic injury in the dog.
2. Development of a continent ileostomy in dogs through the use of abdominal wall muscle conditioning.
3. A new technique for evaluating cutaneous vascularity in conjoined twins.
4. Splenic autotransplantation.
6. Protein-calorie malnutrition and the immunologic reflex.
7. Influence of primary tumor site on lymphocyte antitumor activity.
8. Tumor immunogenicity—the prime determinant of the nutritional influence on the host-tumor relationship.
9. Hepatic and small bowel transplantation in the rat.

The research programs of two individuals, Dr. William Norwood and Dr. Moritz M. Ziegler, merit special mention here.

Dr. William Norwood came to CHOP from Harvard in 1983 to head the Cardiothoracic Division. He is an internationally respected cardiac surgeon who is well known particularly for development of the operation for hypoplastic left heart ("Baby Fay Syndrome"). In addition to building an active clinical service, he has a major research program funded through the NIH, including studies such as those described below.

Protective Effects of Hypothermia During Altered Perfusion States

Myocardial bioenergetics are being assessed using NMR and correlated with systolic and diastolic ventricular function before, during, and after periods of altered perfusion. The current model includes neonatal lambs and pigs that undergo sternotomy, cannulation of the ascending aorta and right atrium, and placement of a surface NMR coil for evaluation of high-energy phosphates and bulk tissue sodium.

The influence of hypothermia on alternations in complex I, II, III, IV, and V of mitochondria derived from brain, heart, and liver subjected to varying periods of ischemia is being studied to elucidate the primary alterations in mitochondrial function that are brought about by periods of ischemia. Further investigation in this area may permit interventions that will attenuate the alterations seen with ischemia.

The Influence of pH and PCO2 on Systemic and Pulmonary Vascular Resistance

The influence of pH and PCO2 on systemic and pulmonary vascular resistance is being studied in an animal model of a single ventricle with a systemic to pulmonary artery shunt. This research is being carried out in neonatal pigs with interarterial communications and these pigs undergo creation of pulmonary atresia with placement of a systemic to pulmonary artery shunt.

Dr. Moritz M. Ziegler, who trained in General Surgery at HUP and Pediatric Surgery at CHOP, is one of the most promising young pediatric surgeons in the country and is the Division's Research Director. He trained in the Harrison Department in transplantation biology and at Fox Chase with Rich Prehn in tumor immunology. He is an active member of the HUP transplant team, rotating as the service chief for kidney transplantation on a regular basis. He recently obtained further training in liver transplantation with Dr. Thomas Starzl in Pittsburgh in preparation for heading the projected liver and kidney transplant programs for children.

Several of Dr. Ziegler's research projects are summarized below.

Immunobiology of Murine Neuroblastoma

Treatment of murine neuroblastoma by surgery, electrocoagulation, laser therapy, radiation, and adjuvant chemotherapy has been evaluated as has immunotherapy with BCG, *Corynebacterium parvum,* and Levamasole. Operative resection of C1300 murine neuroblastoma was found to be effective, but fails to cure the less immunogeneic, widely metastasizing TBJ neuroblastoma clone. Radiation is also an effective therapy that in itself does not suppress the host antitumor immune response if delivered locally. Adjuvant chemotherapy using cell cycle analysis, as a supplement to cytoreductive operation, is also effective but only if cyclophosphamide is used. All other cell cycle specific and nonspecific agents were ineffective whether given before or after cytoreductive surgery. Thus, cell cycle analysis did not lead to development of an effective antitumor regimen. The antitumor activity of cyclophosphamide was noted only in immunocompetent animals, and the antitumor effect was abrogated by immunosuppression of the tumor-bearing host. The antitumor activity of cyclophosphamide was transferable by spleen cell suspensions from treated mice, suggesting that the antitumor effect might be based on an antisuppressor T-cell activity that allowed the host's own cytotoxic T-cells to exert antitumor activity.

In a fortuitous observation, a clone of immunizing C1300 neuroblastoma was identified as TBJ neuroblastoma, which is characterized by rapid local tumor growth and a propensity for metastasis. These two tumors allowed the testing of the hypothesis that the influence of host nutritional status on tumor growth is limited to its influence on the host's antitumor response, *i.e.,* in systems in which the host can mount no antitumor activity or may even accentuate growth of the tumor. This observation was supported by previously reported (but unreconciled) data suggesting that nutritional support had varied effects on the host–tumor relationship, an influence that had not previously been attributed to host antitumor immune activity.

Neonatal Malnutrition and Ischemic Bowel Disease

Because patients in whom necrotizing enterocolitis develops are often iatrogenically malnourished, Dr. Ziegler attempted to develop an animal model of necrotizing enterocolitis based on the malnourished neonate's exposure to hypoxic–hypothermic stress. Maternal malnutrition was induced in the last trimester of pregnancy by protein restriction of the dam, and her small-for-gestational-age offspring were then stressed by hypoxia hypothermia. Ischemic bowel disease histologically similar to human necrotizing enterocolitis developed in one third of the stressed, malnourished neonates. Foster nursing by normally nourished dams abrogated the susceptibility of the neonates. Whether inbred animals were foster nursed by dams of the same or differing MHC compatibility, the protection afforded was the same. These data suggest that leukocytes in breast milk are not the protective element that can prevent the development of enterocolitis. Another model of neonatal nutritional manipulation is currently being studied in which one side of the bicornuate uterus of a pregnant dam is devascularized. The SGA newborns and AGA newborns from the two sides of the bicornuate uterus were compared in a hypoxic–hypothermic stressed model.

In another study of ischemic bowel disease, multiple factors have been analyzed that may protect the host from ischemic intestinal injury when provided by interruption of the mesenteric circulation. Dr. Ziegler found that when the mesenteric circulation of adult animals was temporarily interrupted preischemia nutritional status was an important determinant of outcome, with normally nourished animals faring best. He found proton NMR to be a sensitive index of intestinal ischemic injury, an index even more sensitive than electron microscopy of tissues. He also demonstrated that oxygenated perfluorochemical administered either intraperitoneally or into the gut serves as an effective vehicle for oxygen delivery and prevents progression of ischemic disease. Low molecular weight dextran also is of benefit to ischemic-injured intestine.

Nuclear Magnetic Resonance (NMR) and Organ Transplantation

Accessory cardiac isografts and allografts were transplanted to the neck, a location that permitted their direct assessment by phosphate NMR that was found capable of identifying early cardiac allograft rejection. In rabbits, renal isografts and allografts also have been studied by NMR to distinguish rejection from chemical nephrotoxicity and cyclosporine toxicity.

The following research fellows who were trained by Dr. Ziegler participated in these studies: Arthur Cooper, Irwin Krasna, Charles G. Howell, Haruhiko Naito, Suzanne Topalian, John L. Ricci, Andrew Fox, James E. Miller, Thomas Floyd, Khalil Abu-Dalu, Jane Kugaczewski, and Martin Karpeh.

This summary is far from complete† but may give you some idea of current activity in our laboratories, so much of which is attributable to the attention Dr. Rhoads gave to his responsibilities as Director of the Harrison Department of Surgical Research from 1959 to 1972. Now we must proceed with the main program of this scientific symposium, which will be devoted to presentations by our visitors, Dr. Rhoads' trainees.

† The published summary is in fact more complete than the one delivered on May 9, and was derived from summaries prepared several months earlier by the individual investigators for a departmental report.

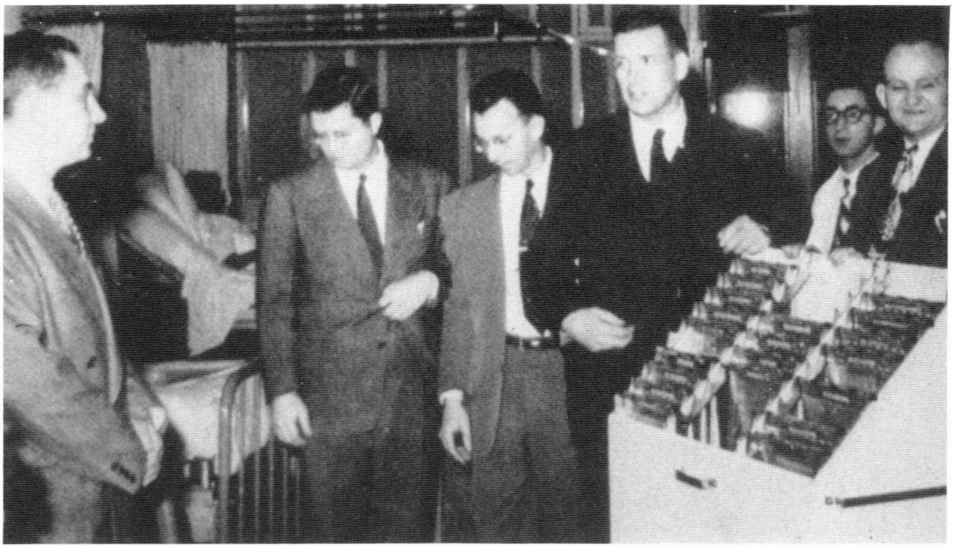

Introduction of Dr. John Howard

Dr. Clyde Barker: We should now get to the major business of the day which is to hear from our outstanding panel of speakers, all of whom are Penn trainees. Our first speaker, John Howard, is seen here with Dr. Rhoads, Jim Hardy, Hal Barker, and Harold Zintel in a photograph taken about 1950, the year that John finished as Chief Resident at HUP. In more recent pictures, Dr. Rhoads possibly looks a bit older, but John looks almost exactly the same.

Since the days of his residency, John has been interested in pancreatitis, which will be the subject of his talk this morning. Dr. Rhoads, as we all know, has also been quite interested in the pancreas and has written about it often. His favorite topic has been treatment of pancreatic tumors, but he has also published papers with Dr. Howard and others on pancreatitis, such as "Death Due to Delayed Hemorrhage in Acute Pancreatitis" (*Surg Gynecol Obstet* 100:458–462, 1955). I have a hunch that John may refer to some of the experiences he shared with Dr. Rhoads in the old days as he speaks this morning on "Pancreatitis 1947–1987."

Dr. Howard's Introductory Remarks

Dr. Rhoads, Dr. Barker, and colleagues, how nice for Nina and me to join you today. Our host of honor has recently written a history of surgery of the pancreas,* but I would like to point out a few things that he didn't include. In 1947, when I was 2 years into my surgical training, I reviewed the experience in acute pancreatitis at HUP from 1922 to 1946, a period of 25 years during the surgical leadership of Drs. Muller, Eliason, and Ravdin. During this 25-year period, 80 patients were diagnosed as having acute pancreatitis. The accuracy of this diagnosis wasn't very good at that time. Smogyi had only recently described his assay for amylase. Although I have not validated this in the literature, I always gave credit to Dr. Robert Elman for adapting this laboratory test to a surgical setting, since at that time, serum amylase determinations were not available in the hospital's clinical laboratory. Dr. Rhoads gave me the opportunity to set up the Smogyi method in the laboratories of the Department

* The history referred to is a chapter in Dr. Howard's book, which has for many years been the standard text on pancreatic disease: *Surgical Diseases of the Pancreas,* (Eds.) J. M. Howard, G. L. Jordan and H. A. Reber, Lea & Febiger, 1987.

of Surgery. I was given a bench up in the Harrison Department, and I made up all of my own reagents. Everything was done by hand, and most of it was done at night or on weekends. One Saturday night, Nina and I were out at a residents' party. She well remembers it. We thought that our whereabouts was known only to the baby-sitter when the telephone rang at 11:00 PM "John, Jonathan Rhoads speaking, I have a patient in the Hospital and it would be awfully helpful to get a serum amylase". And there went that Saturday night. I also remember being asked by Julian Johnson to go to Bethlehem, Pennsylvania, to see a patient in consultation. I was a junior resident. The patient, a student at Bethlehem, was the son of wealthy South American industrialist. My role was to go with Julian, get a blood sample, and bring it back to Philadelphia for an amylase determination. The amylase level was equivocally high, but the patient turned out to have a superior mesenteric vein thrombosis. It was several years more before the test was set up in the laboratories of the Hospital.

Acute Pancreatitis 1947–1987

JOHN M. HOWARD, M.D.

IN 1947, 2 years into residency training, the author reviewed the experience with acute pancreatitis in the Hospital of the University of Pennsylvania over the preceding 25 years: 1922 to 1946.[1] During that 25-year period, acute pancreatitis had been diagnosed in 80 patients, approximately three patients per year. The correct diagnosis had been made before operation or autopsy in only 14 patients (18%). The serum amylase determination had been developed only recently. But as a result, the correct preoperative diagnosis had been made in 60% of the last 20 patients. The determination of amylase levels had been described by Somogyi a few years earlier but the assay was only then being adapted to the clinical setting.

Dr. Rhoads had given the author the research opportunity to develop the serum amylase determination at this institution. The determination was not available through the hospital laboratories. The Somogyi method was set up on a laboratory bench in the Harrison Department, with all reagents and determinations being made by hand.

It took a number of years before the amylase determination became available through the clinical laboratories.

I suspect that 80, the number of patients with acute pancreatitis seen over the 25-year period, are now seen here within a year or two, and the diagnosis must be made by clinical, roentgenographic, and enzyme determinations close to 100% of the time.

In 1947, acute pancreatitis was a single disease insofar as we recognized it. Careful attention, however, was paid to whether or not the patient had biliary tract disease. Gallstone pancreatitis was not recognized as a distinct entity. It or related syndromes appeared in approximately 62 patients, 77.5%, of the 80 patients. Only 18 of the patients (22.5%) appeared to have a normal biliary tract. Table 1 demonstrates the relationship to biliary tract diseases. No clear-cut distinction was made between the biliary disease patients and the nonbiliary disease patients in terms of prognosis. This period was two to four decades after the two (1901) reports by Opie.[2,3] It is clear that the presence of gallbladder disease entered into the thinking at that time, but gallstone pancreatitis, *per se*, was not considered a distinct entity. No other etiologic consideration was given.

Since the diagnosis was made chiefly at operation or autopsy, the pathologic aspects of the pancreatitis were better documented than they would be today. The classification was nonhemorrhagic *versus* hemorrhagic pancreatitis with nonhemorrhagic being subdivided into edematous pancreatitis or pancreatitis with fat necrosis.

Looking back to 1947 and before, it was recognized that of the 80 patients with acute pancreatitis, 37 (41%) had had previous attacks of acute abdominal pain which had been considered acute biliary tract disease, and 11 of the patients (14%) had been diagnosed previously as having an acute attack of pancreatitis.

The mortality rate for the overall series of 80 patients was 29% with the mortality of the nonhemorrhagic form of the disease being 12% of 59 patients and the hemorrhagic form resulting in a mortality rate of 76% among 21 patients (Table 2). Table 3 demonstrates the mortality rate of the two forms of the disease among those patients who underwent laparotomy *versus* those who did not. Among the patients with nonhemorrhagic disease, the operative mortality was 11% among 53 patients, and 17% among six nonoperative patients. Among the patients with hemorrhagic pancreatitis, the operative mortality was 69% among 16 patients, and 100% among five nonoperative patients.

Of the 53 patients with nonhemorrhagic disease who underwent operation, 35 had a cholecystostomy with or without drainage of the pancreas. This constituted 66% of the

Professor of Surgery, Medical College of Ohio, Toledo, Ohio.

TABLE 1. *Acute Pancreatitis (1922–1946)*

Biliary tract disease	No. of patients
Acute cholecystitis: gallstones	18
Chronic cholecystitis: gallstones	35
Acute cholecystitis: no gallstones	4
Other (*e.g.*, common duct stone with previous cholecystectomy)	5
Subtotal	62 (77 5%)
Normal biliary tract	18 (22 5%)

TABLE 2. *Acute Pancreatitis: Mortality Rates (1922–1946)*

	No. of patients	Mortality
Nonhemorrhagic	59	12%
Hemorrhagic	21	76%
Total	80	29%

operative group. Others had the common bile duct drained or had cholecystectomy, or simple drainage of the pancreas.

While following this early group of patients, it was found that five of the patients, after a definitive diagnosis had been made, had recurrence of the pancreatitis, resulting in the death of two of the patients (Table 4). Two patients with nonhemorrhagic disease experienced recurrences of the hemorrhagic form.

Since 1947, most of the advances in management of patients with acute pancreatitis have resulted from clinical studies. Much has been learned about the metabolic, mechanical, and genetic factors associated with pancreatitis, and a great deal of progress has been made in treatment, but perhaps less fundamental knowledge has accrued in understanding the fundamental mechanisms underlying the etiology of pancreatitis.

The etiologic mechanisms, as currently understood from clinical associations, consist of at least a dozen categories with their numerous subdivisions (Table 5). Information is quite incomplete, for seldom are the more esoteric factors systematically sought after hospital admissions. Consider "viral pancreatitis," for instance. When the author reviewed the literature in 1960, only mumps was considered a possible viral form of pancreatitis.[4] Since that time, mumps pancreatitis has been demonstrated clearly and repeatedly to be an etiologic factor. Coxsackie B and echoviruses in association with pancreatitis have been documented. Mycoplasma pneumoniae have been demonstrated. Pancreatitis associated with infectious hepatitis has been described repeatedly. The possible pathogenecity of cytomegalovirus in the development of acute pancreatitis has been raised by several groups. Herpes simplex

TABLE 3. *Mortality Rates* Versus *Management (1922–1946)*

Pancreatitis	No. of patients	Operative	Nonoperative
Nonhemorrhagic	59	11% of 53 patients	17% of 6 patients
Hemorrhagic	21	69% of 16 patients	100% of 5 patients

TABLE 4. *Acute Pancreatitis (1922–1946)*

	No. of patients
Survivors followed (1–24 yr)	47
Recurrent acute pancreatitis	5
Death from recurrence	2

TABLE 5. *Acute Pancreatitis: Probable Etiologic Mechanisms*

Obstruction
Induced ductal hypertension
Ischemia, including chronic low flow
Chemical, toxin, or drug injury
Allergic inflammation
Metabolic, endocrine, or electrolyte disturbance
Nutritional disturbances
Hereditary factors
Bacterial infection
Viral infection
Parasitic infestation
Postirradiation inflammation
Perhaps trauma

virus has been demonstrated with pancreatitis, as has smallpox and the virus of the common cold. Acute pancreatitis complicating rubella encephalitis has been described. Acute pancreatitis associated with Reyes syndrome has been detected repeatedly, the Reyes syndrome resulting from Influenza B, less often Influenza A, and occasionally chickenpox[5] (Table 6). Surgeons seldom study patients with acute pancreatitis for specific evidence of viral diseases, so the frequency of associated viral infections is quite unknown.

Considerable experimental data exists to show that the pancreas does not tolerate acute ischemia or chronic low-flow states well. The incidence of acute pancreatitis after resection of aortic abdominal aneurysms, particularly ruptured aneurysms, is quite high as is acute pancreatitis after extracorporeal bypass of the heart. Hypothermia, either induced or accidental, has been associated repeatedly with acute pancreatitis. Collagen diseases, perhaps reflecting low-flow states in association with pancreatitis, have included lupus erythematosus, periarteritis nodosa, scleroderma, and erythema nodosum (Table 7).

In a recent survey of the world literature, the author identified approximately 115 clinical or laboratory syndromes which may have been etiologically related to pancreatitis.[5] Each may be a specific, separate disease entity, each with its own natural history, and each may eventually require a different form of therapy.

Whereas the causation of the acute pancreatitis is not sharply defined, the results of treatment have been spectacular. Gallstone pancreatitis has clearly evolved as a separate disease entity with the incidence of migration of a stone through the ampulla of Vater being very high, perhaps a universally associated factor in this specific disease. The author reported a series (1951–1984) of 429 patients with only four deaths (0.9%) (Table 8). During the period 1962 to 1984, 178 consecutive patients had been treated without a fatality. Readmission for operation had gradually given way to delayed operation on the first hospitalization, unless the patient had had a life-threatening illness. Including all types of patients with acute pancreatitis, except drug-induced or postoperative pancreatitis, 613 patients were treated from 1962 to 1984 with two fatalities, a mortality rate of 0.3% (Table 9).

Patients are being salvaged today who would certainly have died 40 years ago. By supporting the plasma volume and capillary perfusion, by maintaining adequate ventilation, by supporting nutrition *via* intravenous hyperalimentation, and by withholding or delaying

TABLE 6. *Acute Pancreatitis: Viral Diseases*

Mumps
Enteroviruses
Coxsackie B
Echovirus
Mycoplasma pneumoniae
Infectious hepatitis (various forms)
Infectious mononucleosis
Cytomegalovirus
Herpes simplex, smallpox, "common cold"
Rubella
Influenza B and A, chicken pox

TABLE 7. *Acute Pancreatitis: Ischemia and Low-Flow States*

Atherosclerosis: aneurysms
Cardiac bypass
Hypothermia
Vasculitis of collagen diseases
Lupus erythematosus
Periarteritis nodosa
Scleroderma
Erythema nodosum

TABLE 8. *Acute Gallstone Pancreatitis**

	No. of patients	Deaths
1951–1961	251	4 (0.6%)
1962–1984	178	0
Total	429	6 (0.9%)

* Howard *et al.*[5]

TABLE 9. *Acute Pancreatitis**†

	No. of patients	Deaths
1962–1984	613	2 (0.3%)

* All forms except drug-induced or post-operative.
† Howard *et al.*[5]

operative intervention, patients are surviving the most catastrophic forms of acute pancreatitis. In a recent series (1987) of 35 patient with massive necrosis of peripancreatic or pancreatic tissue, delayed operation has been necessary in 30 patients. Operation was withheld for weeks or months until dead tissue had clearly sequestrated and laparotomy seemed necessary to overcome life-threatening complications such as secondary infection, gastroduodenal obstruction, bleeding, or rupture. Of 35 such patients, 17 required delayed laparotomy on the first hospitalization and 13 required readmission and operation. Only one patient died due to the result of an overlooked stone at the ampulla of Vater associated with a failure of gastroduodenal emptying.

REFERENCES

1. Howard JM, Ravdin IS. Acute pancreatitis: A study of 80 patients. Am Practitioner 1948;2:385–395.
2. Opie EL. Etiology of acute hemorrhagic pancreatitis. Johns Hopkins Hosp Bull 1901;12:182.
3. Opie EL. The relation of choledocholithiasis in disease of the pancreas and to fat necrosis. Johns Hopkins Hosp Bull 1901;12:19.
4. Howard JM, Jordan GL Jr. Surgical Diseases of the Pancreas. Philadelphia: JB Lippincott, 1960.
5. Howard JM, Jordan GL Jr, Reber HA. Surgical Diseases of the Pancreas. Philadelphia: Lea and Febiger, 1987.

Dr. Howard's Concluding Remarks

Dr. Rhoads, the understanding of the clinical ramifications of acute pancreatitis and its treatment have greatly expanded during your career. There is one thing of which I'm sure and that is that in 1947, patients who were critically ill with pancreatitis died, while in 1987, the same critically ill patients live. They live because of the support of intensive care units, house staff, ventilators, departments of respiratory therapy, antibiotics, and a lot of very hard work. But one thing I'm sure of, Dr. Rhoads. Without your contribution which allows us to give them nutritional support intravenously, if necessary even for a period of months, these patients would not survive. For that, our patients and we are very grateful. Thank you, Dr. Rhoads.

DISCUSSION

DR. WILLIAM LONGMIRE: I'd like to ask Dr. Howard about the cases he showed in which he had to operate repeatedly to remove necrotic material. Is this due to the damage of the initial attack of pancreatitis or is it due to a continuing process of some kind, either infection or autodigestion?

DR. JOHN HOWARD: Dr. Longmire, I am not sure which ones are infected. For example, on the Hungarian lady I showed, with the pus exuding, the culture was negative and the gram strain was negative except for many polys. She, of course, had been on antibiotics. I don't know whether this material represents "pus" in the sense of an exudate from bacteria or instead represents liquifying fat. It would be interesting to determine the lipid content of such material. One patient had a stone in the common duct that had been overlooked. He had continuing pancreatitis which I didn't recognize for sure. He was operated on three times. He didn't empty his stomach, and even when we did a gastroenterostomy, he still didn't empty his stomach. He died with continuing illness and the inability to eat.

When you go in to debride, you are frightened of getting into the major vessels. You really can't dissect. You debride very carefully, but the pockets go like the fingers of a glove. You don't know whether you are overlooking some of the necrotic tissue. You think you have it all and whether this reforms, I don't really know, but I think it is there from the beginning.

DR. STAN DUDRICK: Regarding your work on amylase, do you have any thoughts about the hyperamylasemia of salivary gland origin which is sometimes seen? Have you made a correlation between hyperamylasemia of salivary glands *vs.* that of the pancreas? Is there any connection in terms of susceptibility to pancreatitis later on? Sometimes troublesome patients that we think we're treating almost solely for the abnormal chemical determination have surprisingly died.

DR. JOHN HOWARD: This week we had a patient convalescing from multiple intra-abdominal abscesses who developed an increased amylase. We thought maybe he had a pancreatic abscess, but the patient was asymptomatic and it turned out to be salivary gland amylase. I don't think the salivary gland amylase has much to do with pancreatitis except as a differential diagnosis. As you know, the Japanese have written a good bit about it. They say that many trauma patients have an increased serum amylase on admission and that this is characteristically salivary amylase. They also say that when patients with coronary bypass develop amylase elevation, it is often of salivary origin. However, anyone who does a lot of cardiac bypass work recognizes that there is also a high incidence of acute pancreatitis in these patients. I think it is basically a laboratory distinction that we should make and that perhaps, Dr. Rhoads, hospital laboratories should make salivary amylase tests available on Saturday night.

DR. FRANK ROSATO: Have you any feeling about the possible role of peritoneal lavage therapy in the management of severe pancreatitis?

DR. JOHN HOWARD: You are postulating that there is a toxin associated with acute pancreatitis that you can wash out by lavage. This is still a dubious hypothesis. If you take pancreatic juice from a dog and infuse it intravenously, you can carry the dog's serum amylase up to 100,000 Smogyi units, but he tolerates it quite well. Even if you activate the proteolytic enzymes, the dog still doesn't find it very toxic. On the other hand, if you take the peritoneal exudate from a dog with acute pancreatitis and infuse that intravenously, it does make him sick. I am not sure whether this is a bacterial factor. We went through this, some of you may recall, with thermal burn patients. The basic scientists found a toxin, but we recognized after awhile that we were basically dealing with hypovolemia and secondary bacterial infection. I personally don't use lavage and have no experience with it.

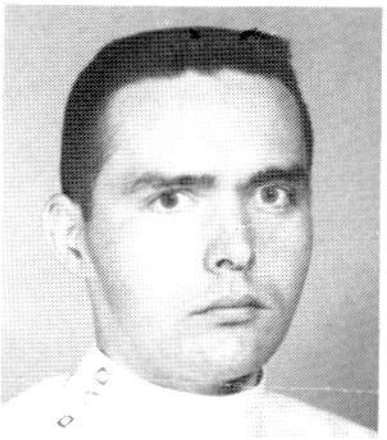

Introduction of Dr. Scott Jones

Dr. Clyde Barker: Scott Jones is a Texan who, after finishing his residency at HUP in 1967, went to Los Angeles for training in GI physiology under Morton Grossman. He then moved to Dr. Dunphy's department in San Francisco to direct his own research program at the VA Hospital, where he became Chief of Surgery before being recruited by Dave Sabiston to Duke where he headed the program in GI surgery. In 1982, he became Professor and Chairman of the Department of Surgery at the University of Virginia.

An article entitled "The Results of Sulfonamide Prophylaxis in the Surgery of Large Bowel" (*Surg Clin North Am* 22:1585–1591, 1942) was written by Drs. Ravdin, Lockwood, and Rhoads in 1942. As you can see from the title, Dr. Rhoads has been writing about Scott's topic of today, colon cancer, for at least 45 years. He was one of the first investigators to use anti-bacterial agents in bowel preps. I am sorry there is not time today to show a movie that Dr. Rhoads and Dr. Ravdin made on abdominoperineal resection. Dr. Schwegman was Dr. Rhoads' collaborator on the operation shown in that movie, as well as on many other AP resections. They described their technique in "One-Stage Combined Abdomino-perineal Resection of the Rectum (Miles) Performed by Two Surgical Teams (*Surgery,* 58:600–606, 1965). Clete has some absolutely fascinating recollections of the operation that was filmed. I advise you to catch him during the coffee break for his account of this.

Dr. Scott Jones' Introductory Remarks

I appreciate the opportunity to participate in this symposium which gives all of us the opportunity to savor the feeling of pride we felt as residents. This is the 20th anniversary of my graduation from the program, and I see several of my cohorts here in this room: Ed Kaplan, Stan Dudrick, and Leonard Weiner. First of all, I want to say Happy Birthday and thank you to Dr. Rhoads and to say that he's blessed everything he's touched. He's blessed this community and this University. He's blessed his profession, and he's blessed every one of us in this room, and for it, we are deeply grateful. Dr. Rhoads has had many accomplishments that everyone in the room knows as well as I do. He has clearly been one of the great leaders in our profession, and those of us who trained under Dr. Rhoads see him as a role model. That term, which has kind of surfaced lately, is one we didn't use much 25 years ago. But even then, we tried to emulate all of the accomplishments and all of the good qualities that Dr. Rhoads demonstrated to us and that we are here today to celebrate. If we had a list of all of Dr. Rhoads' accomplishments, there are many I would personally try to reproduce, but enjoying a nice 80th birthday wouldn't be last on the list.

As the other speakers have done, I will talk about work started here at the Hospital of the University of Pennsylvania a few years ago. I'll begin by reporting a series of patients who were treated at HUP for carcinoma of the colon. The authors on this paper were Drs. Copeland, Miller, and Jones. I don't know how my name ended up last because I did all of the work! But I'll have to be careful what I say because some of the other folks on that paper are going to follow me on this program and I might get hurt a little bit.

I have to turn around here so that I can see the screen. After seeing the other speakers struggle to do this, Ted Copeland told me I should move the podium. But he didn't tell me it was bolted to the floor. Now, if Dr. Rhoads told me to move it, I'd move it!

Prognostic Factors in Carcinoma of the Colon and Rectum

EDWARD M. COPELAND, M.D., LEONARD D. MILLER, M.D., AND RAYFORD S. JONES, M.D.

GILBERTSEN[1] HAS POINTED OUT that the apparent improvement in survival from cancer of the colon is related to the use of selected patients in statistical analysis. He reports an absolute five year survival rate of 32 per cent in an analysis of 840 unselected patients with carcinoma of the colon. Welch and Burke[2] obtained a 38 per cent over-all five year survival rate in a similar group of patients from the New England area. Griffin, Judd, and Gage[3] reported a gross five year survival of 40.1 per cent for a series of patients with cancer of the ascending colon, and Glenn and McSherry[4] arrived at a similar figure (40.2 per cent) for carcinoma of the distal part of the descending colon. In an attempt to further elucidate the absolute five year survival rate for carcinoma of the colon and rectum, all patients with this disease seen at the Hospital of the University of Pennsylvania between 1941 and 1956 were studied. All parameters affecting gross yearly survival were examined. This time interval was chosen for completeness of follow up, and because chemotherapeutic agents, used sparingly throughout this period, can be eliminated as a cause of prolonged survival in any age group.

Since carcinoma of the colon affects an older age group, many patients operated upon for cure die before a five year period and have no detectable disease at death. In other series, patients in this category have been handled in various ways. In this study, the number of patients in this group is stated for each parameter investigated.

General Survey

One thousand eighty-four patients with carcinoma of the colon and rectum treated between 1941 and 1956 were studied. The disease was most prevalent in the sixth and seventh decade. The majority of the lesions were in the sigmoid and rectum, locations consistent with those reported by other observers. Seventy-six per cent of the patients had disease which was estimated to be curable at the time of operation. (Table 1.) All but 6.5 per cent of the patients underwent resection.

One hundred eighty-six patients had palliative resection; results of follow-up in 177 patients in this group appears in Table 2. One half of these patients died within the first twelve postoperative months and 87 per cent were dead at the end of three years. The 8.4 per cent of patients living at the end of five years did not have any evidence of recurrent disease clinically. It is probable that the tumor tissue thought left behind was inflammatory rather than neoplastic. The operative mortality was 4.0 per cent in those having palliative resection, which compares very favorably with present day mortality figures and with the mortality rate for the entire series (4.4 per cent). Patients who underwent exploration for palliation alone (with procedures including colostomy, side to side bypass, and the like) and who did not have resection had a somewhat less favorable prognosis. (Table 2.)

Survival

The over-all five year survival figures are somewhat more encouraging than other published results.[1] There has been a recurring debate in the literature concerning the relative

From the Harrison Department of Surgical Research, School of Medicine, University of Pennsylvania, Philadelphia, Pennsylvania.
This work was supported in part by a Clinical Fellowship of the American Cancer Society.
This article has been reproduced with permission from the *American Journal of Surgery*, Vol. 116, December 1978.

TABLE 1. *Estimate of Curability at Operation*

Status	No. of Patients	Per cent of Total
Curable	826	76.4
Resectable but not curable	186	17.1
Not resectable	26	2.4
Not resected for clinical reasons	45	4.1

TABLE 2. *Survival of Patients Thought Incurable at the Time of Operation*

Survival	Resectable but Not Curable (177 patients)	Unresectable (Palliative Procedure) (71 patients)
Operative deaths	4.0%	7.0%
1–12 mo.	53.5%	66.3%
1–2 yr.	20.4%	18.3%
2–3 yr.	9.0%	5.6%
3–4 yr.	3.6%	1.4%
4–5 yr.	1.1%	0
5 yr. or more	8.4%	1.4%

effectiveness of abdominoperineal resection versus anterior resection for low-lying lesions. In our series, patients with lesions 5 to 14 cm. from the anus had an especially poor over-all prognosis. The lesions in this area were treated by both technics. The five year survival of those patients with lesions estimated curable, and who were treated by abdominoperineal resection, seemed somewhat better than that of a similar group treated by low anterior resection (Table 3), results which conform with the observations of others.[4,5]

The gross five year survival for all patients with carcinoma of the colon and rectum was 37.3 per cent. (Table 4.) Ten per cent of the patients were dead with no carcinoma before a five year period had elapsed. One cannot comment on whether recurrent disease would have appeared in these patients had they survived for the five year period. It is probable that the differing five year survival figures published by other observers result from the difference in handling of this category of patient. Five year survival for patients with estimated *curable* lesions was 48.1 per cent. Another 13.9 per cent of these patients died within five years after treatment with no manifestation of recurrent tumor. Only 3.4 per cent of all the patients were alive at five years with proved recurrent carcinoma of the colon. Consequently

TABLE 3. *Five Year Survival for Patients With Estimated Curable Lesions Treated by Abdominoperineal Resection or Low Anterior Resection*

Status	Abdominoperineal Resection	Low Anterior Resection
Alive with no carcinoma	39.6%	31.6%
Alive with carcinoma	3.8%	1.7%
Dead with no carcinoma	9.8%	16.7%
Dead with carcinoma	45.0%	50.0%

TABLE 4. *Status at Five Years After Treatment*

Status	Gross Survival (1,084 patients)	Estimated Curable (826 patients)
Alive; no details available	0.0%	4.1%
Alive with no carcinoma	34.4%	40.6%
Alive with carcinoma	2.9%	3.4%
Dead with no carcinoma	11.5%	13.9%
Dead with carcinoma	51.2%	38.0%

TABLE 5. *Accumulative Time of Postoperative Occurrence of Distant Metastases in 197 Patients With Lesions Originally Estimated Curable*

Time	Per cent
0–12 mo.	38%
1–2 yr.	64%
2–3 yr.	76%
3–4 yr.	91%
4–5 yr.	94%
5 yr. or more	100%

the disease can recur before the five year period and not be uniformly fatal by this time; this situation, however, is rare.

The time of occurrence of later distant metastases in patients originally estimated curable is evaluated in Table 5. If recurrent disease is to occur after a curative resection, fully three quarters of the cases will have appeared by the end of three years and 94 per cent by the end of five years. Thus a five year survival is virtually equivalent to a cure in this disease.

The liver is the most frequent site of later distant metastases in patients estimated curable, followed by the lung and distant nodes. (Table 6.) Approximately one half of the patients with later distant metastases have no nodal involvement at the time of the original procedure. However, 75 per cent of the patients with metastatic disease to the brain and vertebral column did have nodal involvement at the original procedure. (Table 6.) A significant number of patients in this series fell into a group undergoing an estimated curative operation where one margin of the resected specimen was measured at less than 5 cm. from either or both edges of the tumor. The ensuing suture line recurrence rate was correspondingly high (18.4 per cent). As a result, perhaps, the survival in this group was significantly less than in a similar group of patients in whom at least 5 cm. of normal colon was excised proximal and distal to the lesion. (Table 7.) The suture line recurrence rate for the entire series of 1,084 patients was 10.1 per cent, essentially confirming Cole's data.[6]

Welch and Burke[2] believe that tumors which are highly malignant rapidly produce symptoms and demand urgent care. Those of his patients with long delays between onset of symptoms and treatment had a better prognosis, indicating that these lesions manifested lower malignant potential, and were more amenable to surgical cure. A similar pattern was

TABLE 6. *Site of Later Distant Metastasis in Patients With Lesions Originally Estimated Curable*

Site	Per cent	Original Nodal Involvement
Liver	64.5%	50%
Lung	28.4%	57%
Vertebral column	10.2%	70%
Bowel	11.3%	41%
Brain	4.1%	75%
Distant nodes	14.2%	59%
Adrenal	4.1%	50%
Carcinomatosis	11.2%	52%

TABLE 7. *Five Year Follow-up Data in Patients Undergoing Local Resection for Lesions Estimated Curable*

Status	Local Resection Margin Greater than 5 cm. (141 patients)	Local Resection Margin Less than 5 cm. (206 patients)
Alive with no carcinoma	51.1%	38.4%
Alive with carcinoma	5.7%	2.4%
Dead with no carcinoma	10.6%	17.4%
Dead with carcinoma	32.6%	41.8%

TABLE 8. *Time of First Symptom to Operation* Correlated With Five Year Survival*

Status	Duration: 0 to 5 Months (493 patients)	6 to 12 Months (335 patients)	12 Months or More (152 patients)
Alive with no carcinoma	31%	37%	36%
Alive with carcinoma	3%	2%	2%
Dead; no details available	1%	1%	1%
Dead with no carcinoma	10%	10%	8%
Dead with carcinoma	55%	50%	53%

* The median was 5 months.

noted in this series, in that 37 per cent of the patients having symptoms for six months or longer survived five years without recurrence, whereas only 31 per cent of those with symptoms existing six months or less were alive without recurrence at the end of a five year period. (Table 8.) Obviously a purposeful delay in treatment would not increase survival, but it does seem that the innate virulence of the tumor and the resistance of the host are at least as important as "early diagnosis and treatment." An abdominal mass, obstruction, and anemia have been correlated with a rapidly progressing tumor. The presence of a palpable mass or anemia (symptomatic or asymptomatic) in this series, was not indicative of a poorer prognosis. (Table 9.) Thus a tumor present long enough to produce symptomatic anemia or a mass does not necessarily possess a greater tendency to metastatic spread. Obstructing carcinoma, however, uniformly carried a poor prognosis. (Table 9.)

Vein invasion, nodal and bowel wall involvement, and pathologic differentiation had direct effect upon the five year survival of patients with carcinoma of the colon. The res specimens were examined microscopically venous invasion by special staining techniques (Verhoeff-Van Gieson) in 597 instances. 19 per cent of the patients with vein invasion were alive at five years and free of tumor whereas 40 per cent of those free of vein invasion survived for five years without recurrence. (Table 10.) Thus vein invasion, an isolated phenomenon, carries a poor prognosis and when correlated with other evidence of local spread, further decreases the chance of five year cure. The over-all five year survival for patients with no nodal involvement in 51.5 per cent. (Table 11.) Having one nodule involved reduced the chances of survival, but a further fall in survival rate was not noted until five or more nodes were involved. (Table 11.) Depth of penetration of the bowel wall with or without nodal spreading delineated by an Astley-Coller classification integrally related to

TABLE 9. *Five Year Survival Correlated With the Presenting Signs and Symptoms of Mass, Obstruction, and Anemia*

Status	Mass (220 patients)	Obstruction (133 patients)	Symptomatic Anemia (115 patients)	Asymptomatic Anemia (197 patients)
Alive with no carcinoma	33%	21%	35%	31%
Alive with carcinoma	2%	3%	2%	2%
Dead with no carcinoma	8%	13%	8%	14%
Dead with carcinoma	57%	63%	55%	53%

TABLE 10. *Five Year Survival Related to Vein Invasion*

Status	Without Vein Invasion (482 patients)	With Vein Invasion (115 patients)
Alive with no carcinoma	40%	19%
Alive with carcinoma	3%	3%
Dead with no carcinoma	12%	3%
Dead with carcinoma	45%	75%

TABLE 11. *Correlation of Nodal Involvement and Five Year Survival of Patients With Carcinoma of the Colon*

Status	No Nodes Involved (584 patients)	One Node Involved (112 patients)	Two Nodes Involved (68 patients)	Three Nodes Involved (40 patients)	Four Nodes Involved (24 patients)	Five or More Nodes Involved (110 patients)
Alive with no carcinoma	48.5%	26.8%	25.0%	15.0%	29.1%	9.1%
Alive with carcinoma	3.0%	3.5%	2.9%	2.5%	4.2%	0.9%
Dead with no carcinoma	17.6%	6.2%	5.9%	2.5%	4.2%	4.5%
Dead with carcinoma	31.9%	63.5%	66.2%	80.0%	62.5%	85.5%

TABLE 12. *Bowel Wall Involvement With and Without Nodal Metastasis as Related to Five Year Survival*

Status at Five Years	Involvement of Mucosa without Nodes (66 patients)	Involvement of Mucosa with Nodes (3 patients)	Involvement into but not through Muscle without Nodes (150 patients)	Involvement into but not through Muscle with Nodes (58 patients)	Involvement through Muscle without Nodes (379 patients)	Involvement through Muscle with Nodes (329 patients)
Alive; no details available	0	0	1%	0	1%	0
Alive with no carcinoma	71%	67%	61%	48%	39%	13%
Alive with carcinoma	3%	0	3%	5%	3%	2%
Dead; no details available	0	0	0	0	1%	2%
Dead with no carcinoma	20%	33%	16%	0	16%	3%
Dead with carcinoma	6%	0	18%	47%	40%	80%

prognosis. (Table 12.) Extension of the tumor was most frequently through the muscle of the bowel wall), with a five year survival of 43 per cent when no nodes were involved, and 15 per cent when nodal metastasis was present. Similarly, bowel penetration alone was an important prognostic factor. Tumors that had penetrated into but not through the muscle carried a 65 per cent five year survival, as compared to 43 per cent when the entire muscular coat was invaded. Well differentiated lesions were relatively rare in this series, but when they occurred, they carried a good prognosis. (Table 13.) The majority of the well differentiated lesions were confined to the mucosa with no nodal involvement. The more poorly differentiated the lesion, the greater was the correlation with nodal involvement and bowel wall penetration. These lesions generally produced more disturbing symptoms, shortening the time interval between the first onset of symptoms and definitive therapy. Despite this, as indicated previously, the five year survival was relatively poor.

Comments

It seems to us that the gross five year survival rate is the most accurate indicator of the true virulence of carcinoma of the colon and rectum. The absolute five year survival of 37.3 per cent in this series is somewhat higher than that reported by Gilbertsen[1] and significantly higher than that reported by Grinnell[7] and Floyd, Stirling, and Cohn.[8] The results are consistent with the 38 per cent overall five year survival reported by Welch and Burke.[2] The over-all five year survival for each anatomic site was somewhat better than that reported by Gilbertsen.[1] The reason for this apparent improvement resides in the difference in resectability rates between the two series. The resectability rate in our series was 93.5 per cent, whereas during a similar chronologic period (1940–1950), the resectability rate for patients in Gilbertsen's series was only 76 per cent. The patients in our series had lesions seemingly more amenable to surgical correction when they first presented themselves for treatment. It is also conceivable that a more aggressive approach to resection may yield a significant increment in survival without a concomitant increase in operative mortality. Often, fixation of these lesions to other structures is on the basis of inflammation rather than neoplasm, giving rise to undue pessimism as to curability.[9]

The liver was the most frequent site of later distant metastases in patients with or without local spread at the time of operation. Lymph node involvement, vein invasion, or penetration of the tumor through to the serosa halved the five year survival in patients otherwise operated upon for cure. It is in these patients with tumor spread to the pericolonic fat and mesenteric lymph nodes that the resection for cure by the no-touch isolation technic of Turnbull et al.[10] has doubled the five year survival for lesions proximal to the rectum. There can be little question that once tumor has invaded venous channels, dissemination by surgical manipulation is likely. Since it is impossible to determine venous invasion, and frequently lymph node involvement, at the time of operation, the no-touch isolation technic appears to be a logical and potentially productive refinement of operative technic. It seems unfortunate, therefore, that it is most difficult to apply no-touch principles to lesions of the true rectum, the most common single site of occurrence of carcinoma and the area from which the poorest prognosis may be expected. It seems feasible to us to attempt at least a partial application of the technic for lesions amenable to abdominoperineal resection. Although many patients with rectal carcinoma die of local recurrence and ureteral obstruction, a significant group in our series have died of liver metastases after a seemingly curative

TABLE 13. *Five Year Survival Based on the Pathologic Differentiation of Lesion Found at Surgery*

	Lesion		
Status	Well Differentiated (33 cases)	Moderately Well Differentiated (462 cases)	Poorly Differentiated (159 cases)
Alive with no carcinoma	51.5%	39.4%	20.1%
Alive with carcinoma	6.1%	3.0%	1.3%
Dead with no carcinoma	15.2%	12.3%	9.4%
Dead with carcinoma	27.2%	45.3%	69.2%

procedure. Although tumor embolization through venous channels emptying directly into the systemic circuit is difficult, if not impossible, to control, it is possible that early ligation of the inferior mesenteric vein at the level of the bifurcation of the inferior mesenteric artery would be an aid in preventing dissemination through the portal system.

Summary

The clinical and pathologic findings in 1,084 patients with carcinoma of the colon and rectum have been analyzed. The five year survival for the entire group of patients was 37.3 per cent. The five year survival for patients operated upon for cure was 48.1 per cent. The resectability rate was 93.5 per cent, and the over-all operative mortality 4.4 per cent.

If recurrent disease was to occur after curative resection, 94 per cent of the cases appeared by the end of five years.

In patients operated upon for cure, suture-line recurrence was high unless 5 cm. or more of normal colon was excised proximal and distal to the lesion.

The presence of a palpable mass or symptomatic anemia was not indicative of a poorer prognosis.

Vein invasion, nodal involvement, and deep penetration of the bowel wall halved the five year survival in patients operated upon for cure. A plea is made for widespread application of Turnbull's no-touch isolation technic, and for partial application of it in abdominoperineal resection.

REFERENCES

1. Gilbertsen VA. Adenocarcinoma of the large bowel; factors seemingly responsible for unrealistically optimistic appraisals of current curative achievements, and a suggestion for improvement of therapeutic results. JAMA 1960;174:1789.
2. Welch CE, Burke JF. Carcinoma of the colon and rectum. New England J Med 1962;266:211.
3. Griffin GDJ, Judd ES, Gage RP. Carcinoma of the right side of the colon: operability, resectability, and survival rates. Ann Surg 1956;143:330.
4. Glenn F, McSherry CK. Carcinoma of the distal large bowel: 32 year review of 1,026 cases. Ann Surg 1966;163:838.
5. Gilbertsen VA. The results of surgical treatment of cancer of the rectum. Surg Gynec & Obst 1962;114:313.
6. Cole WH. Recurrence in carcinoma of the colon and proximal rectum following resection for carcinoma. Arch Surg 1952;65:264.
7. Grinnell RS. Results in the treatment of carcinoma of the colon and rectum. Surg Gynec & Obst 1953;96:31.
8. Floyd CE, Stirling CT, Cohn I. Cancer of the colon, rectum, and anus. Ann Surg 1966;163:829.
9. Miller LD, Boruchow IB, Fitts WT. An analysis of 284 patients with perforative carcinoma of the colon. Surg Gynec & Obst 1966;123:1212.
10. Turnbull RB, Kyle K, Watson FR, Spratt J. Cancer of the colon: the influence of the no-touch isolation technique on survival rates. Ann Surg 1967;166:420.

Discussion

DR. CLYDE BARKER: You mentioned that the margins of the tumor were very important in the series you reported. With regard to distal lesions, this could be an important but more controversial issue now, since newer techniques and stapling equipment allow anastomosis and preservation of the rectum and anus even after resection of very distal lesions. Is there still a mandatory minimum margin for adequate resection?

DR. SCOTT JONES: That's an important question. Since this paper dealt with lesions distributed throughout the colon, it was difficult to advocate a different margin for some than for others. In addition to considerations of margin, lymph node metastasis and other factors also may influence outcome. But to be specific about your question on the distal lesions, we believe that the preponderance of lymphatic spread from the distal rectum is upward rather than downward, and this has caused some surgeons to accept narrower and narrower margins. To my knowledge, this has not necessarily been followed by disaster. I'm prepared to be convinced differently, but my current belief is that for mid-rectal lesions, one probably can accept half the margin I mentioned without sacrificing anything. The other factor that should be stressed is the necessity of talking to the patient before making the decision between anterior resection and abdominoperineal resection. Patients should be given as clear a view as possible about what the issues are. We should then listen to the patient to a certain extent. I am not saying that we should put the decision on the patient, but he or she has to be informed.

DR. CLAUDE WELCH: I wonder if you'd comment on radiation therapy.

DR. SCOTT JONES: Yes, that was one of the things that I left off of the slides and I recognized I did so.

There have been a number of reports, including some from your institution, that patients with both rectal and colon lesions may show some improvement in 5-year survival, particularly in certain categories of patients with Duke's B and C lesions. As you know, the earlier radiation trials, such as the VA cooperative trial, didn't demonstrate significant differences between the treated and control groups; however, more recent studies indicate that with radiation, perhaps an additional 10 to 15% survival can be accomplished in certain situations.

DR. CLYDE BARKER: Dr. Copeland, do you wish 30 seconds for rebuttal of Dr. Jones' account of the writing of this paper?

DR. SCOTT JONES: That's too much.

DR. TED COPELAND: The discussion of the papers at this meeting potentially can be a little different than the discussion of papers at any other meeting we'll ever go to. For example, the actual history of that paper is quite interesting. Lennie Miller had looked up the cases and had done the chart work on all 1084 patients. As near as I could tell, Len had gotten very tired of that data. We had no computers in those days, so when Scott came along, he put all the data that Leonard had gotten by hand from the charts—some 80 different responses from each case—on a bunch of punch cards. Scott had then gotten tired of fooling with all of those cards, so when I came along, my chore was to go up on the second floor, run the punch card sorter, and figure out the questions to ask of all that data. Scott and I did research on all of the responses on all of the punch cards to come up with that paper, which is actually a much more popular paper today than it was 20 years ago. At least, it is a lot more popular with me. However, there are a few interesting things buried in that paper. For example, one thing that is being talked about now is doing local excisions for Duke's A and B-1 lesions. Morris' paper of 1966 stated that B-1 lesions only have a 10.6% incidence of lymph node metastasis and his is almost the only study that ever investigated that. However, as Scott showed you, the B-1 lesions in this series had 27% lymph node metastases. Therefore, before people advocate local excision of B-1 lesions or the use of intracavitary radiation therapy for them, more series than just Morris' (which was based on very few patients) should be studied, including this one in which at least a quarter of the patients had lymph node metastasis.

DR. CLYDE BARKER: Ted, we could reminisce about this paper for quite a while. There is something to be said for being in the right place at the right time.

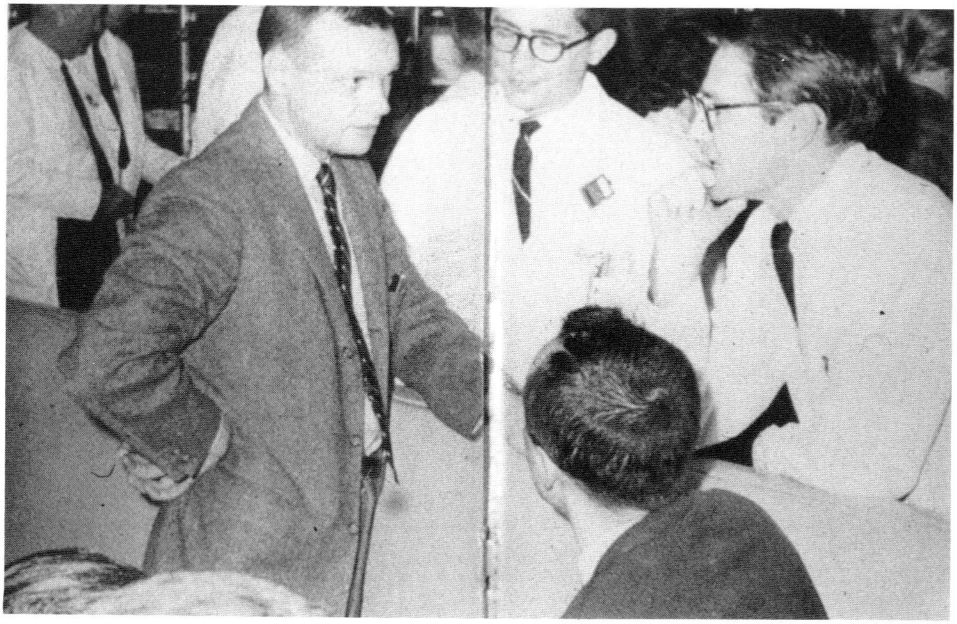

Introduction of Dr. Francis Rosato

Dr. Clyde Barker: Seen here in a yearbook photo from 1966, the year he finished his residency, is our next speaker, Frank Rosato. The caption reads, "You medical guys better keep off our turf." Frank was a very effective resident, and following his residency, he was here on the faculty until 1974 when he moved to Norfolk to become Chairman. Now, of course, he is Professor and Chairman at Thomas Jefferson University. The topic today is "Intraoperative Ultrasound of the Liver: An Important Adjunctive Tool for Decision Making in the Operating Room."

Dr. Rhoads also has had an interest in surgery of the liver. Those of us who know Dr. Rhoads realize that his approach in any given area is likely to be a little more aggressive than that of most, an observation illustrated by the title of his paper with Dr. Warren, "The Hepatic Origin of the Plasma-prothrombin Observations after Total Hepatectomy in Dog" (*Am J Med Sci* 198:193–197, 1939).

Dr. Rosato's Introductory Remarks

Happy Birthday, Dr. Rhoads. You may have noticed in the photo Clyde showed that one of the medical guys I was advising to keep off our turf happens to be the Dean here right now. The year of 1974 was indeed a personally sad time for me when I left Penn to take the Chairmanship at what was then the newest school in the United States, Eastern Virginia Medical School. Before I left, Dr. Rhoads gave me a little bit of his time on a Sunday morning for some advice. He nailed down two major points. He said, "First of all, in your dealings with people in your department, as you sit across the desk from them try your best to put yourself in their position, to understand what their goals, worries, fears and ambitions might be. After you've done that, then make the best decision you can for both your department and for the University as a whole." His second bit of advice was: "Try your best during that first year not to operate upon anybody who might have even the remotest possibility of dying." I think I did better with the first bit of advice than I did with the second. This is a picture of my office (slide) after I uncluttered the desk. When I am talking to somebody across that desk, I've not unintentionally placed the old portrait (Thomas Eakins' *The Gross*

Clinic) behind it so that my guest might have an impression of the long history of surgery and so they might also consider as we speak what the larger issues and institutional goals might be. At the same time, from where I sit, I can always see on the opposite wall (over the shoulder of whomever I am talking to) my photograph of Dr. Rhoads. It not only brings back pleasant memories but also reminds me of the important principles for which Dr. Rhoads stands.

Intraoperative Ultrasound of the Liver: An Important Adjunctive Tool for Decision Making in the Operating Room

MATTHEW D. RIFKIN, M.D.,* FRANCIS E. ROSATO, M.D.,†
CPT. H. MITCHELL BRANCH, M.D.,‡ JONATHAN FOSTER,*
SHUIN-LIN YANG, M.D.,† AND DONNA J. BARBOT, M.D.†

Forty-nine patients operated on for liver or other pathologic processes were examined intraoperatively with special ultrasound transducers during surgical exploration of the abdomen. Subjects were evaluated because of known or suspected disease of the liver. All patients were examined utilizing sterile technique. Prospective diagnosis and retrospective analysis of data were used. In 55% of subjects, no new information was obtained. In 19%, new information was gathered that changed the surgical approach. In 14% of patients, new information was obtained but it was such that no change in the therapeutic approach was needed. In 12% of patients, although no new information was gathered by the use of intraoperative ultrasound, a change in the surgical approach and management of the patient was still possible because of intraoperative ultrasound. These studies show that the routine use of ultrasound during intraoperative procedures, particularly when involving hepatic structures, is a clinically useful technique. In many instances, it will change the course of management.

THE USE OF intraoperative ultrasound was established in the 1960s but the technique was not employed extensively because the available equipment was difficult to use. Thus, the technique did not attract much attention for the first two decades after its introduction. In the early 1980s, with refinement in machinery, intraoperative ultrasound became a useful diagnostic technique, particularly in neurosurgical procedures.[1-4] Intraoperative guidance for renal calculi removal, a previously important use of intraoperative ultrasound, is not employed as frequently today because of the percutaneous treatment of kidney stones. More recently, intraoperative ultrasound has been utilized as a complementary procedure for many routine, as well as complicated general surgical procedures. Delineation of hepatic, biliary, and pancreatic tissue now can be clearly demonstrated and the efficacy of the technique is becoming more widespread.[5-10]

Although the use of intraoperative ultrasound has been established as an effective tool to delineate liver pathology, its ability to alter the therapeutic (surgical) approach to the patient's problem has not been as clearly delineated.[11-15] We undertook a study using prospective diagnosis and retrospective analysis of data to evaluate the benefits of intraoperative ultrasound of the liver in a group of patients with possible hepatic pathology.

Materials and Methods

Forty-nine patients were included in this study. Although not every subject undergoing surgery was studied by intraoperative ultrasound, all patients that were examined are included in this analysis but are not a consecutive series. Patients were selected because of the following: (1) known liver disease, *i.e.*, known or suspected space-occupying lesions or duct dilatation; or (2) unproven liver pathology but with a high possibility of involvement, *i.e.*, patients with rectal or colonic carcinoma with possible metastatic lesions to the liver.

From the *Department of Radiology and †Department of Surgery, Thomas Jefferson University Hospital, Philadelphia, and the ‡Department of Radiology, Williard Hall USAF Medical Center 40013, San Antonio, Texas.

This article has been adapted from *Annals of Surgery*, Vol. 205, No. 5, May 1987.

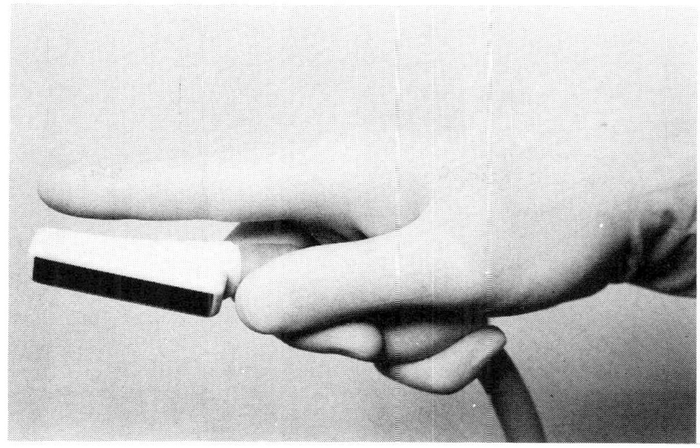

FIG. 1. Intraoperative transducer. The intraoperative transducer is smaller than the finger.

All patients underwent routine preoperative right upper quadrant imaging studies including conventional ultrasound, computed tomography, and/or angiography.

The patients were examined intraoperatively with a 7.5-MHz linear array transducer (Fig. 1) attached to a specially produced intraoperative ultrasound machine, the Aloka 330 (Tokyo). The ultrasound machine was manufactured with simplified controls for use in the operating suite. All controls were minimized and access was *via* the top of the machine covered with a disposable sterile sheath (Fig. 2). Theoretically the surgical team alone could activate and run the apparatus without a break in sterile technique. The intraoperative probe was small enough to fit between two fingers of the palpating hand (Fig. 3). Whereas the transducer and the transducer cable could be gas sterilized, this would require 48 hours aeration; therefore, we used disposable, sterile sheaths to cover the transducer. This allowed repeated use on sequential patients without the lengthy period required by gas sterilization. Acoustic gel was used to interface the transducer crystals to the sterile covering. Commercially available intraoperative latex sheathing was utilized in all cases. Sterile rubber bands secured the covering to the transducer cable. An arthroscope drape was used to cover the full length of the cable (10 feet). Permanent recording of the ultrasound images was made on a video cassette recorder which was incorporated into the ultrasound machine. The ultrasound image was 4 cm wide with a maximum 8 cm depth.

The entire liver was imaged in both a longitudinally oriented (sagittal) and transaxial orientation. The liver was scanned starting from the lateral aspect of the right lobe. The transducer was placed inferior and lateral and moved toward the left to the round ligament with continuous ultrasound scanning. The lateral segment of the left lobe was imaged similarly. When needed, particularly in an enlarged organ, the transducer was placed on the underside of the liver and scanning was commenced with the transducer angled cephalad. Contact between transducer and the liver was by natural peritoneal fluid or sterile saline.

When unsuspected nonpalpable lesions were imaged, ultrasound-guided biopsies were performed as indicated. In these cases, the biopsy needle was positioned adjacent to the transducer and the needle placed into the area of abnormality under continuous ultrasound control.

In this series, an experienced sonologist and surgeon were present during intraoperative sonography. The technique required an average of 10 to 15 minutes additional operating time. No complications were encountered. No contamination of the sterile field was noted.

Results

Of the 49 patients in this study, 18 ultimately proved to have liver tumors. Of these ten were malignant and 8 benign (Table 1). The remainder had no evidence of hepatic involvement and received appropriate treatment for their underlying surgical problems, which were most often tumors of the large intestine. The essential component of this review was the delineation of the influence that operative hepatic ultrasonography would have on the

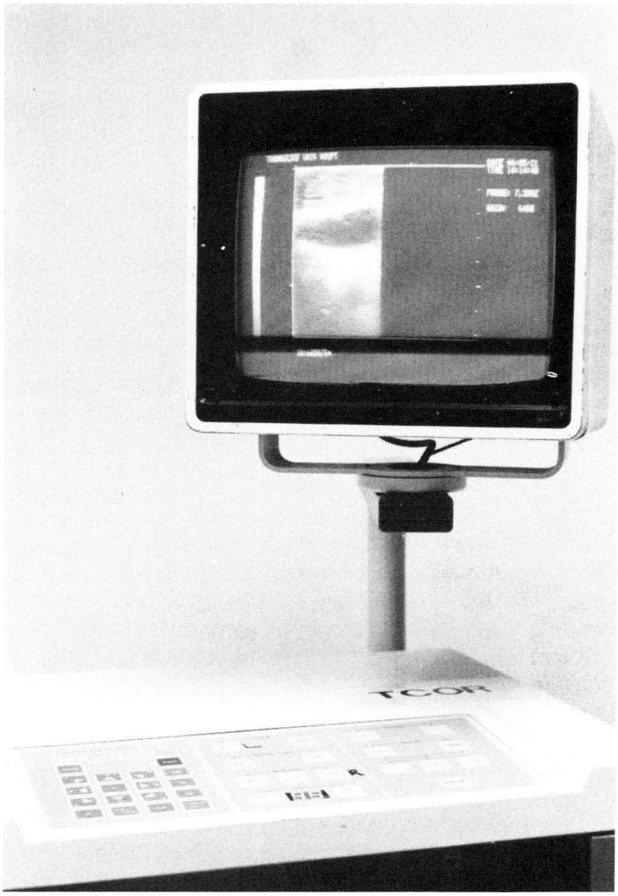

FIG. 2. Intraoperative ultrasound machine. Although conventional ultrasound equipment can be used, a specially produced unit was used for this study. The machine has single touch controls that can be easily covered by a sterile sheath.

extent and type of surgery performed. To analyze this, we divided all the patients into four groups, as follows (Table 2).

Group 1: Patients in whom no new information was obtained by operative ultrasound. The intraoperative ultrasound findings were consistent with preoperative imaging, and

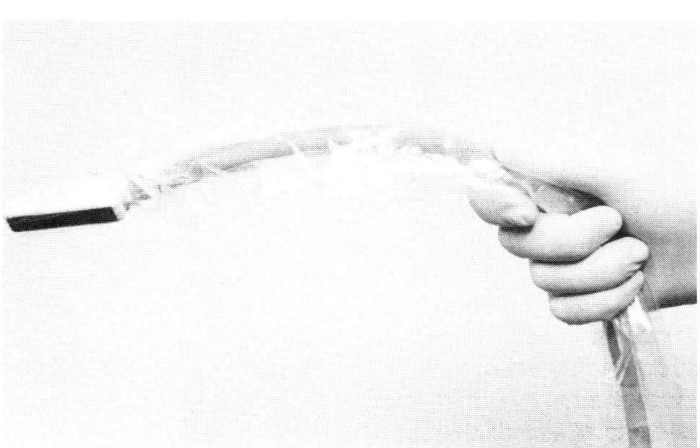

FIG. 3. Sterilized ultrasound transducer. A disposable sterile latex cover is used to ensure sterility over the transducer and the flexible cable.

TABLE 1. *Distribution of Tumors*

Benign (N = 8)	
Hemangioma	2
Granuloma	2
Simple cyst	3
Adenoma	1
Malignant (N = 10)	
Primary	2
Metastatic	8

TABLE 2. *Effectiveness of Intraoperative Ultrasound*

Group		No. of Patients	%
1	No new information: *no change* in therapeutic approach	27/49	55
2	No new information: *change* in therapeutic approach	6/49	12
3	New information: *no change* in therapeutic approach	7/49	14
4	New information: *change* in therapeutic approach	9/49	19

intraoperative evaluation (*i.e.*, palpation and visual inspection) and operation was performed as planned. Twenty-seven of 49 patients (55%) were included in this group.

Group 2: Patients in whom the intraoperative ultrasound demonstrated no new information but the planned surgical treatment was altered because of the sonogram. Included here are those patients with a lesion known by preoperative studies but in whom the abnormality could neither be seen nor felt at operation. Thus, ultrasound guidance for biopsy and/or excision was utilized making the operation more precise and usually less extensive than it would have been without the ultrasound. This group included six of 49 (12%) patients.

Case Report

A 43-year-old woman on birth control pills 12 years was studied because of chronic right upper quadrant pain. A preoperative arteriogram and computed axial tomography (CAT) scan were suggestive of hemangiomas of the right lobe but the technectium-labeled autologous erythrocyte scan was inconclusive. At surgery the exact location could not be seen or palpated. The ultrasound indicated its subcapsular location and allowed liver incision for enucleation of this vascular tumor.

Group 3: Patients where new information was obtained from the intraoperative ultrasound. However, this information produced no change in the planned approach. Seven of 49 (14%) were included in this category. These were mostly benign tumors, simple cysts, or granulomas.

Case Report

A 72-year-old woman had 18 months previously undergone curative resection of a Dukes C-1 left colon lesion. Because of a rising carcinoembryonic antigen (CEA) a CAT scan was performed demonstrating a single right lobe lesion which by arteriogram appeared highly suspicious for metastatic tumor. At operation a second lesion was detected by intraoperative ultrasound on the left lobe and this small lesion on biopsy was a granuloma. A right hepatic lobectomy then was performed.

Group 4: Patients where new information was obtained during the intraoperative sonogram which changed the surgical approach. This group included those patients with negative preoperative studies who by operative ultrasound turned out to have hepatic metastases, usually from colon cancer. It also included patients with a preoperative suspected single lesion, where multiple lesions were identified and either resection had to be abandoned or multiple segmental resections or formal lobectomy performed. Additionally, this group included patients where preoperative studies suggested the presence of a liver lesion, but the intraoperative ultrasound demonstrated the liver to be normal and free of disease. There were nine of 49 subjects (19%) included in this category.

In comparing the effectiveness of the various imaging techniques, we see that overall, operative ultrasonography is the most sensitive (Table 3).

The comparative sensitivity and specificity of the other imaging studies are presented in Table 4. For this analysis, a study was called false positive if a lesion was suspected by a diagnostic technique and not corroborated at operation. A false negative included those cases where a lesion was found at surgery but the given diagnostic technique failed to detect

TABLE 3. *Comparative Studies*

	Patients examined	True positive	True negative	False positive	False negative
Intraoperative ultrasound	49	18	31	0	0
Conventional ultrasound	20	5	12	0	3
Computed tomography	31	6	13	4	8
Angiography	8	4	0	2	2

its presence. These definitions are based on the simple presence or absence of tumor but not on the detection of the absolute number of lesions.

Discussion

Intraoperative ultrasound is a highly sophisticated tool requiring specialized equipment. Although conventional ultrasound machinery can be used, the more flexible dedicated equipment allows rapid and accurate scanning in the operating suite. Although our study utilized a dedicated instrument manufactured by one company, many other commercial firms are now producing either specialized machinery or special transducers to be used on existing conventional equipment. This broad development allows easy access for intraoperative ultrasound.

The equipment is relatively expensive, depending upon the manufacturer, with each transducer costing approximately $7500 in addition to the basic machinery. However, if disposable sterile covers are used, only a single probe is required. Thus, a single piece of equipment can be utilized in the operating suite of a general purpose hospital for a variety of intraoperative sonographic procedures.

The technique can be learned readily and is a valuable tool when an experienced surgeon and an experienced sonologist work together. The diagnostic criteria are similar to conventional ultrasound. However, the orientation, because of the small field of view, may be difficult to understand, particularly for the inexperienced sonologist. Our study, performed on patients undergoing abdominal exploration, has confirmed previous reports of the benefits of intraoperative ultrasound of the liver. These previous studies have shown that clinically known lesions are better defined by intraoperative ultrasound. Secondary abnormalities that are previously unsuspected can be seen, and although it may not be prudent to treat these at the time of surgery, certainly, knowledge of the abnormalities is important.

The technique is safe for patients and for the operating room personnel. Since no radiation

TABLE 4. *Accuracy of Imaging Studies*

	Sensitivity*	Specificity†
Intraoperative ultrasound	100	100
Conventional ultrasound	62	100
Computed tomography	42	76
Angiography	66	0

$$* \text{ Sensitivity} = \frac{TP}{TP + FN}.$$

$$† \text{ Specificity} = \frac{TN}{TN + FP}.$$

TP: true positive; FN: false negative; TN: true negative; FP: false positive.

is emitted, there is less concern in obtaining repeat examinations. When unsuspected, non-palpable lesions are found with intraoperative sonography, it can also be utilized to perform the biopsy.

Although liver function studies have been performed routinely in preoperative evaluation of the liver status, recent reports have shown the sensitivity and specificity of percutaneous ultrasound to be uninfluenced by liver chemistry abnormalities.[16] We have not looked at the precise effect of liver chemistry abnormalities and how they might correlate with operative sonography, but probably one would expect they have little effect on the sensitivity and/or specificity of operative sonography.

Operative ultrasound is of great help in the performance of many hepatic procedures. It can give precise localization of tumors and be used to selectively tamponade the afferent portal branch to minimize operative bleeding and prevent central retrograde tumor embolic migration in the course of tumor resection.[17]

The sonogram can be very helpful in decisions as to the appropriate surgical procedure. Since the depth of a tumor can be measured by operative ultrasound, it can help decide between a wedge resection or a formal lobectomy. When additional occult lesions are found, biopsies can be performed. The results may alter or curtail a planned procedure.

Since the liver is so large, visual or manual assessment constitutes only a part of hepatic evaluation. Routine use of operative sonography is strongly advised to more completely assess liver status.

REFERENCES

1. Knake JE, Chandler WF, Gabrielson TO, Latack JT, Gebarski SS. Intraoperative sonography in the nonsterotaxis biopsy and aspiration of subcortical brain lesions. Am J Neuroradiol 1983;4:672–674.
2. Rubin JM, Dohrmann GJ. Intraoperative neurosurgical ultrasound in the localization and characterization of intracranial masses. Radiology 1983;148:519–524.
3. Braun IF, Raghavendra BN, Kricheff II. Spinal cord imaging using real-time high-resolution ultrasound. Radiology 1983;147:459–465.
4. Quencer RM, Morse BMM, Green BA, Elsmont FJ, Brost P. Intraoperative spinal sonography: Adjunct to metrizamide CT in the assessment and surgical decompression of posttraumatic spinal cord cysts. Am J Radiol 1984;142:593–601.
5. Plainfosse MC, Merran S. Work in progress: Intraoperative abdominal ultrasound. Radiology 1983;147:829–832.
6. Norton JA, Sigel B, Baker AR *et al.* Localization of an occult insulinoma by intraoperative ultrasonography. Surgery 1985;381–384.
7. Sigel B, Coelho JCU, Machi J *et al.* The application of real-time ultrasound imaging during surgical procedures. Surg Gynecol Obstet 1983;157:33–37.
8. Sigel B, Machi J, Ramos JR, Duarte B, Donahue PE. The role of imaging ultrasound during pancreatic surgery. Ann Surg 1984;200:486–493.
9. Herbst CA, Mittelstaedt CA, Staab EV, Buckwalter JA. Intraoperative ultrasonography evaluation of the gallbladder in morbidly obese patients. Ann Surg 1984;691–692.
10. Bowerman RA, McCracken S, Silver TM, Knake JE. Abdominal and miscellaneous applications of intraoperative ultrasound. Radiol Clin North Am 1985;23:107–119.
11. Sheu JC, Sung JL, Chen DS *et al.* Ultrasonography of small hepatic tumors using high-resolution linear-array real-time instruments. Radiology 1984;150:797–802.
12. Castaing D, Kunstlinger F, Habib N, Bismuth H. Intraoperative ultrasonographic study of the liver. Am J Surg 1985;149:676–682.
13. Gozzetti G, Mazziotti A, Bolondi L *et al.* Intraoperative ultrasonography in surgery for liver tumors. Surgery 1986;99:523–530.
14. Sheu JC, Lee CS, Sung JL, Chen DS, Yang PM, Lin TY. Intraoperative hepatic ultrasonography: An indispensable procedure in resection of small hepatocellular carcinomas. Surgery 1985;97:97–103.
15. Igawa S, Sakai K, Kinoshita H, Hirohashi K. Intraoperative sonography: Clinical usefulness in liver surgery. Radiology 1985;156:473–478.
16. Tempero MA, Williams CA, Anderson JC. The value of hepatic ultrasound and biochemical liver tests in screening for liver metastases. J Clin Oncol 1986;4:1074–1078.
17. Castaing D, Emond J, Kunstlinger F, Bismuth H. Utility of operative ultrasound in the surgical management of liver tumors. Ann Surg 1986;204:600–605.

DISCUSSION

DR. ROBERT CRICHLOW: I wonder if you've found intraoperative ultrasound useful in mapping out the anatomy of the liver as you do major hepatic resections.

DR. FRANK ROSATO: Critch, I haven't. I have seen the Japanese literature at the College of Surgeons, and I have attended the movie showing how they map out the portal venous system in planning a resection for a hepatoma—with the most beautiful background music. We have had no experience with this, but I was impressed with it. During a right hepatectomy, we can trace the course of the left hepatic vein that we may wish to save, and we can get a very good idea of its relationship to the tumor. We can even reapply the ultrasound probe from time to time as we develop a plane through the liver. So, it has been a help to us sometimes in anticipating where the major veins are, but in terms of preoperative mapping, we have had no experience.

DR. JOHN HOWARD: Can it demonstrate the point of portal or mesenteric vein occlusion?

DR. FRANK ROSATO: Yes, it definitely can. You can see flow in the vessel, and that is the other thing I should have mentioned: not only does it identify the vessels, but it also gives you an idea whether there is restricted flow in them.

DR. STAN DUDRICK: It is useful in the diagnosis of pancreatic lesions?

DR. FRANK ROSATO: We have not applied it to the pancreas, but Bernie Sigel at MCP hospital has begun to do that.

DR. EDWARD KAPLAN: Bernie Sigel and others are even using it in diagnosis of small islet cell tumors that show up as hypoechogenic areas.

DR. HARVEY SUGERMAN: It is also very helpful for pancreatic cysts.

Introduction of Dr. Marshall Orloff

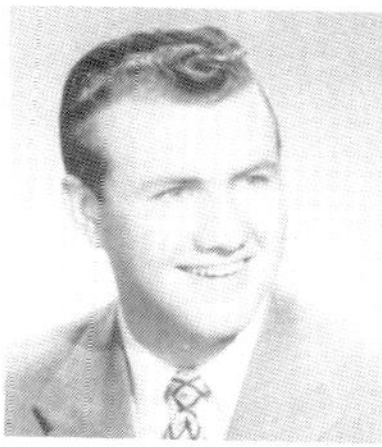

Dr. Clyde F. Barker: Our next speaker, Marshall Orloff, was chief resident at HUP in 1957–58. He then accepted a faculty appointment at the University of Colorado. In 1961, he joined Dr. Longmire's department as Chief of Surgery at Harbor General, and in 1967, he became Chairman of his own department at the University of California at San Diego. From the beginning of his career, he has had an interest in hepatic physiology. Some of his classic experiments in this field helped carry him to the presidency of The Society of University Surgeons. In recent years, he began to work on pancreatic transplantation, and I have followed closely his important contributions in this field. Today, because of his well-known interest in the procedure and controversial advocacy of it, it is most appropriate that he will describe "Three Decades of Experience with Emergency Portacaval Shunting."

If one peruses Dr. Rhoads' bibliography of 300 or 400 papers with enough diligence, it is possible to find one on almost any subject. For example, he included a chapter in Dr. Bockus' *Postgraduate Gastroenterology* (W. B. Saunders Co., Philadelphia, 1950, pp. 1–7) entitled "Indications for and Results of Surgical Procedures in Pronounced Portal Hypertension."

Dr. Orloff's Introductory Remarks

Dr. Rhoads, it is, of course, a great honor and an enormous pleasure for me and for my wife Ann to be here on this momentous occasion, celebrating what is now the second hour of your 80th birthday. I don't feel too badly in seeing my high school graduation picture projected this morning. Two of this morning's speakers have already showed one particular photograph of Dr. Rhoads that hangs on the wall in their offices or studys. I have that same picture in my office, as does Jim Hardy, and many others. As I look back over a period of 25 years, it is the same picture and the same Jonathan Rhoads. Of course, he hasn't really changed that much, has he?

I am really indebted to Jonathan Rhoads in more ways than you will ever know for that interest and for the beginnings of my professional career. When I arrived in Philadelphia, the first service to which I was assigned was Dr. Koop's at Children's Hospital, which was then located in South Philadelphia on Bainbridge Street. Chick Koop was given the assignment of preparing me for Dr. Rhoads. So, after I mastered the two major operations that the residents were allowed to do at Children's Hospital, circumcision and *left* inguinal herniorraphy, I finally rotated to my first service at HUP. That first service was the service of Jonathan Rhoads. I arrived at HUP to find that Dr. Rhoads had scheduled, would you believe, 14 elective cases on a Saturday morning! The very first operation in which I participated at the University of Pennsylvania was as assistant to Dr. Rhoads.

I am also indebted to Dr. Rhoads for introducing me to gourmet cooking and eating. After we finished the Saturday schedule at 5:00 in the afternoon, it was Dr. Rhoads' general custom to take the boys to Horn and Hardart. Now, some of you probably don't know about Horn and Hardart, but those who are old enough to remember it know that it was certainly one of THE gourmet eating places in Philadelphia.

Dr. Rhoads, I want to thank you for being here to celebrate your 80th birthday and for the stimulation you provided and the help you've provided to allow these lifelong studies that we hope will continue to go forward. Thank you.

Emergency Portacaval Shunt: Three Decades of Experience From Philadelphia to San Diego

MARSHALL J. ORLOFF, M.D.

The fertile environment created in the 1950s at the University of Pennsylvania by such giants as Jonathan Rhoads and I. S. Ravdin stimulated the author to study liver disease and portal hypertension, both at the bedside and in the research laboratory. The interest that was nurtured in those early days of his surgical career in Philadelphia, has held his attention throughout his professional life. What the author learned in Philadelphia still holds true, namely, that the mortality rate of bleeding esophageal varices in alcoholic cirrhosis is very high and, therefore, emergency therapy is of paramount importance. The only definitive therapy of portal hypertension and bleeding varices is decompression of the portal system by some form of portal-systemic shunt. From 1963 to 1983 a prospective study was conducted of emergency portacaval shunt performed within 8 hours in 264 unselected patients with alcoholic cirrhosis, all comers included. For purposes of analysis, these patients were divided into an Early Group of 180 patients and a Recent Group of 84 patients. Operative and 5-year survival rates in the Early Group were 58% and 38%, respectively, and in the Recent Group were 83% and 72%, respectively. The survival rate after emergency portacaval shunt in unselected patients during the last 9 years has been at least as high as the survival rates reported for elective shunt in highly selected patients. Comparison of the results of emergency shunt with the author's previous prospective, randomized clinical trial in unselected patients of emergency medical treatment and emergency transesophageal varix ligation (both followed by elective portacaval shunt in survivors) showed that long-term survival is far better in patients treated by emergency shunt. Encephalopathy, the major complication of portacaval shunt, occurred in one third of patients before the shunt, in 31% of the Early Group, and 16% of the Recent Group after the shunt, and was severe in only 7%. Of 153 patients who were operated on 10 or more years ago, 45 (29%) are alive 11 to 23 years after operation. In a recent prospective randomized trial of emergency portacaval shunt and emergency medical therapy followed by elective portacaval shunt, operation resulted in over a two-fold greater survival rate, a markedly lower requirement for blood transfusions, and confirmed all of the earlier results. Similarly, comparison of these results of emergency shunt with results of a prospective study of endoscopic sclerotherapy that the author performed recently showed a survival rate after emergency shunt that was over four-fold greater than that of sclerotherapy. These results show that emergency portacaval shunt, by preventing death from varix hemorrhage in alcoholic cirrhosis, makes it possible for a substantial number of patients to live a normal life span and enjoy an acceptable quality of life.

MY CAREER AS A SURGEON began in 1952, when I came to Philadelphia from San Francisco for my residency in surgery at the University of Pennsylvania. It was at the University of Pennsylvania that the seed of my interest in hepatobiliary disease and its treatment, which has continued throughout my professional life, was planted and nurtured. The first service to which I was assigned at the Hospital of the University of Pennsylvania (HUP) was the service of Dr. Jonathan Rhoads, and the very first operation in which I participated at HUP was as an assistant to Dr. Rhoads on a Saturday morning in a patient who was thought to have obstructive jaundice due to gallstones, but turned out to have the cholestatic phase of viral hepatitis, at that time a poorly understood and not well-recognized condition. Early in my residency, I was given the opportunity to work at night and on

TABLE 1. *Mortality Rate of First Episode of Bleeding From Esophageal Varices in Patients With Cirrhosis*

Reference	Yr reported	Type of hospital	No. of patients	Mortality (%)
Ratnoff and Patek[1]	1942	Five private teaching	106	40
Higgins[2]	1947	City indigent	45	76
Atik and Simeone[3]	1954	City indigent	59	83
Nachlas *et al.*[4]	1955	City indigent	102	59
Cohn and Blaisdell[5]	1958	City indigent	456	74
Taylor and Jontz[6]	1959	Veterans	102	45
Merigan *et al.*[7]	1960	City indigent	74	76
Orloff[8]	1962	City indigent	87	84
		Total	1031	Mean 73

weekends in the Harrison Department of Surgical Research, of which Jonathan Rhoads was the Director. In 1955, Dr. Rhoads arranged for me to receive a seed grant of $10,000 from the Harrison Department. The title of the grant was simply "Hepatic Physiology." On the basis of the pilot experiments performed in the Harrison Department, I obtained my first National Institutes of Health (NIH) research grant while a surgical resident in 1956. It was grant number USPHS H-2757 and was entitled "Studies in Cirrhosis Ascites and the Hepatic Circulation." Jerry Peskin, a co-resident, was the co-investigator.

At the time of my training, HUP was a clinical and research center for hepatobiliary disease. As a result, I was given the opportunity to participate in the care of a large number of patients with cirrhosis of the liver and bleeding esophageal varices. Most of these patients were treated by the portacaval shunt operation, which had been introduced in the United States only a few years earlier by Whipple and by Blakemore and Lord, all working at Presbyterian Hospital of Columbia University. In fact, Whipple came to HUP from New York to present surgical grand rounds and I was assigned the duty of taking him to the train station for his return trip, during which I had the exciting opportunity of hearing first hand of his experience with the treatment of portal hypertension. In 1956, I participated in my first emergency portacaval shunt operation, and that was the beginning of three decades of experience with emergency portacaval shunt. That experience has taken me from Philadelphia, to Denver, to Los Angeles, and finally to San Diego. It has involved the participation and help of many teachers, colleagues, residents, research fellows, nurses, and other health care personnel.

The most frequent cause of death from upper gastrointestinal bleeding is rupture of an esophageal or gastric varix with hemorrhage. Until recently, approximately three of four cirrhotic patients who entered the hospital with their first episode of bleeding varices failed to leave the hospital alive. Table 1, which shows the results of a number of studies conducted during the last 40 years, indicates that as of 1962 the immediate mortality rate of the first variceal hemorrhage averaged 73%.[1-8] From these statistics, it is apparent that the emergency treatment of bleeding esophagogastric varices is the single most important aspect of the therapy of portal hypertension.

The precipitating cause of rupture of esophageal varices is uncertain. It has been proposed that erosion of the mucosa by reflux acid-peptic esophagitis is involved. However, in a gross and microscopic study of the distal esophagus in 20 patients at the time of bleeding we found esophagitis in only one patient.[9] Moreover, bleeding from esophageal varices has been reported in patients with proven gastric achlorhydria. The evidence strongly suggests that increased hydrostatic pressure is responsible for "blowout" rupture of esophageal varices.[9,10] It is important to point out that finding esophageal or gastric varices in a patient with cirrhosis does not mean that the patient will develop bleeding. In fact, only 25% to 35% of patients with proven varices ultimately bleed from the varices.[11] However, once bleeding has occurred, the patient has a 95% probability of bleeding again, usually within a year of

From the School of Medicine, University of California, San Diego, and the Department of Surgery, University of California, San Diego, Medical Center, San Diego, California.

the first bleeding episode, and a 90% to 100% likelihood of dying within 5 years unless he or she receives specific, definitive treatment to relieve portal hypertension.[12,13] The prognosis and therapeutic implications of esophagogastric varices depend on whether or not bleeding has occurred.

The only definitive treatment for portal hypertension and bleeding esophageal varices in patients with cirrhosis is some form of portal-systemic shunt. There are three circumstances in which the shunt operation has been used in patients with esophageal varices, namely, as a prophylactic measure, as elective treatment, and as emergency therapy. Each of these circumstances is different from the other and involves a distinctive group of patients, so that it is inappropriate to compare the results of shunt therapy in one group with those in another or to lump them together in evaluating the effectiveness of the shunt operation.

Prophylactic portal-systemic shunt has been shown by three prospective clinical trials[14–16] to be of no value in prolonging life. Since approximately two thirds of patients with esophageal varices never bleed from their varices, the outcome of these studies was predictable. Good results can hardly be expected from performance of a serious operation designed to prevent a complication that would not occur in two thirds of the subjects if they did not have the operation. However, it cannot be emphasized too strongly that the results of prophylactic shunt have no bearing on what might be expected of therapeutic portal-systemic shunt in a patient who has bled from varices.

Elective therapeutic portal-systemic shunt, used in patients who have recovered from an episode of varix hemorrhage, still is a matter of controversy even though it has been the type of shunt most frequently performed during the last 40 years. There is no question that by carefully selecting patients it is possible to obtain a low operative mortality rate and a substantial long-term survival rate after elective therapeutic shunt. In a series of 612 highly selected patients who were referred to us after having survived a bleeding episode at another hospital, the operative mortality rate of elective shunt was 2%, the 5-year survival rate is 60% and only three patients have rebled from varices.[17] However, there are two problems associated with elective therapeutic portal-systemic shunt. The first is the lack of acceptable prospective studies of any magnitude that have compared elective therapeutic shunt with other forms of therapy in similar groups of patients. The second, and more important problem is that the mortality rate of acute varix hemorrhage in patients with alcoholic cirrhosis is so high that few patients, not many more than 20% to 25% of those who bleed, have survived the bleeding episode and then qualified for elective shunt. Considerable evidence indicates that the traditional approach involving use of temporary, nonsurgical emergency measures to control the bleeding in hopes of permitting methodical preparation of the patients for elective surgery has had little influence on the overall survival of the bleeding cirrhotic population. It is for this reason that we have focused our attention on the third form of shunt therapy, specifically, emergency portacaval shunt.

Prospective Study of Emergency Portacaval Shunt

In 1963, we initiated a prospective study of emergency portacaval shunt.[18] The study was distinguished from all other reported studies of emergency treatment in two respects: (1) it involved every cirrhotic patient admitted with varix bleeding, regardless of his or her condition on admission; and (2) all of the patients were operated upon within 8 hours of admission to our emergency room or, in the occasional patient who started bleeding while in the hospital, within 8 hours of the onset of bleeding. Between 1963 and 1983, 264 consecutive, unselected patients underwent emergency portacaval shunt.[18–27] Follow-up study has been conducted in a special clinic, and the current status of 97% of the patients is known.

We divided our 264 unselected patients into two groups: an Early Group of 180 patients operated upon from 1963 up to 1978, and a Recent Group of 84 patients operated upon from 1978 through 1983. The characteristics of the two groups were similar and are shown in Table 2. Almost all of the patients were chronic alcoholics, and all had cirrhosis on liver biopsy. On admission, about 50% of the patients in each group had jaundice and ascites, 19% had frank encephalopathy or coma, 30% and 42%, respectively, had severe muscle wasting, and 82% and 90%, respectively, had a hyperdynamic state. Systemic intravenous pituitrin temporarily controlled the varix bleeding in 95% of the patients and allowed sufficient time to complete the diagnostic workup. Emergency portacaval shunt promptly

TABLE 2. *Emergency Portacaval Shunt in Unselected Patients With Cirrhosis: Characteristics of Early Group (n = 180) and Recent Group (n = 84)*

	Early Group (%)	Recent Group (%)
Pathologic manifestations		
Hematemesis	98	94
Jaundice on admission	49	48
Ascites on admission	53	42
Encephalopathy on admission	19	18
Severe muscle wasting	30	42
Hyperdynamic cardiovascular state	82	90
Liver dye retention ≥21%	95	92
Varices on endoscopic study	98	100
Varices on x-ray	95	97
Cirrhosis on liver biopsy	100	100
Portal hypertension by direct measurement	100	100
Treatment		
Temporary control by IV vasopressin	95	95
Permanent control by portacaval shunt	98	100
Blood transfusions		
<5000ml	61	69
5000–7000 ml	16	21
>7000 ml	23	10
Type of shunt		
Side-to-side	83	74
End-to-side	15	26
Other	2	0
Skin-to-skin operating time		
<4 h	45	57
4–5 h	42	31
>5 h	13	12
Gradient across shunt <50 mm	86	98

IV: intravenous.

and permanently stopped the varix hemorrhage in 98% and 100% of the patients, respectively. The requirement for blood transfusion before and during operation for the two groups averaged 5.1 l and 3.7 l, respectively. Side-to-side portacaval shunt was performed in 83% and 74% of the patients, respectively, end-to-side shunt in 15% and 26%, respectively, and another type of shunt in three patients in the Early Group. There was no difference in survival rate between patients with side-to-side anastomosis and those with end-to-side anastomosis. The skin-to-skin operating time, which included various measurements of splanchnic pressures and blood flows, averaged 4.1 hours, and was less than 5 hours in 87% and 88% of each group, respectively. All patients had portal hypertension with corrected free portal pressures, obtained by subtracting the inferior vena cava pressure, that averaged 267 mm saline. The portacaval anastomosis reduced the portal pressure to normal in all patients.

Table 3 summarizes the long-term results of emergency portacaval shunt. In the Early Group, 58% of the 180 patients survived the operation, and the 5-year and 12-year survival rates were 38% and 30%, respectively. In contrast, 83% of the Recent Group of 84 patients survived the shunt, and the 5-year survival rate is 72%. One third of the patients in each group had a documented history of encephalopathy before the shunt.[28] After the shunt, 31% of the Early Group and 16% of the Recent Group have had encephalopathy at one time or another. Severe encephalopathy requiring chronic dietary protein restriction occurred in only 7% of the patients. At the time of discharge, 95% of patients in the Early Group, and 99% of patients in the Recent Group could tolerate a diet containing 80 g of protein per day.

Long-term shunt patency has been demonstrated by yearly angiography in 99% of the early patients and 100% of the recent patients. The two thrombosed shunts in the Early Group were of the end-to-side type. Forty-eight percent of the survivors in the Early Group and 70% of the Recent Group have not consumed alcohol at any time during the follow-up period. The lower incidence in the Recent Group may be due to the fact that it has not been

TABLE 3. *Emergency Portacaval Shunt in Unselected Patients With Cirrhosis: Results of Long-Term Follow-Up of Early Group (n = 180) and Recent Group (n = 84)*

Results	Early Group (%)	Recent Group (%)
Operative survival (30 d or longer)	58	83
5-yr survival	38	72
Actuarial 12-yr survival	30	—
Encephalopathy		
Before shunt	33	36
After shunt	31	16
Patency of shunt by yearly catheterization	99	100
Abstinence from alcohol	48	70
General status after 5 yr		
Excellent or good	62	69
Fair	29	24
Poor	9	7
Liver function after 5 yr		
Improved	44	52
Unchanged	33	35
Worse	22	13

followed up for as many years as the Early Group. After 5 years, the general status of the survivors in the Early Group and Recent Group, respectively, is excellent or good in 62% and 69%, fair in 29% and 24%, and poor in 9% and 7%; all but one patient in the poor category have resumed heavy alcohol consumption. Sixty percent of the survivors have been gainfully employed or doing full-time housework during part or all of the follow-up period. Five years after the shunt operation, results of liver function tests showed an improvement over preoperative results in 44% of the Early Group and 52% of the Recent Group, no change in 33% and 35%, respectively, and worsening in 22% and 13%, respectively.

Beginning with the moment of admission and continuing through the lifelong follow-up visits, detailed data on every patient were recorded on standard forms and entered continuously into a computer analysis program. Since our study involved unselected patients, we carefully analyzed all factors present on admission that might have influenced survival, in the hope of identifying criteria for future selection of patients for operation.

Table 4 summarizes the preoperative findings obtained from the history, physical exami-

TABLE 4. *Preoperative Risk Factors That Significantly Decreased Survival of the Early Group of 180 Unselected Cirrhotic Patients Treated by Emergency Portacaval Shunt*

Risk factors	Percent of Group	Survival (%)	Significance (*P*)
Ascites			
Present	53	46	<0.01
Absent	47	72	
SGOT			
$\geq$100 U/dl	34	43	<0.01
$<$100 U/dl	66	70	
BSP retention			
$>$50%	21	36	<0.01
$\leq$50%	79	66	
Hypokalemic alkalosis			
pH >7.5, $K^+ <3.5$	29	42	<0.05
pH ≤7.5, $K^+ \geq3.5$	71	67	
Blood transfusion			
$\geq$5 l before and during operation	39	41	<0.001
$<$5 l before and during operation	61	70	
Last drank alcohol			
$\leq$7 d before admission	71	53	<0.05
$>$7 d before admission	29	71	

SGOT: serum oxaloacetic transaminase; K^+: potassium.

TABLE 5. *Results of Emergency Portacaval Shunt, Transesophageal Varix Ligation, and Medical Treatment in Unselected Patients With Cirrhosis and Bleeding Varices*

Clinical factors and survival rates	Medical treatment*	Varix ligation*	Emergency shunt: Early Group	Emergency shunt: Recent Group
No. of patients	59	28	180	84
Jaundice on admission (%)	42	57	49	48
Ascites on admission (%)	41	50	53	42
Encephalopathy on admission (%)	25	25	19	18
Mean liver index on admission	2.8	2.8	2.4	2.6
Admission hemoglobin 11 g/dl or less (%)	70	71	71	74
Varices demonstrated (%)	95	100	100	100
Mean volume of blood transfused (l)	7.2	4.2	5.0	3.7
Early survival (30 d) (%)	17	54	58	83
5-yr survival (%)	3	21	38	72
12-yr survival (%)	0	11	30	—

* Followed by elective portacaval shunt when possible.

nation, and diagnostic workup that were associated with a statistically significant decrease in survival rate in the Early Group and, therefore, can be considered to be risk factors. Six such risk factors were identified as follows: (1) presence of ascites on admission; (2) serum glutamic oxaloacetic transammase (SGOT) level of 100 U/dl or higher; (3) BSP retention greater than 50% in 45 minutes; (4) hypokalemic alkalosis with an arterial blood pH of 7.50 or greater and a serum potassium level below 3.5 mEq/l; (5) requirement of 5 l or more of blood transfusion before and during operation; and (6) consumption of alcohol within 7 days before admission. Because the presence of these risk factors was associated with survival rates of from 36% to 53%, they cannot be considered contraindications to emergency shunt. Age, sex, jaundice, encephalopathy, severe muscle wasting a small liver, a large spleen, a history of delirium tremens, and the blood levels of bilirubin, albumin, and prothrombin did not have a statistically significant influence on survival.

In 17 patients (9% of our series), jaundice, ascites, encephalopathy, and severe muscle wasting were present concurrently on admission. All of these patients had markedly disturbed liver function, and nine had an SGOT level above 100 U/dl. The operative survival rate of these patients with the most advanced stage of alcoholic cirrhosis was 47%, a rate similar to that of patients with ascites alone. However, 1 year after operation only 18% were still alive, and 5 years postoperatively, the survival rate was only 12%, so the outlook for these patients is grim under any circumstances. Nevertheless, without portacaval shunt, these preterminal cirrhotics rarely survive beyond 2 years.

Table 5 compares the results of three forms of emergency treatment of bleeding varices that we have evaluated prospectively in unselected patients over a period of 25 years: (1) emergency medical treatment followed by elective portacaval shunt in survivors; (2) emergency transesophageal varix ligation followed by elective portacaval shunt in survivors[29]; and (3) emergency portacaval shunt. Figure 1 compares the cumulative survival curve of the Early Group of shunted patients with the survival curves resulting from the other two types of emergency therapy. Although these three groups of patients were not studied concurrently, they are similar from every standpoint. Early survival rates produced by the two forms of surgical therapy were substantially greater than that resulting from emergency medical treatment. Five-year and 12-year survival rates, both actual and actuarial, were significantly greater after emergency shunt than after either of the other two types of emergency therapy.

Figure 2 compares the cumulative survival curve of the 84 patients in the Recent Group with that of the 180 patients in the Early Group. As our experience with emergency portacaval shunt has increased, there has been a striking improvement in results. In unselected patients, all comers included, operative survival rate has increased from 58% to 83%, and 5-year survival rate has almost doubled from 38% to 72%. It should be emphasized that no patient who came to us with bleeding varices was excluded from the emergency shunt

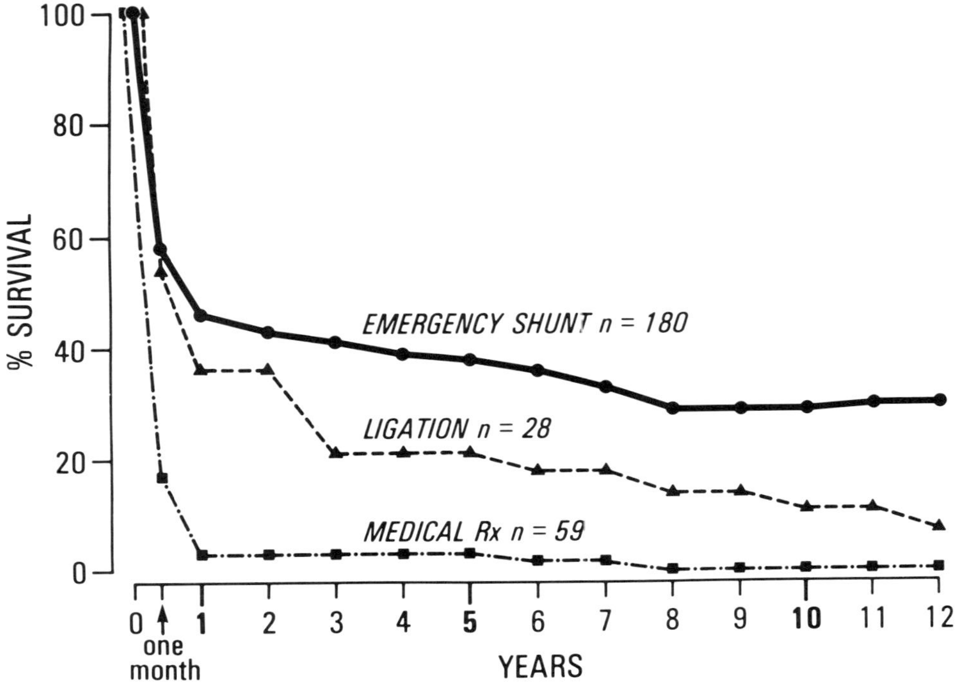

FIG. 1. Cumulative 5-year survival rates of patients with cirrhosis and hemorrhage from esophageal varices after emergency portacaval shunt (Early Group), transesophageal varix ligation, and medical treatment.

program. Nonetheless, the 5-year survival rate of emergency shunt in unselected patients is now the same as or better than the 5-year survival rate of elective shunt in highly selected patients reported by others.

Many patients with alcoholic cirrhosis have not yet reached 50 years of age and, in the absence of liver disease, would have a life expectancy of more than 25 additional years. However, little information is available about survival beyond 5 years after treatment, and almost no information about the quality of life after any form of therapy. Of our 264 patients who underwent emergency portacaval shunt, 153 were operated on ten or more years ago, and 45 survived for from 11 to 23 years. These 45 patients have undergone regular follow-up and the status of all of them is known.[30]

Of the 45 long survivors, 20% were in Child's class A, 73% were in class B, and 7% were in class C at the time of operation. There was a substantial incidence of the six preoperative risk factors that we have found to adversely affect survival.

Table 6 presents data on the quality of life in the patients who survived for 11 to 23 years. All of the patients were shown to have a patent portacaval anastomosis by yearly angiography, and no patient had gastrointestinal bleeding. Eight patients, or 18%, had portasystemic encephalopathy. Four of these patients had a single episode of encephalopathy early in their course, so that the incidence of significant, recurrent encephalopathy was 9%, and it was directly related to use of alcohol. Stated differently, encephalopathy played no role in the lives of 91% of the patients. It should be noted that 22% of the patients had encephalopathy before shunt.

Abstention from alcohol was total and continuous in 58% of the long survivors, and the abstainers had an excellent record of freedom from encephalopathy and productive living. Remarkably, 31% of the patients drank alcohol occasionally and 11% resumed regular use, yet they survived for many years. After 10 years, liver function had improved in 53%, was unchanged in 29%, and was worse in 18% compared to the function at the time of bleeding and operation. Excluding four patients who were 65 years or older at the time of operation and were classified as retired, 68% of the patients were gainfully employed or doing full-

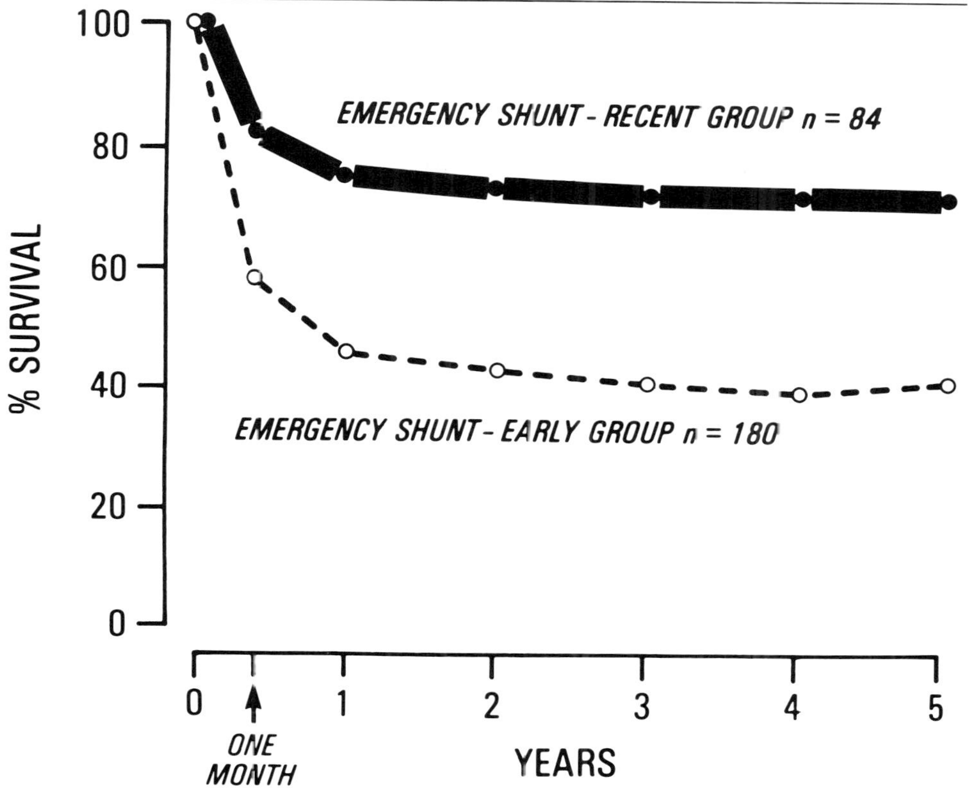

FIG. 2. Cumulative survival rate of 84 unselected patients with cirrhosis who underwent emergency portacaval shunt in the Recent Group, as compared with the cumulative survival rate of 180 patients in the Early Group.

time housework for part or all of the follow-up period. Eleven years after emergency shunt, the general status of the patients was judged to be excellent or good in 73%, and fair in 27%, almost all of whom had resumed use of alcohol. Not surprisingly, and in confirmation of our previous studies, the single factor that appeared to influence long-term survival was resumption of regular alcohol intake.

The results of our studies indicate that emergency portacaval shunt has improved both the immediate and long-term survival rates of cirrhotic patients with bleeding esophageal varices. As is true of survival statistics for cancer and other lethal disorders, the absolute survival rate is of limited meaning unless it is viewed in the context of the natural history of the disease. The 5-year and 12-year survival rates in our experience to date are many times greater than those associated with emergency medical therapy followed by elective portacaval shunt in the relatively small number of patients who survive. Undoubtedly, some patients with advanced cirrhosis will not survive with any form of therapy currently available. The problem is that criteria for identifying such patients are not yet known. The development of sound criteria for selecting patients for various forms of treatment unquestionably will improve the results of operative management. Until such guidelines are developed by well-controlled, prospective studies, or until alternative effective therapy is devised, emergency portacaval shunt appears to be the therapy of choice for most cirrhotic patients who bleed from esophageal varices.

Recent Prospective Randomized Comparison of Emergency Portacaval Shunt and Emergency Medical Therapy

Although our studies showed that emergency portacaval shunt produced a much higher survival rate and much better quality of life than any other form of emergency therapy, a potential shortcoming in the comparisons described above, is that they were not conducted concurrently in a randomized clinical trial. Therefore, in 1978 we initiated a prospective randomized trial comparing emergency portacaval shunt (EPCS) and emergency medical therapy (EMT) involving every patient, without selection, admitted to one of our hospitals with cirrhosis and bleeding esophagogastric varices.[31,32] Survivors of EMT underwent an elective portacaval shunt within 2 to 6 weeks. All patients underwent exactly the same diagnostic workup described previously, and all patients received the same initial therapy. Randomization was done after the diagnosis of bleeding varices was made by drawing a card from an opaque, sealed envelope prepared by the biostatistician according to a randomization design. Randomization resulted in 21 patients receiving EPCS and 22 patients receiving EMT. The EPCS was performed within 8 hours of initial contact, and EMT consisted of a continuation of initial therapy plus continuous systemic intravenous vasopressin and esophageal balloon tamponade. Randomization ended in 1983, and the follow-up rate to date has been 100%.

Table 7 shows the characteristics of the two groups. The only significant differences between them were as follows: (1) a higher incidence of severe muscle wasting in the EPCS group, and (2) fewer Child's risk class A patients and more class C patients in the EPCS group. If anything, these differences would tend to favor emergency medical therapy.

Table 8 shows control of bleeding in the two groups of patients. As we have found consistently in the past, 90% or more of patients responded initially to systemic intravenous vasopressin. However, after the initial response, the differences between the two groups were highly significant. Both early control and permanent control of bleeding were achieved in 100% of the shunted patients, but in only 45% and 30%, respectively, of the medically treated patients. Furthermore, the mean requirement for blood transfusions was three times greater in the EMT group than in the EPCS group, a very important difference in this day when every blood transfusion carries a substantial risk.

Table 9 shows the survival rates in the two groups. Almost twice as many patients in the EPCS group survived to leave the hospital than in the EMT group. Actual survival after 1, 2, and 3 years was two-fold or more greater in patients treated by EPCS than in patients treated by the combination of EMT and elective shunt. Five-year actuarial survival was almost three times greater after EPCS than after EMT elective shunt. The difference in early survival rate between EPCS and EMT elective shunt was particularly striking in Child's risk class B and C patients: 100% *versus* 33% in class B, and 64% *versus* 14% in class C.

TABLE 6. *Quality of Life in 45 Unselected Cirrhotic Patients Who Survived for 11 to 23 Years After Emergency Portacaval Shunt*

Criteria	Patients (%)
Shunt patency	100
Gastrointestinal bleeding	0
Encephalopathy at any time	18
Recurrent	9
Mild (single episode)	9
Existed before and after shunt	11
Alcohol intake	
None	58
Occasional	31
Regular	11
Liver function	
Improved	53
Worse	18
Unchanged	29
General health at 11 yr	
Excellent or good	73
Fair	27
Poor	0
Work status	
Working	68
Not working	32

TABLE 7. *Prospective Randomized Comparison of Emergency Portacaval Shunt and Emergency Medical Therapy Followed by Elective Shunt in Unselected Patients With Cirrhosis and Bleeding Varices: Characteristics of the Emergency Portacaval Shunt Group (n = 21) and Emergency Medical Therapy Group (n = 22)*

Pathologic manifestations	EPCS (%)	EMT (%)
Drank alcohol ≤7 d before admission	62	59
Jaundice on admission	48	50
Ascites on admission	52	54
Encephalopathy on admission	43	27
Severe muscle wasting	81*	32
Hyperdynamic cardiovascular state	90	95
Liver dye retention ≥50%	33	14
SGOT ≥100 U/dl	33	32
Varices on endoscopic study	100	100
Elevated WHVP	100	100
Child's risk class		
A	10	41*
B	38	27
C	52	32

EPCS: emergency portacaval shunt; EMS: emergency medical therapy.
* $P < 0.01$.

When we compared the 21 patients assigned to the randomized EPCS group with the 84 unselected patients in our recent unrandomized series of EPCS, we found that the two groups were very similar from the standpoint of historic data, physical findings, laboratory data, operative data, portal pressure data, and requirement for blood transfusion. Furthermore, survival rates in the randomized series and the unrandomized series were quite similar. In addition, quality of life has been similar in the two groups of patients treated by

TABLE 8. *Prospective Randomized Comparison of Emergency Portacaval Shunt and Emergency Medical Therapy Followed by Elective Shunt in Unselected Patients With Cirrhosis and Bleeding Varices: Control of Bleeding*

	EPCS (n = 21)	EMT (n = 22)	P
Initial response to IV vasopressin (%)	90	91	NS
Response to esophageal balloon tamponade (%)	—	50	—
Early control of bleeding (%)	100	45	<0.001
Permanent control of bleeding (%)	100	36	<0.001
Blood transfusions during emergency period (mean U)	6.6	19.5	<0.001

EPCS: emergency portacaval shunt; EMT: emergency medical therapy; IV: intravenous.

TABLE 9. *Prospective Randomized Comparison of Emergency Portacaval Shunt and Emergency Medical Therapy Followed by Elective Shunt in Unselected Patients With Cirrhosis and Bleeding Varices: Survival Rates*

Survival rate	EPCS (n = 21) (%)	EMT (n = 22) (%)	P
To leave hospital	81	45	0.03
1 yr actual	71	36	0.03
2 yr actual	67	32	0.03
3 yr actual	67	27	0.01
5 yr actuarial	54	19	0.01
By Child's risk class to leave hospital			
A	100	78	NS
B	100	33	<0.02
C	64	14	<0.02

EPCS: emergency portacaval shunt; EMT: emergency medical therapy.

EPCS. All patients have had permanent control of varix bleeding, more than two thirds have abstained from alcohol, and the incidence of encephalopathy at any time (29% in the randomized group, 16% in the unrandomized group) has not been significantly different. Therefore, our results of EPCS over the last 9 years have been confirmed by our prospective randomized clinical trial.

REFERENCES

1. Ratnoff OD, Patek AJ Jr. Natural history of Laennec's cirrhosis of the liver: Analysis of 386 cases. Medicine 1942;21:207–268.
2. Higgins WH Jr. The esophageal varix: A report of 115 cases. Am J Med Sci 1947;214:436–441.
3. Atik M, Simeone F. Massive gastrointestinal bleeding: A study of 296 patients at City Hospital of Cleveland. Arch Surg 1954;69:355–365.
4. Nachlas MM, O'Neil JE, Campbell AJ. The life history of patients with cirrhosis of the liver and bleeding esophageal varices. Ann Surg 1955;141:10–23.
5. Cohn R, Blaisdell FW. The natural history of the patient with cirrhosis of the liver with esophageal varices following the first massive hemorrhage. Surg Gynecol Obstet 1958;106:699–701.
6. Taylor FW, Jontz JG. Cirrhosis with hemorrhage. Arch Surg 1959;78:786–790.
7. Merigan TC Jr, Hollister RM, Gryska PF, Starkey GWG, Davidson CS. Gastrointestinal bleeding with cirrhosis: Study of 172 episodes in 158 patients. N Engl J Med 1960;263:579–585.
8. Orloff MJ. Emergency treatment of bleeding esophageal varices in cirrhosis. In: Longmire WP Jr, ed. Portal Hypertension. Curr Probl Surg 1966.
9. Orloff MJ, Thomas HS. Pathogenesis of esophageal varix rupture: A study based on gross and microscopic examination of the esophagus at the time of bleeding. Arch Surg 1963;87:301–307.
10. Liebowitz HR. Pathogenesis of esophageal varix rupture. JAMA 1961;175:874–879.
11. Garceau AJ, Chalmers TC, and the Boston Inter-Hospital Liver Group. The natural history of cirrhosis: I. Survival with esophageal varices. N Engl J Med 1963;268:469–473.
12. Orloff MJ, Duguay LR, Kosta LD. Criteria for selection of patients for emergency portacaval shunt. Am J Surg 1977;134:146–152.
13. Mikkelsen WP. Therapeutic portacaval shunt: Preliminary data on controlled trial and morbid effects of acute hyaline necrosis. Arch Surg 1974;108:302–305.
14. Conn HO, Lindenmuth WW. Prophylactic portacaval anastomosis in cirrhotic patients with esophageal varices: Interim results with suggestions for subsequent investigations. N Engl J Med 1968;279:725.
15. Jackson FC, Perrin EB, Smith AG *et al.* A clinical investigation of the portacaval shunt: II. Survival analysis of the prophylactic operation. Am J Surg 1917;115:22.
16. Resnick RH, Chalmers TC, Ishihara AM *et al.* A controlled study of the prophylactic portacaval shunt: A final report. Ann Intern Med 1969;70:675.
17. Orloff MJ. Elective therapeutic portacaval shunt. In: Orloff MJ, Stipa S, Ziparo V, eds. Medical and Surgical Problems of Portal Hypertension, London: Academic Press, 1980;67–78.
18. Orloff MJ. Emergency portacaval shunt: A comparative study of shunt, varix ligation, and nonsurgical treatment of bleeding esophageal varices in unselected patients with cirrhosis. Ann Surg 1967;166:456–478.
19. Orloff MJ, Halasz NA, Lipman CA, Schwabe AD, Thompson JC, Weidner WA. The complications of cirrhosis of the liver. Ann Intern Med 1967;66:165–198.
20. Orloff MJ. Emergency treatment of bleeding esophageal varices. In: Markoff NG, ed. The Therapy of Portal Hypertension. Stuttgart: Georg Thieme Verlag, 1968.
21. Orloff MJ. Emergency treatment of bleeding esophageal varices in alcoholic cirrhosis. In: Sardesai VM, ed. Biochemical and Clinical Aspects of Alcohol Metabolism. Springfield: Charles C. Thomas, Publisher, 1969.
22. Orloff MJ, Chandler JG, Charters AC *et al.* Emergency portacaval shunt for bleeding esophageal varices: Prospective study in unselected patients with alcoholic cirrhosis. Arch Surg 1974;108:293–299.
23. Orloff MJ, Chandler JG, Charters AC *et al.* Portacaval shunt as emergency procedure in unselected patients with alcoholic cirrhosis. Surg Gynecol Obstet 1975;141:59–68.
24. Orloff MJ. Emergency portacaval shunt for bleeding esophageal varices. In: Fiddian-Green RG, Turcotte JG, eds. Gastrointestinal Hemorrhage. New York: Grune & Stratton, 1980.
25. Orloff MJ. Emergency treatment of variceal haemorrhage. Can J Surg 1979;22:550–553.
26. Orloff MJ, Bell RH Jr, Hyde PV, Skivolocki WP. Long-term results of emergency portacaval shunt for bleeding esophageal varices in unselected patients with alcohol cirrhosis. Ann Surg 1980;192:325–340.
27. Orloff MJ, Bell RH Jr. Improved survival of unselected cirrhotic patients with bleeding esophageal varices treated by emergency portacaval shunt. Gastroenterology 1983;84:1389.
28. Bell RH Jr, Hyde PVB, Skivolocki WP, Brimm JE, Orloff MJ. Prospective study of portasystemic encephalopathy after emergency portacaval shunt for bleeding varices. Am J Surg 1981;142:144–150.
29. Orloff MJ. A comparative study of emergency transesophageal ligation and nonsurgical treatment of bleeding esophageal varices in unselected patients with cirrhosis. Surgery 1962;52:103–116.

30. Orloff MJ, Bell RH Jr. Long-term survival after emergency portacaval shunting for bleeding varices in patients with alcohclic cirrhosis. Am J Surg 1986;151:176–183.
31. Orloff MJ, Bell RH Jr, Greenburg AG. Prospective randomized trial of emergency portacaval shunt and medical therapy in unselected cirrhotic patients with bleeding varices. Gastroenterology 1986;90:1754.
32. Conn HO. Emergency portacaval anastomosis (EPCA): The long-awaited trial. Hepatology 1986;6:1058–1060.

Discussion

DR. CLYDE F. BARKER: I don't imagine anyone here finds Dr. Orloff's comments provocative! Are there any questions for Dr. Orloff?

DR. CLARENCE DENNIS: Has Dr. Orloff tried arterialization of the hepatic stump of the portal vein in dealing with encephalopathy?

DR. ORLOFF: No, I've never tried that. Of course, arterialization of the hepatic stump of the portal vein has been tried as treatment for portal hypertension combined with a portacaval shunt, and I'd have to say that the results of that have really been unsatisfactory. The longest series comes from Maillard in France, and the vast majority of those have thrombosed over the long haul, so I would have to say that I don't regard that as an acceptable form of therapy.

DR. HAROLD BARKER: Marshall, I think you're to be complimented on being able to keep your patients from going back to drinking. I don't know of any other series in which this has been accomplished so well, which might partially explain your excellent results. Do you have tricks in keeping the patients from returning to drinking?

DR. MARSHALL ORLOFF: I think that the trick is a typical Pennsylvania one, simply dogged determination and absolute tenacity in following the patients. The main reason why the treatment of alcoholism is not as good as it could be in this country is because most physicians don't like to deal with alcoholics and therefore don't follow the patients. This unfortunately is also true of surgeons. They too don't really follow the patients and focus on this issue over the lifetime of the patients. What we've tried to do is to follow the patients closely and simply try a nonpunitive approach to get them to stop drinking.

DR. WILLIAM CURRERI: Marshall, I think we are all envious of your success with emergency portacaval shunt, but I wanted to ask you about the rebleeding rate you report with sclerotherapy because it is certainly much higher than in our own or any published series. I've noticed that since the surgeons at our institution now do all the sclerotherapy that the rebleeding rate is way down as compared with its incidence when the medical endoscopists used to do it. We believe this is probably because the surgeons are a little more aggressive in getting adequate control of bleeding. I wonder whether you wouldn't get better results from emergency sclerotherapy if the surgeons were doing it.

DR. MARSHALL ORLOFF: It is possible. It is true that the gastroenterologists in our institution (and in the vast majority of institutions in the world) are the ones who do endoscopic sclerotherapy. But I can't really comment upon that other than to say that they are expert endoscopists. However, our sclerotherapy experience is a little different from that of others since every single patient coming down the pike receives emergency endoscopic sclerotherapy and then long-term sclerotherapy. This has not been done by others who, in fact, have taken patients that have already stopped bleeding and then subjected them to short and long-term sclerotherapy. That may be a difference, but I don't know. I can only describe our own experience.

Introduction of Dr. Edwin Kaplan

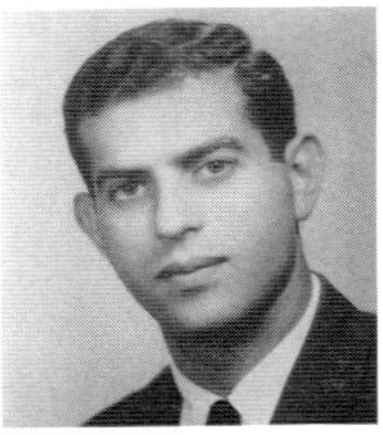

Dr. Clyde Barker: I recall one rotation I had as chief resident on the ward service at HUP during which the junior residents were Ed Kaplan and Scott Jones and the intern was Ted Copeland. One patient was a robust black lady who had suffered a burn of her chest and was in the Hospital for many weeks. She never could get Ed's name right, but instead called him Dr. Castle, as we then all began to do. That Ed still remembers and answers to the name of Castle indicates what a good time we had. After finishing his residency in 1967, Ed went to Michael Reese with Jerry Peskin and then to the University of Chicago where he has had a distinguished career and remains as Professor of Surgery, despite several attempts over the years to recruit him back to Philadelphia and Penn. He is clearly one of the world's experts on endocrine surgery and will speak today on his paper entitled "Nuclear DNA Analysis of Insulinomas and Gastrinomas."

A few days ago I happened to be going through Dr. Rhoads' bibliography and found several interesting titles which bear a relationship to Ed's subject. One is titled "Gastric Hyperchlorhyrdia with Three Primary Jejunal Ulcers and Hypoproteinemia" by Machella, T. E., Rhoads, J. E., and Hobler, R. E. (*Gastroenterology* 13:357–366). It was published in 1949 and makes an interesting association that has since been emphasized by others. Later, in 1950, Dr. Rhoads recorded (along with John Howard and Henry Moss) a large number of cases of islet cell tumors of the pancreas in an article entitled "Hyperinsulinism and Islet Cell Tumors of the Pancreas" (*Surg Gynecol Obstet* 90:417–455, 1950).

Dr. Kaplan's Introductory Remarks

Dr. Rhoads, it is such a pleasure for me to be here today. I'm happy that my brother, sister in law, and mother can also be here to join me in honoring you. Scott Jones spoke earlier about role models. When I think of role models I think primarily of two people in my life. One is my father and the other, truly, is Dr. Rhoads. When I was growing up my Dad, who was a physician, had in his office this etching of Dr. Ravdin done by Harry Moskowitz, a dear friend of our family, which is inscribed, "To my friend Joseph Kaplan, from I. S. Ravdin." When I was growing up my father said, "If you want to do something very good in life, go into Surgery at the University of Pennsylvania Hospital." He said, "That is the greatest team of surgeons that I ever knew."

I will now show some pictures from my medical school yearbook of 1961. Here you see Rav, Julian Johnson, Charlie Kirby, Billy Fitts, and Brooke Roberts (wearing ultraviolet protective garb). Underneath this one it said, "We move on Tel Aviv in the morning." Dr. Royster, Clete Schwegman (as elegant as ever), Bill Blakemore, Jack Mackie, Bob Ravdin, Bugs Lehr, and finally, the man of the hour, Dr. Rhoads, vintage 1961. You see him here holding a patient's hand, tall and straight, compassionate and understanding—exemplifying all the fine virtues I've admired so much.

I remember several conversations I had with Dr. Rhoads during my years as a medical student. I met him in the hallway one day, and he told me that I had done well on the National Boards and should consider surgery as a career. He said, "If you become a surgeon, you are not going to be home much, especially while your children are young. During those years, people may be upset with you. But, if your children turn out as well as mine did, people may say, 'Thank God the old fellow stayed away.' " When I was a senior med student (during my 8th year at Penn), I remember Dr. Rhoads saying, "We can teach you all the surgery you need to know in five years. Go away and study as much medicine as you possibly can." So, I went away to intern at Mt. Sinai Hospital. One day during my internship year, I answered a page and the person on the line said, "This is Jonathan Rhoads. I couldn't come to New York City without calling to say hello." I was a young man, an intern, and I just couldn't believe it. These are the things I've thought back on over the years, which were so inspiring to me as a young person.

Nowadays, at Chicago we speak of "clustering" our patients. If one of my interns gets a patient on another floor, he's upset. But in the old days at HUP, we had patients, perhaps 50, scattered all over the Hospital. To start rounds, we'd go up to the roof of the Gates Pavilion where Dr. Rhoads would look around the territory of West Philadelphia and point out what was going to be built and things like that. Then we would make rounds. When I was a student, Hilary Timmis (who is here today) was our chief resident. Hilary was so careful that everything was perfect. He used to sit down and map out the route we were going to take. He would go along this corridor and down this stairway. We would finish rounds in the basement, and frequently, Dr. Rhoads would treat everybody to a Coke from the machine. Once in a while, if he was not rushed or we had finished a bit early, Dr. Rhoads would say, "Let's all go into the coffee shop and sit down." Dr. Rhoads liked vanilla cokes, and he'd say, "I'll have a vanilla coke." Hilary would say, "I'll have a vanilla coke," and we'd order vanilla cokes—right on down the line. If one was particularly brave and courageous, he might say "I'll have a lemon coke." I remember once we had a new intern on the service. We were in the coffee shop, and it went the usual way, vanilla cokes down the line. Then the intern said, "I'll have two scrambled eggs, coffee, milk, etc." Dr. Rhoads looked up with a twinkle in his eye, and Hilary just about fell off his seat.

Another story exemplifies the controlled manner that Dr. Rhoads always had, which I have tried to emulate. We were operating on a patient who had a sigmoid obstruction, and as we opened the abdomen, we found that the cecum was quite distenced. In fact, it was necrotic. As we opened, the thing sort of burst right before our eyes, and Dr. Rhoads said calmly, "May I have the suction please." He took the suction, and it immediately got clogged. The nurse said, "Dr. Rhoads, I am trying to fix it, I am trying to fix it!," and without a change in inflection, Dr. Rhoads calmly said, "Oh my, how we could use suction now." This may not impress those of you who are not surgeons, but a manner this calm is not usual in dealing with such problems.

I have always been very proud of the years I spent here, and I think back most warmly on those who inspired me to study endocrine surgery—Dr. Rhoads, Dr. Mackie, Dr. Peskin, and Claude Arnaud (who worked with Harold Rasmussen, whom I met when I was a senior resident at HUP). I later went to the Mayo Clinic and studied for a year with Arnaud as his first research fellow, working on parathyroid hormone and calcitonin.

Nuclear DNA Analysis of Insulinomas and Gastrinomas

FRANCESCO STIPA, B.A., MARCO ARGANINI, M.D.,
MARLUCE BIBBO, M.D., FRANCIS STRAUS II, M.D., HARVEY DYTCH, B.S.,
GEORGE WIED, M.D., KEITH HORVATH, M.D.,
AND EDWIN L. KAPLAN, M.D.

The potential for malignancy of an islet cell tumor of the pancreas is difficult to cytologically judge when one evaluates only the primary lesion, because a malignant condition is usually determined by the presence of regional or distant metastases. Nuclear DNA cytometric measurements have proved helpful both in the evaluation of the malignant potential of other endocrine and nonendocrine lesions and in the determination of the "aggressiveness" of these tumors. Thirty-six islet cell tumors or their metastases from 25 patients were studied. Eleven patients had insulinomas and typical insulinoma syndromes, and 14 others had gastrinomas with the Zollinger-Ellison syndrome. Tissue from each tumor was stained by the Feulgen technique, and nuclear DNA cytometry was performed by means of the micro TICAS system designed by the Cytopathology Laboratory of the University of Chicago. Ploidy measurements of insulinomas, taken alone, did not discriminate well between benign and malignant states. However, the single malignant insulinoma could be clearly recognized, for it was one of only two lesions in that group with 5N-exceeding rate (5N-ER) values of 1% or greater. (5N-ER is defined as the percentage of aneuploid nuclei with nuclear DNA content greater than 5N.) On the other hand, seven of eight malignant gastrinomas had ploidy values of 2.5N or greater (our definition of an aneuploid state) and/or had 5N-ER values of 1% or greater, while five of six benign gastrinomas had ploidy values of less than 2.5N and had 5N-ER values of 0%. In addition, the two most aggressive tumors had the highest ploidy and 5N-ER values. Nuclear DNA cytometric studies appear to offer promise as an aid in the evaluation of pancreatic islet cell tumors, particularly gastrinomas.

THE DIFFERENTIATION BETWEEN benign and malignant pancreatic islet cell tumors is dependent primarily on the recognition of lymph node, liver, or other distant metastases. Cellular morphology or pleomorphism is not important in this evaluation in most cases. DNA ploidy analysis has been used as both an adjunct to diagnosis of malignancy and a prognostic factor in analysis of other endocrine tumors.[1-9]

For several years, the Section of Cytology at the University of Chicago has used various computer systems for rapid DNA ploidy evaluation on tissues and smears.[10-13] This method is useful because it yields quantitative information about the nuclear DNA content in addition to data on other cytometric parameters. This article presents the results obtained when this technique was used on specimens from patients with insulinomas and gastrinomas.

From the Section of Cytology, Department of Obstetrics and Gynecology, and the Departments of Surgery and Pathology, University of Chicago School of Medicine, Chicago, Illinois.

Presented at the Eighth Annual Meeting of the American Association of Endocrine Surgeons, Chicago, Illinois, March 30–31, 1987.

This study was supported in part by Grant CA37352-04 and The Nathan and Frances Goldblatt Society for Cancer Research.

This article has been reproduced with permission from *Surgery*, Vol. 102, No. 6, December 1987.

Material and Methods

Pathologic data from 25 patients with islet cell tumors were studied. Twenty-one patient histories were obtained from the files of the Department of Pathology of the University of Chicago Medical Center and four were obtained from corresponding files of the Michael Reese Hospital. Eleven tumors were from patients with insulinomas, each of whom had been diagnosed because of a typical clinical syndrome as well as the documentation of an inappropriately elevated insulin level in the face of severe hypoglycemia. One of these tumors (9%) was classified as malignant on the basis of the presence of a single lymph node metastasis; the others were benign (Table 1).

Fourteen patients with gastrinomas were evaluated; these patients had typical manifestations of the Zollinger-Ellison syndrome. Most manifested severe gastric hyperchlorhydria as well as hypergastrinemia. The primary site of the gastrinomas was pancreatic in seven patients, including two with multiple endocrine neoplasia type I syndrome (MEN-I); within the duodenal submucosa in five patients; and extrapancreatic in two patients, one periduodenal and a second from the gastric antrum. Eight patients (57%) had malignant lesions: three had lymph node metastases, four had liver metastases or liver and lymph node metastases, and one had lung metastases without other evidence of spread. The tumors from six other patients (43%) were considered to be benign because of the absence of identifiable metastatic spread. In all, 26 tumor specimens were available for analysis from this gastrinoma group of 14 patients, since in four patients multiple specimens were obtained. These included 10 pancreatic, seven duodenal, and one extrapancreatic primary tumors as well as four lymph node and four liver metastases.

The tumor tissues had been fixed in 10% buffered formol saline solution and embedded in paraffin. For this study, paraffin sections were cut at 4 μm thickness; these were deparaffinized and stained by both the standard hematoxylin and eosin (HE) technique and the Feulgen reaction.[13] which stains nuclear DNA. The slides were then mounted in Permount (Fisher Scientific Co., Fairlawn, N.J.) and coverslipped. The appearance of the nuclei of a benign insulinoma, which was prepared with a Feulgen stain, is shown in Fig. 1.

The DNA measurements of the Feulgen-stained nuclei were performed at the Cytopathology Laboratory of the University of Chicago with the MicroTICAS system.[11,12] This DNA cytometry system for the IBM PC comprises hardware and software subsystems that, coupled with a user-supplied, ordinary light microscope, enable the measurement of the total nuclear optical density (extinction) and various other cytometric parameters, including nuclear size and roundness, on tissue cell specimens. Since the material in this study was Feulgen stained, the total optical density and the average optical density could also be expressed in terms of the ploidy value (N).

The ploidy value and other parameters of at least 150 cells from each islet cell tumor were recorded and stored in a computer file. Nuclei of at least 50 normal cells from normal pancreatic, duodenal, or lymph node tissue from each of the 25 cases were used to establish the diploid value.

Statistical analyses were performed on these data to examine the significance of differences in group means of the following parameters: mean ploidy, mean nuclear size, mean nuclear roundness, 2N-deviation index (2N-DI), and the 5N-exceeding rate (5N-ER).[14] The 2N-DI, a measure of the deviation of the cells from the diploid number, is defined as the sum of the squares of the differences between the ploidy value of each nucleus and the diploid reference divided by the number of measured nuclei. The 5N-ER is defined as the percentage of aneuploid nuclei with a nuclear DNA content greater than 5N.

In all, 37 tumor specimens were analyzed from the 25 patients with insulinomas and gastrinomas. Mann-Whitney U tests were performed on the data collected from (1) each separate tumor, 37 in all, and (2) from a single tumor specimen from each patient that had the highest ploidy and 5N-ER values. Within these two categories, insulinomas and gastrinomas were considered together, and then the gastrinoma group was evaluated separately. The primary group differences investigated were those based on tumor type (insulinoma versus gastrinoma), metastases (any or none), and aggressive metastases (liver or lung metastases versus nodal metastases or none).

TABLE 1. *Pathologic and Morphometric Data of Pancreatic Islet Cell Tumors*

Patient	Age (yr)	Sex	Primary tumor	Diagnosis	Site of metastases	Site of analysed tumor	Follow-up: Status	Follow-up: Years	Mean ploidy (N)	Mean nuclear size (sq. μm)	Mean nuclear roundness	5N-ER (%)	2N-DI
A. Gastrinomas													
1. M.B.	53	F	Duodenal tumors ×3	Benign	—	Duodenum ×2	A	10	1.70	25.40	1.03	0.00	0.16
						(2 sections of			2.30	25.60	1.01	0.00	0.30
						one tumor)			3.00	19.80	1.01	1.39	1.24 ←
2. A.B.	45	M	Duodenal	Benign	—	Duodenum	A	1	1.90	23.00	1.02	0.00	0.16
3. M.S.	44	F	Duodenal	Benign	—	Duodenum	D*	8	2.40	42.20	1.10	0.00	0.48
4. F.W.	49	M	Duodenal	Benign	—	Duodenum	D*	0.5	2.40	29.10	1.02	0.00	0.41
5. J.S.	55	M	Pancreatic	Benign	—	Pancreas	A	1	2.40	20.10	0.98	0.00	0.38
6. E.T.	36	F	Periduodenal	Benign	—	Periduodenal tumor	A	12	1.90	36.80	1.05	0.00	0.26
7. O.B.	29	M	Duodenal	Malignant	Lymph node	Lymph node	D†	2	2.30	20.50	1.00	0.00	0.38
8. E.H.	50	F	Pancreatic	Malignant	Lymph node	Lymph node	A	18	2.60	39.20	1.01	1.68	0.85
9. R.E.	53	F	Probable pancreatic	Malignant	Liver	Liver (autopsy specimen)	D‡	2 days	2.70	26.00	1.06	0.00	0.70
10. M.M.	53	F	Pancreatic	Malignant	Liver	Liver	A	18	2.60	34.40	1.07	0.00	0.59
11. L.M.	51	F	Probable	Malignant	Lymph nodes	Lymph node	A	1	2.80	28.10	1.03	0.72	1.55
			pancreatic		Liver	Liver			2.20	35.20	1.04	1.12	0.40
						Lymph node			3.30	41.60	1.03	1.80	2.70 ←
12. C.M.	57	M	Gastric antrum	Malignant	Lymph nodes Liver	Liver (autopsy specimen)	D‡	no op	2.10	24.80	1.01	1.23	0.25
13. J.M.	24	F	MEN-I syndrome,	Malignant	Lung	Pancreas ×6	D†	11	2.60	30.30	1.03	0.00	0.74
			pancreatic						2.10	26.10	1.03	0.00	0.32
			(multiple)						2.00	24.00	1.02	0.00	0.21
									2.40	43.30	1.04	0.79	0.57
									2.30	27.10	1.06	1.03	0.60
									3.00	34.60	1.08	5.60	2.31 ←
14. N.P.	32	M	MEN-I syndrome,	Malignant	Lymph node	Pancreas ×3	A	6	1.80	26.40	1.01	0.00	0.23
			pancreatic			Lymph node			1.80	28.70	1.04	0.00	0.25
			(multiple)						2.00	30.40	1.04	0.00	0.30
									2.50	25.50	1.01	0.00	0.54 ←

TABLE 1. *Pathologic and Morphometric Data of Pancreatic Islet Cell Tumors (Continued)*

Patient	Age (yr)	Sex	Primary tumor	Diagnosis	Site of metastases	Site of analysed tumor	Follow-up Status	Follow-up Years	Mean ploidy (N)	Mean nuclear size (sq. μm)	Mean nuclear roundness	5N-ER (%)	2N-DI
B. Insulinomas													
1. M.A.	24	M	Pancreatic	Benign	—	Pancreas	A	4	2.50	41.30	1.04	0.88	0.44
2. L.C.	63	F	Pancreatic	Benign	—	Pancreas	A	11	2.00	28.80	1.06	0.00	0.17
3. W.C.	61	M	Pancreatic	Benign	—	Pancreas	D*	6	2.10	31.10	1.05	0.00	0.17
4. A.F.	67	M	Pancreatic	Benign	—	Pancreas	A	9	2.20	25.50	1.00	0.00	0.16
5. J.G.	27	F	Pancreatic	Benign	—	Pancreas	A	5	2.50	42.30	1.08	0.00	0.46
6. K.G.	22	F	Pancreatic	Benign	—	Pancreas	D*	2	2.50	46.90	1.13	0.00	0.76
7. J.L.	68	F	Pancreatic	Benign	—	Pancreas	A	10	2.20	27.00	1.03	1.32	0.41
8. J.P.	53	M	Pancreatic	Benign	—	Pancreas	A	7	2.60	28.10	1.03	0.00	0.59
9. S.R.	53	F	Pancreatic	Benign		Pancreas	A	3	2.80	35.80	1.06	0.00	1.09
10. P.W.	28	M	Pancreatic	Benign	—	Pancreas	A	8	2.70	36.00	1.03	0.00	0.70
11. W.D.	23	M	Pancreatic	Malignant	Peripancreatic lymph node	Lymph node	A	11	2.20	41.00	1.07	1.02	0.41

5N-ER, 5N-exceeding rate; 2N-DI, 2N-deviation index; ←, in patients in whom multiple tumors were analyzed, the highest grade lesion was used for statistical analysis in the "selected" group.

* Died without evidence of islet cell tumor.

| Died with evidence of islet cell tumor but not because of tumor spread.

‡ Died of perforated ulcer.

Results

An analysis of patient data as well as mean ploidy, mean nuclear size, mean nuclear roundness, and 2N-DI and 5N-ER values is summarized in Table 1. Significant ($p < 0.05$) differences in group means were noted in several of the measured karyometric parameters. Nuclear size of the gastrinomas was somewhat smaller than that of the insulinomas (a mean of 29.6 μm^2 versus 34.9 μm^2, respectively, for all the tumors measured, $p < 0.04$). Of greatest importance is that the 5N-exceeding rate (5N-ER) seems to be significantly higher in the more aggressive tumors. Of the 37 tumors, both gastrinomas and insulinomas, tumors with any metastatic spread (regional or distant) had an average 5N-ER of 0.79% compared with 0.20% for tumors without metastases ($p < 0.06$); tumors with distant metastases (liver or lung) had an average 5N-ER of 1.02% compared with 0.25% for those with local or no metastases ($p < 0.03$). In the gastrinomas only, the average 5N-ER for all tumors in the group with distant metastases was 1.02% compared with 0.22% for those without ($p < 0.04$), whereas if we consider only the "selected tumors" (the highest-grade tumor when multiple tumors were present) this difference becomes 1.73% to 0.34%.

Analyses of ploidy measurements of individual tumors are of further interest. A histogram of normal pancreatic tissue is demonstrated in Fig. 2. Note the sharp bell-shaped curve of these cells, which have a mean ploidy value of 2.0N. In Fig. 3, A and B the histologic appearance of a benign insulinoma stained by standard HE techniques is seen. The histogram of this tumor is shown in Fig. 3C. Note that the mean ploidy value of cells of this tumor is 2.1N and the 5N-ER value is 0%. Fig. 4, A and B shows the histologic appearance of a malignant insulinoma. The diagnosis of malignancy was based not on the histologic characteristics of the primary tumor but, rather, on the presence of a single lymph node that contained metastatic tumor. The histogram of this tumor is shown in Fig. 4C. Its cells are diploid, 2.2N; however, a 5N-ER value of 1.02% was obtained.

An example of a benign gastrinoma, in this case from the duodenal submucosa, is seen in Fig. 5, A and B. A histogram (Fig. 5C) demonstrates a mean ploidy value of 2.4N and a

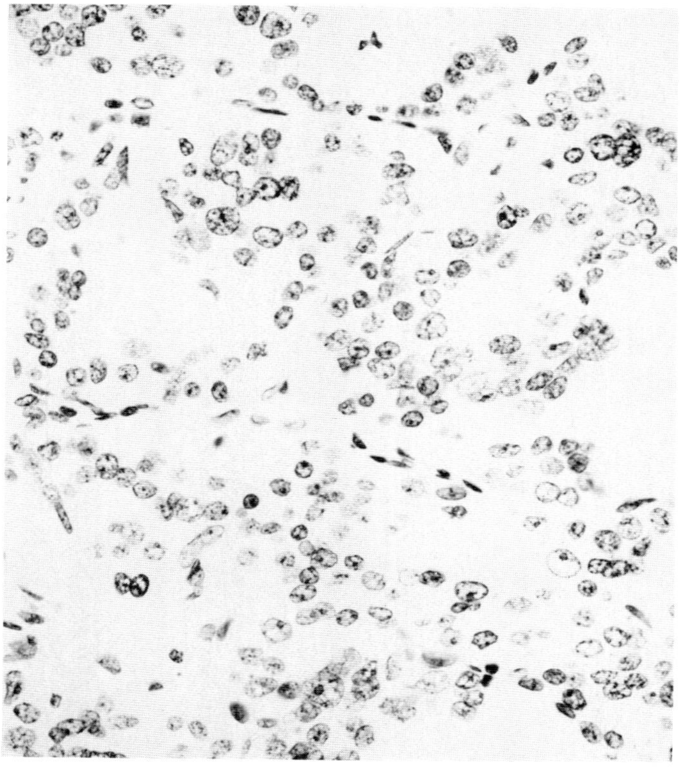

FIG. 1. Benign insulinoma shows variation in nuclear size and shape. Only non-overlapping tumor nuclei are used for analysis. Fibroblast and endothelial nuclei can be used for control analysis. (Feulgen stain; original magnification ×400.)

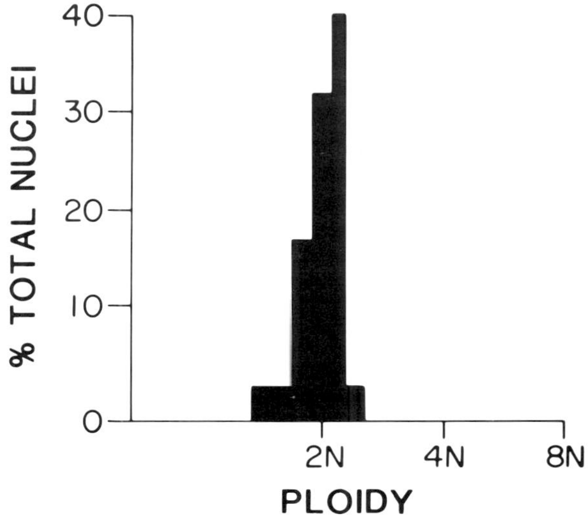

FIG. 2. Histogram of normal pancreatic tissue.

5N-ER value of 0%. In contrast is a lymph node metastasis from a pancreatic gastrinoma, which is demonstrated in Fig. 6, A and B. A histogram (Fig. 6C) shows that the mean ploidy value of this lesion is 3.3N, which is clearly aneuploid, and the 5N-ER value is 1.80%.

An evaluation of the DNA measurements of all eleven insulinomas is shown in Fig. 7. Of note is that six tumors exhibited mean ploidy values of 2.5N or greater, our arbitrary value of an aneuploid state.[10] However, only two tumors manifested 5N-ER values of 1.0% or greater, and one of these two was the only malignant insulinoma in the group.

A compilation of data on gastrinomas is demonstrated graphically in Fig. 8. Seven of eight malignant gastrinomas had ploidy values of 2.5N or greater (aneuploid) and/or had 5N-ER values of 1.0% or greater; on the other hand, five of six benign gastrinomas exhibited ploidy values of less than 2.5N and had 5N-ER values of 0%.

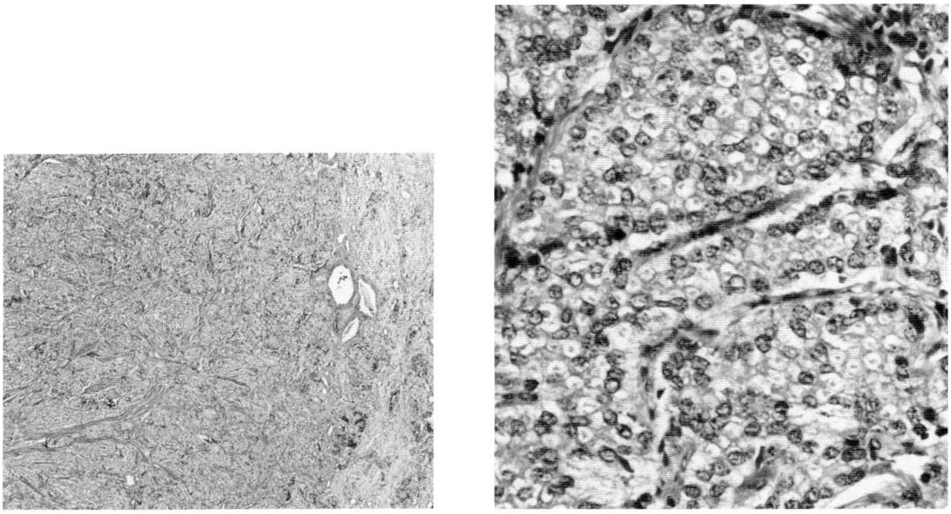

FIG. 3. A (*left*), Benign insulinoma with apparent capsular invasion and islet cells growing in broad alveolar nests. (Hematoxylin-eosin stain; original magnification ×40.) B (*right*), Higher magnification shows regular islet cell nuclei and secretory cytoplasmic structures. (Original magnification ×400.)

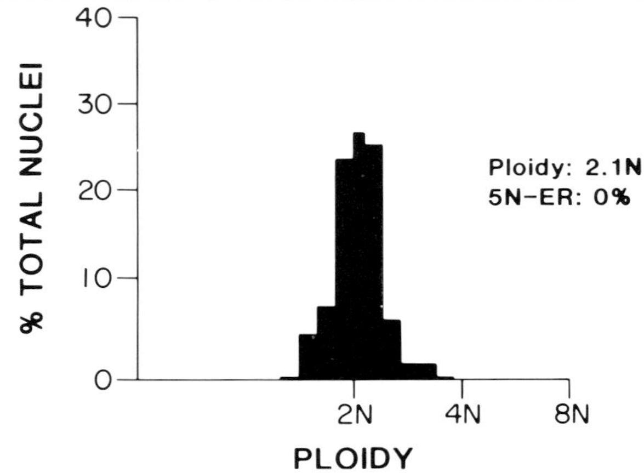

FIG. 3C. Histogram of the benign insulinoma. Ploidy value, 2.1N, and 5N-ER, 0%.

Discussion

As is the case with other endocrine tumors, the difficulties in differentiating benign from malignant islet cell tumors by evaluating the histologic characteristics of the *primary tumor* are well established.[15] The analysis of nuclear DNA has been used in the study of other endocrine tumors, thyroid cancers,[1,4–6,8,9] carcinoid tumors,[16–20] pheochromocytomas,[2,7] and adrenal cortical carcinomas.[3,7] Hürthle cell tumors have been previously evaluated in this manner in our laboratory.[5] These techniques show promise both as a means of recognition of a malignant state before lymph node or distant metastases are present and as a prognostic tool whereby aggressive tumors can be separated from others with less virulence.

It is well known that about 90% of insulinomas are benign.[21] Among the tumors examined for this study only one of 11 manifested evidence of metastatic spread at the time of operation. In that case, a single lymph node with metastatic spread was found adjacent to the primary tumor. Despite this categorization by light microscopy, six of 11 of the insulinomas manifested ploidy values of 2.5N or greater—the arbitrary definition of an aneuploid state that has been used previously in our laboratory in the study of Hürthle cell tumors of

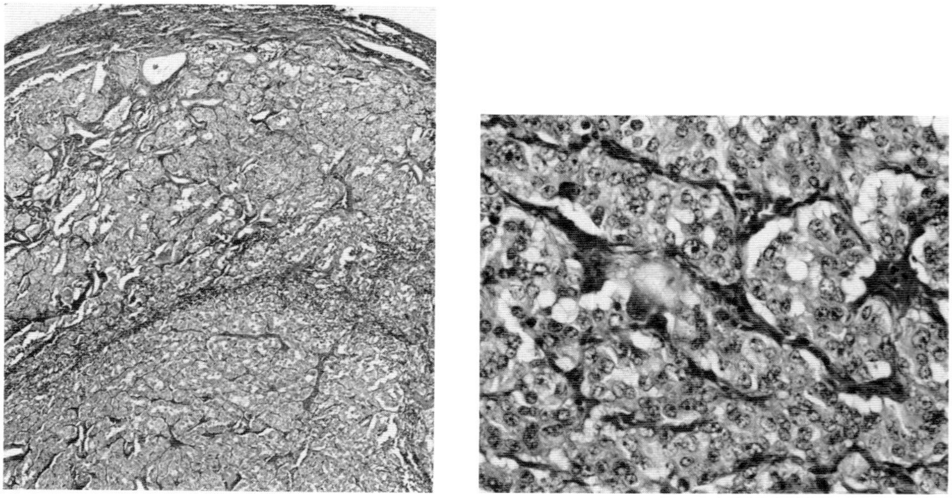

FIG. 4. A (*left*), Malignant insulinoma with sharp peripheral demarcation and variable sized alveolar cell clusters. (Hematoxylin-eosin stain; original magnification ×40.) B (*right*), Higher magnification shows alveolar nests, varying sized tumor cell nuclei, and prominent nucleoli. (Original magnification ×400.)

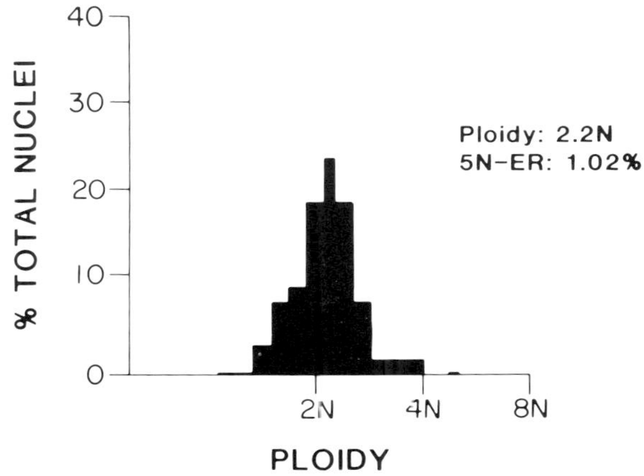

FIG. 4C. Histogram of the only malignant insulinoma (patient W.D.) demonstrates diploid value, 2.2N, but abnormal 5N-ER value of 1.02%.

the thyroid.[5] Of note, however, is that only two of the insulinomas had 5N-ER values of 1.0% or greater and that one of these two tumors was the malignant insulinoma. Thus while ploidy values per se, do not appear to discriminate between benign and malignant insulin-

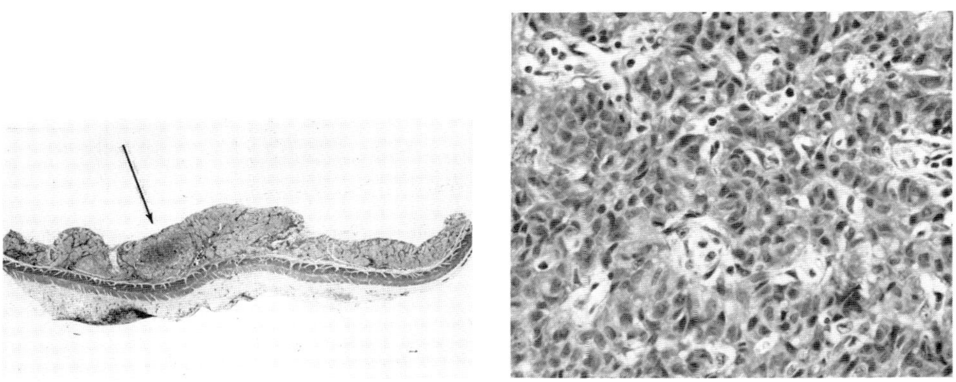

FIGS. 5A AND 5B. A (*left*), Intramucosal and submucosal benign duodenal gastrinoma (*arrow*). (Hematoxylin-eosin stain; original magnification ×10.) B (*right*), Anastomotic trabecular pattern of a benign gastrinoma with some variation in nuclear chromisity and outline. (Hematoxylin-eosin stain; original magnification ×40.)

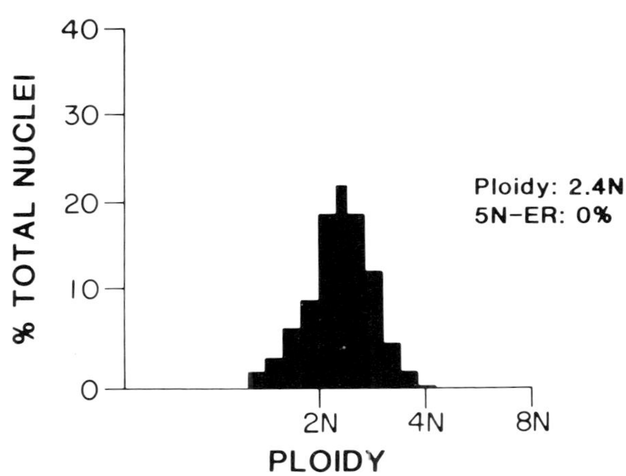

FIG. 5C. Histogram of benign duodenal gastrinoma demonstrates normal ploidy value, 2.4N, and 5N-ER, 0%.

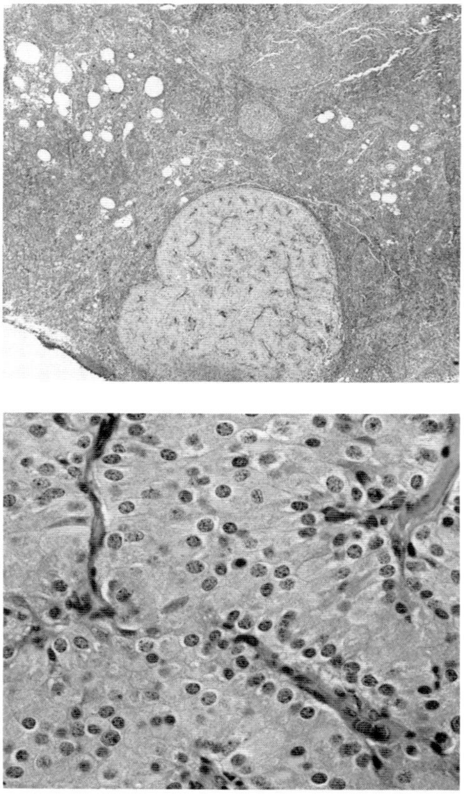

FIGS. 6A AND 6B. A (*left*), Metastatic gastrinoma in a peripancreatic lymph node. (Hematoxylin-eosin stain; original magnification ×40). B (*right*), Higher magnification of the same metastatic focus showing an anastomosing trabecular pattern with large granular acidophilic tumor cells containing regular round nuclei with prominent clumped chromatin patterns. (Original magnification ×400.)

omas, the finding of a 5N-ER value of 1% or greater may prove to be a significant indicator of a malignant state when greater numbers of these tumors are evaluated.

About 60 percent of gastrinomas are known to be malignant.[22] These tumors typically spread first to regional lymph nodes. Then the more aggressive lesions spread to the liver and to other distant sites. While many deaths are known to be due to complications of the

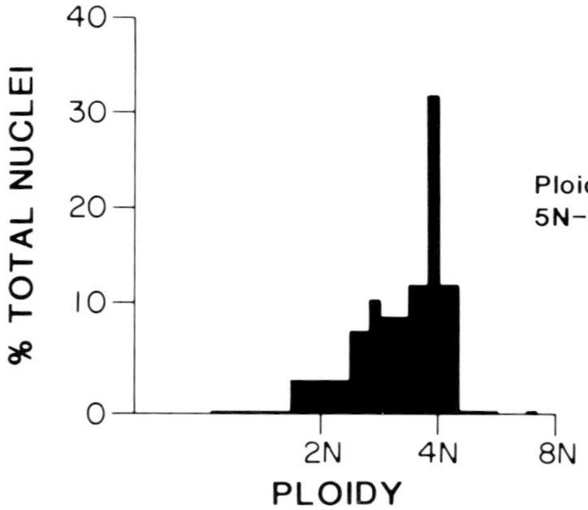

FIG. 6C. Histogram of pancreatic gastrinoma with lymph node metastases demonstrates ploidy value of 3.3N (aneuploid) and 5N-ER value of 1.80%.

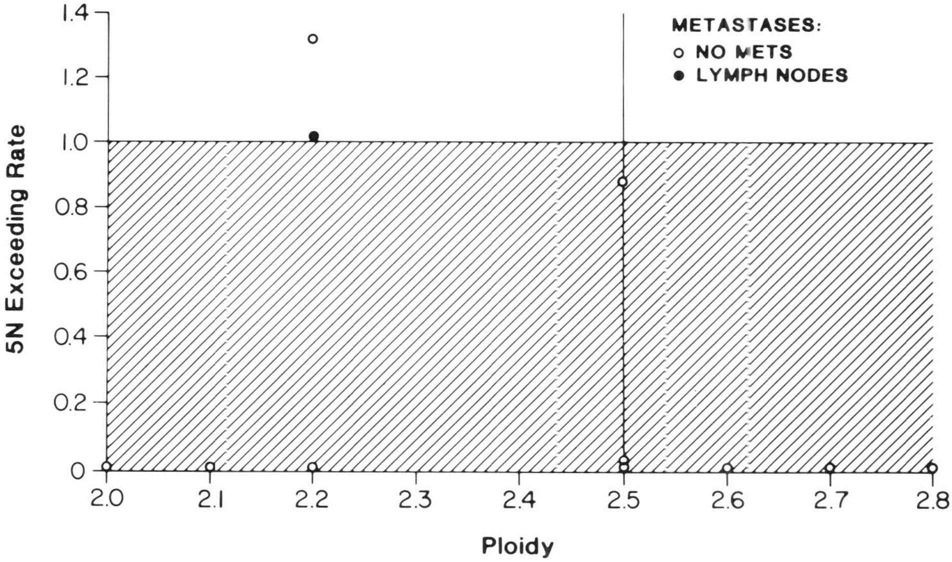

FIG. 7. Graphic display of data from 11 insulinomas. Of importance is that the malignant insulinoma was one of two tumors that had a 5N-ER value of greater than 1%.

virulent ulcer diathesis, which is caused by the hypergastrinemia and gastric hyperacidity of the Zollinger-Ellison syndrome, other deaths from tumor growth are well documented.[23] Tumor virulence among these lesions is variable. In some cases aggressive tumor growth occurs and leads to rapid demise, whereas in many persons with metastatic lesions tumor growth is slow, and if the consequences of gastric hyperacidity are controlled, the prognosis for prolonged survival is good. A means of differentiating these lesions would be helpful.

The evaluation of gastrinomas by DNA measurements demonstrated that seven of eight

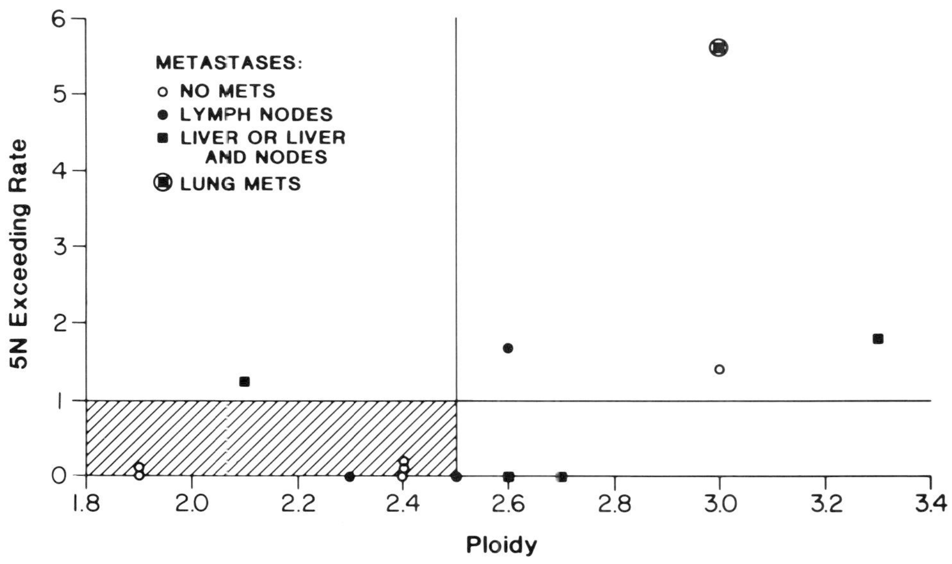

FIG. 8. Plot of ploidy and 5N-ER values of the "most aggressive" tumors of 14 gastrinoma patients. Note that five of six benign gastrinomas had ploidy values of less than 2.5N and 5N-ER values 0%. On the other hand, seven of eight malignant gastrinomas exhibited mean ploidy values of 2.5N or greater (aneuploid) and/or had 5N-ER values of 1% or greater. Finally, the two most aggressive tumors clinically exhibited the highest ploidy and the highest 5N-ER values.

malignant gastrinomas exhibited ploidy values of 2.5N or greater, our definition of an aneuploid state,[5] and/or had 5N-ER values of 1% or greater. Furthermore, the two patients with most aggressive tumors—one (J.M.) with multiple lung metastases and the second (L.M.) with progressive liver metastases, which required chemotherapy—exhibited the highest 5N-ER and ploidy values, respectively.

Finally, values of 5N-ER were shown to be greater in the group of gastrinomas that demonstrated metastatic spread than in those lesions that were benign. The highest 5N-ER values were found in those gastrinomas that had metastasized distally to either the liver or the lungs.

Larger numbers of patients with gastrinomas must be studied in the future; however, this pilot nuclear DNA cytometric study is very promising. If "aggressive" gastrinomas can be recognized by means of this technique, radical cancer operations might be reserved for this group.

ACKNOWLEDGMENT

We thank Dr. Wendy Recant for providing four tumor specimens and Ms. Noreen Fulton for technical assistance.

REFERENCES

1. Backdahl M, Carstensen J, Auer G, Tallroth E. Statistical evaluation of the prognostic value of nuclear DNA content in papillary, follicular, and medullary thyroid tumors. World J Surg 1986;10:974–980.
2. Hosaka Y, Rainwater LM, Grant CS, Farrow GM, vanHeerdern JA, Lieber MM. Pheochromocytoma: nuclear deoxyribonucleic acid patterns studied by flow cytometry. Surgery 1986;100:1003–1010.
3. Bowlby LS, DeBault LE, Abraham SR. Flow cytometric analysis of adrenal cortical tumor DNA. Relationship between cellular DNA and histopathologic classification. Cancer 1986;58:1499–1505.
4. Bondeson L, Azavedo E, Bondeson AG, Caspersson T, Ljungberg O. Nuclear DNA content and behavior of oxyphil thyroid tumors. Cancer 1986;58:672–675.
5. Galera-Davidson H, Bibbo M, Bartels PH, Dytch HE, Puls JH, Weid GL. Correlation between automated DNA ploidy measurements of Hürthle-cell tumors and their histopathologic and clinical features. Anal Quant Cytol Histol 1986;8:158–167.
6. Backdahl M, Auer G, Forsslund G, et al. Prognostic value of nuclear DNA content in follicular thyroid tumours. Acta Chir Scand 1986;152:1–7.
7. Klein FA, Kay S, Ratliff JE, White FK, Newsome HH. Flow cytometric determinations of ploidy and proliferation patterns of adrenal neoplasms: an adjunct to histological classification. J Urol 1985;134:862–866.
8. Bengtsson A, Malmaeus J, Grimelius L, Johansson H, Ponten J, Rastad J, Akerstrom G. Measurement of nuclear DNA content in thyroid diagnosis. World J Surg 1984;8:481–486.
9. Cohn K, Backdahl M, Forsslund G, et al. Prognostic value of nuclear DNA content in papillary thyroid carcinoma. World J Surg 1984;8:474–480.
10. Bibbo M, Bartels PH, Bytch HE, Wied GL. Ploidy measurements by high-resolution cytometry. Anal Quant Cytol Histol 1985;7:81–88.
11. Dytch HE, Bibbo M, Puls JHA, Bartels PH, Wied GL. Software design for an inexpensive, practical, microcomputer-based DNA cytometry system. Anal Quant Cytol Histol 1986;8:8–18.
12. Puls JH, Bibbo M, Dytch HE, Bartels PH, Wied GL. MicroTICAS: The design of an inexpensive video-based microphotometer/computer system DNA ploidy studies. Anal Quant Cytol Histol 1986;8:1–7.
13. Wied GL, Bartels PH, Dytch HE, Pishotta FT, Bibbo M. Rapid high-resolution cytometry. Anal Quant Cytol Histol 1982;4:257–262.
14. Bocking A, Adler CP, Common HH, Hilgarth M, Granzen B, Auffermann W. Algorithm for DNA-cytophotometric diagnosis and grading of malignancy. Anal Quant Cytol Histol 1984;6:1–8.
15. Franz VK. Atlas of tumor pathology (Fascicles 27 and 28 Tumors of the pancreas). Washington, DC: Armed Forces Institute of Pathology; 1959:99.
16. Cohn G, Erhardt K, Cedermark B, Hamberger B, Auer G. DNA distribution pattern in intestinal carcinoid tumors. World J Surg 1986;10:518–551.
17. Wilander E, Bengtsson A, Norheim I, Oberg K. Interferon-induced nuclear DNA alterations in malignant carcinoid tumors in vivo. JNCI 1986;76:429–433.
18. Wilander E, Glimelius B, Kraaz W, Ponten J, Pahlman L, Scheibenpflug L. Nuclear DNA record in a malignant rectal carcinoid. A case report. Acta Pathol Microbiol Immunol Scand [A]. 1984;92:339–343.
19. DeCaro LF, Paladugu R, Benfield JR, Lovisatti L, Pak H, Teplitz RL. Typical and atypical carcinoids within the pulmonary APUD tumor spectrum. J Thorac Cardiovasc Surg 1983;86:528–536.
20. Blondal T, Arnorsson T, Bengtsson A, Wilander E. Nuclear DNA in carcinoid tumours of the lung. Eur J Respir Dis 1983;64:298–305.

21. Kaplan EL, Arganini M, Kang S-J. Diagnosis and Treatment of Hypoglycemic Disorders. Surg Clin North Am 1987;395–410.
22. Ellison EH, Wilson SD. The Zollinger-Ellison syndrome. Re-appraisal and evaluation of 260 registered cases. Ann Surg 1964;160:512–530.
23. Fox PS, Hoffman JW, DeCosse JJ, Wilson SD. The influence of total gastrectomy on survival in malignant Zollinger-Ellison Tumors. Ann Surg 1974;180:558–566.

Dr. Kaplan's Concluding Remarks

In concluding, I will make one observation and tell one final story. The observation reflects the greatness of this residency program, particularly at the time I went through. I note that of the 16 speakers on today's program, nine were either in my residency year or only a few years behind or ahead of me. It was just a wonderful time—a spectacular time—to be with so many fine individuals.

The final story, I think, tells us a great deal about Dr. Rhoads' dedication. At the time of the story, Dr. Rhoads was on the School Board and was spending much of his time downtown in meetings. We used to make rounds at 6:00 in the morning, and then he would come in around midnight or whenever and it was hard for the residents to keep up with him. We had one very ill patient, and Dr. Rhoads said, "If this patient dies, I want to be present." The junior resident, Henry Berkowitz, called me about 2:30 or 3:00 in the morning, and I came in and saw the patient who was about to breathe his last. I called Dr. Rhoads, and he asked, "How far away is the family." After I told him, he said, "Wait fifteen minutes so I can get there and then call the family." And he came in and spoke with the family. After everything was settled, and this was perhaps 5:00 in the morning, Dr. Rhoads asked me to come to breakfast with him. As we were walking out, I said, "Gee, that was a very tough one." Dr. Rhoads said, "Ed, life is really great if you don't weaken." I have always remembered those words and tried not to weaken. But I know that Dr. Rhoads has never weakened!

Introduction of Dr. James Thompson

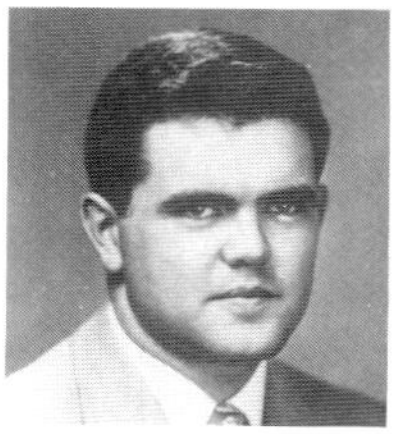

Dr. Clyde Barker: In everyone's life, there are a few heroes. Of course, Dr. Rhoads is a hero for us all, but in my life, Jim Thompson was a special hero, possibly because when I was an intern at HUP, he was my first chief resident. However, apparently, not everyone was as impressed as I was, and in fact, Jim told me that during his residency Dr. Ravdin fired him many times. Being curious about the reasons for this, I looked up his record in the Department's files. On March 22, 1958, Dr. Ravdin dictated a note saying, "in some ways Dr. Thompson is a rough diamond. He has a tendency to talk back constantly but I think I have broken him of this." Dr. Ravdin wasn't often wrong, but he was wrong that time! I teased Jim once before, while I was in Galveston, by reading to Jim's own residents this letter of Dr. Ravdin's. So, today, I'll try to compensate for this by reading another evaluation of him as a resident that was written by a man I know Jim greatly admired, Bob Ravdin, who said this: "Thompson is a remarkable and excellent man with a keen mind, stubborn curiosity and a quick wit. Thompson is one of the most individualistic residents we have. His interests range well beyond medicine and deeply too. He is skeptical but not obnoxiously so. Stimulating is the best word from my point of view." Mark Ravitch, in his book entitled *A Century of Surgery*, describes Jim in a word that I find even more apt, "iconoclastic." Robert Ravdin continues, "He wants to know what you are up to and how you justify it, he practically forces teaching while at the same time working hard at things himself. His judgement is good, his manner with patients at times breezy but in general very much appreciated and his medical knowledge excellent. I rate him with our very best." Bob Ravdin was perceptive, wasn't he?

After graduating from our program in 1959, Jim went to work at the old Pennsylvania Hospital where he's told me he founded the Philip Syng Physick Society, an exclusive organization for which I've often hoped he might someday propose me. I think there are only two members. In 1963 he joined Bill Longmire's faculty where he became Chief of Surgery at Harbor General and in 1970 went home to his own medical school, the University of Texas Medical Branch at Galveston, where he has been Chairman since then. He has made his subject of today one that he owns in surgery: the clinical significance of gastrointestinal hormones.

Dr. James Thompson's Introductory Remarks

First of all, I would like to comment that there is something almost eerily significant about this podium. It exemplifies almost everything I remember about Pennsylvania. It is massive, beautiful, and it faces the wrong direction. But it works just fine. Everybody learns how to use it and takes it to be absolutely natural. The Chairman of the Department stands here in front of it and leans across it to push the control buttons. I don't know where in the world Clyde got that goddamn Bar Mitzvah picture of me.

I am here entirely by accident. I am a great believer in planning, but the results of my life give it no substantiation. Everything that is worth a nickel to me was an accident. I had always wanted to be a surgeon, and when I was a senior medical student, I applied to the Mayo Clinic like everybody did in that part of the world, because that's where all the great surgeons came from. I was accepted the first week in December of my intern year. I was interning in Galveston because I had to finish the thesis I was writing on "The Age of Beginning Reactivity of the Pituitary Adrenal Cortical System in the Newborn Rat." Anyhow, I later got a wire from the Mayo Clinic saying that they were having a terrible time replacing people going off to Korea so they'd decided not to take anybody who had not already fulfilled his military requirement and would I please do that and then they would be happy to have me. Well, I knew to take orders so I sent away to the Air Force and got a great big application and filled it all out. On New Year's Day, it was sitting on my desk all filled out ready to go in and my daughter spilled a bottle of ink on it. I reflected on that . . . and thought that was probably a message from God. So, I quickly changed my plans and wrote everybody listed in the AMA directory asking for a residency. But, of course, everybody was filled by then. Dr. Ravdin, however, wrote back, *wired back*, and said, "We're filled! However, any descendent of the great James Thompson of Galveston is welcome in my program. You just come here and we'll put you in the Harrison Department for a year and we'll work you in." That faced me with a moral dilemma. I was not related to James Thompson. I reflected on that for some time, accepted the residency, waited six months, and told Dr. Ravdin. Nothing was ever said about this until the graduation banquet (about 30 years later) when Dr. Ravdin got up and announced that I had gotten into the program by subterfuge.

I'll have to say that everything that's ever been of any good to me intellectually or clinically or investigatively has come as a result of being here. I came from Hebbronville, Texas, and I went to Texas A&M and then to Galveston. I did not have any money at all, and I had to get into a medical school before I got drafted. I got into medical school when I was 17. That shows that if you're really impelled, you can do anything. Anyhow, I finally finished there in Galveston and I came here. I was never so startled in all my life to see all of these bright—you'd call them Yuppies now, but they didn't have a name for them then and I just called them wonderful—hard working guys that just never went to bed, and I was scared absolutely to death. I was sure that somebody would find out that I was a phony that had gotten into this outfit, so I figured the only way I'd ever handle it was to stay up and work all the time, and I did that. There was a competition here to see how long you could stay up. I didn't win it, but I was a finalist. I think maybe the greatest resident I ever knew was Jack Mackie, because he'd figured a way to go home at 4:30 in the afternoon. Really efficient! It really got my attention to see how hard everybody worked. I was here two years before anyone told me I could unpack. That was Billy Fitts who was immediately reprimanded by the Professor who said it was still under advisement.

I also spent a long, long time on the service "gastronomique" under Dr. Rhoads. We used to go over to the Horn and Hardart across Woodland Avenue, across the streetcar tracks. Except that when our service was working (we worked a lot harder than when Dr. Orloff was on), we usually didn't get finished until about 6 or 7 o'clock. Often Horn and Hardart was closed at that time, so we would hie across Walnut Street to a bar that served a very good corned beef sandwich. Dr. Rhoads loved that bar for many reasons, one of which was the corned beef sandwiches but the most important of which was the sign over the bar. Every time we walked into the bar he would start chuckling. The sign said, "Work is the Curse of the Drinking Class."

Ted Shohl was my mentor here, and he kept me out of trouble as well as he could, but that was just about a full-time job. You all probably know that Dr. Rhoads hates cancer. In fact, this is an absolutely visceral response for him. He had a patient one time that had a very large mass in the tail of the pancreas, a mass sufficient to inhibit any ordinary surgeon. But it proved to be a stimulus to Dr. Rhoads, and after considerable maneuvering, he got this mass up on the anterior abdominal wall, to everyone's absolute surprise. Now, at a certain time that day, Dr. Rhoads had to be in Washington at a meeting of the National Research Council, so he kept glancing nervously at the clock. Just as he got this huge mass up on the anterior abdominal wall—I'll phrase it delicately, sort of like Dr. Kaplan did—the portal vein took the opportunity to commit suicide. Now, again, that would inhibit almost anybody else. But Dr. Rhoads just put two big sponges in and said, "Where is Clete"? And everything went just fine. As far as I know, that patient is still alive and walking around. It went very well and many things went very well.

While I was here, I did spend my first year in the Harrison Department. I occupied a corner of Harry Vars' desk. It was the greatest year, I guess, of my whole life, learning from that great and saintly man. Nearly everything I know, I think I learned from him. He was a walking encyclopedia.

Now, for just a little while, I am going to give a general survey of gastrointestinal hormones. My group has been very productive, and this is largely due to them. My genius has been in choosing them and stimulating them to work hard. That's about all. I am not a great scientist, but we have chosen great people (I don't know how) who are smart and who work hard and are productive. We have just written a book on this field, which for me has been the labor of a lifetime. I give that book to Dr. Rhoads as my birthday present.

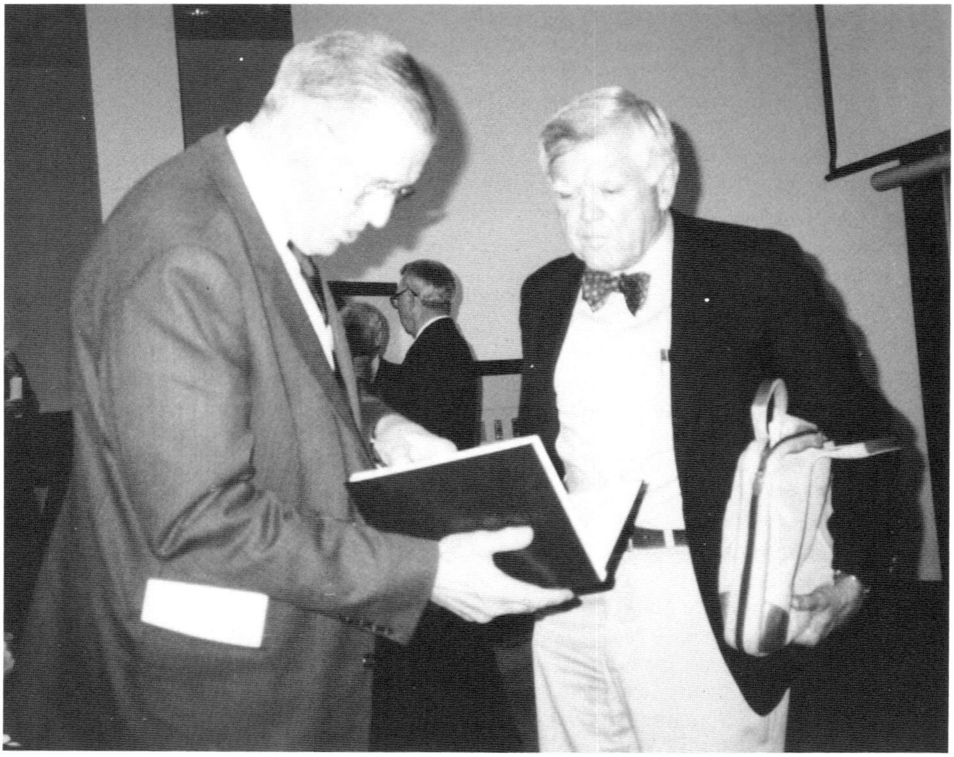

Dr. Thompson presenting Dr. Rhoads with a copy of his book *Gastrointestinal Endocrinology* (Thompson JA, Greeley GH Jr, Rayford P, Townsend CM Jr, eds. New York: McGraw-Hill, 1987).

Gastrointestinal Hormones

JAMES C. THOMPSON, M.D.

In this report the author gives a brief historical introduction regarding gastrointestinal (GI) hormones, summarizes some of their roles in gut physiology, discusses his clinical studies with gastrin and cholecystokinin, and then individually describes the GI hormones, considering their roles in disease syndromes.

ALTHOUGH GASTROINTESTINAL (GI) hormones are called "hormones," they do not always function in a truly endocrine fashion, *i.e.*, the active peptides are not always discharged into blood to act at a distant site. Sometimes they are discharged and act locally in a paracrine fashion. They also may serve as transmitting agents for nerve impulses or they may be discharged into the bloodstream after nerve stimulation in a neuroendocrine fashion. But the truth is that the field of endocrinology includes all of these functions, and we do not always know, nor is it always possible to determine by current methods, when an agent acts locally as well as at a distant site. That makes many of our observations somewhat unreliable. For example, when we measure increased concentrations of a peptide in the blood, we say that indicates that an observed activity may be a result of the action of that agent. In fact, some agents, particularly somatostatin and prostaglandins, act locally, and the concentrations in the blood may represent merely an overflow and bear scant temporal relationship to their physiologic activity.

Whereas true endocrinologists are often reluctant to admit it, the entire field of endocrinology began with gut hormones. It began on the afternoon of January 16, 1902, when Bayliss and Starling, working at the University College Hospital in London, demonstrated that the introduction of hydrochloric acid into a denervated loop of small intestine elicited the brisk secretion of pancreatic juice. Contrary to most such events, they understood the significance of this observation immediately, and they suggested that some unidentified, blood-borne chemical messenger was released from the acidified intestine to mediate the response. (They actually presented their report on this subject at the Royal Society 3 weeks later. Currently it would take at least a year to get a similar article into publication.) To describe this chemical messenger, Starling, on the advice of his philologist friend Sharpeg-Shaeffer, coined the word "hormone," which comes from the Greek word ormos, which means "I arouse to activity."

Three years later in 1905, Edkins, working at St. Bartholomew's Hospital in London, prepared extracts of antral mucosa, which, when injected into cats, stimulated gastric secretion. Edkins called this activity "gastrin."

Komorov was Pavlov's last resident. He left St. Petersburg, went to Berlin, to Montreal, where he worked at McGill with Babkin, and then he came to Philadelphia to Temple University, where he worked with Shay. There I got to know him and his cats well. Komorov decided that gastrin was probably a polypeptide and that it should be studied by methods applicable to polypeptide chemistry. While at McGill, Komorov described the isolation of a crude gastrin in the *Revue Canadienne de Biologie* in 1942, but the extraction was difficult and the results capricious.

The physiologic evidence that gastrin was released by distention of the antrum was provided by Dragstedt and Woodward. They showed that the release of gastrin was suppressed by acidification of the antrum and suggested that this was a biologic feedback mechanism, the first time that this classic endocrine phenomenon had been implicated in control of gastric secretion.

In 1960, Gregory in Liverpool set about to prepare some gastrins from the then-existing recipes. He wanted to stimulate gastric secretion and test for enterogastrone activity. He and

From the Department of Surgery, The University of Texas Medical Branch, Galveston, Texas.

his colleague, Tracy, became so embroiled, however, when they found out that they could not make gastrin from any of the published methods, that they dropped the original idea and worked for 4 years, which resulted in the isolation and chemical characterization and synthesis of pure gastrin. This initiated the biochemical era of GI endocrinology in 1964.

Yalow and Berson learned how to measure the infinitesimally small quantities of peptides that bring about all of these activities. They created the technique of radioimmunoassay, which allows us to measure what are called femtomolar quantities of circulating peptides. A femtomole is a billionth of a trillionth part of a gram molecular weight. A molar solution is a gram molecular weight of a compound dissolved in a liter of fluid. After Berson's death, Yalow received the Nobel Prize for the development of the radioimmunoassay method.

Gastric Secretion: A Model of Neurotendocrine Control

We might next summarize the neurohumoral events that occur when we eat a meal. Pavlov in 1892 divided the mechanisms for stimulation of acid secretion into three so-called phases: cephalic, gastric, and intestinal. When we first see food and chew it and swallow it, the vagal nuclei in the medulla send out efferent impulses along the peripheral vagi, which result in release of acetylcholine, some of which is released in the wall of the stomach and stimulates the parietal cell to secrete acid.

Distention of the stomach after a meal releases histamine, and when food comes into contact with the antral mucosa, the hormone gastrin is released. Gastrin, acetylcholine, and histamine stimulate the parietal cell to secrete acid. When acid flows down and coats the antrum and causes the luminal pH to drop below 3.5, output of gastrin is diminished, and when the pH reaches 1.5, output of gastrin is completely halted. This feedback mechanism can be summarized in a typical endocrine closed-loop relationship between gastrin and acid. Gastrin stimulates the release of acid, and when a sufficient concentration of acid is achieved, it blocks the further release of gastrin. Acidified chyme coming through the pylorus stimulates the release of secretin, which in turn stimulates the release of pancreatic bicarbonate.

Gastrointestinal Hormones

The hormones that we will consider consist of two families: the gastrin-cholecystokinin family and the secretin-glucagon family, which also contains gastric inhibitory polypeptide (GIP) and vasoactive intestinal peptide (VIP). These are grouped together because of similarities of their amino acid composition and of some of their actions. There also is a group of newer agents which are impatiently clamoring for recognition and adoption as full-fledged GI hormones.

We now know that gastrin and probably all peptide hormones exist in several molecular forms. These always seem to include a small active form and one or more larger forms, which contain the small active molecule plus extra peptides whose function is unknown. They probably act to protect the smaller active form from rapid catabolic destruction.

Gastrin

Gastrin is a linear peptide whose amino acids, when written, are conventionally listed in a straight line from left to right, *i.e.*, from the so-called nitrogen, or N-terminus to the so-called C-terminus, or carboxyl-terminus. The C-terminal four peptides are called tetragastrin. These peptides—tryptophan, methionine, aspartic acid, and phenylalanine—possess all of the properties and activities of the entire gastrin molecule. Everything else seems to exist to protect this C-terminal peptide segment. This fragment is particularly important biologically because it also forms a C-terminal tetrapeptide unit of cholecystokinin (CCK), and it accounts for many of the similarities that we find between gastrin and CCK.

The first form of gastrin, isolated by Gregory and Tracy, had 17 amino acids and is now called "little gastrin." There is a minigastrin that has 14 amino acids, a big gastrin with 34 amino acids, another with 58 amino acids, and an intermediate sized form called Component I. Yalow isolated a form about the size of albumin, which she called big-big gastrin.

Gastrin was first described in 1905, but it was not purified until 1964. Gastrin is apparently synthesized and is certainly stored in specific gastrin or G-cells located in the mucosa of the gastric antrum and of the upper small bowel.

Although almost three dozen actions have been described, certainly the most important action of gastrin is stimulation of acid secretion from the parietal cell. Gastrin releases pepsin and stimulates gastric mucosal blood flow. It has a most important function as a growth hormone for the stomach mucosa and the mucosa of the proximal small bowel and for the pancreas. It does not stimulate the growth of antral mucosa itself.

As clinicians, we are interested in gastrin because it is a major stimulant of normal acid secretion, and because it is the etiologic agent in the Zollinger-Ellison (ZE) syndrome. Since gastrin stimulates acid secretion, and since the duodenal ulcer diathesis is associated with increased secretion of acid, it has been tempting to relate gastrin to peptic ulcer, but so far this has been unsuccessful.

One should obtain a measurement of serum gastrin whenever the ZE syndrome is suspected. I think the determination should be made in any patient who has a duodenal ulcer sufficiently serious to require an operation, and certainly in a patient whose ulcer recurs after operation. One should order a gastrin measurement in any patient who seems to have a particularly virulent form of ulcer disease, a form associated with great hypersecretion of acid with basal acid secretory levels that are greater than 15 mEq/hour, or patients who develop ulcers in the postbulbar area of the duodenum or in the proximal jejunum. Patients with chronic diarrhea associated with acid hypersecretion should have measurements of serum gastrin because many patients with the ZE syndrome may initially complain of diarrhea. Patients with duodenal ulcer and hypercalcemia should be studied to rule out the possibility of a multiple endocrine neoplasia syndrome.

There are, of course, many causes of elevated gastrin levels. Hypergastrinemia may be caused by increased stimulation of gastrin release, by decreased inhibition of gastrin release, by decreased destruction of gastrin, and by unknown causes. The most important of all these, of course, is a gastrinoma, which must be differentiated from all others. Antral G-cell hyperplasia is so rare that I have never seen it, although I am convinced that it exists . . . sort of like Katmandu for me. Patients with pyloric obstruction may cause real confusion. Some postvagotomy patients are worrisome. When performing a vagotomy, serum gastrin levels rise, apparently because the vagal fibers in man carries inhibitory messages for the release of gastrin. The key to diagnosis in our hands is the secretin challenge, which will almost always successfully distinguish patients with the ZE syndrome. The disease that most clearly typifies GI endocrinopathy is the ZE syndrome.

Cholecystokinin

In 1928, Ivy reported that fat in the small intestine stimulated the release of a substance that caused contraction of the gallbladder. He named that hormone, CCK. Later, in 1947, Harper and Raper in England found that a hormone released from the duodenum stimulated secretion of enzymes by the pancreas. They called that activity, pancreozymin. In the early 1960s, Mutt and Jorpes at the Karolinska found that the two agents were identical, and we now call the peptide CCK, because that was the first name given Cholecystokinin is present in special CCK cells in the mucosa of the proximal small bowel. It is released on contact of these cells with amino acids and fatty acids. Like gastrin, CCK circulates in several molecular sizes, varying as far as we know from eight to 58 amino acids, and there are suggestions of intermediate forms. There is good evidence that there may be a CCK-12. The small forms again possess all of the activities of the larger forms. The original form isolated had 33 amino acids. Cholecystokinin-octapeptide (CCK-8) has been found in high concentrations in the brain, where it functions as a neurotransmitter. This activity is apparently important in the function of certain brain cells and circuits. Cholecystokinin also probably functions as an appetite suppressant. Caerulein is a 10-amino acid analogue of CCK that is found in the skin of the European blue frog, *Hyla caerulea,* truly only God knows why.

Cholecystokinin is a strong stimulant of contraction of the gallbladder and of the release of digestive enzymes by the pancreas. It has been shown recently to be a powerful stimulant of small bowel motility. Cholecystokinin is a potent growth hormone for the pancreas.

For the last several years, we have been interested in the correlation of release of CCK in man, with demonstration of its activity in causing gallbladder contraction. This project began just after Phil Rayford in our group had developed and validated an excellent radioimmunoassay for CCK. Our assay reacts fully with CCK-33 and CCK-39, and with CCK in plasma and duodenal extracts. It reacts poorly with gastrin-17 and gastrin-34 and with various fragments of the CCK molecule. The significance is that our radioimmunoassay apparently requires nearly the entire CCK-33 molecule to react and that it does not cross-react with gastrin, which makes it worthwhile in studying the differential effects of gastrin and CCK.

Whenever one wants to study the metabolism of any hormone, one must first develop an assay and then correlate the evidence of its release, measured by radioimmunoassay or some other assay, with evidence of its biologic activity. That is, it must be clear that the active principle, and not some artifact, is measured, not some innocuous or inactive fragment of a molecule. We had a fine assay for CCK, but we needed to correlate its activity with biologic action in man. I had read an article in which gallbladder size had been measured with accuracy by ultrasonography, and it struck me that we could use that as a bioassay. We enlisted eight colleagues from among our investigators and placed a tube into the duodenum under fluoroscopic guidance. Through this duodenal tube, we administered liquid corn oil, Lipomul (Upjohn, Kalamazoo, MI). We did this in the ultrasound unit and obtained frequent blood samples for CCK measurements and simultaneously performed ultrasonograms before and after the Lipomul administration.

The ultrasonograms showed maximum contraction at 18 minutes after the intraduodenal administration of Lipomul. There was a decrease in the calculated volume from 33 cm^3 to about 11 cm^3, or to about one third the original volume. The first significant contraction of the gallbladder occurred at 6 minutes after administration of Lipomul. There was a progressive diminution of gallbladder size, reaching maximum contraction at 18 minutes, at which time the volume was one third the original. Refilling of the gallbladder was normal at about 25 minutes after Lipomul. Basal concentrations of CCK were about 80 pg/ml, and this concentration rose rapidly and progressively after Lipomul was given. The peak concentration of CCK was achieved at 16 minutes, which is 2 minutes before the maximum contraction of the gallbladder. We subjected the data to linear regression analysis, which showed highly significant correlation during both the period of contraction and of relaxation. We next wanted to see if we could reproduce this correlation using oral administration of Lipomul. In fact, we obtained nearly identical results, and the correlation was again highly significant.

We next wanted to be sure that the gallbladder contraction was actually due to CCK itself, and not due to something else which just happened to be released at the same time that CCK was released, so we administered the pure CCK-33 intravenously to five of our investigators, which produced an immediate rise in peripheral plasma CCK. After 1 hour, the infusion was halted and plasma CCK fell to baseline quite rapidly. During the high plateau of CCK concentration, the gallbladder contracted and remained small. Again, there was an excellent negative correlation between CCK concentrations and gallbladder volume on linear regression analysis, which allowed us to conclude that the contraction was due to CCK itself.

It appeared that this technique might provide a way to study patients with gallstone disease to determine whether an abnormality in CCK metabolism might be involved in the pathogenesis of gallstones. We studied gallbladder contraction in 24 patients. Four were found to have hydrops, with huge, noncontracting gallbladders. There were an additional six patients whose normal sized gallbladders failed to contract and 14 patients whose gallbladders contracted. The pattern of contraction in these 14 patients was nearly identical to that of 12 volunteers.

However, release of CCK in 12 normal volunteers compared with 14 gallstone patients whose gallbladders contracted showed a significant difference in CCK release at each point. The integrated release of CCK over the 1-hour period showed that gallstone patients release less than 50% of the total amount of CCK compared with controls.

When we subjected the relationship between gallbladder volumes and plasma CCK levels in the control group and in the gallstone patients to linear regression, both showed a high degree of statistical correlation. Interpretation of these lines indicates that for a given dose of CCK, the diseased gallbladders underwent less contraction than the controls. The diminished release of CCK and the increased gallbladder sensitivity to CCK in these gallstone patients is evidence that an abnormality exists. After looking at this, we suggested that there may be two separate groups of gallstone patients, one in whom gallbladder motility is diminished as exemplified by the six patients whose gallbladders did not contract, so that they have stasis as a major factor in the pathogenesis of stones. In the other group, gallbladder motility is normal, but release of CCK is diminished and gallbladder sensitivity increased. How does that lead to pathogenesis of stones? We do not know It may alter hepatic secretion of bile. Perhaps there is less bile, or perhaps, as a result of diminished gut motility, there is a diminution in the enterohepatic circulation of bile salts.

Secretin

Secretin arises from "S" cells scattered throughout the duodenum, jejunum, and ileum. This distribution of secretin is an enigma, because the mechanism for release of secretin is chiefly acidification, and as far as we know, the requisite level of acidification is achieved, only in the proximal duodenum. That is, the intraduodenal pH must fall to less than 4 and actually to less than 2 to provoke any significant release of secretin. It is not yet known what all of this remaining secretin is doing, and how it is released (perhaps by fat or bile), and why it is there.

Although secretin activity was discovered in 1902 by Bayliss and Starling, it was not until 1966 that Mutt and Jorpes described the amino acid sequence. The most important action of secretin is stimulation of secretion of water and bicarbonate from the pancreas. Bicarbonate secretion is roughly equivalent to the amount of acid secreted by the stomach, so that secretin truly functions as a natural antacid. Secretin also stimulates bile secretion, it diminishes gut motility, it diminishes acid secretion by the stomach, and it inhibits food-stimulated release of gastrin. Clinically, secretin is used as a standard stimulant of pancreatic function, and most important, as a discriminatory test for the ZE syndrome, since secretin has a unique property of causing rapid release of gastrin from ZE tumors.

Pancreatic Secretion

Studies on the endocrine control of the pancreas have served as a prototype for investigations of gut hormones. When acid, stimulated by a meal, flows into the duodenum, it causes a fall in duodenal pH and secretin is liberated and carried by the blood to the pancreas, where it stimulates pancreatic ductal cells to release bicarbonate. Bicarbonate flows into the duodenum and neutralizes gastric acid. When the intraduodenal pH rises above 4, further secretin release is halted. This can be summarized in the typical endocrine closed-loop relationship between secretin and bicarbonate. Acid causes release of secretin, secretin causes release of bicarbonate, and bicarbonate flows into the duodenum, and raises the intraduodenal pH. When the pH rises above 4, further release of secretin is halted.

Food, in the early process of digestion in the stomach, is propelled into the duodenum, and certain amino acids, particularly phenylalanine and tryptophan and certain fatty acids, with chain lengths between carbon (C)10 and C18, bring about release of CCK from specialized CCK cells lying within the duodenal mucosa. We know the mechanisms for release of CCK, and studies by Owyang in Michigan and by Gómez in our laboratory have shown that feedback inhibition of CCK release depends on the presence of, respectively, pancreatic enzymes and bile. For a while, we thought that presence of trypsin in the duodenum was that mechanism, but we now know that that mechanism apparently exists only in rats, and not in man.

Two different types of exocrine secretions are elaborated by the pancreas. The pancreatic acinus releases a juice that is high in enzyme concentration, but low in volume and low in bicarbonate. The ductal or tubular cells of the pancreas secrete a juice that is very low in enzymes, but high in volume and high in bicarbonate. Outflow of pancreatic juice after a meal is, of course, a mixture of these two secretions.

The pancreatic acinus is stimulated to secrete primarily by CCK and by gastrin, and probably also by vagal acetylcholine, although this has been extraordinarily difficult to prove. Without question, the most important hormone for stimulation of the ductal cells is secretin. There is evidence that the peptide hormone, somatostatin, acts to diminish pancreatic secretion by two routes. It directly inhibits secretion of the pancreatic cells and depresses release of CCK and secretin. Pancreatic polypeptide is released in the pancreas by vagal stimulation and by CCK. It is a strong inhibitor of the action of CCK and secretin in stimulating pancreatic secretion, but its physiologic significance is unknown.

Glucagon

Pancreatic glucagon is the hormone of energy release, as insulin is the hormone of energy storage. There is a peptide called gut glucagon in the intestinal tract of man and animals which is identical with pancreatic glucagon. In addition, there is a smaller gut peptide, which cross-reacts with specific glucagon antiserum. Glucagon is a powerful inhibitor of bowel motility and is used clinically in x-ray studies for hypotonic duodenography. One, both, or sometimes all three forms may be secreted by endocrine tumors of the gut, but rarely.

The clinical syndrome of glucagonoma is characterized by a severe, often generalized, eczematoid dermatitis. Most cases are referred to surgeons by dermatologists. These patients have a specific skin lesion called necrolytic migrating erythema. One such patient was recently found to have a serum glucagon level of nearly 3000 pg/ml (the upper limit of normal is 200). She was found to have a tumor of the tail of the pancreas on computed axial tomography (CAT) scan, and was cured by excision of that tumor. Glucagon levels fell to 120 pg/ml after excision.

Gastric Inhibitory Polypeptide

Gastric inhibitory polypeptide was first isolated from duodenal mucosa by Brown and Mutt in 1969. After a meal, there is an early release caused by glucose and a late release due to fat. Initially, GIP was thought to have its major action as an inhibitor of gastrin secretion. Recently, however, it has been shown to be involved in the physiologic release of insulin, almost certainly the most important action. In a series of studies, Anderson showed that GIP has a major role in the hepatic metabolism of glucose.

Vasoactive Intestinal Peptide

Vasoactive intestinal peptide was first isolated from the mucosa of the proximal small bowel by Said and by Mutt in 1972. Vasoactive intestinal peptide has many important and potent metabolic effects, but its physiologic role is a mystery. The mechanisms for its release are not well understood. It is released by distention. Studies in our lab by Chayvialle show that it is also released by ischemia. Vasoactive intestinal peptide is the usual etiologic agent for the Verner-Morrison syndrome, the so-called watery diarrhea, hypokalemia, and achlorhydria (WDHA) syndrome. This condition, this watery diarrhea, is caused by a non-beta cell tumor of the pancreas, and may be cured by excision of the tumor.

Pancreatic Polypeptide

Pancreatic polypeptide (PP) is found chiefly in the pancreas. It is released by vagal stimulation and by CCK. It sharply curtails pancreatic secretion of water, bicarbonate, and enzymes. Its physiologic actions are not now clear. Many have suggested that PP levels, because they are elevated in some patients with a variety of pancreatic tumors, might be important as a marker for pancreatic tumors.

Candidate Hormones

There is an additional group of candidate hormones awaiting introduction into the club. Grossman suggested that a true hormone should meet three criteria: (1) the agent should be present in endocrine cells; (2) it should be released by feeding or by some other physiologic event and produce its characteristic biologic action; and (3) its effect should be reproduced by infusion of the exogenous peptide in doses which achieve plasma concentrations that are found with endogenous release. Furthermore, this dose of exogenous peptide should reproduce the biologic actions.

When Guillemin gave his distinguished address before the Society of University Surgeons at its meeting in San Diego in 1976, he suggested that there were local agents, physically adjacent to most endocrine cells, that functioned as on–off switches for the release of these hormones. He called these local agents cybernins, and his prediction may have been correct for most gut hormones. We now know that somatostatin functions as an "off" switch for nearly all gut hormones, and bombesin, or gastrin-releasing peptide, functions as an "on" switch for gastrin, CCK, PP, GIP, insulin, glucagon, and neurotensin. Bombesin does not release secretin, according to our findings, and its effects on somatostatin itself and on VIP and substance P are, as far as I know, unknown.

We are greatly interested in neurotensin, a small peptide with 13 amino acids and a molecular weight of about 1600 daltons. It is found in both the brain and gut, with about 90% coming from the small bowel mucosa, especially the distal end. It is released by a fatty meal, by bombesin (BBS), and by the gastrin-releasing peptide. Its major actions seem to be vasodilatation, stimulation of pancreatic secretion of water and bicarbonate, and decreased bowel motility. We have shown that it stimulates gallbladder contraction in dogs, but causes gallbladder relaxation in humans, and is therefore an example of endocrine nonparallelism. That is, it duplicates some of the actions of CCK, but not others. Neurotensin is a potent inhibitor of gastrin-stimulated gastric secretion, it has been found elevated in many patients with the Verner-Morrison syndrome, and it is released in patients with the dumping syndrome, but on injection, it does not itself produce dumping.

I might simply list the most currently promising candidates (some of which, serotonin and prostaglandins, for example are not even peptides) BBS, chymodenin, enkephalins and endomorphins, intestinal phase hormone (entero-oxyntin), motilin, neuromedin B, neuromedin C (GRP-10), neurotensin, peptide YY, prostaglandins, serotonin, somatostatin, substance P.

Brain–Gut Axis

One of the most startling discoveries in the last decade has been the demonstration that several gut peptides are present in high concentrations in the central nervous system (CNS), particularly in the brain. These peptides include gastrin, CCK, secretin, glucagon, VIP, neurotensin, somatostatin, and many others. Intraventricular injection of gut peptides causes peripheral effects. Several of us have recently shown that gastrin and CCK, however, do not pass the blood–brain barrier. Intraventricular injections of BBS, cause an increase in plasma gastrin, but they do not cause any increased concentrations of gastrin within the cerebrospinal fluid (CSF). Zhu, a surgeon from Peking in our laboratory, has shown that injection of CCK-8 into the CSF causes an increase in pancreatic polypeptide in plasma peripherally and that this increase can be abolished by vagotomy. This means that CCK injected into the ventricle causes vagal stimulation. Many of these agents function as neurotransmitters, and CCK may suppress appetite.

Calcium Interrelations

I would like to discuss briefly interrelations between calcium and certain gut hormones. We have shown that calcium releases gastrin and later that it releases CCK. Calcium releases calcitonin, which stimulates uptake of calcium by bone, and parathormone stimulates resorption from bone. Not only does calcium stimulate release of CCK, but it is also a requisite for pancreatic enzyme secretion. Both calcitonin and somatostatin inhibit gallbladder function and pancreatic enzyme secretion. Calcium stimulates gastrin release, whereas calcitonin inhibits it. Gastrin stimulates release of calcitonin, a function that is utilized in the pentagastrin-infusion test of medullary carcinoma of the thyroid devised by Wells and Cooper. A group from the National Institutes of Health has reported that a new peptide, isolated from the fundus of the stomach, stimulates release of parathormone, and another group suggests that long-term administration of secretin also may stimulate release of parathormone.

We have recently studied the effects of intraduodenal instillation of divalent cations, magnesium and zinc, as well as calcium, on the output of pancreatic polypeptide, gastrin, CCK, and protein from the pancreas. All three cations—magnesium, zinc, and calcium—stimulate release of all three agents—pancreatic polypeptide, gastrin, and CCK—as well as the release of enzymes from the pancreas.

Clinical Roles for Gastrointestinal Hormones

Are there any therapeutic uses for all these hormones? Cholecystokinin and its analogues, caerulein and CCK-8, have been used successfully in treatment of ileus. They have been proposed by several investigators for treatment of obesity, but preliminary reports are discouraging. Somatostatin has been used widely for a variety of serious conditions, patients with GI hemorrhage and the Verner-Morrison syndrome and the carcinoid syndrome. Most reports so far are anecdotal, but they are encouraging. We have made the hypothetical suggestion that gastrin may be used as a growth hormone for the proximal gut in patients with the short-bowel syndrome, especially children with midgut volvulus. Stimulation of acid secretion in those patients could be blocked by H_2-antagonists.

We have discussed various syndromes associated with GI hormones. The prototype is the ZE syndrome, caused by gastrin. The Verner-Morrison syndrome of watery diarrhea is caused by VIP. The carcinoid syndrome is associated with 5-hydroxytryptamine and with substance P. Excess secretion of glucagon by pancreatic tumors causes the glucagonoma syndrome. Several studies show low values of CCK and secretin in patients with chronic pancreatitis and with sprue. We should mention that there are no known syndromes involving excess quantities of secretin, CCK, or GIP.

The relationship of gut hormones with cancer has recently undergone careful scrutiny. If epidermal growth factor, which is a gut hormone, is removed, there is a stimulation of the rate of induction of carcinoma in mice by exogenous carcinogens. Townsend and colleagues in our department and others have provided evidence that human colon and stomach cancer cells have receptors on them for gastrin and for VIP. Human pancreatic carcinoma has been shown to possess receptors for secretin. Townsend and others in our laboratory also have shown that administration of secretin and caerulein will stimulate the growth, both weight and DNA content, of hamster pancreatic carcinoma.

Townsend and I have asked ourselves whether, in an analogy with breast cancer, we can affect the growth of gut cancers by altering the levels of certain gut hormones that act normally to stimulate growth of gut mucosa and pancreas, specifically gastrin, CCK, and secretin. We have embarked on a major study of this possibility.

Addendum

Just recently, Sakamoto, a young man from Osaka who has spent 2 years in our laboratory, studied the differential effects on pancreatic protein output of portal and systemic administration of two forms of CCK: CCK-33 and CCK-8. These are injected in dogs prepared with pancreatic fistulas and with portacaval transpositions. In these dogs, hind-leg injection results in hepatic transit before reaching the systemic circuit, whereas foreleg injection gives immediate systemic access. When we injected CCK-33, there was no difference in the amount of pancreatic proteins secreted, whether we injected it into the portal or through the systemic circuit. But injection of CCK-8 into the portal vein cut the activity by 50%. The small form of CCK was metabolized by the liver, and the larger form was protected against this catabolism. (Sakamoto *et al.* J Clin Invest 1985;75:280–285).

BIBLIOGRAPHY

Bethge N, Diel F, Usadel KH. Somatostatin: A regulatory peptide of clinical importance. J Clin Chem Clin Biochem 1982;20:603–613.

Bloom SR, Polak JM. Gut Hormones. New York: Churchill Livingstone, 1981.

Brown JC, Dryburgh JR, Ross SA *et al.* Identification and actions of GIP. Recent Prog Horm Res 1975;31:487–532.

Grossman M, Speranza V, Basso N *et al.* Gastrointestinal Hormones and Pathology of the Digestive System. New York: Plenum Press, 1978.

Hacki WH. Secretin. Clin Gastroenterol 1980;9:609–632.

Lilja P, Fagan CJ, Wiener I *et al.* Infusion of pure cholecystokinin in humans: Correlation between plasma concentrations of cholecystokinin and gallbladder size. Gastroenterology 1982;83:256–261.

Lonovics J, Devitt P, Watson LC *et al.* Pancreatic polypeptide: A review. Arch Surg 1981;116:1256–1264.

Krieger DT. Brain peptides: What, where and why? Science 1983;222:975–985.

Morley JE. The ascent of cholecystokinin (CCK): From gut to brain. Life Sci 1982;30:479–493.

Rayford PL, Miller TA, Thompson JC. Secretin, cholecystokinin and newer gastrointestinal hormones. N Engl J Med 1976;295:1093–1101, 1157–1164.

Rayford PL, Thompson JC. Gastrin. Surgery 1977;145:257–268.

Rehfeld JF: Cholecystokinin. Clin Gastroenterol 1980;9:593–607.

Said SI. Vasoactive Intestinal Peptide. New York: Raven Press, 1982.

Sakamoto T, Fujimura M, Newman J, Zhu X-G, Greeley GH Jr, Thompson JC. A comparison of hepatic elimination of different forms of cholecystokinin in dogs: Bioassay and radioimmunoassay comparison of CCK-8 and CCK-33. J Clin Invest 1985;75:280–285.

Schwartz TW. Pancreatic polypeptide: A hormone under vagal control. Gastroenterology 1983;85:1411–1425.

Thompson JC. Gastrointestinal Hormones. Austin: University of Texas Press, 1975.

Thompson JC, Fried GM, Ogden WD *et al.* Correlation between release of cholecystokinin and contraction of the gallbladder in patients with gallstones. Ann Surg 1982;295:670–676.

Thompson JC, Greeley GH Jr, Rayford PL, Townsend CM Jr. Gastrointestinal Endocrinology. New York: McGraw Hill, 1987.
Thompson JC, Marx M. Gastrointestinal hormones. Curr Probl Surg 1984;21:1–80.
Walker JP, Khalil T, Wiener I, Fagan CJ, Townsend C, Greeley GH, Thompson JC. The role of neurotension in human gallbladder motility. Ann Surg 1985;201 678–683.
Walsh JH, Lam SK. Physiology and pathology of gastrin. Clin Gastroenterol 1980;9:567–591.
Wiener I, Inoue K, Fagan CJ, Lilja P, Watson LC, Thompson JC. Release of cholecystokinin in man: Correlation of blood levels with gallbladder contraction. Ann Surg 1981;194:321–327.

Dr. Thompson's Closing Remarks

I think my time is up, and I would like to say first of all, "Happy Birthday, Dr. Rhoads!" I am honored to be here. I have always been honored to have come from this program.

I've always been amazed at Dr. Rhoads' versatility. One day when we were making rounds, running up the Gates pavilion, we got out on the roof and it was the day of a solar eclipse. I don't know how Dr. Rhoads knew about it, but he handed out four pieces of smoked glass, and we all stood there in great awe and watched the solar eclipse.

I'm always impressed also by Dr. Rhoads' thoughtfulness. I've received postcards from him that were written in airplanes over Saudi Arabia. When I was here two weeks ago for the College meeting, Dr. Rhoads sidled up to me at a cocktail party and said, "Jim (that always gets me), I see you are giving some talks in Perth." I said, "Yes, sir, I am." He said, "Thought I might drop by." I always wonder how in the world Dr. Rhoads does all of this. He is going to be in Japan visiting his sister, which is only about 1000 light years from Australia.

Thank you, Dr. Rhoads, for everything.

Discussion

Dr. Clyde Barker: Those were two great talks. There are probably only a couple of people in the audience, or the country, who could actually discuss them. Maybe Dr. Kaplan and Dr. Thompson can discuss them at lunch, if there's time for lunch. We are so far behind schedule that we really have no time for questions.

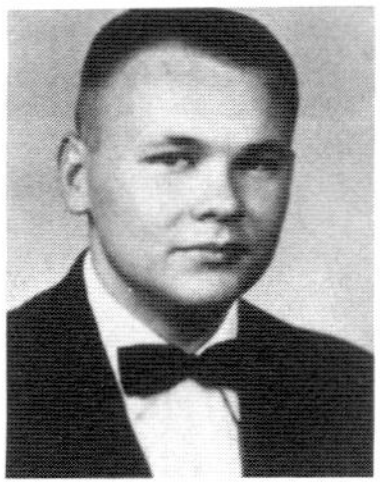

Introduction of Dr. Carter Nance

Dr. Clyde Barker: Carter Nance is seen here a few years before he graduated from this program in 1966. He then went to New Orleans where for many years he seemed to be a fixture on Isidore Cohn's faculty at LSU. Just recently he moved to become Professor and Chairman of the Department of Surgery at St. Barnabas in New Jersey where I have visited him, finding St. Barnabas to be an elegant Medical Center. Carter's work entitled "Abdominal Trauma at the Southern Surgical Association, 1888–1987" suggests that he will be giving a historical paper but I suspect that it will have something to do with the modern treatment of trauma, in which he is one of the country's leading experts.

Dr. Rhoads (who was a co-founder of the Trauma Society) has of course written about trauma over a period of many decades. Two of his papers are "Problems of Fluid Balance in the Traumatized Patient" (*Ann Intern Med* 18:988–990, 1943) and "The Metabolic Response to Trauma" (*Ann Rev Med* 7:141–156, 1956).

Dr. Nance's Introductory Remarks

I first want to establish my endocrine credentials by giving an informal report on the first patient at HUP with the Zollinger–Ellison syndrome (at least this was the first patient operated on here with a preoperative diagnosis of Zollinger–Ellison syndrome and this was within a few months of the meeting in which the Zollinger–Ellison syndrome was first described). I found this case when Dr. Rhoads sent me to the record room to look up all of the gastrectomies that had been done at HUP. This case had a preoperative diagnosis of Zollinger–Ellison syndrome but a postoperative diagnosis of Ravdin–Machella syndrome, which was a case in which you operated on a patient thinking that you were operating for Zollinger–Ellison but you could not find the tumor. I do not think that that case was ever reported.

I want to say how glad I am to join the others in wishing Dr. Rhoads a Happy Birthday. I did not realize how important this meeting was until I realized that Dr. Rhoads was giving up a Saturday operating day. But I cannot give a talk on trauma without acknowledging another person at HUP who had a profound influence on me, Dr. William T. Fitts. Billy's enthusiasm for trauma was incredible in an institution that had a Quaker-like approach to trauma (that is, we never saw any) and he imbued in me some of the same enthusiasm. I remember well the time that I spent as chief of the trauma service that Billy put together during my senior year. I think we had one patient. This was a patient with a gunshot wound. We salivated over him, thought over him, and learned about him. Billy was totally enthusiastic about the whole thing. Billy took me to my first meeting of the Association for the Surgery of Trauma and always told me that this was the greatest organization in the world.

I also remember the time when I, having been influenced by an internship at Dr. Dragstedt's institution, the University of Chicago, did a vagotomy and pyloplasty on a patient from Dr. Fitts' ward service. We presented the patient at grand rounds and it need hardly be said that this particular operation was not regarded with much enthusiasm at that time by any of the attending staff at HUP, where the standard procedure was subtotal gastrectomy. Actually, I did not do the vagotomy and pyloroplasty. Stan Dudrick stole the case, but he let me present it to the staff. After my presentation Dr. Rhoads began the discussion, expressing less than total enthusiasm. Then Dr. Fitts, who also did not have much enthusiasm for the operation, got up and said that if that was the operation his boys had done it must have been the right thing to do. That was the kind of person Billy Fitts was.

When I finished my residency I went down to New Orleans where I found myself surrounded by gunshot wounds. A few years ago I began to look up the history of Charity Hospital and its relationship to gunshot wounds and abdominal trauma. As Mark Ravitch has said, Charity Hospital was a fertile area for the study of abdominal trauma. This slide indicates that the Americans at the Battle of New Orleans in 1815 did not get much experience in trauma because our guys were all protected behind cotton bales. But the British got a lot of experience. 2,000 casualties including the commanding general. In New Orleans we adopted the principles of Benjamin Rush in treating abdominal trauma: putting leaches on, giving them a little morphine to keep them from complaining, and reporting only the survivors, which were not very many.

Abdominal Trauma at the Southern Surgical Association, 1888–1987

FRANCIS C. NANCE, M.D., F.A.C.S.

Since 1888 98 papers have been presented to the Southern Surgical Association (SSA) dealing directly or indirectly with abdominal trauma. The papers reflect the progress over the century in the management of this injury. Almost two-thirds of the papers have originated from the major city hospitals of the south. An interest in abdominal trauma has been manifest among the officers of SSA. Twenty-two presidents have presented papers or taken part in discussions. Four 25-year eras were identified. In the earliest, exploration of abdominal wounds was firmly established as a principle. The second period was characterized by consolidation of principles and strengthening of supportive care. The third era encompassing World War II marked a nadir in productivity. In the last 25 years a reawakened interest has resulted in a marked increase in the number and quality of presentations, which have increasingly focused on specific organ injuries.

THE LOVE AFFAIR of the Southern Surgical Association (SSA) with the subject of abdominal trauma began at the first meeting in 1888 and has continued with undiminished ardor to the present day. Ninety-eight papers dealing directly or indirectly with abdominal trauma have been presented and many of these have profoundly influenced the management of trauma as it has been practiced in the United States. The presence of large public teaching hospitals in most of the major southern cities undoubtedly has contributed to the large number of reports that have come out of the South. Institutions such as Charity Hospital in New Orleans, the Hillman Hospital of Birmingham, Grady Hospital in Atlanta, the Louisville General Hospital, Parkland Hospital in Dallas, and the Ben Taub Hospital in Houston have provided the opportunity for young surgical investigators to make important contributions in the study of trauma and, of course, have served as a training ground for innumerable southern surgeons. The importance of these great institutions can hardly be underestimated. Almost two-thirds of the total number of papers on abdominal trauma had their origin in the records of these great institutions (Fig. 1). The New Orleans Charity Hospital, with its 11 papers, may well have had the most single-minded devotion to abdominal trauma. Since 1893 case records of more than 10,000 patients with abdominal injury have been reported in the literature from that institution alone.

The story of abdominal trauma at the SSA may be conveniently divided into four 25 year eras (Table 1). The first, extending from 1888 to 1912, could be characterized as one that defined the role of surgery in the management of abdominal trauma. The sense of excitement and adventure that permeated the papers and the discussions of that period is almost palpable. The second era, which includes the first World War, was one of consolidation of principles. Attention was focused on individual management of specific lesions and the general support of the patient before and after operation. The third era encompassed World War II and represented the nadir of productivity with only 15 papers presented to the SSA during this period. The Lessons of War appear to have been taken to heart by most surgeons with uncritical enthusiasm and no one seemed willing to question apparently settled issues. The last era has been characterized by the presentation of 33 papers (Fig. 2), many of them reexamining old dogmas, with nothing left sacred. These papers have played an important

From the Department of Surgery, Saint Barnabas Medical Center, Livingston, New Jersey.

Presented at the 100th Anniversary Meeting of the Southern Surgical Association, Hot Springs, Virginia, December 6–9, 1987.

This article has been reproduced from *Annals of Surgery*, Vol. 207, No. 6, June 1988.

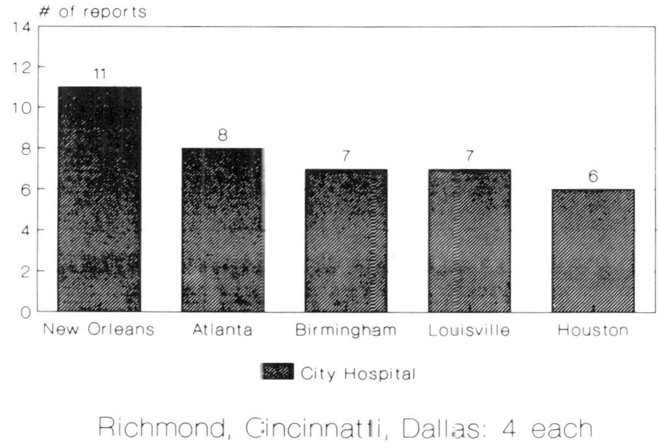

FIG. 1. Contributions on abdominal trauma from major city hospitals. Almost two-thirds of the presentations on abdominal trauma have had their origin in the major city hospitals of the South.

role in shaping the modern management of abdominal trauma and continue to open new pathways. While presentations of the earlier eras tended to dwell on the general topic of abdominal trauma, the latter era has focused on specific intra-abdominal lesions (Fig. 3).

The enthusiasm of the membership for abdominal trauma has been shared over the years by our officers. Twenty-two of our past presidents have manifested major interests or have presented papers on abdominal trauma at a meeting of the SSA (Fig. 4).

Discovery and Excitement, 1888–1912

The surgical management of abdominal trauma had its origins just prior to the founding of the SSA. Prior to 1880, no formal laparotomies had been performed for gunshot wounds of the abdomen, and during the Civil War (1861–1865) such wounds were managed by expectant therapy. In 1881 the death of President Garfield from an assassin's abdominal gunshot wound focused attention on the possible role of surgery in this lesion. Garfield had been managed without operation, but by 1882 Professor R. A. Kinloch of Charleston (Fig. 5), a founding member of the SSA, had explored a patient and sutured five intestinal wounds. Unfortunately, the patient had seven intestinal wounds and did not survive.[1] This preliminary attempt was followed shortly by Kocher's successful suture of a stomach wound and Bull's successful closure of an intestinal wound (the first in the United States). In 1887 three papers were presented to the American Surgical Association discussing the propriety of laparotomy for gunshot wounds, among them a paper by Kinloch. A long discussion ensued with important contributions from a number of southern surgeons. By the time of the first meeting of the SSA, the utility of laparotomy for penetrating wounds of the abdomen, in particular gunshot wounds,[3,4] was becoming fairly firmly established.

The first presentation on this topic to the SSA was at the first meeting, by R. M. Cunningham[2] of Pratt Mines, Alabama, who reported on the case of a Scotch miner who had shot himself with a .38 caliber pistol. He was managed expectantly. Eighteen hours later, signs of peritonitis appeared and the patient died at 52 hours.

The following year, two papers were presented in tandem, dealing with anastomotic techniques for the small bowel. Much of the discussion of these two papers was in the context of the application of these techniques to the management of gunshot wounds. The general tenor of the discussion that followed was that laparotomy should be strongly

TABLE 1. *Four 25-Year Eras of Abdominal Trauma at the SSA*

1888–1912	Discovery and Excitement
1913–1937	Consolidation
1938–1962	The Lessons of War
1963–1987	Reexamination and Discovery

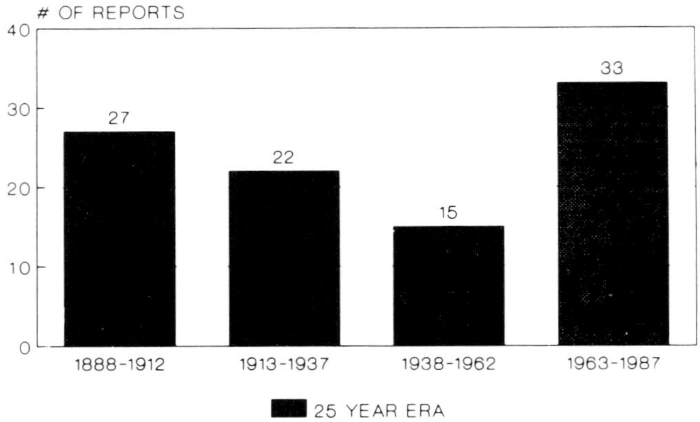

FIG. 2. Papers presented to the SSA by 25-year eras. A nadir of productivity was reached following WW II, but in recent years, there has been a vigorous reawakening of interest with a marked increase in the number and quality of presentations.

considered for patients with penetrating gunshot wounds. President Hunter H. McGuire (Fig. 6) of Richmond was perhaps most succinct in reminiscing about his days as a military surgeon in the Civil War: "I look back with horror on the days of the war when I practiced surgery on gunshot wounds to the abdomen. We gave them opium, etc. and waited until they died. Now a man has no right to do this."[5]

Four years later, at the meeting in New Orleans, W. F. Westmoreland of Atlanta came down on the side of laparotomy in his paper on the treatment of gunshot wounds.[6] Westmoreland seemed particularly incensed about some of his less radical colleagues: "The

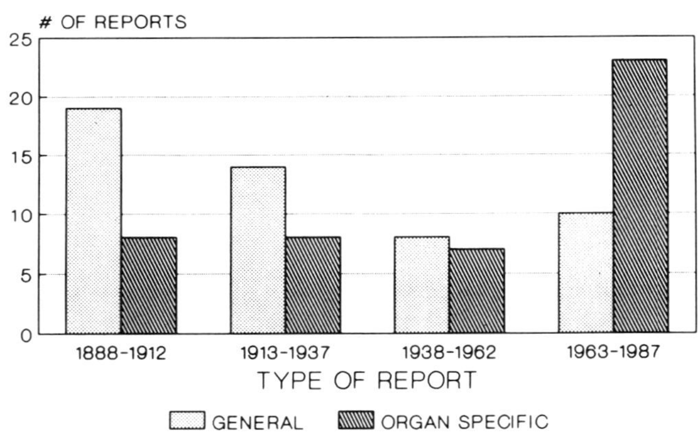

FIG. 3. General *versus* organ-specific reports on abdominal trauma (by era). In recent years an increasing proportion of papers has focused on specific organ injuries. In the earliest era general papers on the suitability of laparotomy dominated the discussions.

1888-1912	1913-1962	1963-1987
WD Haggard	*JY Brown	*JD Martin
HH McGuire	A Singleton	*H Wilson
*B Brown	A Ochsner	*JD Rives
*LM Tiffany	JD Rives	*RS Sparkman
WEB Davis		*WD Warren
*FW McRae		*I Cohn, jr
HA Kelly		A Mansberger
FW Parham		JL Sawyers
*WO Roberts		
R Matas		

FIG. 4. A list of the presidents of the SSA who manifested major interests in abdominal trauma. *Made presentation on trauma at an annual meeting of the SSA.

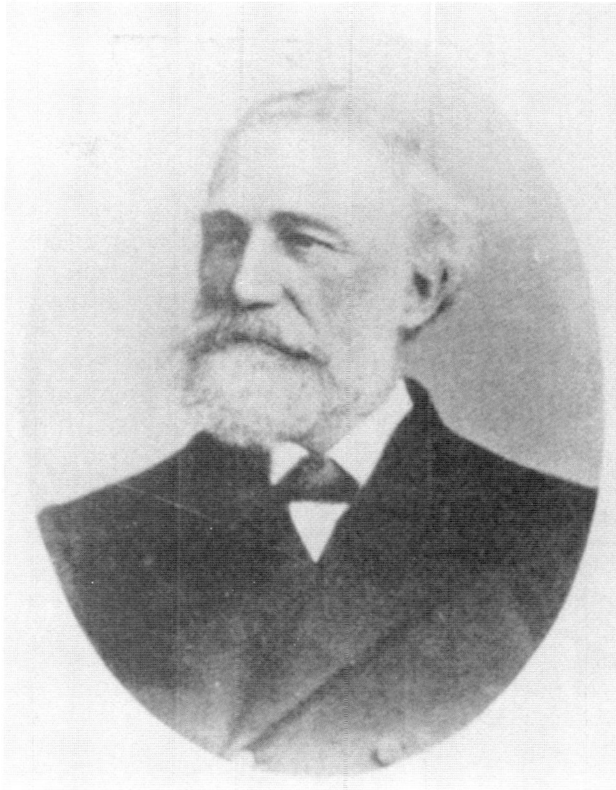

FIG. 5. Professor R. A. Kinloch of Charleston, a founding member of the Southern Surgical and Gynaecological Association. He was the first American to explore a patient with a gunshot wound of the abdomen.

physician calls in the abdominal surgeon and, although he expresses himself very radically about operations involving the removal of ovaries and tubes, when he comes to these cases [abdominal trauma] it is *opium and wait.* When he comes to the bedside and sees the case before him, he does not have the courage of the convictions he has so openly avowed. Particularly, this is true of those gynaecologists and coeliotomists who, like toadstools, spring up in a night." Westmoreland was supported in his views by A. B. Miles of New Orleans, Cunningham of Alabama, and J. McF. Gaston of Atlanta, but J. D. S. Davis of Birmingham expressed some caution about routine laparotomy.[7]

Papers by Tiffany of Baltimore in 1894,[8] and by Bradford Brown of Alexandria in 1895[9] continued the colloquy, climaxed by the paper of W. E. Parker of New Orleans, Louisiana at the meeting in Nashville in 1896.[10] Parker reported on 13 personal cases operated upon at Charity Hospital, New Orleans of whom six survived. He provided an extensive summary of the world's literature on the management of bullet wounds to the abdomen published to that date, and provided excellent descriptions on how to manage individual lesions. Parker's paper provoked a long, excited discussion with the vast majority of the individuals strongly supporting an aggressive employment of laparotomy in the management of gunshot wounds.

Finally, Howard A. Kelly of Baltimore rose and made the following proposal: "Would it not be well, Mr. President, in view of the serious medico-legal complications that arise in these cases, to pass a resolution favoring immediate operative interference whenever any of us come in contact with these cases? I, therefore, offer the following: Resolved, that it is the sense of the members of the Southern Surgical and Gynecological Association that in gunshot wounds penetrating the abdominal cavity the proper routine procedure is to make an immediate exploratory incision. Seconded and carried."

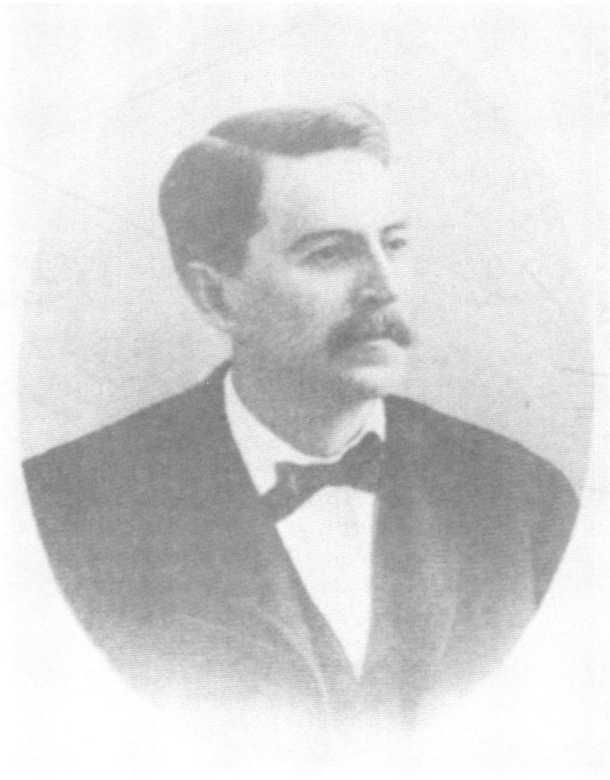

FIG. 6. Hunter H. McGuire of Richmond, a founding member of the SSA and an early proponent of laparotomy for trauma. He had served as Stonewall Jackson's surgeon and was perhaps the most respected and influential trauma surgeon of his day.

One can almost picture Parker being carried from the auditorium on the shoulders of his cheering fellow members! His high standing among his colleagues was to be short-lived.

Two years later Parker returned to the speaker's podium with another paper.[11] In the interim, he had served as a surgeon with the American military forces in Cuba. Parker had entered the conflict with the intention of exploring patients who sustained abdominal wounds, but soon found "surgery with troops in the field is a very different thing from surgery in civil life."[11] He concluded, "Wounds of the abdomen healed without operative interference. When I saw the conditions I strongly advised against surgical management."[11] He had discovered that exploration of abdominal wounds in a military field hospital was too dangerous. His conclusion, it should be stated, was shared by most of the other physicians who had participated in the Cuban expedition and by virtually the entire military surgical establishment. Yet Parker's recantation of his advocacy of laparotomy for penetrating abdominal wounds did not sit well with his audience. One after another of his fellow members rose and denounced him. H. H. Grant of Louisville, who had presented a paper recommending laparotomy for all gunshot wounds,[13] said, "Some of the statements by Dr. Parker are unquestionably astonishing." F. W. McRae[14] from Atlanta had reported on the recent experience at Grady Hospital and reiterated his firm conviction that every case of penetrating wound of the abdomen "where there is reasonable doubt as to injury of the abdominal viscera should be subjected, at least, to an exploratory operation." One or two faint voices were raised in support of Parker, but the discussion continued with a reiteration of Kelly's resolution from the 1896 meeting and the accusation that Parker was advising "masterly inactivity."[2] Westmoreland went further: "It's not 'masterly inactivity,' it is '*criminal inactivity.*' " Parker, in fact, had not changed his position on civilian gunshot wounds. He still advocated exploration for these lesions.

Grant was so incensed that the next year he presented another paper continuing his denunciation of Parker and concluding "With these facts before us, it is clear that to delay, in a delusive hope, until peritonitis shows its folly is almost a crime. The practical management of a suspected penetrating wound is as plain a duty as the tying of a bleeding artery. As soon as possible after injury, the patient is to be transported to a suitable place [and explored]."[15] And lest there be any doubt about how he stood about Parker's recommendations: "Because a man falls out of a balloon from a considerable height . . . without sustaining injury is that any reason why we should encourage others to undertake similar experiences?"

Undaunted, Parker stood his ground saying that he had not operated on a gunshot wound to the abdomen for about 3 years and reiterating the firmly held belief by the military that operations in the field could not be performed safely. (This conclusion of the military surgeons, shared by the British, continued until 1915.)

Another dozen papers over the ensuing years[16–23] continued the argument with ill-tempered comments about the military surgeons and about Parker continuing until 1915. The most important of these subsequent papers was that of E. D. Fenner[17] of New Orleans who updated the Charity statistics presenting 152 cases (which was a larger series than that experienced by the army during the Spanish American War). Parker, in the meantime, resigned from the SSA and retreated to Hot Springs, Arkansas.

An interesting sidelight of this era was the formidable presence of Nicholas Senn. Senn was elected to membership of the SSA in 1893 and was a member until he resigned in 1905. No evidence could be found that he actually attended a meeting, but the rise and fall of his influence at the meetings makes an interesting story.

Senn was perhaps the most prolific intestinal surgeon of his era, with a deep interest in abdominal trauma. He had developed a variety of techniques of intestinal anastomosis, had invented the Nicholas Senn hydrogen gas insufflation test for diagnosis of abdominal visceral penetration,[24] and was the founder of the Association of Military Surgeons (Fig. 7). Senn's hydrogen gas test consisted of insufflating hydrogen through a tube inserted into the anus of a wounded patient. The patient was then examined for abdominal distention and tympani. A lighted taper was placed near the wound of entrance. A small explosion accompanied by a flaring blue flame was a positive test, indicating penetration of the intestines. The value of this test was stressed by Cunningham in his first paper on abdominal trauma in 1888 when he expressed his opinion that the Senn test would have made the diagnosis in his patient and led him to earlier exploration.[2] The papers on intestinal anastomosis the following year paid tribute to Senn's seminal contributions in intestinal anastomosis.[3,4] There were repeated favorable references, both to the hydrogen gas test and to Senn's contributions in these papers and in the discussion which followed. McGuire was typical: "I think the whole profession is greatly indebted to Dr. Senn" and J. D. Davis emphatically said: "I don't open up the abdomen when I have the hydrogen gas with me until I have used it." Senn's ascendency continued through Parker's presentation of 1896,[10] but when Senn supported Parker's views about the management of abdominal wounds in the military,[25] he might as well have written his epitaph. By the next year, Grant was calling the Senn test "worse than useless." McRae went further: "the gas test of Senn is worse than useless. It is dangerous" And W. E. B. Davis, who in previous years had made complimentary remarks about Senn, was moved to say, "Dr. Senn's influence has been harmful. Every Community has suffered from his writings." Senn's opinions and writings disappeared from the transactions and no further favorable reference to him can be found. Senn's name does not appear in any subsequent discussions. He resigned in 1905, whether or not at the instigation of the council is not recorded. It is notable that in a presentation celebrating the 50th anniversary of the SSA, Hubert Royster spoke as if Senn had actually attended a meeting. This is strong evidence of his forceful influence.

Seventy-five years later, a young perhaps foolish member* had the temerity to advocate again "masterly inactivity" in the management of gunshot wounds of the abdomen.[26] Perhaps, if he had known at that time the fate of Parker and Senn he would have been more cautious!

* The author is referring to his own epochal work in this field (Ed).

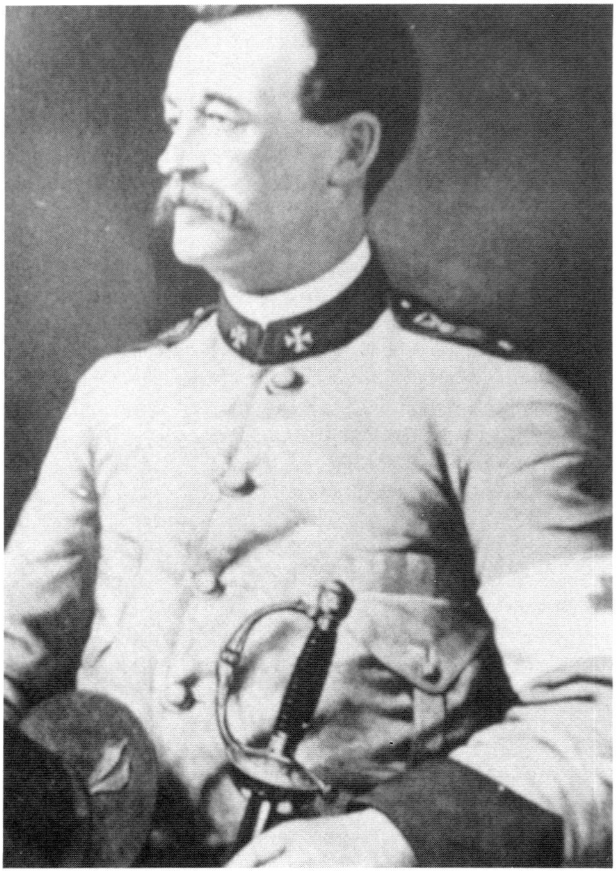

FIG. 7. Nicholas Senn of Milwaukee, a prolific student of abdominal trauma whose presence was very much felt during discussions of abdominal trauma in the first decade, founder of the Association of Military Surgeons.

Consolidation, 1913–1937

This era was marked by considerably more civility in the discussions about abdominal trauma. Just prior to the beginning of this era, W. D. Roberts of Louisville had given a presidential address on Southern Surgeons, reminding his audience that he himself had performed the first successful exploration of a stab wound in 1884.[27] John W. Brown's presidential address of 1913 was a superbly comprehensive paper on the management of acute abdominal conditions, including abdominal trauma.[28]

With the coming of the World War, there was a renewal of interest in the military aspects of trauma. The 1914 meeting had three papers dealing with military surgery.[29] The paper of H. D. Marcy of Boston was an affectionate reminiscence, 50 years later, of his experiences as a young military surgeon in the Yankee Army during the occupation of Charleston, South Carolina.[30] His description of the hardships endured by the Yankee soldiers apparently fell on deaf ears and the paper was not discussed. Colonel Charles Richard of the U.S. Army, a guest speaker, reiterated the military's continuing position that formal exploration of the abdomen for penetrating gunshot wounds should not be undertaken unless there was evidence of uncontrolled hemorrhage.[31] This position of military surgeons still rankled and Colonel Richard was subjected to pointed questioning during the discussion. The members of the SSA were, of course, right on this issue and the military abandoned its position shortly following the start of the war.

W. L. Haggard of Nashville was moved to wax patriotic in his presidential address of 1917.[32] C. H. Peck of New York returned from the front in 1918 to describe the treatment of war wounds in the hospitals of the expeditionary forces.[33] The 1920s brought a focus of interest in improving the supportive care of patients with abdominal injuries. A. M. Willis of Richmond reported on some clinical and experimental observations in the use of saline irrigations in diffuse peritonitis due to trauma.[34] Mason presented a paper on the influence of hemorrhage in the mortality of gunshot wounds of the abdomen.[35] Mason and the program committee were so impressed by this paper that he gave a second one with the same title the following year.[36] Mason divided his series into two groups, a large hemorrhage group of patients, and a small hemorrhage group. The large hemorrhage group had a mortality rate of 90%, whereas the small hemorrhage group had a mortality rate of only 30%. He concluded that hemorrhage was an important factor in the mortality rates of these patients and strongly advised the use of blood transfusions, a conclusion that was supported by many of the discussants.

Later in the era, there occurred a brief infatuation with shotgun wounds of the abdomen, beginning with the report of G. H. Bunch, of Columbia in 1928[37] of four patients who sustained close-range shotgun wounds; three died. Of three with long range shotgun blasts, two died. Bunch advocated early exploration, a position seconded by most of his discussants. Mason was back again during the discussion giving a minipaper reiterating the increase in mortality associated with hemorrhage in gun shot wounds of the abdomen.

Willis[38,39] followed Bunch's paper in 1931 with a report on penetrating wounds of the abdomen from pistol, rifle, and shotgun missiles and emphasized that long-range shotgun wounds with scattered shots could be managed nonoperatively, a position he soon supported with a paper in 1934 reporting a series of animals wounded with long-range shotgun blasts in which more than one-half of the animals survived without operation. Willis' 1931 report was also notable: 63 cases, all treated in the tiny hamlet of Rocky Mount, North Carolina. L. H. Landry, from New Orleans, in discussing Willis' paper, brought the audience up to date on recent Charity Hospital statistics, which included a total of 3141 gunshot injuries treated from 1914 to 1924.[40]

Perhaps the most important major presentation from this era was that of Heuer[41] who reported on 7000 cases of major trauma seen at the Cincinnati General Hospital, among which there were 334 patients with abdominal injury treated with a mortality rate of 50% for gunshots and 13.2% for stabs. This paper stimulated a general discussion on the importance of establishing trauma as a specialty and the need for establishment of special training in trauma surgery.

The Lessons of War, 1937–1962

The war in Europe had begun when Storck[42] presented his paper on penetrating wounds of the abdomen. It was a series of 46 cases operated on personally, with a mortality rate of only 40% among the gunshot wounds. This very long, impressively documented paper extensively described the proper management of penetrating wounds of the abdomen and served as the basis for his manual on the management of abdominal trauma, which became an official army document. The following year, with war raging in Europe, a symposium on war injuries was given, with Storck[43] again making the presentation on abdominal wounds. During the war, there were papers by M. E. DeBakey and B. N. Carter[44] on war surgery, DeBakey and F. A. Simeone[45] on vascular injuries, and Lt. Col. L. G. Lewis[46] on pelvic injury, a remarkably small output considering the number of surgeons who participated in the war. In the early postwar period, there was a marked drop-off of interest in trauma, perhaps reflecting a general conviction that war surgery had provided all of the answers for the management of abdominal trauma. This view clearly was reflected in the paper of D. H. Poer of Atlanta in 1947, which strongly recommended applying military surgical principles to civilian trauma.[47]

The era closed with an important paper by Wilson and Sherman.[49] This presentation was a harbinger of things to come in a later era and set the stage by raising questions about the appropriateness of universal application of military principles to civilian trauma.

Only 15 papers were presented during this era, representing a nadir of interest and productivity perhaps reflecting a post-war attitude that all of the important issues had been answered.

Reexamination and Discovery, 1963–1987

The most recent era has been characterized by a marked increase in the interest in the general subject of abdominal trauma and a focus on the more specialized aspects of specific organ injury. Heated discussions, new ideas, and a willingness to challenge old precepts returned in full force to the forum of the SSA. J. E. Pridgen's[50] presentation in 1966 on penetrating wounds of the abdomen reported on 776 cases from the University of Texas in San Antonio and provoked discussions on the advisability of exploration for stab wounds. F. C. Nance's[26] paper in 1973 extended this discussion. By this time, the concept of selective management of stab wounds was being grudgingly accepted in a number of trauma institutions, but Nance's inclusion of gunshot wounds as candidates for selective nonoperative management was greeted with deep suspicion, if not hostility. The discussion was continued in 1983 when W. C. Lee, J. F. Uddo, and Nance presented the Charity Hospital experience with selective management of stab wound reiterating the conviction of the LSU group in New Orleans that clinical criteria alone were sufficient to decide whether or not a patient with a stab wound needed exploration. These authors reported a negative laparotomy rate of 7.8% and a mortality rate of 2.2%. One death from inappropriate application of their protocol was acknowledged.[51] D. V. Feliciano of Houston, in discussing this paper, reiterated the reliance at Ben Taub Hospital on local wound exploration, a policy also followed by L. M. Flint Jr. in Louisville. A. V. Donovan of Los Angeles supported the authors, saying that clinical criteria were utilized in Los Angeles in the evaluation of patients.

Specific Organ Injuries

An important aspect of the bibliography of abdominal trauma of the SSA has been the papers that have focused on specific organ injuries. As laparotomy became firmly established, a concentration on management of individual lesions became inevitable. The trend has become much more pronounced as very large series of patients from the major trauma centers became the subject of comprehensive study.

Diaphragm

Three case reports constitute the total discussion of diaphragmatic injuries at the SSA. The first report was given in 1904 on a patient who had sustained gangrenous changes to the bowel; the patient died.[52] The other two cases were patients diagnosed 6 and 7 weeks postinjury in whom successful elective repairs had been accomplished.[53,54] All of the authors emphasized the difficulty in making the diagnosis of ruptured diaphragm (which is perhaps understandable because in all of the case reports the diagnosis had been delayed).

Vascular

Past presentations on vascular injuries have been made nine times beginning with LaRoque's report of an A-V fistula following a bullet wound to the external iliac artery and vein that he managed by ligation of both vessels.[55] The patient and his extremity survived. In describing his concern about the vascular supply to the leg, G. P. LaRoque of Richmond comments that a week after the operation, "I took the liberty of sticking a pin in his toe to see if it would bleed. It bled."[55] LaRoque finished his paper by including a thorough review of the available literature on the lesion, paying tribute in particular to the contributions of Halsted and Matas. LaRoque returned the next year with another paper.[56] At least LaRoque had the modesty to quote a "distinguished American surgeon" as having "prayed to be delivered in time of illness from the care of a doctor who has had a case. Might he not with equal fervency pray to be delivered from the surgeon who's opinions are firmly fixed after the successful management of *another* case."[56] This patient was also treated by ligation and survived with an intact leg.

In 1928, an aortic injury was reported by J. G. Sherrill of Louisville in a patient who sustained severe blunt trauma. He developed a thrombosis of the distal aorta. Sherrill had attempted thrombectomy but, unfortunately, his patient did not survive.[57] He was congratulated for his courage by the members during the discussion.

The modern papers on vascular injury began with DeBakey and Simeone's review of arterial injuries encountered during World War II, presented at the meeting in 1945.[45] This classic presentation reviewed 2471 cases of arterial injury and has served as a milestone for all subsequent reports on arterial injuries. The paper included a discussion of 47 intra-abdominal arterial injuries.

Most other presentations on arterial injuries have dealt in passing with the abdominal vessels. The presentation of Hardy et al.[58] in 1974 described their experience in Jackson with 22 abdominal aortic and 44 other abdominal vessels among 360 arterial injuries. Reynolds et al. reviewed 20 abdominal vessels among 191 patients with arterial injuries.[59] Feliciano et al.[60] reported on 408 patients with vascular injuries seen in 1 year, among them being 130 patients with abdominal arterial injuries. Many of the patients in this series were treated with prosthetic bypass or insertion of a venous conduit.

McCune et al.[61] dealt with the specialized problem of mesenteric thrombosis following blunt trauma. They emphasized the high mortality rate associated with the lesion, having observed three deaths among the four reported cases.

In 1974 Mattox et al.[62] presented a series of 22 patients with injury to the portal vein of whom 11 survived. The authors recommended lateral repair, end-to-end anastomosis, or portacaval shunt because ligation was associated with a 100% mortality rate.

The consensus of opinion regarding vascular injuries to the major abdominal vessels revolves around the need for early diagnosis and control of hemorrhage. Virtually all reports and discussion confirm the need for direct arterial repair and/or anastomosis where feasible, or insertion of a variety of prostheses where primary repair is not possible.

Urology

Six presentations before the SSA have dealt with trauma to the urogenital tract. Two papers presented in successive years, 1917 and 1918, reported on injuries to the kidney. J. M. Mason's paper reviewed the literature and presented three cases.[63] Mason and the majority of the discussants of the paper favored nephrectomy or suture of the injury.[63] There was considerable discussion about the virtues of suture with a general consensus that the kidney should be preserved if possible. The following year, S. G. Ledbetter[64] also presented a case of kidney rupture treated by suture with survival, and in the discussion, T. S. Cullen, among others, strongly supported his view.

Wounds of the urinary bladder were first discussed by R. Douglas of Nashville in 1893.[65] He described a patient who had had a bladder ruptured by the shaft of a buggy. After determining that it was an extraperitoneal injury, Douglas managed the patient by simple drainage apparently without a bladder catheter; the patient recovered fully.

Other papers have dealt with bladder injuries associated with pelvic fractures.[66] In 1944, a guest speaker, Lt. Col. L. G. Lewis[46] described four severe war injuries and W. L. Weems of Jackson[67] discussed a series of 86 GU injuries identified in 282 patients with pelvic fractures. Both authors recommended suprapubic cystostomy through a small lower abdominal transverse incision with appropriate drainage. Weems' paper made an excellent case for delayed repair of urogenital lesions, relying initially on suprapubic cystostomy and drainage and making a formal repair at a later time.

Pelvis

Only one paper over the years has dealt specifically with pelvic injuries, that of Flint et al.[68] of Louisville, which was presented in 1978. (Two other papers dealing with the pelvis focused on genitourinary injuries.) Flint's paper defined a subgroup of patients with pelvic fractures who had severe extraperitoneal hemorrhage and described the use of a G-suit with inflation to control hemorrhage from this severe complication. One of their patients was managed by angiography, a method that might well be regarded as the method of choice at the present time.[68]

Spleen

Four papers on splenic trauma have been presented to the SSA. They reflected the cyclic evolution of the management of splenic trauma over the past century. Tiffany's presentation in 1894 discussed a patient with a gunshot wound of the spleen managed by suture. The tenor of the discussion was that splenic trauma could be managed either by suture of splenectomy.[8]

W. P. Carr's presentation in 1906 also described management of splenic trauma by suture of splenectomy, but Carr recommended a splenorrhaphy only for "injuries that can be safely repaired."[69] By 1917, A. M. Willis of Richmond was advocating splenectomy for all splenic trauma.[34] This rather rigid approach continued and was epitomized by the discussion of J. H. Morton's paper on blunt trauma in 1956 in which one of the members stated "the treatment for ruptured spleen is, of course, splenectomy."[70]

The report in 1952 by King and Shumacker[71] first called attention to the risk of overwhelming infection following splenectomy in infancy. Subsequently, other reports led to a reevaluation of the management of splenic trauma. A history of this reevaluation was summarized by R. T. Sherman of Tampa in 1980.[72]

By 1984 Feliciano et al.[73] presented a series of 305 patients with splenic injury managed by selective splenorrhaphy and splenectomy. Forty-five percent of the patients had splenorrhaphy and 55% of the patients had splenectomy; they concluded that splenectomy would be generally required in patients with multiple associated intra-abdominal injuries and the more severe grades of splenic injuries and that splenorrhaphy could be performed in patients with a smaller number of associated intra-abdominal injuries and less severe grades of splenic injury.[73]

The operative management of splenic injury had thus come full circle to the point where it existed in 1894, namely, splenic injuries are treated selectively, either by suture when possible, splenectomy, or by nonoperative management.

Liver

Martin's presentation in 1946 marked the first time that a paper dealing specifically with wounds to the liver had been given to the SSA.[74] Martin's paper dealt with an experimental injury inflicted to dog livers by hitting each liver 50 times. He reported that hemorrhage following this type of injury could be controlled by packing and debridement.[74] Discussion included a comment by DeBakey reporting on his war experiences with liver trauma and emphasizing external drainage and control of shock.

Sparkman and Fogelman[75] of Dallas presented a summarized series of liver trauma patients from the Parkland Hospital in 1953. The series was subsequently updated by Trunkey et al.[76] in 1973; 811 patients were managed primarily by suture and drainage. However, almost 6% of the total were managed by major resection. A subsequent report by Flint et al.,[77] and the discussion following it, reiterated the importance of less aggressive treatment of hepatic injuries utilizing hepatic artery ligation, selective debridement, drainage, and packing.

Sandblom et al.[78] presented an experimental study in 1975 on healing of liver wounds, demonstrating that the presence of bile greatly slowed the rate of healing of liver wounds.

The paper presented by Busuttil et al.[79] in 1979 dealt with extrahepatic injuries to the portahepatis, including bile duct and portal vein injuries. A total of 28 patients was presented with a variety of repairs recommended as would be expected in this diverse group of injuries.

The most recent paper, that of Pachter et al.[80] emphasized the use of finger fracture technique to allow local control of hemorrhage from hepatic injuries. This paper reiterated the more modern view that these injuries should be treated selectively with minimal reliance on major resections. The discussion that followed emphasized the use of packing in patients with massive hepatic hemorrhage.

The presentations on hepatic trauma at the SSA have reflected changes in attitude that have evolved since 1945. In the 1950s and 1960s there was enthusiasm for aggressive approach to hepatic trauma utilizing major resections. This has gradually changed to one that calls for minimal debridement of necrotic tissue and simple repair by any means that will effectively control hemorrhage. A brief interest in hepatic artery ligation and in common duct drainage appears to have been abandoned by most recent authors.

Pancreas and Duodenum

The first presentation dealing specifically with injuries to the duodenum and pancreas was not made until 1963, which is perhaps understandable considering the complexity of pancreatic and duodenal trauma. Moore and Erlandson dealt with intramural duodenal hematoma.[81] They presented two cases and reviewed 33 others in the literature. Surprisingly, they made no mention of conservative, nonoperative, treatment, nor did they make any mention of serosal incision as a method of management of duodenal hematoma. These issues, however, were brought up during the discussion and by the time of a second presentation on the same subject by Fuller et al.,[82] nonoperative management in selected patients had become well established and was recommended.

Barnett et al.[83] reviewed the experience of the University of Mississippi in the management of pancreatic injury yielding an overall mortality rate of 13%. Barnett's group relied primarily on drainage. One-third of the 18 patients were treated by distal pancreatectomy and drainage; only one death had occurred.

Several groups have presented large series of patients with duodenal, pancreatic, or combined injuries. The recommended therapies have generated significant controversy in the discussions that followed the presentations. Flint,[84] in discussing duodenal injury, recommended tube decompression of the duodenum through an enterotomy stating that no duodenal fistulas had been observed in any of the ten patients so treated. The majority of duodenal injury patients were treated by suture with a few being treated by other means, such as anastomosis, pancreaticoduodenectomy or duodenojejunostomy.

Jones' report[85] emphasized his preference for anastomosing a Roux-en-Y limb of jejunum to the injured pancreas, which he had employed in 38 of his 274 patients. Drainage alone, either by Penrose or sump, was performed in 197 of the 274 patients.

The presentation by Feliciano et al.[86] emphasized their preference for "duodenal diverticulization" in which the pylorus is closed by absorbable or nonabsorbable sutures and a proximal gastrojejunostomy is constructed. This method was utilized in 68 of 129 patients with combined pancreaticoduodenal injuries. In discussions following this paper, H. H. Stone from Grady Hospital in Atlanta emphasized his preference for triple intubation (gastrostomy, jejunostomy tube extending proximally into the duodenum, and jejunostomy tube extending distally into jejunum for feeding) and F. C. Nance expressed his discomfort with all of these methods, preferring simple reliance on sump drainage, distal pancreatic resection, and occasional pancreaticoduodenectomy.

The controversy over the role of pancreaticoduodenectomy for trauma raised in other forums has seldom been a cause for discussion at the SSA. Salaam et al.[97] reviewed four patients who had been followed 3 years after surviving Whipple procedures for trauma and reported that all were biochemically and physiologically normal. Most large series have included a few patients who were managed by pancreaticoduodenectomy with mortality rates ranging from 20% to 40%.

It seems clear that the management of pancreatic and duodenal injuries is in a state of flux and will be a continuing subject of discussion at future meetings of the SSA.

Esophagus, Stomach, Small Bowel and Colon

There have been ten papers over the years that have dealt with wounds of the hollow viscera. Symbas et al.[87] report in 1979 included seven patients, among 48 with esophageal injuries who had gunshot wounds of the abdominal esophagus. Four patients were managed by primary repair, or by repair and plication with survival and no sequelae. Two patients had exteriorization of the esophagus because of the extensive injury. These two patients also survived. Symbas et al.[87] recommended early exploration with primary repair of the esophageal wound and plication with adjacent serosa if possible.

W. M. Jordan's report from Birmingham in 1904[88] was the only one to deal solely with stomach injuries. He reported two patients, one of whom had survived. He recommended purse string suture of the stomach wound and appropriately advised searching for the wound of exit in the retrogastric space.[88]

At the second meeting of the SSA, in 1889, two major papers on intestinal anastomosis based on experimental studies were presented.[3,4] Both dealt extensively with repair of small bowel injuries following penetrating trauma. Davis had done an experimental study utilizing a catgut mat as partial support of the anastomosis. A. V. L. Brokaw from St. Louis, presented a series of experiments utilizing rubber rings. Both authors made it clear that the utility of these techniques was primarily for penetrating trauma to the gut. An extensive discussion of both papers followed, including comments by Hunter McGuire of Richmond

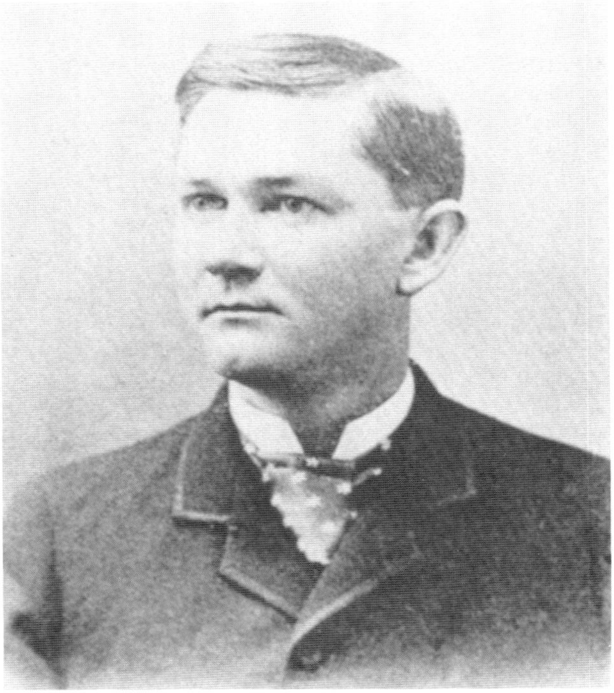

FIG. 8. A. B. Miles of New Orleans, an early vigorous participant in the discussions on abdominal trauma until his untimely death in 1893 at the age of 42.

(perhaps the most respected trauma surgeon of his day), W. O. Roberts of Louisville, and W. E. B. Davis of Birmingham. A striking feature of both the presentations and the discussion is the repeated reference to Nicholas Senn and his pioneering efforts in developing anastomotic techniques. Both Davis and Brokaw acknowledged Senn's contributions in their papers and in their closing remarks.

Three other papers dealing with intestinal injury took the form of case reports. The most notable of these papers was that of A. B. Miles[89] of the New Orleans Charity Hospital wherein lies an interesting story (Fig. 8). Miles reported on a patient who shot himself while carelessly handling his own pistol. The Charity Hospital ambulance brought him to the hospital and he was on the operating table within a half hour of injury. Sixteen small bowel lacerations and three mesenteric wounds were identified and repaired by suture. He made an essentially uneventful recovery. Miles first reported this case to the SSA in 1890. As a young professor of surgery at Tulane, he was undoubtedly aware of the need to publish or perish and this case report appeared in no fewer than four additional publications. Moreover, the patient was mentioned on at least four subsequent occasions during meetings of the SSA. In 1907 during a clinical visit to Charity Hospital, the members of the SSA were given the opportunity to meet the sturdy survivor some 18 years after his injury!

The SSA has had three important presentations on colonic injury, all subsequent to 1970. During World War II, mandatory colostomy for all colonic injuries, no matter how trivial, had been introduced as a method of therapy and had been largely credited for the improvement in survival noted among patients who sustained injuries to the colon. The principle of mandatory colostomy was enthusiastically adapted to civilian practice and became firmly ingrained in clinical protocols at major trauma institutions.

The enthusiasm for the use of colostomy for all colonic injuries continued despite a number of reports beginning with that of Woodhall and Ochsner[90] suggesting that many civilian colonic injuries could be more safely managed by primary suture repair. These reports had little impact on surgical practice.

The 1971 paper by Beall et al.[91] continued a series of reports from Houston strongly endorsing selective employment of primary suture for colonic injury. This was followed in

1981 by Flint et al.,[92] who strongly endorsed selective utilization of primary suture.[92] In a discussion of this last paper, Harlan H. Stone's prospective study on colon injury was favorably commented upon and a number of the discussants strongly advocated a wider application of primary suture for colonic injury.

The most recent paper presented by Burch et al.[93] in 1985 was a further update of the Houston series, continuing to reiterate the virtues of selective employment of primary suture. These three papers, and others in the recent trauma literature, have served to modify slowly the approach away from the army's mandatory colostomy for all injury towards a more selective approach to colonic trauma.

Blunt Trauma

Four papers have dealt specifically with blunt trauma, although many others have included patients who sustained nonpenetrating injury. Landry's paper in 1934 on football injuries included eight patients who had experienced hematuria, two of whom required nephrectomy.[94] In 1938, F. W. Baily[95] of St. Petersburg presented 100 cases in whom a 34% mortality rate had occurred. The majority of patients were transportation injuries. In 1956, Morton et al.[48] reported on 120 cases treated in Rochester, NY. The most commonly injured organ was the spleen, which these authors felt should be routinely managed by splenectomy. Davis et al.[96] reviewed 437 patients from the Charity Hospital in 1975. A mortality rate of 13.3% was observed, mostly in patients with concomitant head injury. Clinical criteria for evaluation were recommended.

Summary

One cannot come away from a reading of these 98 papers without acquiring a sense of the gusto, enthusiasm, and downright enjoyment that the members of the SSA have had in wrestling with the topic of abdominal trauma. Discussions have been spirited and tough, occasionally boisterous, but usually gentlemanly. New ideas have been presented and challenged, accepted, or rejected. Young men have questioned long-held established principles, and older men have freely shared their wisdom. As a result, the forum of the SSA has been one of the important sources of progress in the field of trauma management. Members of the SSA may be perhaps forgiven if they concur with one of their former presidents, F. W. McRae of Atlanta, who in 1908 said: "When the history of gunshot wounds of the abdomen shall have been written, chief credit must be given to Southern surgeons. Most of the papers on this subject that are worthwhile have been written by fellows of this Association and have been printed in its Transactions."[22]

REFERENCES

1. Kinloch RA. Pistol shot wounds of the abdomen treated by laparotomy and suturing the intestines. Ann Surg 1888;5:183–192.
2. Cunningham RM. Cases in surgery. Trans South Surg Gynecol Assoc 1888;1:102–113.
3. Brokaw AVL. Intestinal anastomotic operations with segmental rubber rings. Trans South Surg Gynecol Assoc 1889;2:174–191.
4. Davis JDS. Intestinal anastomosis. Trans South Surg Gynecol Assoc 1889;2:142–153.
5. Discussion Paper by Brokaw.[3]
6. Westmorland W. Treatment of gunshot wounds. Trans South Surg Gynecol Assoc 1893;6:177–192.
7. Discussion Paper by Westmoreland.[6]
8. Tiffany LMcL. Gunshot wounds of spleen and kidney; abdominal section; hemostasis by deep suture; recovery. Trans South Surg Gynecol Assoc 1894;7:83–91.
9. Brown B. Stab wounds in the peritoneum. Trans South Surg Gynecol Assoc 1895;8:40–62.
10. Parker WE. Bullet wounds of the abdomen. Trans South Surg Gynecol Assoc 1896;9:272–310.
11. Parker WE. Gunshot wounds. Trans South Surg Gynecol Assoc 1898;11:15–21.
12. Discussion Paper by Parker.[11]
13. Grant HH. The practical management of bullet wounds of the abdominal viscesa. Trans South Surg Gynecol Assoc 1898;11:39–49.
14. McRae FW. Penetrating wounds of the abdomen with reports of cases. Trans South Surg Gynecol Assoc 1898;11:22–38.
15. Grant HH. The practical management of bullet wounds of the abdominal viscera. Trans South Surg Gynecol Assoc 1899;12:37–52.
16. Wysor JC. Report of a case of a gunshot wound of the abdomen. Trans South Surg Gynecol Assoc 1901;14:178–179.

17. Fenner ED. Penetrating wounds of the abdomen. Trans South Surg Gynecol Assoc 1901;14:180–200.
18. Neff W. Gunshot wound of the abdomen. Trans South Surg Gynecol Assoc 1901;14:365–372.
19. Johnson RW. Five recent successful laparotomies for gunshot wounds of the abdominal viscera. Trans South Surg Gynecol Assoc 1903;16:339–348.
20. Caldwell CE. Penetrating wounds of the abdomen. Trans South Surg Gynecol Assoc 1904;18:398–411.
21. Guerry LeG. The report of eight consecutive cases of gunshot wound of the abdomen with one death. Trans South Surg Gynecol Assoc 1907;20:348–360.
22. McRae FW. Penetrating wounds of abdomen. Trans South Surg Gynecol Assoc 1908;21:236–254.
23. Price J. A brief discussion of some of the surgical junk demanding further surgical interference. Trans South Surg Gynecol Assoc 1909;22:17–28.
24. Senn N. Rectal insufflation of hydrogen gas. An infallible test in the diagnosis of visceral injury of the gastrointestinal canal in penetrating wounds of the abdomen. JAMA 1888;1:680–688.
25. Senn N. The modern treatment of gunshot wounds in military practice. JAMA 1898;2:46–55.
26. Nance FC, Wenner WH, Johnson LW, et al. Surgical judgement in the management of penetrating wounds of the abdomen. Experience with 2212 patients. Trans South Surg Assoc 1973;85:117–124.
27. Roberts WO. Southern surgeons and surgery. Trans South Surg Gynecol Assoc 1910;23:1–24.
28. Brown JY. Diagnosis and surgical technique to be employed in the handling of acute abdominal conditions. Trans South Surg Gynecol Assoc 1913;26:1–18.
29. Bloodgood JC. What the civilian surgeon can do for military surgery. Trans South Surg Gynecol Assoc 1914;27:157–166.
30. Marcy H. The surgical service of the civil war then and now. Trans South Surg Gynecol Assoc 1914;27:138–156.
31. Richard C. Military surgery. Trans South Surg Gynecol Assoc 1914;27:166–187.
32. Haggard WD. The medical professor and the great war. Trans South Surg Assoc 1917;30:1–11.
33. Peck C. Treatment of war wounds in hospitals of the American expedition. Trans South Surg Assoc 1918;31:227–234.
34. Willis AM. Traumatic rupture of the spleen. Trans South Surg Assoc 1917;30:74–88.
35. Mason JM. The influence of hemorrhage on the mortality in gunshot wounds and other injuries of the abdomen. Trans South Surg Assoc 1922;35:36–56.
36. Mason JM. The influence of hemorrhage on the mortality in gunshot wounds and other injuries of the abdomen. Trans South Surg Assoc 1923;36:499–507.
37. Bunch GH. Shotgun wounds of the abdomen. Trans South Surg Assoc 1928;41:38–48.
38. Willis BC. Penetrating wounds of abdomen received from pistol, rifle and shotgun missiles. Trans South Surg Assoc 1931;44:114–131.
39. Willis BC. Shotgun wounds of the abdomen. Trans South Surg Assoc 1934;47:215–236.
40. Landry L. Discussion of paper by Willis.[39]
41. Heuer GJ. Observations in traumatic surgery. Trans South Surg Assoc 1930;43:377–394.
42. Storck AH. Penetrating wounds of the abdomen. Trans South Surg Assoc 1939;52:103–147.
43. Storck AH. Abdominal injuries. Trans South Surg Assoc 1940;53:79–88.
44. DeBakey ME, Carter BN. Current considerations of war surgery. Trans South Surg Assoc 1944;56:160–179.
45. DeBakey ME, Simeone FA. Battle injuries of the arteries in World War II: An analysis of 2471 cases. Trans South Surg Assoc 1945;57:65–110.
46. Lewis LG. Cases of severe pelvic injury. Trans South Surg Assoc 1944;56:86–94.
47. Poer DH. Management of penetrating abdominal injuries comparative military and civilian experiences. Ann Surg 1947;127:1092–1102.
48. Morton JH, Hinshaw JR, Morton JJ. Blunt trauma to the abdomen. Ann Surg 1957;145:699–711.
49. Wilson H, Sherman R. Civilian penetrating wounds of the abdomen: factors in mortality. Ann Surg 1961;53:639–649.
50. Pridgen JE, Herff AF, Watkins HO, et al. Penetrating wounds of the abdomen. Ann Surg 1967;165:901–907.
51. Lee WC, Uddo JF, Nance FC. Surgical judgement in the management of abdominal stab wounds utilizing clinical criteria from a 10 year experience. Trans South Surg Assoc 1983;95:59–64.
52. Brown GS. A case of rupture of the diaphragm. Trans South Surg Gynecol Assoc 1904;17:425–430.
53. Beall FC. Rupture of the diaphragm. Trans South Surg Assoc 1925;38:77–82.
54. Strode EC, Vance CA. Herniation of right diaphragm secondary to trauma. Ann Surg 1953;137:609–615.
55. LaRoque GP. Ligation external iliac artery above and below a communicating bullet wound. Trans South Surg Assoc 1920;33:420–457.
56. LaRoque GP. Another case of bullet wound of the femoral artery and vein. Trans South Surg Assoc 1921;34:318–323.
57. Sherrill JG. Traumatism to the abdominal aorta. Trans South Surg Assoc 1928;41:48–57.
58. Hardy JD, Raja S, Neely WA, Bary DW. Aortic and other arterial injuries. Trans South Surg Assoc 1974;86:154–167.
59. Reynolds RR, McDowell HA, Diethelm AG. The surgical treatment of arterial injuries in the civilian population. Trans South Surg Assoc 1978;90:170–179.

60. Feliciano DV, Bitondo CG, Mattox KL, et al. Civilian trauma in the 1980's: a one year experience with 456 vascular and cardiac injuries. Trans South Surg Assoc 1983;95:227–234.
61. McCune WS, Keshishien JM, Blades BB. Mesenteric thrombosis following blunt abdominal trauma. Ann Surg 1952;135:606–614.
62. Mattox KL, Spade RE, Beall AC. Traumatic injury to the portal vein. Trans South Surg Assoc 1974;86:33–37.
63. Mason JM. Management of subparietal injuries of the kidney. Trans South Surg Assoc 1917;30:183–197.
64. Ledbetter SI. Suture of ruptured kidney. Trans South Surg Assoc 1918;31:13–18.
65. Douglas R. The recognition and management of wounds of the urinary bladder. Trans South Surg Gynecol Assoc 1893;5:350–358.
66. Smith PG. Urogenital injuries. Trans South Surg Assoc 1940;53:89–91.
67. Weems WL. Management of genitourinary injuries in patients with pelvic fractures. Trans South Surg Assoc 1978;90:187–193.
68. Flint LM, Brown A, Richardson JD, Polk HC. Definitive control of bleeding from severe pelvic fractures. Trans South Surg Assoc 1978;90:179–186.
69. Carr WP. Splenectomy indications. Trans South Surg Gynecol Assoc 1906;19:379–397.
70. Discussion of paper by Morton.[48]
71. King H, Shumacker HB. Splenic studies susceptibility to infections after splenectomy performed in infancy. Ann Surg 1952;136:239–242.
72. Sherman R. Perspective in management of trauma to the spleen. J Trauma 1980;20:1–13.
73. Feliciano DV, Bitondo CG, Mattox KL, et al. A four year experience with splenectomy versus splenorrhaphy. Trans South Surg Assoc 1984;96:568–575.
74. Martin JD Jr. Wounds of the liver. Trans South Surg Assoc 1945;58:252–264.
75. Sparkman RS, Fogelman MJ. Wounds of the Liver. Ann Surg 1954;139:690–719.
76. Trunkey DD, Shires GT, McClelland R. Management of liver trauma in 811 consecutive patients. Trans South Surg Assoc 1973;85:200–207.
77. Flint LM, Mayo ET, Aaron WS, et al. Selectivity in the management of hepatic trauma. Trans South Surg Assoc 1976;88:121–126.
78. Sandblom P, Markovitch V, Gardial D. The healing of liver wounds. Trans South Surg Assoc 1975;87:227–232.
79. Busuttil RW, Kitahima K, Cerise E, et al. Management of blunt and penetrating injuries of the *porta hepatis.* Trans South Surg Assoc 1979;91:123–130.
80. Pachter HL, Spencer FC, Hofstetter SR, Cooper GF. Experience with the finger fracture technique to achieve intrahepatic hemostasis in 75 patients with severe injuries to the liver. Trans South Surg Assoc 1982;94:277–284.
81. Moore SW, Erlandson ME. Intramural hematoma of the duodenum. Ann Surg 1964;157:798–809.
82. Fuller WD, Sella JG, Martin LW, Altemeier WA. Intramural duodenal hematoma. Trans South Surg Assoc 1973;85:27–34.
83. Barnett WO, Hardy JD, Yelverton RL. Pancreatic trauma. Ann Surg 1966;163:892–901.
84. Flint LM. Duodenal injury: Analysis of common misconceptions in diagnosis and treatment. Trans South Surg Assoc 1979;91:179–184.
85. Jones RC. Management of pancreatic trauma. Trans South Surg Assoc 1977;39:113–122.
86. Feliciano DV, Martin TD, Cruse PA, et al. Management of combined pancreaticoduodenal injuries. Ann Surg 1987;205:673–680.
87. Symbas PN, Hatcher CR, Ulasis SE. Esophageal gunshot injuries. Trans South Surg Assoc 1979;91:185–189.
88. Jordan WM. Gunshot wounds of the stomach. Trans South Surg Gynecol Assoc 1904;17:476–481.
89. Miles AB. Report of a case of gunshot wound of the abdomen; with three mesenteric and sixteen intestinal wounds; laparotomy; recovery. Trans South Surg Gynecol Assoc 1890;3:436–438.
90. Woodhall JP, Ochsner A. The management of perforating injuries of the colon and rectum in civilian practice. Surgery 1951;29:305–320.
91. Beall AC, Bricker DL. Alessi F, DeBakey ME. Surgical considerations in the management of civilian colon injuries. Ann Surg 1971;173:971–978.
92. Flint LM, Vijole GG, Richardson JD, Polk HC. The injured colon: relationships of management to complications. Ann Surg 1981;193:619–627.
93. Burch JM, Gevirteman L, Feliciano DV, et al. The injured colon. Trans South Surg Assoc 1985;97:253–265.
94. Landry L. Injuries peculiar to modern football. Trans South Surg Assoc 1934;47:407–418.
95. Bailey FW. Non-penetrating intra-abdominal injury. Trans South Surg Assoc 1938;51:267–277.
96. Davis JJ, Cohn I, Nance FC. Diagnosis and management of blunt abdominal trauma. Trans South Surg Assoc 1975;87:220–227.
97. Salam A, Warren WO, Kalser M, Laguna V. Pancreaticoduodenectomy for trauma. Clinical and metabolic studies. Ann Surg 1972;175:663–672.

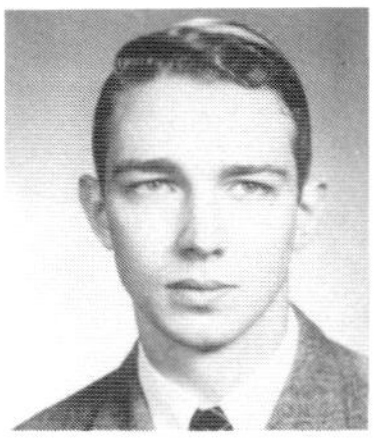

Introduction of Dr. Gordon Danielson

Dr. Clyde Barker: This morning's final speaker, Gordon Danielson, is seen here at the time he began his general surgery residency at HUP. After finishing his general surgery at HUP in 1962, he obtained additional training in cardiac surgery first at HUP and then at the Karolinska (Sweden). He became a Markle Scholar and was a member of Dr. Rhoads' faculty for two years before Ben Eisman recruited him to take Frank Spencer's position as Chief of Cardiac Surgery at the University of Kentucky when Frank went to NYU. Shortly thereafter, Gordon moved to a similar position at the Mayo Clinic and Mayo Medical School, where he is presently Professor of Surgery and Chairman of the Division of Thoracic and Cardiovascular Surgery.

It should be mentioned that Julian Johnson, Dr. Rhoads' second in command while he was Barton Professor, was Dr. Danielson's mentor in cardiothoracic surgery. As you know, Julian died recently, and we all miss him very much.

Dr. Danielson's Introductory Remarks

Thank you Clyde. It is a real honor and privilege to be invited here today to help celebrate Dr. Rhoads' 80th birthday. I apologize that I do not have a general surgery topic to present. Early in my residency, I was enticed away into cardiac surgery. Perhaps Dr. Rhoads was actually responsible in part for this, as he was kind enough to let me rotate for three months on Cardiology in the Robinette Foundation at HUP to learn about cardiovascular diseases and how they affect the surgical patient. This rotation sharpened my interest in surgery of the heart and great vessels. It has been interesting and challenging to work out new ideas and techniques in the fields of congenital and acquired heart disease, and I will discuss one of these today—pulmonary atresia with hypoplastic pulmonary arteries.

Before that, I would like to mention that cardiac surgeons who operate on patients for complex congenital heart disease or severe acquired cardiac disease know that such patients may have long and difficult postoperative courses. For them, the nutritional techniques developed by Dr. Rhoads and his associates have played a very important role in their support through the postoperative period—as much so as for patients with difficult general surgical problems. Thus, I would like to echo Dr. John Howard's comments earlier this morning by saying again that cardiothoracic surgeons are indebted to Dr. Rhoads for his great contributions in this area. I personally am doubly indebted to Dr. Rhoads since I had the privilege of completing my training in his program. Dr Rhoads, thank you and Happy Birthday.

Surgical Management of Pulmonary Atresia, Ventricular Septal Defect, and Hypoplastic Confluent Pulmonary Arteries

GORDON K. DANIELSON, M.D. AND FRANCISCO J. PUGA, M.D.

Continuity between the right ventricle and a pulmonary artery confluence was established in 105 patients with pulmonary atresia, ventricular septal defect, and hypoplastic confluent pulmonary arteries (first-stage procedure). There were 12 hospital deaths (11%). Fifty-seven patients had follow-up cardiac catheterization a mean of 33 months postoperatively. In 31 of these, final repair was deferred because of insufficient pulmonary artery enlargement (14), restricted peripheral distribution (nine), or both (eight). Second-stage complete repair has been carried out in 24 patients. Repair included right ventricular outflow tract reconstruction (n = 18), relief of central pulmonary artery stenosis (n = 14), and ligation of systemic-to-pulmonary collateral arteries (n = 10). The mean postrepair peak systolic right ventricular–left ventricular pressure ratio was 0.67 (range, 0.32–1.0). There was one hospital death (4%). Follow-up of 19 patients showed all are in functional Class I or Class II. A two-stage surgical approach is highly successful in those patients whose pulmonary arteries are too hypoplastic to allow single-stage repair.

SURGICAL MANAGEMENT of pulmonary atresia with ventricular septal defect and hypoplastic pulmonary arteries is difficult and controversial. Although repair of pulmonary atresia with ventricular septal defect in the presence of normal pulmonary arteries can be accomplished with low mortality and excellent results,[1,2] closure of the ventricular septal defect in the presence of hypoplastic pulmonary arteries results in right ventricular failure and often death. We prefer to manage this challenging problem by establishing right ventricular to pulmonary artery (RV-PA) continuity (first stage) followed by subsequent closure of the ventricular septal defect (second stage) if pulmonary arterial growth and distribution are adequate.[3,4]

Patients and Methods

Patients with pulmonary atresia, ventricular septal defect, and hypoplastic confluent pulmonary arteries operated on from 1976 through July 1984 were reviewed. Included were those patients with double-outlet right ventricle and transposition of the great arteries. Excluded were those patients with more complex anomalies such as univentricular heart or double-inlet ventricle. Pulmonary atresia was defined as the absence of continuity between the right ventricle and pulmonary arteries.

During this period 97 patients underwent right ventricular outflow tract construction without closure of the associated ventricular septal defect (first-stage repair). An additional eight patients, initially thought to be candidates for total correction, had ventricular septal defects closed only to be reopened before completion of the initial repair because of elevated right ventricular pressures secondary to poor pulmonary arterial outflow. These individuals thus had the equivalent of a first-stage operation.

From the Department of Cardiovascular Surgery, Mayo Clinic and Mayo Foundation, Rochester, Minnesota.

TABLE 1. *Associated Anomalies (35 Patients)*

Anomaly	No.
Secundum atrial septal defect	16
Transposition of the great arteries	7
Double outlet right ventricle	4
Patent ductus arteriosus	2
Primum atrial septal defect	1
Other	15
Total	45

Ages of these 105 patients at the time of the first stage procedure ranged from 6 months to 54 years (mean, 11.2 years). Fifty-three patients (50%) were male. Eighteen individuals (17%) had a total of 21 previous systemic–pulmonary shunts. Most were cyanotic and all exhibited exercise intolerance. Mean preoperative hemoglobin was 18.2 g percent (range, 12.1–25.4 g percent) with an average oxygen saturation on room air of 62% (range, 49%–89%). Forty-five associated cardiovascular anomalies were encountered in 35 of the patients (Table 1).

Before right ventricular outflow tract construction, delineation of pulmonary arterial anatomy and sources of pulmonary blood flow was accomplished by one or more of the following techniques: (1) aortography, (2) selective opacification of previously constructed systemic-to-pulmonary arterial shunts, (3) selective injection of systemic-to-pulmonary arterial collaterals, and (4) retrograde visualization of pulmonary arteries by pulmonary vein wedge injection. Right and left pulmonary arterial diameters were assessed by direct measurement of the angiographic image, with correction for magnification by a factor derived from measured and known size of the angiographic catheter. The combined area of the right and left pulmonary arteries then was compared to normal main pulmonary artery area for patients of the same body surface area, as derived from standard tables. Accessible pulmonary and systemic pressures were recorded. Pulmonary, systemic, and shunt flows also were calculated when possible.

First-Stage Repair

Eighty-eight individuals had first-stage repair utilizing standard techniques of median sternotomy, cardiopulmonary bypass, and myocardial protection as previously published.[4] The remaining 17 patients had outflow tract construction using a closed technique through a left thoracotomy.[5] Several methods of outflow tract construction were utilized (Table 2). In nearly one fourth of the patients, patch angioplasty techniques were used. In the remaining patients RV-PA conduits were employed. Only 21% of the outflow tract constructions were valved.

There were 12 hospital deaths (11%), all of low cardiac output or hypoxia. An additional 11 patients (10%) died after hospital discharge and before second-stage repair. The principle

TABLE 2. *Methods of First-Stage Right Ventricular Outflow Tract Construction*

Technique	Patient	Percent
Patch		
Autogenous pericardium	21	20
Prosthetic	3	3
Conduit		
Woven nonvalved	29	28
Woven valved	23	22
Knitted nonvalved	15	14
Autogenous pericardial tube	11	10
PTFE nonvalved	3	3
Total	105	100

PTFE: polytetrafluoroethylene.

causes of death were arrhythmia, accidental, and congestive heart failure. Five of these individuals had undergone late cardiac catheterization; two were candidates for complete repair whereas three were deemed unacceptable for second-stage correction at that time.

Late Cardiac Catheterization and Angiography

After first-stage construction of the right ventricular outflow tract, patients were followed serially and evaluated by catheterization and angiography as indicated to determine suitability for complete repair based on pulmonary artery growth and distribution. Patients whose pulmonary arteries were thought to be large enough and whose pulmonary artery distribution was to more than the equivalent of one total lung, in conjunction with a predominantly left-to-right shunt (in the absence of a restrictive RV-PA conduit) were considered candidates for second-stage (complete) repair.

Twenty-five patients currently are awaiting a follow-up evaluation of suitability for complete repair. This subgroup generally represent patients who have undergone first-stage operation most recently. In another 62 patients, follow-up cardiac catheterization and angiography were performed. In 34 of these, final correction was deferred because of anatomic abnormalities.

Thirty-one of these 34 patients are still alive; they had a mean age of 10.6 years at first stage correction (range, 5 months–54 years). The mean interval from first stage operation to latest follow-up catheterization was 33 months (range, 12–60 months). Final repair was considered inappropriate because of insufficient enlargement of the pulmonary arteries (14 patients, 45%), restricted pulmonary artery distribution (nine patients, 29%), or both (eight patients, 26%).

Twenty-eight individuals were accepted for complete repair, and this has been carried out in 24 who are the subject of the remainder of this report.

Second-Stage (Complete) Repair

Twenty-four patients went on to complete repair of their anomaly. Mean age at first stage procedure was 12.2 years (range, 5–26 years) and mean age at second-stage correction was 14.7 years (range, 7–31 years). Average interval between procedures was 32 months (range, 6–48 months). Nineteen patients had no previous palliation before first-stage repair and five had previous systemic-to-pulmonary artery shunts (two Waterston, three Potts).

Everyone in this group had adequate peripheral pulmonary artery distribution (total distribution equivalent to at least one lung) to tolerate complete repair. Eighty-eight percent had good or excellent distribution defined as central flow to the entire pulmonary parenchyma of both lungs or to both lungs minus a single pulmonary segment.

All patients in this group exhibited an increase in pulmonary arterial size to at least 75% of calculated normal except in one who was totally corrected when her pulmonary artery outflow area was 44% of normal. This patient was early in our series and had a right ventricle to left ventricle (RV/LV) peak systolic pressure ratio of 1.0 at the end of the repair. She would not undergo total correction by our current criteria and was the only hospital death among these patients. Over a mean interval of 32 months, average pulmonary size grew from 25% of normal (range, 6%–58%) at the time of first-stage repair to 99% of normal (range, 44%–147%) at second-stage correction. The mean pulmonary-to-systemic flow ratio (Q_p/Q_s) at the time of second-stage repair was 1.28.

Second-stage correction was performed in all cases through a median sternotomy utilizing cardiopulmonary bypass. The sizes of the right and left pulmonary arteries were determined by calibrated probes when possible. Prerepair and postrepair pressure measurements were recorded. Procedures (Table 3) included patch closure of the ventricular septal defect in all 24 patients and placement or replacement of an RV-PA prosthetic conduit in 18 (75%) of the patients. Seventeen of the conduits were valved and one was nonvalved. Of the six patients who did not undergo conduit placement or replacement, five had a valved and one had a nonvalved prosthesis already in place.

Twenty-three patients (96%) survived second-stage repair. The one patient who died (4% mortality), mentioned previously, had a residual RV/LV pressure ratio of 1.0 and died after emergency reoperation for creation of an atrial septal defect. At reoperation, a ruptured tricuspid papillary muscle was found, necessitating a concomitant tricuspid valve replacement. Morbidity included deep (n = 2) and superficial (n = 1) wound infections, reoperation

TABLE 3. *Second-Stage Procedures (24 Patients)*

Procedure	No.		Percent	
Closure ventricular septal defect		24		100
Revision right ventricular outflow tract		18		75
Closure atrial septal defect		16		67
Enlargement pulmonary artery		14		58
Unilateral	9		38	
Bilateral	5		21	
Ligation systemic-to-pulmonary artery collaterals*		10		42
Partial	8		33	
Complete	2		8	

* Eight other patients had previous (interim) ligation of systemic-to-pulmonary artery collaterals.

for bleeding (n = 2), and respiratory insufficiency requiring tracheostomy (n = 1). An additional two individuals developed signs of right ventricular failure which resolved with aggressive medical management. These were the only two patients with nonvalved conduits at the completion of second-stage repair.

The RV/LV pressure ratios recorded at the end of operation ranged from 0.32 to 1.0 (mean, 0.67). The patient who died had a ratio of 1.0, another patient had a ratio of 0.97, and the remainder had ratios less than 0.85.

Of the 23 operative survivors, three overseas patients were lost to follow-up (87% complete follow-up). The remaining 20 patients have been followed for an average of 38 months (range, 4–77 months). There was one late death in a patient who died of sepsis 4 years postoperatively after three operations for pacemaker implantation for atrial arrhythmias, closure of residual ventricular septal defect, and tricuspid valve replacement, respectively. The remaining 19 patients (95%) have required no further hospitalization or additional surgery and are in New York Heart Association Class I or II. Fourteen of the 19 require no cardiac medications and five are taking digoxin only.

Discussion

Surgical repair of pulmonary atresia with ventricular septal defect is associated with good results when central pulmonary arterial size and peripheral distribution are normal.[1,2] In such patients, lack of restriction to pulmonary arterial blood flow allows closure of the ventricular septal defect, and postoperative right ventricular pressures are low. However, significant hypoplasia of central pulmonary arteries, extensive limitations in peripheral pulmonary arterial distribution, or both, preclude ventricular septal defect closure. In this subset of patients with pulmonary atresia, a preliminary procedure which establishes continuity between the right ventricle and pulmonary arterial confluence has both therapeutic and diagnostic significance, achieving three important objectives: (1) palliation of cyanosis by increasing pulmonary arterial blood flow; (2) progressive enlargement of pulmonary arteries thus connected to the right ventricle, and, (3) creation of an anatomic pathway through which direct angiography of the pulmonary arteries is possible. Direct angiography allows precise definition of the complex arterial perfusion of the lungs including distribution of both the central pulmonary arteries and the systemic-to-pulmonary arterial collaterals.

Previous reports have documented achievement of similar goals through the creation of systemic-to-pulmonary arterial shunts.[6–8] However, problems encountered with this approach such as peripheral interruption or distortion of the small pulmonary arteries, limited shunt durability, and inadequate pulmonary arterial enlargement have prompted us, since 1976, to adopt right ventricular outflow tract construction as the procedure of choice for initial surgical treatment of these patients.[3,4] In our experience, this operation has provided more rapid and more complete pulmonary arterial growth and more efficient palliation than systemic-to-pulmonary arterial shunts.

Adequate pulmonary arterial enlargement can be achieved in a significant number of patients after right ventricular outflow tract construction. The average central pulmonary arterial size increased from 25% of normal at first stage to 99% of normal at complete repair. It has not been possible to predict those patients in whom such favorable changes will occur.

Pulmonary arterial growth is rapid and uniform in some patients, is focally incomplete in others (resulting in segmental stenoses), and is diffusely slow in a minority of patients. Nevertheless, all patients have derived excellent palliation from first-stage repair.

The minimal acceptable size of pulmonary arteries for permitting successful second-stage repair is not known. However, when the combined right and left pulmonary arterial area of our patients was 75% of normal or greater, the postoperative RV/LV pressure ratio was less than 0.85 in all but one patient. We believe it is desirable to obtain a postrepair pressure ratio less than 0.85 as this allows some margin for increased right ventricular pressure related to cardiovascular demands of moderate exercise.

If the RV-PA connection is not restrictive, the right-to-left shunt at ventricular level will gradually diminish and become predominantly left-to-right as the pulmonary arteries grow. A ratio of RV-PA blood flow to systemic blood flow of 1.3 or greater suggests the pulmonary arteries are large enough for a second-stage correction. Unfortunately, precise measurement of total pulmonary blood flow and flow exiting through the right ventricular outflow reconstruction usually are not possible due to multiple extracardiac sources of pulmonary flow in these patients. In some borderline cases, interim ligation of systemic-to-pulmonary collaterals facilitates assessment of blood flow through the right ventricular outflow tract. Temporary balloon-catheter occlusion of the major collaterals at the time of cardiac catheterization also facilitates this assessment.

The pulmonary arterial enlargement induced by a first-stage procedure is a time-related phenomenon. We have continued to evaluate serially patients who have yet to show adequate central pulmonary artery growth. Close supervision of the enlargement process is required to prevent the development of advanced congestive heart failure or obstructive plexogenic pulmonary arteriopathy. We currently recommend yearly clinical evaluation, supplemented with angiography and cardiac catheterization as indicated.

Any discrete stenosis of proximal pulmonary artery branches or restriction of right ventricular emptying through the outflow reconstruction must be considered during preoperative evaluation of a candidate for second-stage repair. These problems can be corrected at final reconstruction. Localized proximal left pulmonary stenosis frequently occurs after first-stage outflow tract construction, but this is easily corrected at final repair by patch angioplasty techniques. On the other hand, pulmonary artery distortion resulting from previous systemic-to-pulmonary arterial shunts occurs more peripherally and is more difficult, if not impossible, to correct at the time of final repair.

At second-stage repair, many patients require reconstruction of the right ventricular outflow tract. Three fourths of our patients had RV-PA connections replaced with a prosthetic conduit. Revision generally is performed to remove a small or obstructed conduit and to place a larger, valved conduit to accommodate the enlarged pulmonary arteries. In contrast to repair of pulmonary atresia with normal pulmonary arteries, in which nonvalved RV-PA conduits generally are employed, we recommend the use of a valved prosthesis for second-stage repair in patients with previously hypoplastic pulmonary arteries in order to optimize the postoperative course. The only two patients in our series with a nonvalved RV-PA conduit after second-stage repair developed temporary right heart failure.

In addition to ventricular septal defect closure, complete repair entails management of systemic-to-pulmonary artery collateral vessels. Careful preoperative angiographic evaluation, best obtained with selective collateral arterial injections, is important in planning an appropriate surgical approach. These communications usually are not divided at the first-stage reconstruction as they are necessary to provide adequate pulmonary blood flow, and perhaps they help augment pulmonary arterial growth. Although these vessels usually are stenotic peripherally, excessive blood flow through some of them may prompt interim ligation before pulmonary artery size is adequate for complete repair. Otherwise, these arteries are managed at the time of second stage repair. Collateral communications that supply portions of pulmonary parenchyma shared by branches of the main pulmonary artery generally are ligated. If these vessels represent the sole source of arterial supply to a particular pulmonary segment, they should be left untouched or subtotally ligated, as complete ligation may precipitate pulmonary infarction. If collaterals cannot be approached surgically because of technical reasons, radiographic embolization remains an alternative.[9]

Not all patients undergoing a first-stage procedure who have adequate pulmonary arterial growth have become candidates for complete repair. A subset of patients demonstrates good pulmonary arterial size, but lack sufficient peripheral distribution. In these patients, establishment of lobar pulmonary arterial continuity (unifocalization operations) may increase pulmonary arterial distribution so that complete repair is possible.

Careful selection of patients for final repair is essential. Currently, acceptable candidates include those patients with the following: (1) a calculated central combined right and left pulmonary arterial area as measured from the (anteroposterior) AP angiogram of at least 75% of predicted normal; (2) distribution of unobstructed, confluent pulmonary arteries equivalent to at least one whole lung; and (3) the presence of a predominant left-to-right shunt at ventricular level in the absence of a restrictive RV-PA connection.

REFERENCES

1. Olin CL, Ritter DG, McGoon DC, Wallace RB, Danielson GK. Pulmonary atresia: Surgical considerations and results in 103 patients undergoing definitive repair. Circulation 1976;(Suppl 3)54:35–40.
2. Alfieri O, Blackstone EH, Kirklin JW, Pacifico AD, Bargeron LM Jr. Surgical treatment of tetralogy of Fallot with pulmonary atresia. J Thorac Cardiovasc Surg 1978;76:321–335.
3. Gill CC, Moodie DS, McGoon DC. Staged surgical management of pulmonary atresia with diminutive pulmonary arteries. J Thorac Cardiovasc Surg 1977;73:436–442.
4. Piehler JM, Danielson GK, McGoon DC, Wallace RB, Fulton RE, Mair DD. Management of pulmonary atresia with ventricular septal defect and hypoplastic pulmonary arteries by right ventricular outflow construction. J Thorac Cardiovasc Surg 1980;80:552–567.
5. Puga FJ, Uretzky G. Establishment of right ventricle-hypoplastic pulmonary artery continuity without the use of extracorporeal circulation. J Thorac Cardiovasc Surg 1982;83:74–80.
6. Kirklin JW, Bargeron LM Jr, Pacifico AD. The enlargement of small pulmonary arteries by preliminary palliative operations. Circulation 1977;56:612–617.
7. Alfieri O, Blackstone EH, Parenzan L. Growth of the pulmonary annulus and pulmonary arteries after the Waterston anastomosis. J Thorac Cardiovasc Surg 1979;78:440–444.
8. Gale AW, Arciniegas E, Green EW, Blackstone EH, Kirklin JW. Growth of the pulmonary annulus and pulmonary arteries after the Blalock-Taussig shunt. J Thorac Cardiovasc Surg 1979;77:459–465.
9. Yamamoto S, Nozawa T, Aizawa T, Honda M, Mohri M. Transcatheter embolization of bronchial collateral arteries prior to intracardiac operation for tetralogy of Fallot. J Thorac Cardiovasc Surg 1979;78:739–743.

Introduction of Dr. John Waldhausen

Dr. Clyde Barker: In 1959, John Waldhausen was recruited out of the HUP residency program by Harry Shoemaker with whom he finished his training. In 1966, he was recruited back to the University of Pennsylvania, where he built a premier congenital heart surgery service at Children's Hospital. In 1970, he went to Hershey as Professor and Chairman of Surgery, at Pennsylvania State University College of Medicine. Not only has he been a highly successful chairman there, but he has also served as Provost and Dean in that institution. The photograph that you see here was taken in Philadelphia during a meeting of the Society of Clinical Surgery in 1983, while John was serving as its President. John and Dr. Rhoads (who had been the Society's president in 1965) are examining the Society's interesting gavel, which resides now in the Museum of the College of Physicians of Philadelphia. Its head is fashioned from a doorknob obtained from Pasteur's house in Paris by another member of the Society, Alexis Carrell. The handle is a leg from Lord Lister's dressing table.

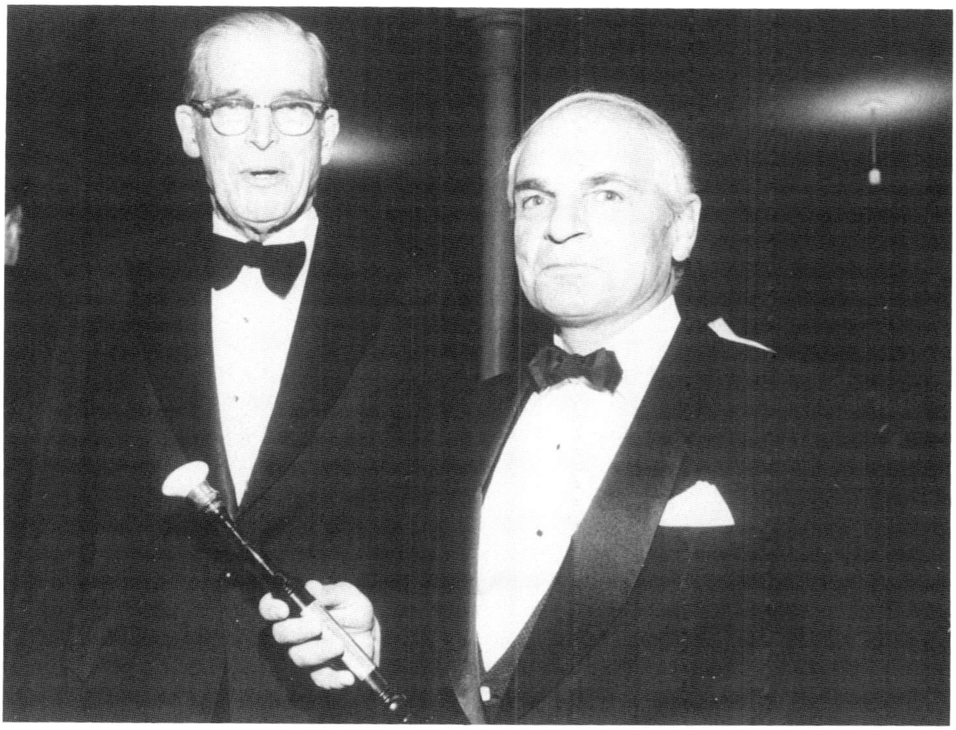

Dr. Waldhausen will speak today on the management of coarctation of the aorta in infants.

Dr. Waldhausen's Introductory Remarks

It is a great privilege and honor for me to be a speaker at this meeting, because, as you heard, I was something of a peripatetic resident and was more or less adopted by this august department. I must say that Dr. Rhoads was probably more responsible for my happiness here than any other individual, and he always went out of his way to help me. When I told Dr. Rhoads that I had made the decision to leave the Penn faculty and go to Hershey, I don't think he was totally pleased. He must have had some other things in mind for me. But he said, "Well if you must go, at least Hershey is on the Boston-Washington axis."

Coarctation of the Aorta in Infancy

DAVID B. CAMPBELL, M.D., JOHN L. MYERS, M.D., AND JOHN A. WALDHAUSEN, M.D.

COARCTATION OF THE AORTA is recognized as a common cause of congestive heart failure and death in infants. In the past it has been classified as either an "infantile" (preductile) or an "adult" (juxtaductal or postductal) type. Studies by Rudolf *et al.*[1] have shown that there are only two types of coarctation and that their development is influenced by hemodynamic molding. The "preductal" type is better described as tubular hypoplasia of the isthmus proximal to a patent ductus arteriosus. It is frequently associated with intracardiac defects in which a left-to-right shunt is present. Thus there is a decrease in the amount of blood that traverses the aortic valve, nearly all of which supplies the cranial vessels. The majority of blood flow to the descending aorta is through the ductus arteriosus. Little flow traverses the isthmus, and causes isthmus hypoplasia. In contrast, juxtaductal coarctation is characterized by a shelf-like narrowing of the aorta opposite the patent ductus and this lesion is less commonly associated with intracardiac lesions. Postductal coarctation may represent a juxtaductal type in which distal migration of the coarctation shelf has occurred with time. It is rarely seen in newborns.

The ductus arteriosus contributes significantly to the pathophysiology of the coarctation complex in both types of coarctation. In patients with hypoplasia of the isthmus, rapid closure of the ductus after birth decreases blood flow to the lower body and kidneys causing hypoxia, oliguria, and acidosis. This, in turn, can cause and perpetuate myocardial depression and congestive heart failure. In juxtaductal coarctation there may be ductile type tissue extending into the aortic wall. Flow from the arch to the descending aorta often is around the coarctation shelf and through the widely patent mouth of the ductus. Narrowing of the ductus then is associated with constriction of the aorta. Lower body hypoxia and acidosis follow because of the increased severity of the coarctation.[2] Only a gradual closure of the ductus, which allows for the development of collateral blood flow around the obstruction, is compatible with life.

Preoperative Preparation

Intensive preoperative preparation is of paramount importance to survival. Neonates and infants with coarctation often are in profound left ventricular failure and have superimposed metabolic acidosis because of inadequate perfusion. The correction of acidosis with sodium bicarbonate, the use of inotropic drugs such as digitalis and catecholamines, and the optimization of fluid status are essential to preparing an ill infant for operation. When there is evidence of heart failure either dobutamine or dopamine is given intravenously at low to moderate doses (continuous infusion < 7 μg/kg/minute) and digoxin is given as well. If the volume status of the patient is excessive, a diuretic, such as furosemide is given.

Intravenous prostaglandin E1 (PGE1, alprostadil) has become a major adjunct to the preoperative therapy of neonates.[3,4] It maintains the patency of the reactive ductus arteriosus and thus increases perfusion of the aorta below the coarctation. The clinical response to its use in newborns often has been dramatic. Prostaglandin E1 is much less effective after the first few days of life since the older child will not have a reactive ductus. In addition to the increased flow beyond the coarctation, the effects of intracardiac left-to-right shunts become less severe because a "popoff" is provided for the pulmonary circulation, which limits excessive blood flow to the lungs. A prostaglandin E1 infusion is started at 0.1 μg/kg/minute and the dose is decreased to the lowest value at which a response can be

From the Department of Surgery, Division of Cardiothoracic Surgery, The Milton S. Hershey Medical Center, The Pennsylvania State University, Hershey, Pennsylvania.

maintained. These modalities should be tried even before cardiac catheterization in any infant with clinical evidence of coarctation. Whereas operative intervention is imperative, several hours of aggressive preoperative care may be required to achieve the best operative results.

Surgical Options for Neonates and Infants

Most commonly, the goal of operation is to remove the obstruction and thereby decrease left ventricular afterload, establish flow to the descending aorta, and to stop the shunting at the level of the ductus. A number of operations have been devised to remedy coarctation of the aorta: resection and end-to-end anastomosis, prosthetic patch angioplasty, and variations of the two.[5–7] It has become clear, in the follow-up of patients treated by these different methods, that favorable results are not always achieved.[8–15] In infants younger than 1 year of age who are treated by coarctectomy and end-to-end reconstruction, the rate of "recoarctation" is reportedly between 16% and 50%. Recent series of reoperations[16,17] document the frequency of failure of the end-to-end method when used in the neonatal age patients. Reconstruction with a prosthetic patch certainly has limited growth potential as well as failure potential of the artificial materials.[18] Balloon catheter angioplasty has been reported,[19] but the early follow-up data indicate that these patients have not been well served by this option. Neonatal and infant cases are to be distinguished from the cases of older children (older than 1 year) and adults, in whom several surgical options are open.

Subclavian Flap Angioplasty

The subclavian flap procedure for the correction of coarctation of the aorta in young patients[20] was developed initially because of the shortcomings of other operative approaches; it has received increasing preference.[21–24] Bergdahl *et al.*,[25] addressing the issue of operative risk in neonates, treated the choice of operation as a variable. Their analysis concluded that use of the subclavian flap procedure was the only variable that correlated significantly with survival. The risks and effects of the loss of the subclavian artery on upper extremity perfusion are recognized from clinical experience with the Blalock-Taussig shunt.[26–28] In this literature and in a recent report on subclavian flap angioplasty,[29] minimal changes in arm growth and strength have been demonstrated.

The operative details of the subclavian flap angioplasty are shown in Figures 1 through 4. A left fourth intercostal space thoracotomy provides optimal exposure and the pleura overlying the proximal descending aorta is incised longitudinally and the aorta, ductus, distal arch, and proximal left subclavian artery are freed and controlled. The limits of the dissection are the left carotid artery at the proximal extent on the arch, and 1.5 to 2 cm of aorta beyond the level of the ductus (Fig. 1). The few intercostal vessels above this level often are thin and dilated and are temporarily controlled with Potts' ties or included in the aortic crossclamp. The left subclavian artery, from its origin to just beyond the vertebral artery posteriorly, is freed of surrounding tissues. An ascending pharyngeal branch occasionally arises from the subclavian artery proximal to the vertebral artery, in which case, it is ligated and divided. The vertebral artery routinely is ligated at its origin to prevent the possibility of subclavian steal. The subclavian vessel is ligated distal to the vertebral artery. If present, the ductus then is ligated. Crossclamps are applied to the aorta distal to the left carotid artery and, inferiorly, below the level of the coarctation.

The subclavian artery is transected proximal to the ties and turned down over the descending aorta to assess the length of the repair. An incision in the lateral wall of the aorta below the level of the coarctation is then made. Using Potts' scissors, this incision is enlarged proximally, cutting across the narrowed segment, into the origin of the subclavian artery, and then through its length. The interior of the aorta at the level of the coarctation then is inspected and the coarctation membrane excised sharply (Fig. 2). The subclavian "flap" is turned down to overlay the aortic defect. The aortotomy is extended inferiorly as the flap length of the subclavian artery allows.

We currently use polydioxanone (PDS, Ethicon, Inc., Somerville, NJ) suture material in a continuous manner. This is an absorbable monofilament product with handling qualities similar to polypropylene, and which has undergone animal trials at our institution.[30,31] The early results of its clinical use for the repair of a variety of congenital anomalies also have

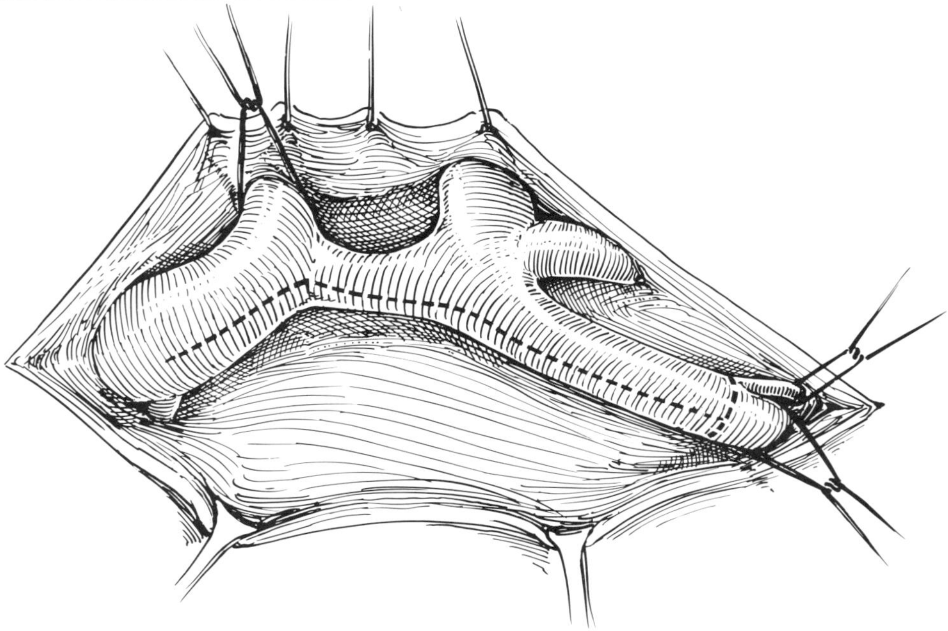

FIG. 1. The operative exposure through a left thoracotomy shows the limits of dissection and the lines of incision.

been reported. The reconstruction is begun by securing the apex of the flap inferiorly with a mattress suture. Simple sutures are placed at the superior corners of the aortic defect and carried down using a continuous simple suture technique to meet the mattress suture, where

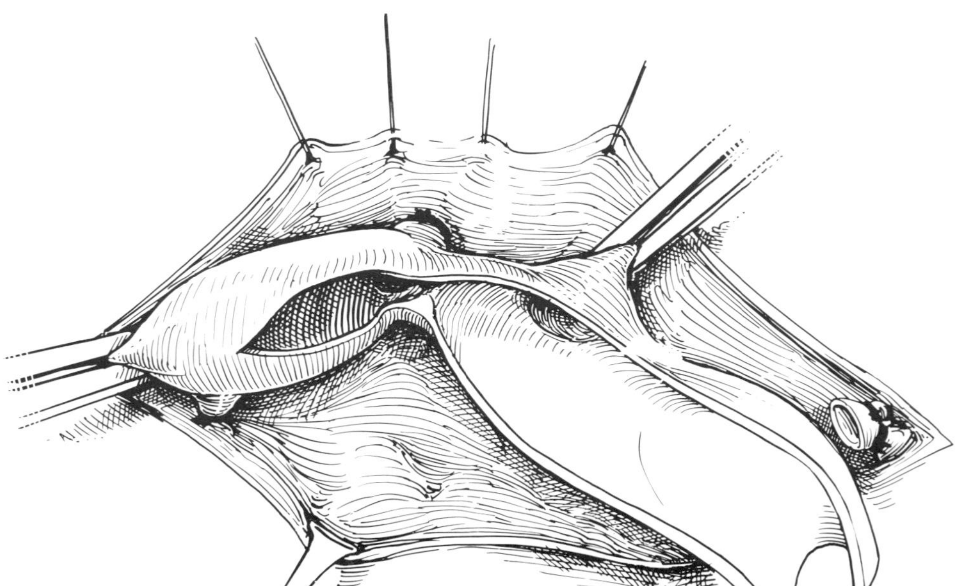

FIG. 2. Aortic crossclamps are in place and the subclavian artery has been transected and opened longitudinally. The incision is carried down through the aortic isthmus, across the coarcted segment, and into the descending thoracic aorta.

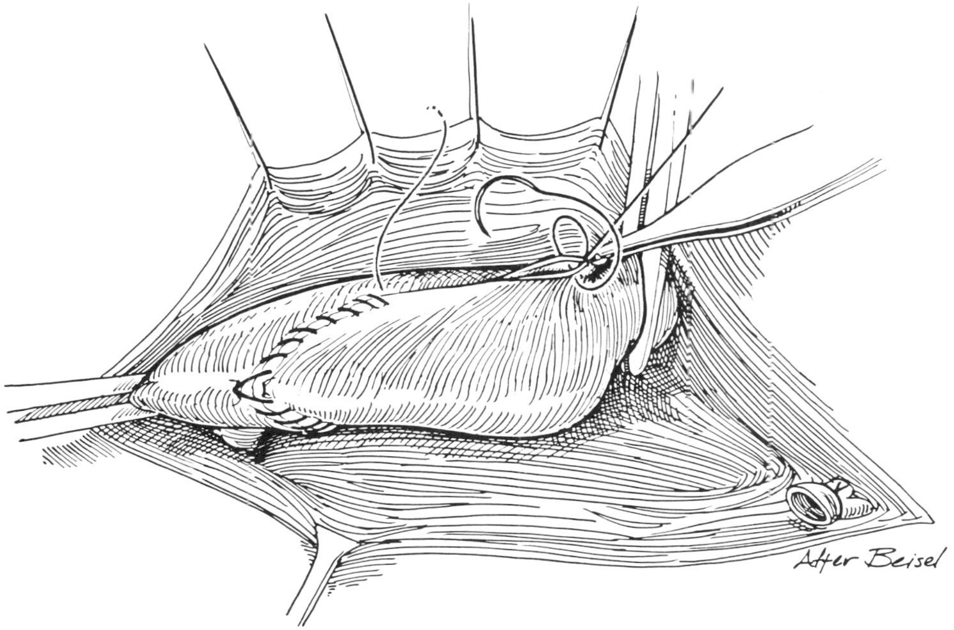

FIG. 3. Following sharp excision of the coarctation shelf, the opened subclavian artery is brought down as a flap across the opened aorta. After the apex sutures are placed, the repair is completed using a continuous absorbable vascular suture.

they are tied (Fig. 3). After completion of the suture lines the distal crossclamp is released slowly to evacuate air and to examine hemostasis. Any required simple sutures are placed. The proximal clamp then is gradually released, allowing resumption of lower body perfusion. The completed repair is illustrated in Figure 4. When hemostasis is achieved, the intercostal ties are released and the pleura is closed over the repair. The chest is closed after the insertion of a single apical–posterior chest tube.

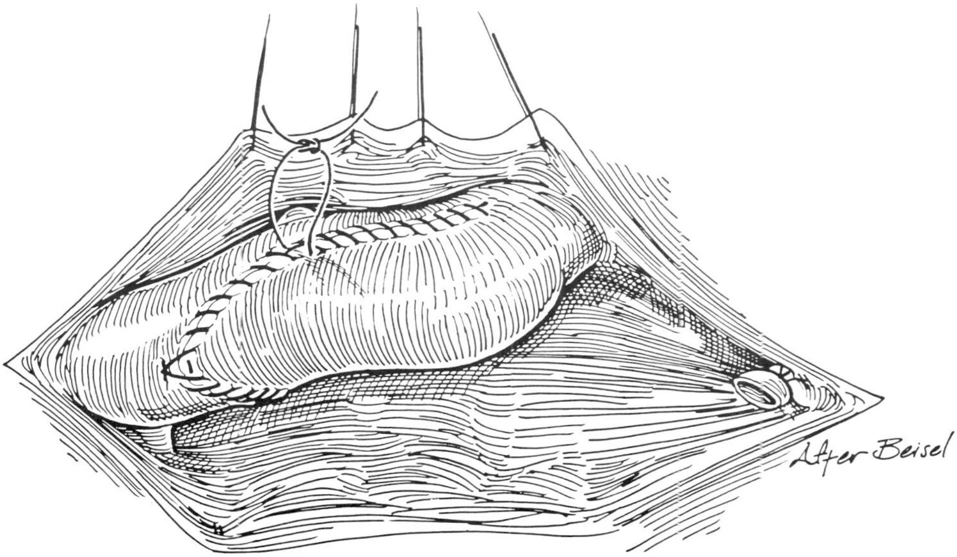

FIG. 4. Air is evacuated from the repaired area as crossclamps are removed before tying the final suture of the reconstruction.

Several technical points of the operation deserve further emphasis. Division of the subclavian artery at the origin of the vertebral artery provides a length which is adequate for the repair of coarctations in the preductal and juxtaductal locations. We have not seen any case which would require more length, and believe that further mobilization is both unnecessary and potentially hazardous to the collateral circulation of the arm. Because of the position of the takeoff of the subclavian vessel this is an anterolateral aortic repair, which must be kept in mind as the aorta is opened. The aortotomy must not be carried too far down on the aorta because of the risks of compromising the repair diameter and placing excessive tension on the flap. The goal of the operation is to enlarge the lumen of the aorta at the level of the coarctation. Providing increased circumference far beyond the narrowed segment serves no useful purpose. No tissue is trimmed from the flap or otherwise discarded.

The use of a continuous absorbable suture has been satisfactory during a follow-up period of up to 4 years, and minimal crossclamp times are a benefit. If nonabsorbable material is used, an interrupted suture technique allows optimal future growth. Continuous suture technique, with nonabsorbable material, is not advocated because of potential problems with intraluminal bowstringing[31] and limited growth.

Pulmonary Artery Banding

Concomitant pulmonary artery banding in patients with ventricular septal defects is a controversial topic.[32,33] In infants with restrictive ventricular septal defects, it is almost certainly not indicated, nor is it in infants with nonrestrictive ventricular septal defects. Recent trends are away from banding. Many small ventricular septal defects will close or become smaller in time, ultimately making the band unnecessary and, possibly, detrimental. If banding is omitted, and should congestive heart failure persist after coarctation repair, then repair of the ventricular septal defect is indicated. Only wider experience will clarify the need for this palliative operation.

On the other hand, infants with ventricular septal defects as part of complex anomalies often should be banded at the time of coarctation repair, since the corrective operation is quite complex and is more safely done after the patients have grown. If pulmonary artery banding is to be carried out, the band should be placed before clamps are applied to the aorta to help prevent flooding of the pulmonary circulation and the attendant intraoperative difficulties and instability. After the repair, the band is properly adjusted to reduce the distal pulmonary artery pressure to about one third of the systemic level.

Results

In our most recent 14-year series (1973–1987), 63 infants of less than 13 months of age have undergone subclavian flap repair of coarctation of the aorta at the Milton S. Hershey Medical Center of The Pennsylvania State University (Hershey, PA). Our indications for operation have been presented previously.[34] Of these patients, 40 were 1 month of age or younger. All coarctation patients were categorized as Group I (with or without patent ductus arteriosus [PDA] only), Group II (associated ventricular septal defect [VSD]) or Group III ("complex" associated intracardiac defects). Table 1 provides the breakdown of patients into these categories. Intracardiac lesions with significant shunting were found in 33 patients (52%) and consisted of ventricular septal defects either alone or in combination with other lesions. Table 1 also provides more specific information about the primary complex associated anomalies in the Group III patients. Significant intracardiac valve lesions were noted in 13 of 23 patients in this group.

There were two operative deaths (30-day mortality, 3%), and both infants had severe cardiac failure and marked systemic acidosis before operation. One was a one-day-old with hypoplastic left heart syndrome who also had an intramyocardial dye injection at the time of catheterization, the other, a gravely ill neonate with an associated PDA. This second child did not have the benefit of prostaglandin therapy before operation.

In the patients with significant intracardiac anomalies, 11 of 41 had concomitant pulmonary artery (PA) banding at the time of the subclavian flap procedure. The indication for banding in all cases was the preoperative assessment of massive left-to-right intracardiac shunting. Four of the Group II patients were banded; of the other seven infants, two had double-outlet right ventricle (DORV), two had transposition of the great arteries (TGA), one

TABLE 1. *Associated Anomalies and Operative Mortality (1973–1987): Sixty-Three Infants 12 Months of Age or Younger*

Coarctation of the thoracic aorta		
Group I		
±PDA only	22	1
Group II		
+VSD	18 (4*)	0
Group III (complex anomalies)		
+DORV	7 (2*)	0
+Mitral abnormalities	2	0
+Aortic valve abnormality	7 (1*)	0
+L-TGA	3 (2*)	0
+Hypoplastic left heart	2 (1*)	1
+A-V canal	2 (1*)	0
	63 (11*)	2 (3%)

DORV: double-outlet right ventricle; L-TGA: left transposition of the great arteries; A-V: atrioventricular.
* Indicates concomitant pulmonary artery banding

had a complete atrioventricular (A-V) canal defect, one had severe subvalvular aortic stenosis (AS) and VSD, and one had a hypoplastic left heart. There were no operative deaths in this combined procedure group.

In the immediate postoperative period, none of the infants in this series required drugs to control hypertension. Neither was there evidence of the abdominal pain syndrome which is seen occasionally in older children.

Nineteen children have undergone repeat catheterization between 2 months and 8 years after the subclavian flap procedure. Aortography has routinely revealed a near-normal appearing contour in the area of repair. A single patient in this series has required reoperation for recurrent aortic obstruction. This child had impressive isthmus hypoplasia and the repair, done at 3 days of age, was believed to have been satisfactory. Recatheterization, 3 years later, was performed to evaluate mitral stenosis, and demonstrated a gradient of 5 mmHg across the repaired coarctation. At the age of 8.5 years the presence of a significant gradient prompted reoperation and repair by resection and end-to-end anastomosis. Two patients have been found to have residual gradients of 20 mmHg or greater. All three of these patients were repaired by the subclavian flap method as neonates and continuous nonabsorbable suture material was used. Another 31 patients have had outpatient systolic blood pressure determinations, only four of which exceeded 100 mmHg. No patient has required long-term management with antihypertensive medication.

In the entire group, interrupted nonabsorbable suture was used in 26, continuous nonabsorbable suture in 17, and continuous absorbable suture (polydioxanone) in the most recent 20 patients. The running technique with absorbable suture now has been adopted as our operation of choice for infants and neonates, as the time required for repair is minimized and the handling qualities of the suture are judged to be quite satisfactory.

Twenty-five patients with associated intracardiac defects have undergone corrective operations after the original repair of the aorta with the subclavian flap; 15 children survived these procedures as listed in Table 2. Late death from pneumonia occurred in two other children with complex associated anomalies at 4 months and 6 months, respectively, after coarctation repair.

Limited follow-up studies on the growth of the arms have demonstrated no significant

TABLE 2. *Corrective Operations and Secondary Operative Mortality*

Group II	11 (2)
Group III	14 (9)

impairment in function and minimal, if any, shortening on the operated side. Exercise tolerance and gradients (noninvasive) after repair have been examined in some of these patients,[35] and no difference has been found between the group which underwent operation and age-matched controls. Seven children also have been closely evaluated in our noninvasive vascular laboratory and have been found to have both normal vascular resistance and normal blood flow in opposite forearms.[36]

Conclusion

The subclavian flap procedure for the repair of coarctation of the aorta has proven to be an effective operation since its introduction in 1966. In our opinion, it is the operation of choice for repair of coarctation in neonates and infants. We have used successfully it in children up to the age of 3 years, especially in cases of long segment coarctation. Intensive preoperative preparation, including the use of prostaglandin E1, results in stabilized infants who tolerate the operation more readily. Excellent growth of the aorta after repair and the low operative mortality is associated with subclavian flap repair of this anomaly. The long-term outlook for patients with complex associated heart disease is guarded, but both morbidity and mortality are determined by the intracardiac anomalies. We believe that the subclavian flap procedure offers the best surgical repair of coarctation of the aorta in infants and has, in follow-up, yielded the best long-term results.

REFERENCES

1. Rudolf AM, Heymann MA, Spitznas V. Hemodynamic considerations in the development of narrowing of the aorta. Am J Cardiol 1972;30:514.
2. Talner NS, Berman MA. Postnatal development of obstruction in coarctation of the aorta: Role of the ductus arteriosus. Pediatrics 1975;56:562–569.
3. Heymann MA, Berman W Jr, Rudolph AM, Whitman V. Dilatation of the ductus arteriosus by prostaglandin E1 in aortic arch abnormalities. Circulation 1979;59:169–173.
4. Graham TP, Atwood GF, Boucek RJ. Use of prostaglandin E1 for emergency palliation of symptomatic coarctation of the aorta. Cathet Cardiovasc Diagn 1978;4:97–102.
5. Crafoord C, Nylin G. Congenital coarctation of the aorta and its surgical treatment. J Thorac Cardiovasc Surg 1945;14:347–352.
6. Campbell J, Delorenzi R, Brown J *et al.* Improved results in newborns undergoing coarctation repair. Ann Thorac Surg 1980;30:273–277.
7. Barbero-Marcial M, Berginelli G, Sirera JC, Ebaid M, Zerbini EJ. Surgical treatment of coarctation of the aorta in the first year of life: Immediate and late results in 35 patients. Thorac Cardiovasc Surgeon 1982;30:75–78.
8. Groves LK, Effler DB. Problems in the surgical management of coarctation of the aorta. J Thorac Cardiovasc Surg 1960;39:60–90.
9. Pennington DG, Lithbertson RR, Jacobs M *et al.* Critical review of experience with surgical repair of coarctation of the aorta. J Thoracic Cardiovasc Surg 1979;77:217–229.
10. Herrmann VM, Laks H, Fagan L *et al.* Repair of aortic coarctation in the first year of life. Ann Thorac Surg 1978;25:57–63.
11. Patel R, Singh SP, Abrahms L, Roberts KD. Coarctation of the aorta with special reference to infants: Long-term results of operation in 1261 cases. Br Heart J 1977;39:1246–1253.
12. Williams WG, Shindo G, Trusler GA *et al.* Results of repair of coarctation of the aorta during infancy. J Thorac Cardiovasc Surg 1980;79:603–608.
13. Shinebourne EA, Tam ASY, Elseed AM *et al.* Coarctation of the aorta in infancy and childhood. Br Heart J 1976;38:375–380.
14. Bjork VO, Bergdahl L, Jhonasson R. Coarctation of the aorta: The world's longest follow-up. Adv Cardiol 1978;22:205–215.
15. Bergdahl L, Jhonasson R, Bjork VO. Late results of operation in children with coarctation of the aorta. Scand J Thor Cardiovasc Surg 1980;14:83–89.
16. Beekman RH, Rocchini AP, Behrendt DM, Rosenthal A. Reoperation for coarctation of the aorta. Am J Cardiol 1981;48:1108–1114.
17. Pollack P, Freed MD, Castaneda AR, Norwood WI. Reoperation for coarctation of the aorta: Follow-up of 26 patients. Am J Cardiol 1983;51:1690–1694.
18. Emmrich K, Herbst M, Trenckmann H, Schultz HG, Wohlgemuth B. Severe late complications after operative correction of aortic coarctation by interposition of prosthesis. J Cardiovasc Surg 1982;23:205–208.
19. Singer MI, Rowen M, Dorsey TJ. Transluminal aortic balloon angioplasty for coarctation of the aorta in the newborn. Am Heart Journal 1982;103:131–132.
20. Waldhausen JA, Nahrwold DL. Repair of coarctation of the aorta with a subclavian flap. J Thorac Cardiovasc Surg 1966;51:532–533.
21. Hamilton DI, DiEusanio G, Sandrasagea FA, Donnelly RJ. Early and late results of aortoplasty with

a left subclavian flap for coarctation of the aorta in infancy. J Thorac Cardiovasc Surg 1978;75:699–704.
22. Thibault WN, Sperling DR, Gazzaniga AB. Subclavian artery patch angioplasty: Treatment of infants and young children with aortic coarctation. Arch Surg 1975;110:1095–1098.
23. Midgley FM, Scott LP, Perry LW, McClenathan JE. Subclavian flap aortoplasty for treatment of coarctation in early infancy. J Pediatr Surg 1978;13:265–268.
24. Pierce WS, Waldhausen JA, Berman W Jr, Whitman V. Late results of the subclavian flap procedure in infants with coarctation of the thoracic aorta. Circulation 1978;(Suppl)58:78.
25. Bergdahl LAL, Blackstone EH, Kirklin JW, Pacifico AD, Bargeron LM. Determinants of early success in repair of aortic coarctation in infants. J Thorac Cardiovasc Surg 1982;83:736–742.
26. Folges GM Jr, Shah KD. Subclavian steal in patients with Blalock-Taussig anastomosis. Circulation 1965;31:241–246.
27. Kent JV. Development of rib notching after surgical intervention in congenital heart disease with a description of two cases. Br J Radiol 1953;26:346–351.
28. Reivich M, Holling EH, Roberts B, Toole JF. Reversal of blood flow through the vertebral artery and its effect on cerebral circulation. N Engl J Med 1961;265:878–885.
29. Todd PJ, Dangerfield PH, Damilton DI, Wilkinson JL. Late effects on the left upper limb of subclavian flap aortoplasty. J Thorac Cardiovasc Surg 1983;85:678–681.
30. Pae WE, Myers JL, Waldhausen JA, Prophet GA, Pierce WS. Subclavian flap angioplasty: Experimental study in growing piglets. J Thorac Cardiovasc Surg 1981;82:922–927.
31. Myers JL, Waldhausen JA, Pae WE, Abt AB, Prophet GA, Pierce WS. Vascular anastomoses in growing vessels: The use of absorbable sutures. Annals Thorac Surg 1982;34:529–535.
32. Myers JL, Campbell DB, Waldhausen JA. The use of absorbable monofilament polydioxanone suture in pediatric cardiovascular surgery. J Thorac Cardiovasc Surg 1986;92:771–775.
33. Neches WH, Park SC, Lenox CC *et al.* Coarctation of the aorta with VSD. Circulation 1977;55:189–194.
34. Leanage R, Taylor JFN, DeLeval MR, Stark J, Macartney FJ. Surgical management of coarctation of aorta with ventricular septal defect: Multivariate analysis. Br Heart J 1981;46:269–276.
35. Waldhausen JA, Whitman V, Werner JC, Pierce WS. Surgical intervention in infants with coarctation of the aorta. J Thorac Cardiovasc Surg 1981;81:323–325.
36. Fripp RR, Whitman V, Werner JC, Nicholas GG, Waldhausen JA Blood pressure response to exercise in children following the subclavian flap procedure for coarctation of the aorta. J Thorac Cardiovasc Surg 1983;85:682–685.
37. Sinoway LI, Shenberger J, Prophet S *et al.* Left forearm vascular function following subclavian flap repair for aortic coarctation (Abstr). J Am Col Cardiol (submitted for publication).

Discussion

Dr. Gordon Danielson: I think John has made a great contribution to our understanding of this problem. John, there has been some evidence that aneurysms might eventually form if a patch is used. One theory is that the ductal tissue you leave behind in this operation might cause problems later on. With the subclavian flap operation, there is a very low incidence of late coarctation, but are you concerned that you might end up with the ductal dilatation?

Dr. John Waldhausen: To my knowledge, there has never been an aneurysm reported with the flap procedure. The aneurysms are primarily related to use of prosthetic patches. The reason for this is not totally clear, but it may be that they stem from a mismatch of the patient's tissue with a rather rigid prosthesis. In any case, I know it is a very common problem with prosthetic patches, but I've not seen one or heard of one with the subclavian flap.

Dr. Stan Dudrick: You mentioned that you might have to go back at a second stage to do something about the pulmonary artery. How often did you have to go back in your series?

Dr. John Waldhausen: All patients that have intracardiac defects ultimately undergo repair. So, once you take one of these kids on and get them through the first stage, you keep operating on them until you correct these intracardiac defects.

Dr. Jim Hardy: What is the longest follow-up of a patient after the subclavian flap operation?

Dr. John Waldhausen: I did the first one in 1963 and that child is still well. By the way, one major concern that has been raised is what is the blood flow to the arm like. We recently did a study that's not yet published in which, interestingly enough, blood flow to the arm was found to be normal compared to the other arm, presumably because the collateral circulation is so good.

Dr. Mark Ravitch: How about the length of the arm and of the bones of the arm?

Dr. John Waldhausen: Surprisingly, that's a difficult thing to answer conclusively because it turns out that we all have unequal arm length. There are probably some minor differences in these patients, and when I say minor, I am talking about a centimeter or so but even that is a little bit shaky because people don't have equal arm length.

Dr. Mark Ravitch: I thought almost certainly that Dr. Taussig wrote a book about the thousand or more blue babies she followed over many years, but it is not mentioned in any of her papers. Dr. O'Neill knows about her material and they never did make those measurements.

Dr. John Waldhausen: The only person I know of who ever did make measurements is a surgeon in Liverpool, England, by the name of Hamilton, a pediatric cardiac surgeon, and his study suggested there may be a slight difference between the two but it is minimal. One accurate way of measuring arm length would be with x-rays. That is what I wanted to do, but the pediatricians wouldn't agree. They said these would be unnecessary x-rays, so we haven't done this.

DR. STAN DUDRICK: John, on the blood flow studies to the arm, are they also normal with exercise?

DR. JOHN WALDHAUSEN: Yes, they respond to exercise normally.

DR. STAN DUDRICK: And did you have aortograms?

DR. JOHN WALDHAUSEN: We have aortograms on a lot of them because they are restudied prior to their intracardiac repair, and although the arm has not been looked at specifically, the arch looks good.

Introduction of Dr. James Hardy

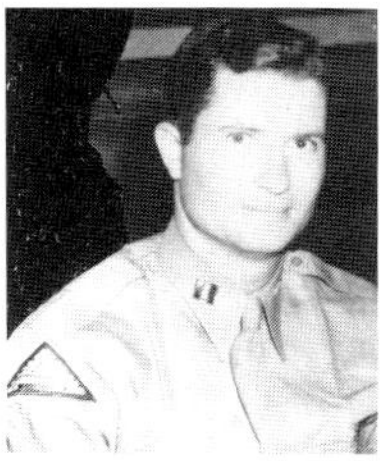

Dr. Clyde Barker: Our next speaker is Jim Hardy whose name has been familiar to me since I was a boy, long before I was in medicine. Jim Hardy and my brother Hal went through the war in Europe together, and Hal's letters home frequently mentioned Jim Hardy. Before the war, Jim was a medical resident at the University Hospital, and the Department files have a letter in which T. Greer Miller (of the Miller-Abbot tube) describes Jim as the best medical resident he ever knew. This slide shows Jim in uniform just after the war when he transferred from the medical program into surgery. He completed the surgical residency here in 1951. He then became Director of Surgical Research at the University of Tennessee, and in 1955, he went to the University of Mississippi as Professor and Chairman of a department there that has flourished remarkably under his guidance. Jim was a boy wonder who never looked back. His major contributions to the fields of cardiac, vascular, and transplantation surgery include the performance of the first heart and the first lung transplant in man. No wonder Mark Ravitch, in his book, *A Century of Surgery,* notes that Jim Hardy is "as multi-faceted a clinician and investigator as there is." His article today is entitled "The First Clinical Lung and Heart Transplants: Scientific Bases and Societal Dimensions in Retrospect."

Some of you might think that however broad his interests, Dr. Rhoads would have had nothing to do with transplantation. However, I can tell you that that is not true. At the time I was working on basic transplantation biology with Rupert Billingham in a lab jointly supported by him and Dr. Rhoads, Dr. Billingham told me of a paper by Dr Rhoads that he considered quite important. It appeared in 1948, long before the importance of the thymus was clearly understood. The article, by Harris, Rhoads, and Stokes, was entitled "A Study of the Role of the Thymus and Spleen in the Formation of Antibodies in the Rabbit" (*J Immunol* 58:27–32, 1948). Another of Dr. Rhoads' publications that has great relevance to transplantation deals with a related strategy for replacement of organ function. It was written in 1938 and describes what I believe to be the earliest experience anywhere with peritoneal dialysis (Rhoads, J. E.: Peritoneal Lavage in the Treatment of Renal Insufficiency. *Am J Med Sci* 196:642–647, 1938).

Incidentally, if it hadn't been for his confidence in me as a very junior faculty member and his generosity and support, I could never have started the transplant program at HUP. I continue to be very grateful for that opportunity.

Dr. James Hardy's Introductory Remarks

Thank you, Dr. Barker, for your most generous introduction. And I am very happy to learn of Dr. Miller's letter to Dr. Ravdin at the time when I was trying very hard to get a residency in surgery, with the disadvantage of still being in the Army.

I am sure that Dr. Rhoads knows what a pleasure and honor it is for me to be here to help celebrate his birthday, for Dr. Rhoads was indirectly responsible for my choosing the academic career. It came about in this way. When in 1950 I began to look for a job to support my new family, I went to Dr. Rhoads for advice. I had been offered a lucrative position in private practice in Dallas. He said, "Well, Jim, you should go down and look the situation over. But let's say you make 50 thousand dollars the first 10 years and put it in the bank. What are you going to do the next 10 years, the same thing? I have watched you since you were a medical student and you are at home in the laboratory, a rarity in a surgical resident. If you could get your heavy water (measurements of total body water) going, I think you would be useful to a good many departments of surgery." I went to Dallas, looked around, and returned to Philadelphia: "Dr. Rhoads, I'm going to make that heavy water work!"

Now, I am going to be talking about research that we began in our laboratory 30 years ago. If some of it looks primitive by today's standards, it was primitive by today's standards. And I ask you to bear this in mind.

When Watts Webb and I arrived in Jackson in 1955, we launched into the development of open heart surgery, and lung and heart (and kidney) transplantation research fit readily into this objective.

The First Lung (1963) and Heart (1964) Transplants in Man: Scientific Bases and Societal Dimensions in Retrospect

JAMES D. HARDY, M.D., F.A.C.S.

THIS IS A VERY SPECIAL DAY for all of us who have so long known and so long admired Jonathan E. Rhoads. I came to know him the first full day I was ever in Philadelphia, in September of 1938. It came about in this way. Members of the Phi Chi medical fraternity had escorted me over to the University Hospital, the mecca for all medical students at the University of Pennsylvania, to watch an operation, this being the favorite medical fraternity rush activity. There Dr. Isidor S. Ravdin was performing a cholecystectomy but, when he saw us in the observation gallery, he stood back from the operating table, introduced Dr. Jonathan Rhoads who was continuing the operation and, as they say, the rest is history. In point of fact, Dr. Rhoads is responsible for the research which I present in this report. For it was he who encouraged me to stay in academic surgery, at that special time when all finishing residents must consider carefully what direction their professional future is to take. For this alone, but also for many other things, I shall always treasure the rich privilege of my almost 50-year association with Jonathan Evans Rhoads.

The work I present here goes back a long time. In the broad sweep of medical history, there come moments when it is possible to perceive the end of one era and the start of a new one. Such a historical watershed is clearly at hand with respect to clinical organ transplantation. Someone has characterized clinical organ transplantation as the general surgeon's tomorrow.

Today heart transplants are performed so commonly that this operation occasions only interested attention in many institutions, as it now does in our own hospital. But it was not always so. In fact, it would not be possible to impart to a young surgeon, just now entering the field of organ transplantation, the huge excitement and challenge which its early pioneers felt in the late 1950s and the early 1960s. It was during such a time that we began to investigate in the laboratory the techniques of lung, heart, and heart–lung transplantation. Our studies of heart transplantation were begun by Watts R. Webb in 1956. He was able to achieve early survival of dogs by the following year. Somewhat later, Fikri Alican and I began studies of lung transplantation in various species of animals, largely dogs, resulting in a number of related publications. Time does not permit detailed documentation here of the remarks I shall make, but pertinent references will appear in the published manuscript. Not all the studies had been published before the clinical transplants, but most were under way. Furthermore, it should also be appreciated that many workers contributed to our studies of heart and lung transplantation at the University of Mississippi, and that similar investigations were being carried out elsewhere.[1–4]

Lung Transplantation

Experimental Studies

Operative technique: The first objective of our single lung transplantation studies was to establish, in our own laboratory, a dependable and consistently successful operative technique for lung reimplantation in dogs. This was achieved by using a left atrial cuff for anastomosis of the pulmonary veins, plus anastomoses of the pulmonary artery and bronchus (Figs. 1A and 1B). Early bronchial leakage or late bronchial stenosis proved to be less

From the Department of Surgery, University of Mississippi Medical Center, Jackson, Mississippi.

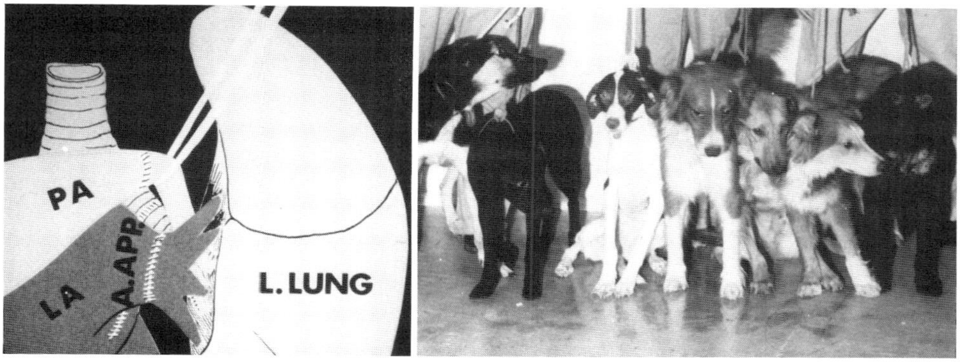

FIGS. 1A AND 1B. (A, left) Operative technique for lung transplantation. (B, right) Colony of dogs surviving on the reimplanted left lung, with ligation of the right pulmonary artery.

frequent than had been expected. Of 68 dogs in which either the right or left lung was reimplanted, 33 were long-term survivors.

Respiratory studies of the reimplanted lung: Once animal survival had been achieved, we proceeded to investigate the function of the reimplanted lung.[5] The colony of 33 chronic survivors was divided into four groups and subjected to further surgical procedures on the contralateral lung, as follows: (1) contralateral pneumonectomy, (2) contralateral pneumonectomy and reimplantation, (3) contralateral pulmonary artery ligation (Figs. 1A and 1B), and (4) contralateral multiple lobectomies.

Respiratory reflexes: The dogs in the first two groups, in which of course the nerves had been divided, displayed characteristic patterns of slow, deep respirations with the participation of accessory muscles. None were long-term survivors. In the third and fourth groups, where the nerves had remained intact, the respiratory pattern remained in the normal range, and long-term survivors were obtained unless severe pulmonary edema had developed. It was concluded that, whereas respiratory reflexes might not always be absolutely essential, the animal without respiratory reflexes was at a very serious disadvantage. Microscopic studies showed that early degeneration of the lung nerve fibers[6] was followed by regeneration at 6 to 18 months. Incidentally, the Hering-Breuer reflex, lost after lung transplantation, later was shown to have been restored in five of six chronic dogs restudied 4 years after bilateral lung reimplantation.[7] Moreover, the function and compliance of these reimplanted lungs at 4 years was almost normal, with normal pulmonary artery pressure and pulmonary vascular resistance; but there was a somewhat higher right to left shunt than normal.

Function of the transplant: Effect of differential division of hilar tissue: It had been found—by differential bronchospirometry and oxygen uptake measurements, lung scans and other modalities—that the function of the reimplanted lung fell to approximately 50% the preoperative value, over the first several days postoperatively, but that commonly its function gradually returned almost to normal by the end of approximately 2 weeks.[8] For this reason, 43 dogs were divided into four groups and differential stripping or division of the following structures at the left pulmonary hilium was carried out: (1) the bronchus, pulmonary artery, and pulmonary veins were freed up from the surrounding tissue but were left intact (ten dogs); (2) the bronchial and hilar adventitial arteries were ligated and divided (ten dogs); (3) the lymphatics were severed (five dogs); and (4) the vagus nerve was severed high in the neck (18 dogs). In brief, the loss of vagal innervation was found to impair both ventilation and oxygen uptake of the lung. Division of the bronchial arteries and the lymphatics did not appear, under the circumstances of this study, to affect function of the reimplanted lung. However, in a later study involving the regeneration of divided bronchial lymphatics, there was at least a positive correlation between the improving lung function and the regeneration of lymphatics at from 7 to 12 days.[9]

Bilateral lung reimplantation: Despite numerous modalities for studying the function of the reimplanted lung, the best test of lung function was achieved by studying animals both of whose lungs had been reimplanted at staged operations or at the same operation.[10] Here there could be no question but that the entire respiratory activity was being provided by reimplanted lung tissue. The virtually normal function of such reimplanted lungs was noted previously. (The operative technique of immediate one-stage bilateral lung reimplantation later was to prove particularly valuable in the assessment of lung function after one-stage bilateral allotransplantation of the lung.) The function of bronchial cilia after lung reimplantation was not studied in our laboratory but was studied elsewhere.[11]

Lung growth in puppies: We were asked by a pediatrician caring for children with cystic fibrosis whether or not a lung transplanted in a child would grow. We reimplanted the left lung in puppies, and the chronic survivors exhibited normal growth in both the size and the function of the reimplanted lung.[12]

Lung storage: A very large number of experiments were directed toward achieving long-term lung storage but, suffice it to say, rather little progress was made in that direction. The lung tolerated cold storage for 2 to 3 hours, but longer storage, even at elevated ambient oxygen concentrations, commonly was followed by a bloody pulmonary edema after reimplantation.

Lung Allotransplantation

Once the essential baseline data for lung reimplantation had been achieved, attention was turned to single-lung allotransplantation.[13] This added, to the pathophysiology of lung transplantation itself, the immunologic factors involved in the homograft or allograft rejection reaction. The left lung was transplanted from an unrelated dog in 107 animals so studied, utilizing various protocols and modalities. The mean survival time of control animals was approximately 7.4 days. In contrast, 20 of 34 surviving animals treated with Imuran (azathioprine) in a dosage of 4.0 mg per kg per day by mouth lived an average of 30.4 days. Two of the 20 were permanent survivors, but when sacrificed many months later it was found that the homografted lung had been rejected at some time in the past and was encased in a fibrous envelope. The angiocardiogram in one of these two permanent survivors had been remarkably normal on the day before sacrifice, and this again emphasized that only by differential lung function studies, or by ligation of the contralateral pulmonary artery, or by sacrifice of the animal could one be certain of the state of the allografted lung. The normal microscopic picture of the lung tissue exhibited a progressive loss of normal architecture (Figs. 2A and 2B). Many other studies of single lung allotransplantation were performed later on, comparing azathioprine, azathioprine–prednisone, azathioprine–actinomycin C, and methotrexate for immunosuppression, but survival times were not increased significantly.

One-stage allotransplantation of both lungs: Despite ligation of the contralateral pulmonary artery, bronchospirometry and oxygen uptake measurements, lung scans and pulmonary arteriograms, the true functional capacity of the allotransplanted lung tissue always re-

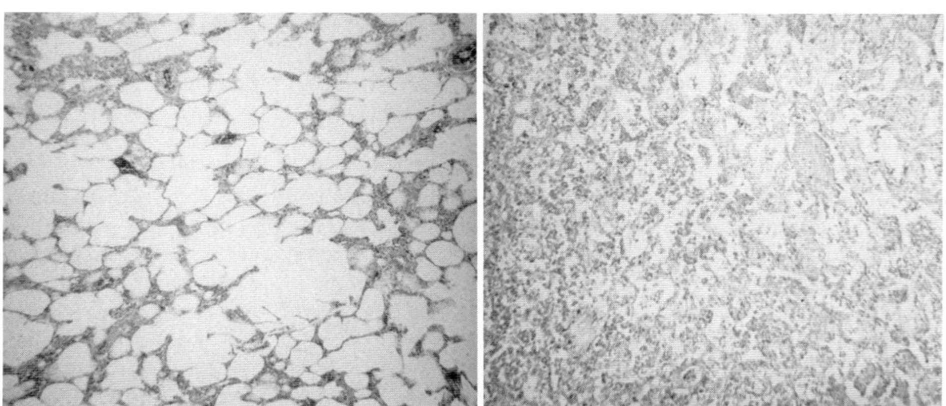

FIGS. 2A AND 2B. (A, left) Microscopic picture of normal canine lung. (B, right) Rejected lung allograft. Notice virtually complete loss of the normal lung architecture. (From: Hardy JD *et al.*[13])

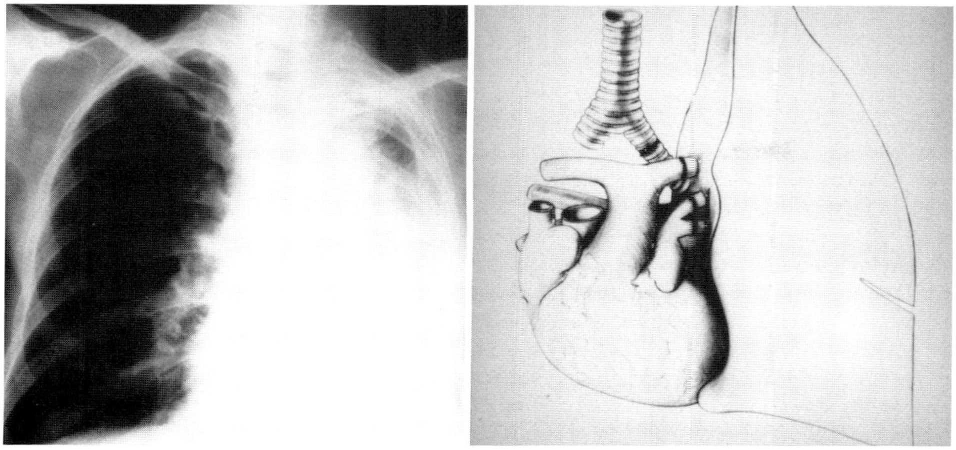

FIGS. 3A AND 3B. (A, left) Almost complete collapse of left lung secondary to carcinoma of the left main stem bronchus. (Reprinted with permission from Hardy JD *et al.* Lung homotransplantation in man: Report of the initial case. JAMA 1963;186:1066. © 1963, American Medical Association.) (B, right) Operative technique employed for transplantation of first human lung (see text). (Reprinted with permission from Hardy JD. The transplantation of organs. Surgery 1964;56:699.)

mained somewhat uncertain until only allotransplanted lung tissue remained in the animal. This desideratum was achieved by one-stage allotransplantation of both lungs in 33 dogs.[14] Eight dogs serving as an untreated control group died of pulmonary edema and early rejection changes within 2 to 5 days. Immunosuppressive treatment in the remaining dogs prolonged survival, but rejection eventually occurred. In a similar study, bilateral allotransplantation in 58 animals resulted in 40 survivors.[15] Two dogs in the treatment group were long-term survivors, the longest survival well over 1 year.

The First Lung Transplant in Man

In the early spring of 1963, my colleague Watts Webb and I went to Dean and Vice Chancellor Robert Q. Marston and reviewed with him our extensive studies in animals. We requested permission to move toward lung transplantation in man if a suitable occasion and need should arise. He agreed.

A number of possible lung recipients were considered and carefully studied over the months, but it was not until June that an acceptable patient presented.[16,17] The 58-year-old man, a long-time heavy smoker, had far-advanced emphysema and respiratory distress even at bed rest. A large carcinoma of the left main stem bronchus had produced extensive infection distal to the obstruction, and this infection had not responded to antibiotic therapy. The left lung was virtually collapsed and contributing little to the respiratory support of the patient (Fig. 3A). Furthermore, it was the left lung that was involved, rendering transplantation more readily achieved technically than had it been the right lung that was involved. Thus, (1) the patient was in chronic pulmonary insufficiency, (2) he had a probably incurable disease (the advanced lung cancer), (3) thoracotomy was required to manage the distal infection, (4) no significant amount of functioning left lung would be removed by left pneumonectomy, (5) there was a reasonable possibility that his respiration would be improved, and (6) the patient and his family were willing to try lung transplantation to relieve his dyspnea.

Three negative considerations were (1) the fact that significant infection existed in the left lung distal to the malignancy, complicating immunosuppressive therapy, (2) he had a considerable degree of chronic renal impairment, and (3) the transplant might not function effectively and relieve his respiratory distress. However, after much deliberation we elected to proceed with transplantation. One surgical team would perform the left thoracotomy on the patient and the other team would remove the cadaver lung in an adjacent operating room. Tissue typing was not available to us at the time.

A number of days elapsed before a cadaver lung became available, but at approximately 7:30 PM on the evening of June 11, 1963, a patient was admitted to the emergency room with acute heart failure due to myocardial infarction and died almost immediately. The family gave permission for autopsy and donation of the left lung. The donor was ABO group B and the recipient ABO group A.[17]

The operative technique employed is shown in Figure 3B. The superior and inferior pulmonary veins of the donor lung were anastomosed to the superior and inferior pulmonary veins of the recipient. The pulmonary artery and the bronchial anastomoses then were carried out. The donor lung had been ventilated intermittently with oxygen throughout the hour that was required to insert the new lung. The patient had been anesthetized using a double-lumened endotracheal tube. The transplant was expanded readily by the anesthesiologist as soon as the bronchus had been unclamped. The transplant functioned immediately as an effective organ of respiration, as reflected in blood samples taken from the pulmonary artery and the pulmonary veins of the transplant. The chest was closed with some initial concern, due to the disparity in size between the chronically contracted left hemithorax and the large donor lung. Nonetheless, this closure was achieved satisfactorily, and the planned tracheostomy was performed.

The early postoperative course was a smooth one (Figs. 4A and 4B). The transplanted lung functioned well immediately and the arterial oxygen saturation remained generally in the ninety-eighth percentile during almost all the 18 days of his life. The immunosuppressive drug therapy consisted of azathioprine and prednisolone, and a total of approximately 875 roentgens of radiation was directed to the mediastinum and thymic area. The cause of death was basically a slow but steady increase in azotemia and renal failure. As previously noted, the patient had had significant renal impairment, with borderline compensation, preoperatively, and the stress of the thoracotomy with the transplantation had precipitated uremia. He was dialyzed and hyperkalemia was never a problem, but the usual poor prognosis of postoperative renal failure eventuated in a fatal outcome. Autopsy revealed virtually no gross or microscopic evidence of rejection of the transplant (Figs. 5A–5D). Of course, the incipient uremia could well have exerted an additional immunosuppressive effect.

In sum, this first lung transplant in man, although not achieving long-term success, did in fact show that the technical procedures of the laboratory were satisfactory for the clinic, that the transplanted lung functioned immediately and effectively as an organ of respiration, and that the current immunosuppression modalities could achieve an abrogation of the allograft reaction for at least the duration of this patient's life. Inasmuch as the carcinoma had been found at operation to involve the hilum and the parietal pleura as well as the bronchus and

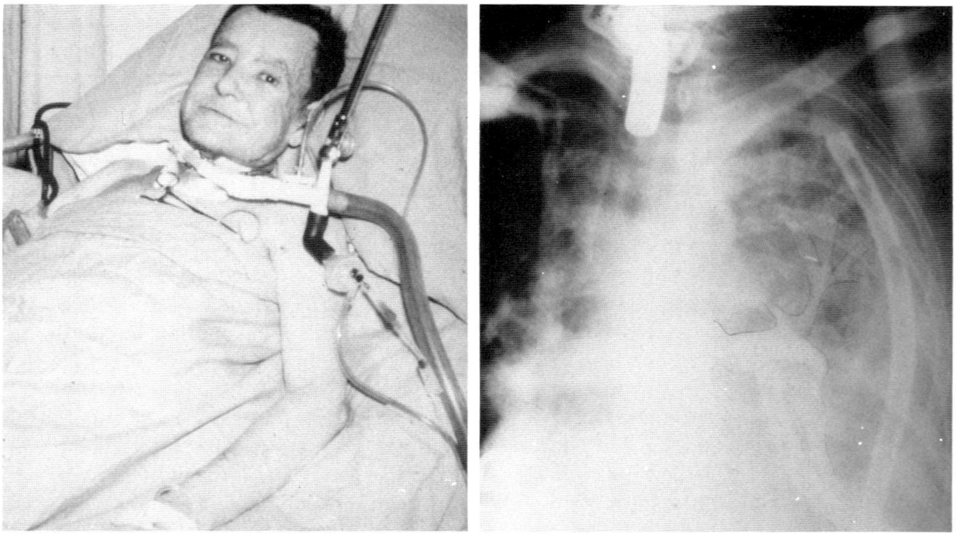

FIGS. 4A AND 4B. (A, left) John R. Russell. The first human lung transplant recipient. (B, right) Postoperative left pulmonary arteriogram. There is slight narrowing of the pulmonary artery at the site of the anastomosis. The lung itself is well expanded. (Reprinted with permission from Hardy JD *et al.* Lung homotransplantation in man: Report of the initial case. JAMA 1963;186:1071. © 1963, American Medical Association.)

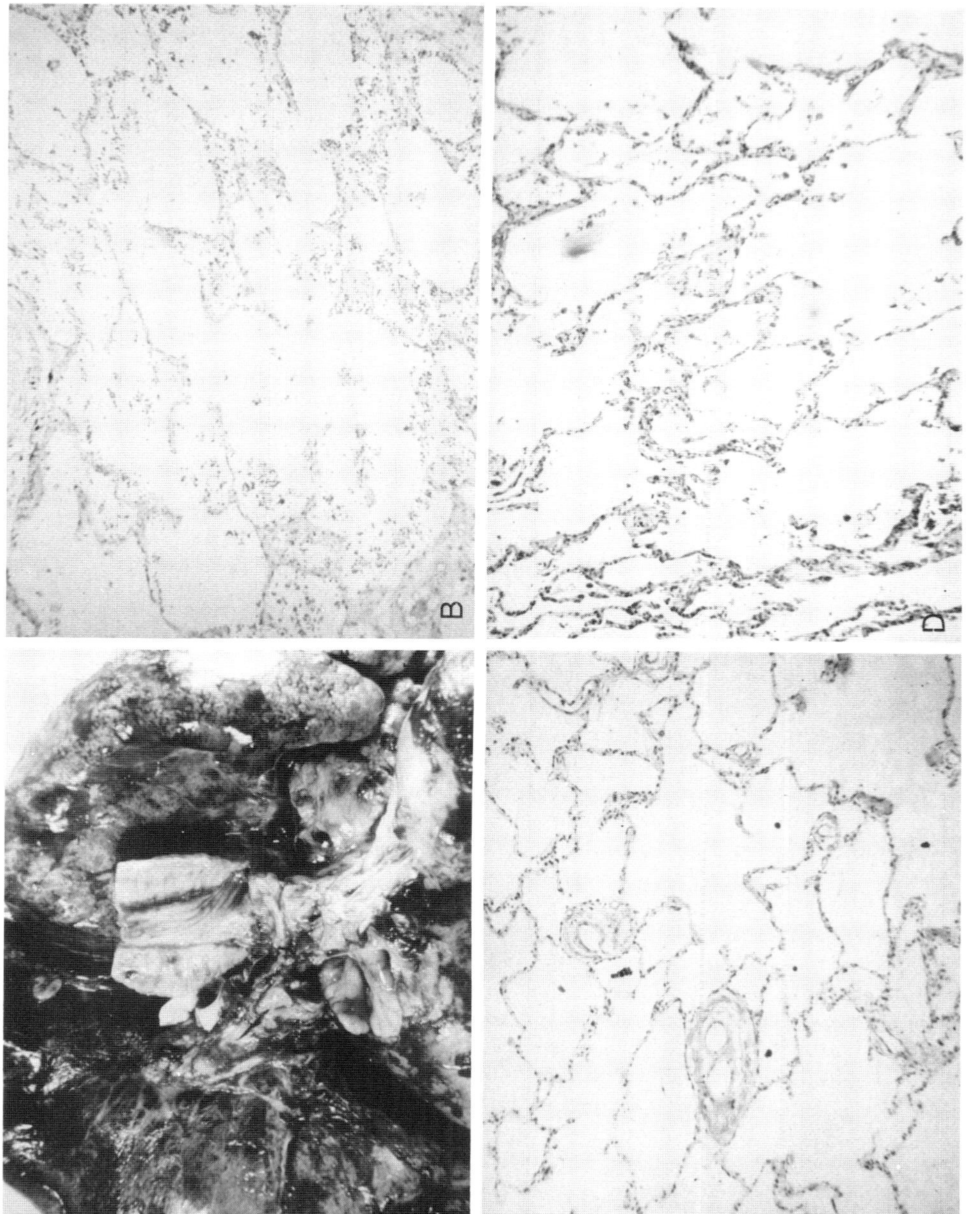
A
B
C
D

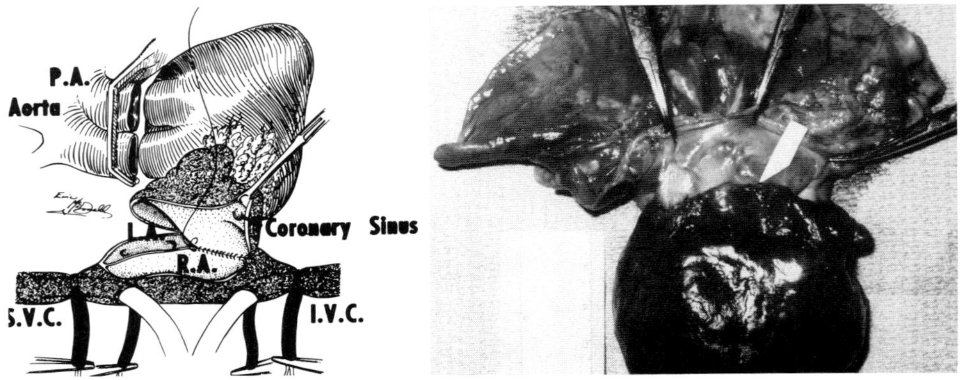

FIGS. 6A AND 6B. (A, left) Operative technique for heart transplantation. The SA node should be preserved. (Reprinted with permission from Hardy JD, Chavez CM. The first heart transplant in man: Historical reexamination of the 1964 case in the light of current clinical experience. Transpl Proc 1969;1:717.) (B, right) The gross appearance of a rejected canine allograft. Notice the healthy, glistening atria above, as compared to the dark, "beefy" appearance of the rejected ventricles. The visible portions of the atria were those of the recipient animal and thus were not rejected.

thus was incurable, we had achieved this transplantation milestone without substantially shortening a patient's life. In this respect, therefore, we considered the transplant a scientific success, achieved under acceptable moral and ethical circumstances.

Heart Transplantation

Heart transplantation was begun by Webb in our laboratories in 1956.[18–20] Emphasis at that time was placed on combined heart–lung transplantation, and these studies involved reimplants and homologous transplants of the heart and both lungs, and transplantation of the heart combined with one lung. These heart–lung transplantations, performed without the pump-oxygenator, were achieved using hypothermia combined with vascular coupling devices to permit rapid restoration of blood flow. Following six technically successful heart–lung transplants, the animals lived from 75 minutes to 22 hours. A movie of one such animal exercising was presented at the Clinical Congress of the American College of Surgeons.

These heart–lung transplants were continued, but in due course the major thrust was directed toward simple heart reimplantation and allotransplantation in various animals, but particularly in dogs and lower primates (monkeys). Basically, our operative technique for heart reimplantation or allotransplantation became that described by Lower *et al.* in 1961.[21] In this technique, anastomosis of the venous structures is avoided by anastomosing left atrium to left atrium and right atrium to right atrium, with the additional anastomoses of the pulmonary artery and the aorta (Figs. 6A and 6B).

First a large number of cardiac reimplantations were performed to study various parameters of operative technique, organ storage, cardiac function (Fig. 7A), and animal survival.[22] As others had shown, eventually we were able to demonstrate return of cardiac innervation in most chronic autotransplant dogs and in some allotransplant dogs.[23] Next, attention was turned to cardiac allotransplantation and the modalities available for preventing rejection. One of the main problems met, in achieving effective immunosuppression, was that only cardiac output values and changes in the electrocardiogram (Fig. 7B) then were available for regulating the immunosuppressive therapy as needed to suppress impending rejection. The electrocardiogram of the rejecting heart exhibited diminished voltage and, not infrequently,

FIGS. 5A–5D. (A, top left) The lungs at autopsy. Notice the full volume of the left (darker) transplanted lung. (Reprinted with permission from Hardy JD *et al.* Lung homotransplantation in man: Report of the initial case. JAMA 1963;186:1072. © 1963, American Medical Association.) (B, top right) The microscopic picture of the right (nontransplanted) lung. Compare this with the transplant immediately below, which exhibits less cellular infiltration. (C, bottom left) Photomicrograph of lung transplant before its insertion. (D, bottom right) The transplant at autopsy. (Reprinted with permission from Hardy JD *et al.* Lung homotransplantation in man: Report of the initial case. JAMA 1963;186:1072. © 1963, American Medical Association.)

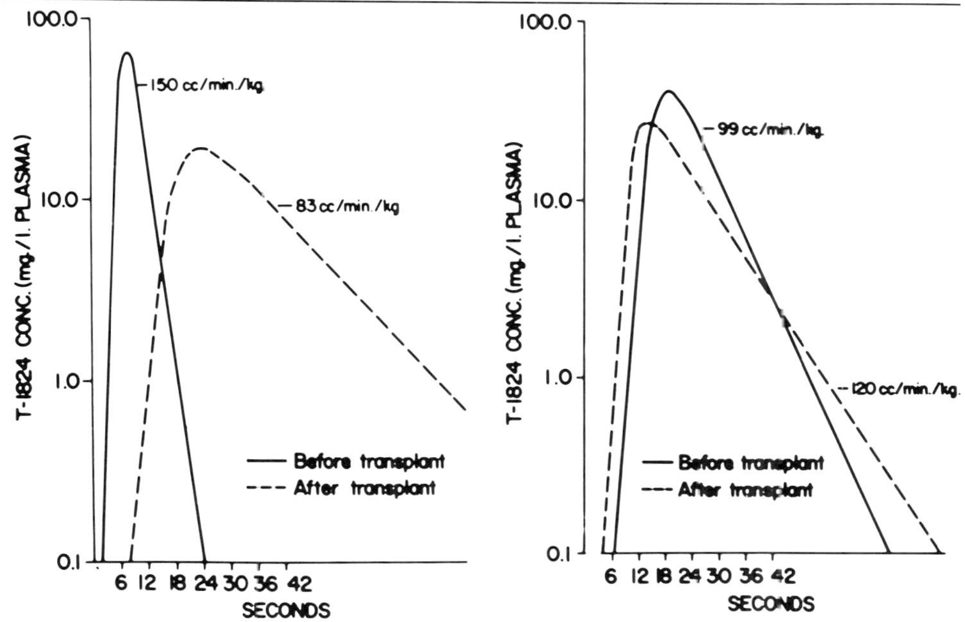

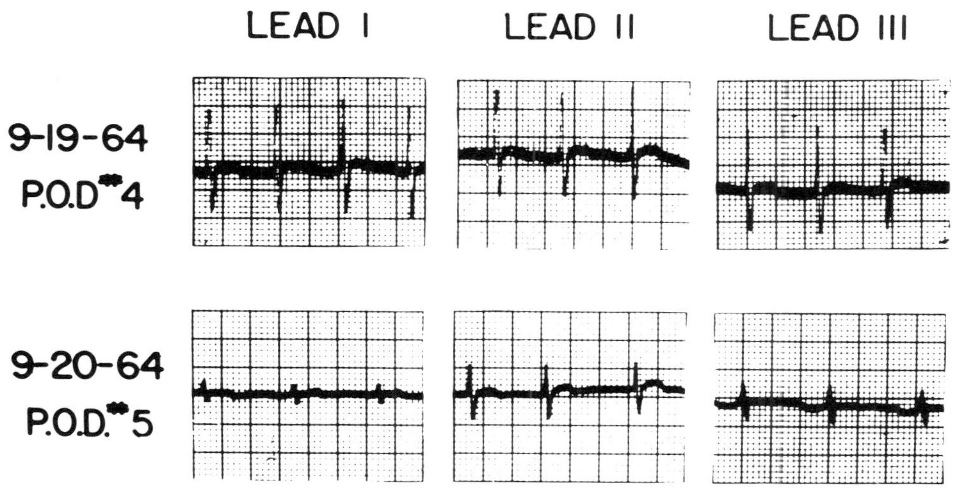

FIGS. 7A AND 7B. (A, top) Cardiac output curves before and after transplantation of the heart [dye dilution curves in (left) Dog 42 and (right) Dog 41]. (B, bottom) Electrocardiograms from Dog 100 (homotransplant; died September 21, 1964). Notice that, with impending rejection of the heart transplant, the voltage of the electrocardiogram declined markedly. (Reprinted with permission from Hardy JD *et al.* Heart transplantation in dogs: Procedure, physiologic problems and results in 142 experiments. Surgery 1966;60:361–367.)

the onset of various arrhythmias, especially bradycardia. The cardiac output of these animals declined and they appeared ill. However, by the time these relatively gross changes had occurred, increased immunosuppressive therapy was usually not effective in preventing rejection. It was to be more than a decade before the group at Stanford was to show that transvenous biopsies of the right ventricle, with microscopic monitoring for signs of rejection, could be performed periodically to modulate successfully the immunosuppressive therapy.[24]

With the technique of heart transplantation in animals well in hand, and in view of the significant scientific success achieved with the first lung transplant some months previously, Webb and I again approached Dean and Vice Chancellor Marston and proposed that we transplant a heart clinically if, again, the appropriate clinical, moral, and ethical circumstances should arise. Meanwhile, we had organized two teams in the laboratory, one team to place the recipient animal on cardiopulmonary bypass and excise the heart, and the other team to excise the heart of the donor animal and initiate rapid cooling of this organ. Several months went by without a suitable occasion having arisen. A number of potential recipients were considered but they then surprisingly improved, whereas others proposed died abruptly and there was no time for transplantation. Thus it became ever more clear that the recipient should most appropriately be a patient with long-standing heart disease now refractory to medical therapy, and not correctable surgically, who was progressing inexorably toward death. At that time coronary angiography and coronary bypass had not been developed.

The First Heart Transplant in Man

Meanwhile, Dr. Webb accepted the chair of cardiothoracic surgery at Southwestern Medical School in Dallas, and Dr. Carlos M. Chavez, who had been working with us in the laboratory, moved up to take Dr. Webb's leadership of the second team.

On January 22, 1964, a 64-year-old man (Fig. 8A) was referred to the surgical service with gangrene of the lower portion of his left leg. He had a long history of hypertension and multiple heart attacks, for which he had been taking digitalis and diuretics. He had been admitted to his community hospital in a comatose state and with no detectable blood pressure. Rapid atrial fibrillation had been recorded there, and drugs had been given in high dosage to elevate the blood pressure and assist in resuscitation of the markedly enlarged heart (Fig. 8B).

The following morning it was possible to maintain his blood pressure with minimal vasopressive drug therapy. His sensorium had cleared slightly. Whether this impaired mental state was secondary to the previous shock, with the resulting brain hypoxia imposed by already atherosclerotic brain arteries, or to intracranial hemorrhage, or to a blood pressure level that remained abnormally low for this previously hypertensive patient was not determined. He was able to move all four extremities, but this motion was limited.

The consulting cardiologist stated that life expectancy could be measured only in hours. There was a prospective "brain dead" donor on the neurosurgical service, but it was apparent that this patient might not "die" within the next few hours. At that time brain death was not accepted as a state permitting organ removal, and it certainly would not have been accepted in our hospital. The heart had first to stop in the donor. We were prepared to insert femoral catheters premortem and to initiate cooling of the cadaver immediately when the

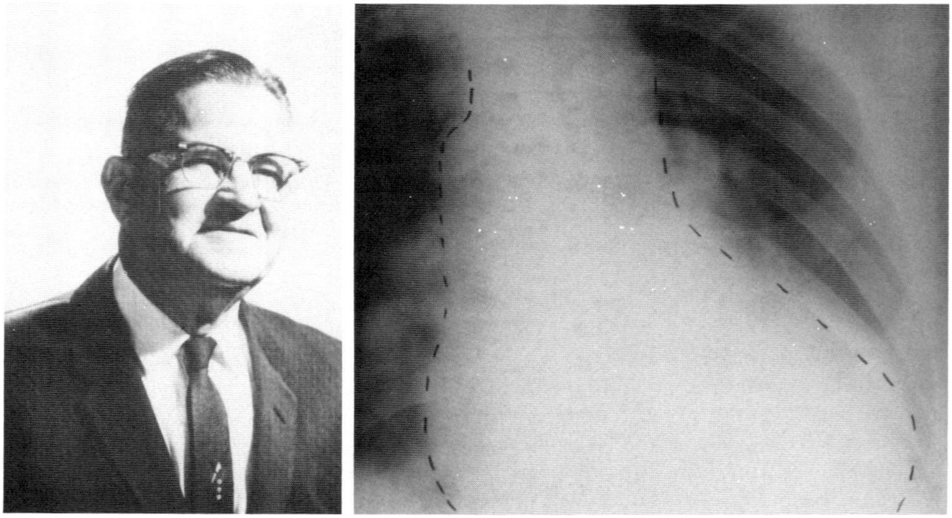

FIGS. 8A AND 8B. (A, left) Boyd Rush. Recipient of first heart transplant in man. (B, right) Notice marked enlargement of the decompensated heart of the prospective heart transplant recipient. (Reprinted with permission from Hardy JD, Chavez CM. The first heart transplant in man: Historical reexamination of the 1964 case in the light of current clinical experience. Transpl Proc 1969;1:720.)

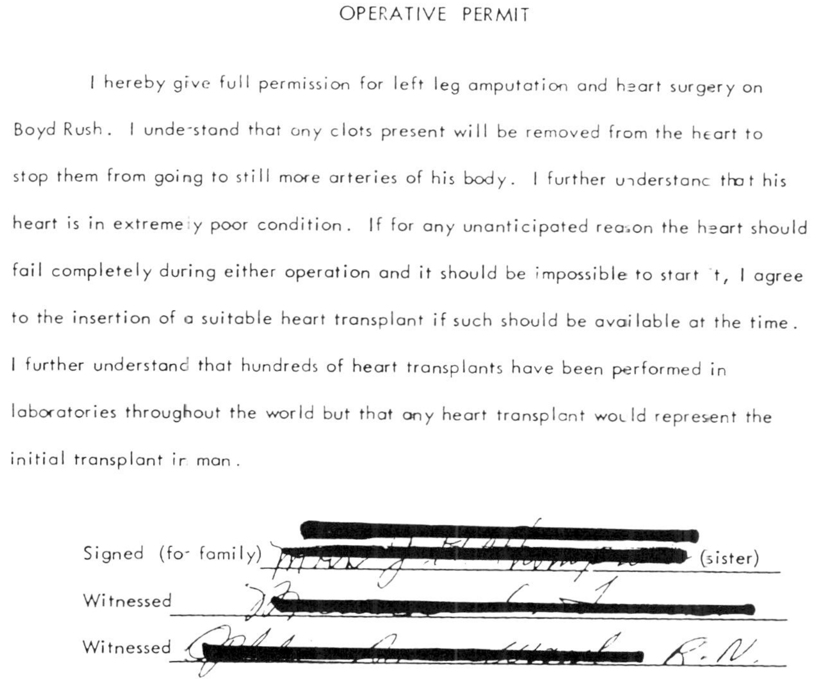
OPERATIVE PERMIT

I hereby give full permission for left leg amputation and heart surgery on Boyd Rush. I understand that any clots present will be removed from the heart to stop them from going to still more arteries of his body. I further understand that his heart is in extremely poor condition. If for any unanticipated reason the heart should fail completely during either operation and it should be impossible to start it, I agree to the insertion of a suitable heart transplant if such should be available at the time. I further understand that hundreds of heart transplants have been performed in laboratories throughout the world but that any heart transplant would represent the initial transplant in man.

Signed (for family) ______ (sister)

Witnessed ______

Witnessed ______ R.N.

FIG. 9. Operative permit for first heart transplant in man. (Reprinted with permission from Hardy JD, Chavez CM. The first heart transplant in man: Historical reexamination of the 1964 case in the light of current clinical experience. Transpl Proc 1969;1:721.)

heart did stop, having previously obtained permission from the family for autopsy and donation of the heart.

Meanwhile, however, we had visited the surgical service at Tulane University of Louisiana, where chimpanzee kidneys had been transplanted clinically with a surprising degree of early success.[25] We had purchased four chimpanzees for this purpose, for we, too, were having much difficulty in securing donations of cadaver kidneys. The largest chimpanzee was a male who weighed approximately 45 kg and his measured cardiac output, under anesthesia, was approximately 4 l/minute.

When the prospective recipient went into shock again, he was rushed to the operating room and placed on the pump-oxygenator just as his heart arrested. The operative permit, signed by the responsible member of the family, stated explicitly that any transplant would represent the first heart transplant in man (Fig. 9). The prospective human donor continued to survive and, with the patient surviving only because of the pump oxygenator, the heart of the largest chimpanzee was transplanted.[26] It was preserved during transplantation by the retrograde perfusion of cold oxygenated blood through the coronary sinus[27] (Fig. 10A). Thus, the blood emerging from the right and left coronary artery orifices at the root of the aorta was cyanotic, having passed through the capillary bed. The donor heart was considerably smaller than the large dilated heart that had been excised. The transplanted heart exhibited strong ventricular fibrillation when rewarmed, and it responded immediately to a single pulse of the defibrillator (Fig. 10B). Digoxin was administered as planned and the transplant immediately reflected the drug's effects with pulsus bigeminus, which was quickly reversed. The beat was regular and forceful, and it supported the patient with a blood pressure of between 90 and 100 mm systolic for approximately 1.5 hours after discontinuation of cardiopulmonary bypass. Ultimately, however, the heart failed. Microscopic studies revealed no evidence of acute immunologic rejection of the xenograft.

Although the donor heart had been smaller than would have been desirable, the advanced state of shock in the recipient was believed to have been the major factor in failure of the transplant, and this was to be proven later in our laboratory. We found that hearts

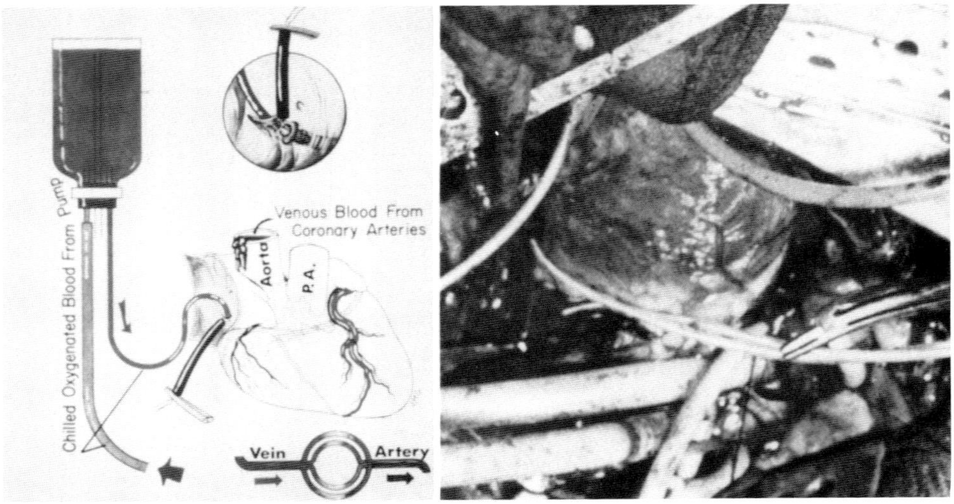

FIGS. 10A AND 10B. (A, left) Retrograde perfusion of the subhuman primate heart through the coronary sinus, with cold and oxygenated blood to preserve the organ during transplantation. (Reprinted with permission from Hardy JD *et al.* Heart transplantation in man: Developmental studies and report of a case. JAMA 1964;188:1135. © 1964, American Medical Association.) (B, right) The first heart transplant in man. (Reprinted with permission from Hardy JD, Chavez CM. Transplantation of the heart. In: Hardy JD, ed. Human Organ Support and Replacement. Springfield, IL: Charles C. Thomas, 1971; 311.)

transplanted from dogs dying from either blood loss shock[27] or from endotoxin shock[28] would support a healthy recipient animal routinely. Incidentally, however, shock induced by norepinephrine infusion damaged the heart itself, and hearts transplanted from animals dying from norepinephrine shock would rarely support the new host.[29]

In summary, it was apparent that the heart could be preserved effectively with cold oxygenated blood for the one hour required for heart transplantation in man, using the standard heart transplant procedures that had been employed in the laboratory. It was concluded that this clinical heart transplantation, performed under a most unusual set of circumstances, did demonstrate the scientific feasibility of clinical heart transplantation. It was further concluded that, given a larger heart from a "brain dead" donor and a human recipient not in shock, heart transplantation could "someday add years of life to many patients."[25]

Societal Dimensions of the First Lung and First Heart Transplants in Man

The first heart and lung transplants in man, in the 1960s, precipitated issues and controversies which greatly transcended the public interest that had been prompted by the first kidney transplants, performed in the 1950s. And, as regards the first lung as compared with the first heart, the latter stimulated a reaction which infinitely exceeded that of the lung.*

First, the heart was an unpaired organ, like the liver which had been transplanted clinically the previous year. However, the liver had been an abdominal organ and carried with it few of the psychological connotations associated with the heart at that time. Such connotations were reflected in phrases such as "fainthearted," or "with all my heart." How would one lover react to a partner whose newly transplanted heart had belonged to a stranger? The very center of the individual's being was commonly accepted as being "in the heart."

Thus, any heart transplant was certain to arouse strong emotions in both physicians and the population at large. Moreover, we had not transplanted merely a human heart, we had transplanted a subhuman heart. Our heart transplant precipitated intense ethical, moral, social, religious, financial, governmental, and even legal concerns. The reaction of the public media—print, television and radio—was enormous. Yet, in point of fact, the chimpanzee is

* Both the first lung transplant and the first heart transplant were requested by, and donated to, the Smithsonian Institute.

very close to human beings genetically, far more so than the baboon. But the sheer magnitude of the public display of the fact that a heart could be transplanted, had been transplanted, set in motion the inexorable process of human imagination and gradual acceptance which has evolved into our current almost casual attitude toward heart transplantation. The more successful an operation becomes, the less immoral it is perceived to be.

Major issues in clinical heart transplantation, other than the condition of the prospective recipient, revolve around donor organ supply and costs. The availability of donor hearts, usually from brain dead donors, has been improved by regional computer networks and jet airplane transport. However, the supply will always be insufficient unless a non-human supply can be made available. In view of the rapid advances in genetic engineering, it has been suggested that the large subhuman primates be rendered genetically more closely related to human beings, so that these lower primates can serve more successfully as organ donors. However, with the highest subhuman primates already closely related to man, any significant degree of genetic rapprochement would pose obvious and profound moral problems and decisions.

To reduce at least a few of the current societal problems precipitated by heart transplantation to practical issues, let me cite a patient in whom we have just recently transplanted a heart. First, he was 58 years old, considerably above the usual upper age limit of 50 years. His selection was controversial even among our transplant team. Should not the heart available for transplantation, many miles away, be directed to a younger recipient? Especially since the heavy smoking prospective recipient had had two coronary operations (in our hospital) and also had pulmonary emphysema, increasing the overall operative risk? Further, the potential donor was 40 years old and, although a woman, her heart could well have been assaulted by disease processes in the past. And what of the expense, who would pay? Our heart transplant program had long been severely retarded by the requirement that the prospective recipient deposit $100,000 with the hospital in advance. And herein lay the crux of the decision in this case. The prospective recipient was well covered by appropriate insurance, he desperately wanted the transplant, the prospective donor heart was a good match, and we felt obligated to him because we had operated upon his heart twice before. Fortunately, his postoperative course has been very satisfactory and he can now look forward hopefully to a substantial period of comfortable life, as compared with the few weeks he had before him preoperatively.

Again, the cost of heart transplantation and the shortage of donors are perhaps the two major societal problems before us: who pays for the transplants, and who gets the transplants? Almost all the lesser, ephemeral issues and criticisms have virtually faded behind us in the distance, and now heart transplants are so common that they hardly evoke comment.

In closing, on this most auspicious occasion, I again tender my fond best wishes to Dr. Rhoads.

REFERENCES

1. Blumenstock DA, Hechtman HB, Jarelzki A III, Hosbein JB, Zingg W, Powers JH. Prolonged survival of orthotopic homotransplants of the heart in animals treated with methotrexate. J Thorac Cardiovasc Surg 1963;46:616–625.
2. Juvenelle AA, Citret C, Wiles CE Jr, Stewart JD. Pneumonectomy with replantation of lung in dog for physiologic study. J Thorac Cardiovasc Surg 1951;21:111–115.
3. Neptune WB, Weller R, Bailey CP. Experimental lung transplantation. J Thorac Surg 1953;26:275–289.
4. Willman VL, Cooper T, Cian LG, Hanlon CR. Autotransplantation of the canine heart. Surg Gynecol Obstet 1962;115:299–302.
5. Alican F, Hardy JD. Lung reimplantation: Effect on respiratory pattern and function. JAMA 1963;183:849–853.
6. Eraslan S, Hardy JD, Elliott RL. Lung replantation: Respiratory reflexes, vagal integrity, and lung function in chronic dogs. J Surg Res 1966;6:383–388.
7. Kondo Y, Culpepper RD, Turner MD, Hardy JD. Cardiopulmonary function studies in long-term survivors of one-stage bilateral lung reimplantation. J Thorac Cardiovasc Surg 1974;68:303–308.
8. Eraslan S, Hardy JD. Differential division of hilar tissue: Effects upon lung function in the dog. Dis Chest 1966;50:449–456.
9. Eraslan S, Turner MD, Hardy JD. Lymphatic regeneration following lung reimplantation in dogs. Surgery 1964;56:970–973.
10. Alican F, Cayirli M, Isin E, Hardy JD. Surgical technique of one-stage bilateral lung reimplantation in the dog. J Thorac Cardiovasc Surg 1971;61:847–856.

11. Marshall R, Gunning AJ. The long-term physiological effects of lung reimplantation in the dog. J Surg Res 1966;6:185–195.
12. Webb WR, Unal M, Cook WA, Eraslan S, Hardy JD. Growth and function of the transplanted lung in puppies. Clin Res 1965;13:49.
13. Hardy JD, Eraslan S, Dalton ML, Alican F, Turner MD. Re-implantation and homotransplantation of the lung: Laboratory studies and clinical potential. Ann Surg 1963;157:707–718.
14. Alican F, Isin E, Cockrell JV. One-stage allotransplantation of both lungs in the dog. Ann Surg 1973;177:193–198.
15. Kondo Y, Isin E, Cockrell JV, Hardy JD. One-stage bilateral allotransplantation of canine lungs: Further studies. Early rejection and prolonged survival with immunosuppression. J Thorac Cardiovasc Surg 1972;64:897–906.
16. Hardy JD, Eraslan S, Webb WR. Transplantation of the lung. Ann Surg 1964;160:440–448.
17. Hardy JD, Webb WR, Dalton ML Jr, Walker GR Jr. Lung homotransplantation in man: Report of the initial case. JAMA 1963;186:1065–1074.
18. Webb WR, Howard HS. Cardio-pulmonary transplantation. Surg Forum 1958;8:313–317.
19. Webb WR, Howard HS. Restoration of function of the refrigerated heart. Surg Forum 1957;8:302–306.
20. Webb WR, Howard HS, Neely WA. Practical methods of homologous cardiac transplantation. J Thorac Surg 1959;37:361–366.
21. Lower RR, Stofer RC, Shumway NE. Homovital transplantation of the heart. J Thorac Cardiovasc Surg 1961;41:196–204.
22. Hardy JD, Chavez CM, Eraslan S, Adkins JR, Williams RD. Heart transplantation in dogs: Procedure, physiologic problems and results in 142 experiments. Surgery 1966;60:361–367.
23. Kondo Y, Matheny JL, Hardy JD. Autonomic reinnervation of cardiac transplants: Further observations in dogs and rhesus monkeys. Ann Surg 1972;176:42–48.
24. Billingham ME, Caves PK, Dong E Jr, Shumway NE. The diagnosis of canine orthotopic cardiac allograft rejection by transvenous endomyocardial biopsy. Transplant Proc 1973;5:741–743.
25. Reemtsma K, McCracken BH, Schlegel JV *et al.* Renal heterotransplantation in man. Ann Surg 1964;160:384–410.
26. Hardy JD, Chavez CM, Kurrus FD *et al.* Heart transplantation in man: Developmental studies and report of a case. JAMA 1964;188:1132–1140.
27. Hardy JD, Kurrus FD, Chavez CM, Webb WR. Heart transplantation in infant calves: Evaluation of coronary perfusion to preserve organ during transfer. Ann NY Acad Sci 1964;120:786–788.
28. Culpepper RD, Kondo Y, Hardy JD, Turner MD. Successful orthotopic allotransplantation of hearts from dogs in irreversible shock. Surgery 1975;77:126–131.
29. Kondo Y, Culpepper RD, Hardy JD, Turner MD. Heart transplantation in endotoxin shock. Surg Gynecol Obstet 1975;140:252–254.
30. Tessler MP, Kondo Y, Cayirli M, Hardy JD. Effect of pretreatment with norepinephrine on survival of cardiac allotransplants in dogs. Surg Gynecol Obstet 1978;147:541–544.

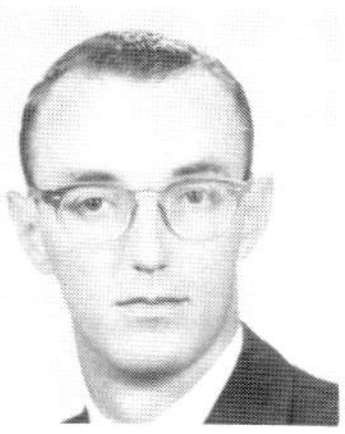

Introduction of Dr. Ted Copeland

Dr. Clyde Barker: Coming up is a group of papers on nutrition and metabolism. To some extent, this introduction pertains to all of them. The first speaker is Ted Copeland who you can see still looks the same as he did as a resident when he finished the program in 1969. After his war-time experience in Vietnam, Ted became a member of Stan Dudrick's faculty at the University of Texas and was very prominent in the program at MD Anderson before moving to Gainesville to become Chairman at the University of Florida. Ted's topic today is hyperalimentation and cancer. Dr. Rhoads has no entry in his bibliography with that exact title, but I thought it would be pertinent to show you just a few of the many, many publications that indicate his long-standing productivity, his breadth of interest, and his tremendous commitment and contributions to the entire field of nutrition. The names of his co-workers over the years are, of course, familiar ones to this group: I. S. Ravdin, Chick Koop, Bugs Lehr, Harry Vars, Stan Dudrick, Doug Wilmore, and many others. They collaborated on papers such as:

1) Thompson, W. D., Ravdin, I. S., Rhoads, J. E., and Frank, I.L.: Use of Lyophile Plasma in Correction of Hypoproteinemia and Prevention of Wound Disruption. *Arch Surg* 36:509–518, 1938.

2) Riegel, C., Koop, C. E., Drew, J., Stevens, L. W., and Rhoads, J.E.: The Nutritional Requirements for Nitrogen Balance in Surgical Patients During the Early Postoperative Period. *J Clin Invest* 26:18–23, 1947.

3) Scott, S. M., Bevilacqua, J. E., Lehr, H. B., Vars, H. M , Rosenthal, O., and Rhoads, J. E.: Clinical Experimental Studies of Fat Emulsions for Intravenous Use. *Trans Southern Surg Assoc* 66:5–7, 1954.

4) Rhoads, J. E.: Diuretics as an Adjuvant in Disposing of Extra Water as a Vehicle in Parenteral Hyperalimentation. *Fed Proc* 21:389, 1962.

I remember Dr. Rhoads' early interest in the use of diuretics in nutritional support in something we called the 5-liter or 10-liter program. If a resident could get on that particular research team, he was assured of a number of publications such as the following one: Rhoads, J. E., Rawnsley, H. M., Vars, H. M., Critchlow, R. W., Nelson, H. M., Spagna, P. M., Dudrick, S. J., and Rhoads, J. E., Jr.: The Use of Diuretics as an Adjunct in Parenteral Hyperalimentation for Surgical Patients with Prolonged Disability of Gastrointestinal Tract. *Bull Int Soc Surg* 24:59–70, 1965. Note that Stan Dudrick's name is now coming into prominence on this team. Finally, this abstract constitutes a landmark in the development of modern nutrition: Dudrick, S. J., Vars, H. M., Rawnsley, H. M and Rhoads, J. E.: Total Intravenous Feeding in Growth in Puppies. *Fed Proc* 25:481, 1966. Now, we'd better give Ted Copeland the floor to tell us about hyperalimentation and cancer.

Dr. Copeland's Introductory Remarks

I know I can have the floor for 40 to 45 minutes because Stan Dudrick follows me, and he never uses more than 10 to 15 minutes. Stan only has two carousels of slides today. Dr. Rhoads, Happy Birthday! I certainly am glad you made it to 80 for all kinds of reasons. One of the most important of the long list of reasons is the chance for all of us to get together again. This is really a great homecoming. I remarked to Terry and Stan Dudrick this morning at breakfast, that it was like a fraternity house, because it was hard to decide which one of your friends you wanted to eat with.

I have been the repository for a lot of stories about Dr. Rhoads along the way, but I don't think I can tell any now since I need two or three drinks before I have the courage to tell them. But, I would like to tell you a couple of things, not necessarily about Dr. Rhoads, but about how I happened to come here. I went to Cornell Medical School. I came originally from Central Georgia, but I had been brainwashed in New York to think that you could only train in New York. This was much as we felt in Philadelphia that you could only train here and as those in Boston felt about training in Boston at that time. I am sure that has changed.

Hasn't it Dr. Welch? Anyway, I came to Penn because they had a straight surgery internship on paper that I knew in reality was a rotating internship, which I wanted. I intended to go back to Columbia, but I had an uncle who told me that this program was superb, so I came down to Philadelphia to look at the rotating internship. When I got here, the first person I met on the wards was a fellow who was studying colon cytology. He had been up all night long, and he had on the outfit of a guy who would be studying colon cytology, and he had on him what you'd expect on someone studying colon cytology and that was Carter Nance. The next person I met was Ralph Hamilton. Ralph had on glasses, and one side of his glasses was broken. So, the whole time I was walking around with him I couldn't help but fixate on why he had on glasses with a big stillate crack in the center of one lens. Well, I was just about to leave when all of a sudden a big handsome man who looked dapper arrived. He was dressed in a tweed coat and professed to be one of the chief residents. That was Bob Critchlow, and I knew I'd be alright.

Anyway, I came here and stayed for the residency. I want to thank Dr. Rhoads for, among many things, having had such a gentlemanly residency. One of the things that I think has helped all of us who have gone on to do anything, but certainly those of us who have become chairmen, has been to have in our minds the kind of training program we went through in a period of time when I think that probably (in fact, not probably) we had the best training program in the country! I apologize to those of you from other places (actually, I don't apologize). But, during that era, we did have the best program, and it is kind of fun to go to Bill Curreri's program, Scott Jones' program, etc., because you see in those programs the same thing you are trying to develop in your own, and it has been a treat for me.

Intravenous Hyperalimentation and Cancer: A Historical Perspective

EDWARD M. COPELAND III, M.D.

I have often thought during my career that I was in the right place at the right time and certainly to have been a surgical resident at the University of Pennsylvania for 1963–1969 emphasizes this point. The faculty and residents under the leadership of Dr. Jonathan E. Rhoads during this era have been proven over time to be the best (although I will admit to being a bit prejudiced). The pursuit of intellectual thought, professional judgement, and collegiality which we learned during the residency have now been extended to multiple other surgical training programs, private practice environments, and research laboratories throughout this country. Dr. Rhoads can be proud to have established such a tradition of excellence, and I am proud to have been a participant in this process as I am proud to be a part of this eightieth birthday celebration.

I was privileged to deliver the annual Jonathan E. Rhoads Lecture before the American Society for Parenteral and Enteral Nutrition in 1986. In honor of Dr. Rhoads, I have elected to have the address published in its entirety herein.

I AM HONORED TO BE ASKED to deliver the 1986 Jonathan E. Rhoads Lecture. I take this opportunity to again thank Dr. Rhoads for having played such a positive and influential role in the development of my moral and ethical fiber as a physician. He provided the leadership for the surgical training program at the Hospital of the University of Pennsylvania, where I was privileged to train from 1963 to 1969. It was there that I formed my most lasting friendship in medicine and was able to observe the development of intravenous hyperalimentation (IVH) by Stanley Dudrick and his co-workers. I am, likewise, honored to be asked to deliver the Rhoads Lecture by your President, Dr. John Daly, the Jonathan E. Rhoads Professor of Surgery at the University of Pennsylvania. Although not much of the work I will relate to you today was done at the University of Pennsylvania, the discipline, motivation, inquisitiveness, desire, and capability to do the investigations sprang from the tutelage of Dr. Rhoads at our parent institution.

By 1968, Drs. Stanley Dudrick, Douglas Wilmore, Harry Vars, and Jonathan Rhoads had demonstrated that long-term total parenteral nutrition would result in growth and development with positive nitrogen balance in both experimental animals and human beings.[1] The safe technique of long-term central venous catheterization in patients with benign diseases had, likewise, been described by these investigators.[2] Few cancer patients, however, had received IVH because of the fear both of stimulating tumor growth by the nutrient solutions and of potential septic complications secondary to indwelling central venous catheters in patients with myelosuppression and induced immune deficiency disorders.

Our group was assembled in Houston, Texas, in 1972, and my responsibility was to run the University of Texas Medical School's surgical service at the M. D. Anderson Hospital and Tumor Institute. Cancer patients were being maintained by multiple and intricate life-support mechanisms in an attempt to treat them with more aggressive antineoplastic agents. We reasoned IVH might, likewise, have a place in this armamentarium, and identified a group of

From the Department of Surgery, University of Florida College of Medicine, Gainesville, Florida.

Received for publication, March 10, 1986.
Accepted for publication, March 10, 1986.
Presented at the 10th Annual A.S.P.E.N. Meeting, February 1986 in Dallas, TX as the Jonathan E. Rhoads Lecture.
This article has been reproduced with permission from the *Journal of Parenteral and Enteral Nutrition,* Vol. 10, No. 4, July/August 1986.

cachectic patients whose tumors were potentially responsive to appropriate cancer therapy but who were being denied treatment because of fear of complications secondary to malnutrition. Aggressive nutritional repletion seemed justified in these patients despite the potential hazards. In 1974, companion publications[3,4] from our group described the use of IVH in over 100 consecutive cancer patients. Catheter-related sepsis was the lowest reported, to date, 2.2%, and no stimulation of tumor growth was detectable clinically. The average duration of catheterization was 25.9 days; the longest single catheter was in place 96 days; the longest continuous period of IVH was 100 days; 1.6% of patients developed subclavian vein thrombosis; and a similar percent developed pulmonary edema. Dr. Bruce MacFadyen and I managed all patients with single lumen, polyvinyl catheters and pediatric microdrip delivery units. Catheters were used solely for delivery of the nutrient solutions.

By 1975, we had amassed 58 patients who received IVH in order to be considered candidates for appropriate chemotherapy.[5] This report served as a springboard for multiple, future randomized trials of IVH as an adjunct to chemotherapy. The safety of the technique in myelosuppressed patients was proven. Twenty-eight patients had leucocyte count depression below 2500 cells/m^3 for an average duration of 7.2 days. No catheter-related sepsis occurred in these patients. Five patients expired during treatment, but a 50% or greater reduction in tumor volume occurred in 21 of the 58 patients (36%). To be a candidate for IVH, patients were required to have tumors that were potentially responsive to conventional chemotherapy; therefore, the 36% response rate represented our ability to choose patients for chemotherapy, not the response rate necessarily associated with IVH.

Patients were treated with multiple chemotherapeutic regimens, allowing for several observations. Positive nitrogen balance was maintained during treatment with 5-fluorouracil (5-FU); gastrointestinal symptoms were reduced; and larger doses of 5-FU were tolerated, thereby confirming an observation made previously by Schwartz et al.[6] The use of Vincristine, however, regularly depressed an established positive nitrogen balance, often below equilibrium. Wilmore's group,[7] several years later, confirmed the difficulty reversing protein catabolism with IVH during intensive chemotherapy for patients with metastatic testicular tumors. The catabolic effects, however, were much more devastating in Wilmore's patients who did not receive IVH.

Fifteen patients of the 58 were among a larger study of patients with non-oat cell carcinoma of the lung treated with a five-drug chemotherapeutic regimen containing Bleomycin. Patients *not* receiving IVH, but responding to chemotherapy, had lost minimal weight (2%) prior to treatment, and further weight loss during chemotherapy did not exceed 2%. Those patients *not* receiving IVH, and likewise not responding to chemotherapy, had lost 11% of body weight prior to chemotherapy and lost another 10% of body weight during treatment. This observation was one of the first to demonstrate that nutritionally intact patients had a significantly greater chance of responding to chemotherapy than did their malnourished counterparts, a fact later to be confirmed by Lanzotti et al.[8] For the non-oat cell cancer patients who did receive IVH, responding patients gained significantly more weight during IVH than did nonresponding patients, and responding patients maintained the weight gained after IVH was discontinued. This same observation of weight gain during IVH and maintenance of it after discontinuation of the nutrient solutions also was made in patients who responded to treatment with radiation therapy.[9]

Our group was eager to make it clear to all audiences that only malnourished patients had been candidates for IVH combined with chemotherapy, and in 1974 wrote the following:

> "If the debilitated patient, who is cachectic because of malignant cell growth, could be repleted nutritionally, he might better tolerate chemotherapy and its toxic effects; immunocompetence and quality of life might be improved; and tumor response might be achieved in a patient who otherwise would have been deprived of adequate antitumor therapy because of malnutrition."[5]

We concluded that our data, at least in part, supported our hypothesis and concluded the following:

> "No physician can be criticized for nutritionally repleting any salvageable patient with benign disease and we have herein presented evidence to support this premise in patients with malignant disease."[5]

Since that time, both nonrandomized and randomized clinical trials of IVH as a nutritional

TABLE 1. *IVH and Chemotherapy Response*

Investigator	Tumor type	Response (difference)*	Randomized	Malnourished
Copeland et al[5]	Mixed	+	No	Yes
Souchon et al[10]	Colon	+	No	Yes
Lanzotti et al[8]	Lung-non oat	+	No	Yes
Issell et al[11]	Lung-non oat	+	Yes	Yes
Jordan et al[12]	Lung-non oat	±	No	No
Valdivieso et al[13]	Lung-oat cell	(±)	Yes	±
Clamon et al[14]	Lung-oat cell	(−)	Yes	No
Popp et al[15]	Lymphoma	(−)	Yes	No
Levine et al[16]	Lymphoma	(−)	Yes	No
Shamberger et al[17]	Sarcoma	(−)	Yes	No
Samuels et al[18]	Testicular	(−)	Yes	No
Nixon et al[19]	Colon	(−)	Yes	Yes

* The symbols in parentheses represent a response difference between IVH and control patients in randomized prospective trials. A negative symbol means no response difference; a positive symbol means a response difference

adjunct during chemotherapy have been published[10–19] (Table 1). Characteristic of these reports is a response advantage for nonrandomized patients who were malnourished uniformly, and no response advantage in the randomized trials for IVH patients who were, for the most part, *not* malnourished. Often, in the latter studies, body weight gain was as water and fat mass, as would be expected when using IVH in nutritionally intact patients. Criteria for identifying an increase in lean body mass was lacking. Also, no response advantage for nutritionally intact IVH patients should be expected. My frustration with many of these randomized studies resulted in a review and update of IVH and chemotherapy published in JPEN in 1982,[20] and for the interested reader, much more detail about these studies may be found in this publication. Suffice it to say that nutritional repletion depends upon the degree of initial malnutrition; the initial and continuing catabolic response from the disease and its treatment; energy exenditure during oncologic therapy; time, content, and method of nutritional repletion; and physician expertise in the technique of nutritional rehabilitation.

A proposed study would include the evaluation of cachectic patients identified by a good definition of malnutrition; randomization of malnourished patients between IVH and conventional nutritional maintenance; control group of well-nourished patients on conventional nutritional maintenance; drugs with moderate systemic toxicity; a cancer that is moderately responsive to the drugs; and, of most importance, correlation between nutritional response (lean body mass) to nutritional therapy and tumor response to chemotherapy. In 1982, Levine and co-workers[16] confirmed our observations of 1975, and wrote the following:

> ". . . studies designed to answer the question of whether TPN is a major adjunct to cancer treatment require that TPN candidates be malnourished (and not able to be renourished enterally), that their tumors be potentially responsive, and that they cannot receive an adequate trial of intensive therapy because of the effects of malnutrition."

A well-designed randomized study by Samuels et al[18] set out to evaluate the use of IVH in *healthy*, young adult males with metastatic testicular carcinoma. The recovery period between cycles of Vinblastine and Bleomycin was predicated upon nutritional recovery and return to normal of bone marrow elements. In IVH patients only bone marrow recovery was necessary; consequently, more cycles of chemotherapy could be given to the IVH patients per unit time. This process was expensive since IVH patients required hospitalization to receive nutritional therapy, whereas the non-IVH patients went home after bone marrow recovery to gain lost weight by standard enteral means. Response rate in the two groups was the same, indicating that IVH was not an adjunct for this particular chemotherapy protocol in *healthy*, young males with metastatic testicular tumors. Previously, we had noted that the survival advantage secondary to IVH was in the testicular tumor patients who did *not* respond to chemotherapy.[21] In 1983, Yamada and colleagues[22] confirmed this observation in

TABLE 2. *IVH and Response to Surgery*

Investigator	Tumor type	Response (difference)*	Randomized	Malnourished
Copeland and Dudrick[21]	GI	+	No	Yes
Mullen et al[23]	Mixed	+	No	Yes
Dioniegi et al[24]	GI	+	No	Yes
Daly et al[25]	Esophagus	+	No	Yes
Copeland et al[26]	H & N	+	No	Yes
Muller et al[27]	UGI	(+)	Yes	Yes
Senivkov et al[28]	H & N	(+)	Yes	Yes
Yamada et al[22]	Gastric & 5-FU	(+)	Yes	±
Heatly et al[29]	Gastric	(±)	Yes	±
Holter and Fischer[30]	GI	(−)	Yes	±

* The symbols in parentheses represent a response difference between IVH and control patients in randomized prospective trials. A negative symbol means no response difference; a positive symbol means a response difference.

patients undergoing treatment for advanced carcinoma of the stomach by palliative gastrectomy and 5-FU with and without IVH. IVH patients had a 54% 3-yr survival *vs* 0% for non-IVH patients.

In a consecutive series of malnourished surgical patients treated with IVH and reported in 1976,[21] we had only a 4% mortality rate, much below the predicted mortality rate, in our opinion. These patients were from my surgical service and IVH was used an average of 12.3 days preoperatively and 13.9 days postoperatively. The decision as to when nutritional repletion was adequate preoperatively was made on clinical judgment based usually on return of strength and general well-being, rather than on any specific test. In this report, we first published our definition of malnutrition as a recent weight loss below 10% or more, a serum albumin level below 3.4 g/dl, and a negative reaction to a battery of recall skin test antigens. Any combination of two of these three criteria was sufficient to indicate the need for preoperative nutritional repletion. During 12.3 days of preoperative IVH, serum albumin might not rise significantly, and if below 2.5 g/dl, exogenous serum albumin was given to raise the level above 3.4 g/dl in order to return serum oncotic pressure to normal by the day of operation. In patients in whom clinical judgment alone would not identify adequate nutritional repletion, reaction to a battery of recall skin test antigens was used. Continued anergy dictated further preoperative IVH. Possibly, the current Veterans Administration randomized clinical trial, attempting to define the value of preoperative IVH, will identify the efficacy of secretory proteins with a short half-life, such as prealbumin, as predictors of nutritional repletion.

In general, nonrandomized and randomized trials of IVH for surgical patients published to date have indicated a reduction in morbidity and/or mortality for the IVH group[21–30] (Table 2). In comparison to IVH-chemotherapy randomized trials, surgical trials have contained more malnourished patients. Usually, IVH was infused empirically for 10 days preoperatively, a time which should nutritionally replete the majority of nonstressed malnourished patients, at least based on our average figure of 12.3 days described earlier. In one negative report by Holter et al[30] IVH was used for only 3 days preoperatively and, as would be expected, no advantage for IVH was identified.

In our surgical series, patients with head and neck malignancies had failed previous attempts at enteral repletion prior to beginning IVH.[26] Malabsorption of ingested enteral nutriments was common. Diarrhea, bloating, and abdominal pain accompanied enteral feeding. It should be pointed out, however, that the majority of head and neck cancer patients can be repleted by gut if adequate time is available to do so, such as during preoperative radiation therapy. During IVH, the decision to continue some enteral nutrition, even though the annoying symptoms of malabsorption might result, was based on studies our group did in conjunction with Drs. Leonard Johnson and Gilbert Castro of the Department of Physiology at the University of Texas Medical School at Houston.[31–34] These investigators noted the small bowel, pancreas, oxyntic gland area of the stomach, and, to a degree, the colon of the rat to atrophy if the animals were maintained solely on IVH with no enteral alimentation. Likewise, disaccharidase enzyme content of the brush border diminished significantly. The addition of pentagastrin to the IVH solutions and bulk to a liquid diet would prevent both gut atrophy and decreased content of brush border disaccharidase enzymes. We postulated that the bulk diet might work by release of endogenous gastrin or other yet to be determined substances and, therefore, continued the head and neck cancer patients on enteral supplements despite adequate calories and nitrogen delivered by vein. In time, symptoms of malabsorption abated and the ability to absorb enteral nutriments returned. The accuracy of this decision is being further evaluated in several laboratories nationwide today.

Since malnutrition depresses delayed cutaneous hypersensitivity, we felt that at least a portion of the suppression of cell-mediated immunity in cancer patients was due to malnutrition and not to a substance produced by the cancer, *per se*. In 1976, we published the results of serial skin testing for 47 malnourished cancer patients who received IVH.[35] A battery of five recall skin test antigens was utilized. A positive test was defined by a 10 × 10 mm or greater area of induration within 48 hr of injection of the skin test into the volar aspect of the forearm. For a test to convert from negative to positive, at least 10 × 10 mm of induration must exist, as well as a doubling of the size of a previous negative test. For example, if a previous negative test was 6 × 6 mm of induration, it must be 12 × 12 mm of induration before being considered a positive conversion. These rather stringent criteria minimized observer error.

In patients treated with chemotherapy, 76% of the negative reactors converted skin test reactions to positive as did 66% of the surgery group, 62% of the supportive care group, and 25% of the radiation therapy group. This data was confirmed in a larger series of 160 patients published in 1980.[36] The chemotherapy group was heterogeneous in both tumor type and drug protocols; nevertheless, 52% of patients who converted skin test reactions from negative to positive had a significant reduction in tumor volume in response to chemotherapy, whereas no individual who converted an initial positive skin test reaction to negative responded to chemotherapy. Patients in the surgery group who maintained positive skin test reactions or converted from negative to positive reactions had significantly less morbidity and mortality (25%) than did patients who failed to manifest positive skin test reactions (69% morbidity and mortality).

The supportive care group is an interesting one, for these patients represent individuals who had become malnourished during aggressive antineoplastic therapy and could not regain lost weight because of anorexia and general debilitation, even though a significant tumor reduction often had been achieved. They were admitted to the hospital for a general "nutritional tune-up" with IVH. Most patients had a small, but definite, measurable tumor burden, yet with nutritional repletion, positive skin test reactivity was restored. Likewise, surgery patients who received IVH preoperatively and converted skin test reactions to positive, did so prior to operation and removal of their cancer. In these patients, the likelihood is remote that a substance produced by the cancer caused the negative skin test reaction, and removal of the tumor or its reduction in size is also eliminated as a reason for positive skin test conversion. Nutritional repletion seems the obvious reason for the positive skin tests, since the patients were not otherwise septic or receiving immunosuppressive drugs. This report demonstrated that cancer-bearing patients who were capable of being nutritionally replenished would have positive skin test reactivity. Delayed cutaneous hypersensitivity can, therefore, be used as one of the tests to determine repletion of lean body mass in patients with measurable malignant disease.

Several animal experiments that evaluated the relationships between host and tumor as competitors for nutrients deserve mention. Dr. John Daly and his co-workers[27] demonstrated that lean body and organ mass could be restored as easily in malnourished rats with subcutaneously implanted Walker-256 carcinosarcomas as in nontumor-bearing, malnourished rats, as long as tumor mass did not exceed 5% of carcass weight. If tumor mass was 25% of carcass weight or greater, nutritional repletion by gut or by vein became impossible. Nixon and colleagues[38] have excellent data in malnourished patients with metastatic malignancies to indicate a metabolic block that may exist and prevent exogenous nutrients from improving lean body mass. Such a situation should be remembered when attempting to

TABLE 3. *Tumor Response to Chemotherapy Based on Methotrexate Dose and Nutritional Maintenance*

	30% Dextrose: 5% amino acids		Oral regular diet
Methotrexate dose (mg/kg)	IV fed tumor wt (g)	Enteral *ad lib* tumor wt (g)	Control tumor wt (g)
20	7.3 ± 2.5*	11.3 ± 2.8	
40	1.1 ± 2.5*	3.7 ± 1.0	
60	0.8 ± 0.2	0.8 ± 0.2	
Saline (control)			19.6 ± 5.2

*$p < 0.05$ IV *vs* enteral *ad lib.*

replenish a patient with multiple metastatic deposits who must undergo a palliative surgical procedure.

Daly's group, again studying Sprague-Dawley rats with transplanted Walker-256 carcinosarcoma, demonstrated that protein-calorie repletion of malnourished animals would accelerate both host and tumor growth within 48 hr, and within 6 days would result in tumor growth patterns similar to those of well-nourished, tumor-bearing animals.[39] If nutritional repletion does stimulate tumor cell metabolism and increased cell replication, there may be an optimal time period during early nutritional repletion when tumor cell growth and division are maximal and the tumor is most susceptible to cell-cycle specific antimetabolites such as methotrexate. To investigate this hypothesis, tumor-bearing, malnourished animals were given methotrexate either 2 or 6 days after protein repletion had begun. Methotrexate administration had no effect on tumor or carcass weight if a protein free diet was continued. The greatest inhibition of tumor growth occurred in rats that were switched from a protein-free diet, initially used to produce protein malnutrition, to a regular diet and were treated with methotrexate 2 days after nutritional repletion had begun. The greatest reduction in tumor weight compared with the largest gain in carcass weight also occurred in this group of rats. Since methotrexate inhibits DNA synthesis, conclusions were that the good response to methotrexate after nutritional repletion had begun was secondary to an increase in tumor cell replication by feeding the regular diet, and, conversely, the poor response to methotrexate in rats that continued to receive the protein-free diet was secondary to depressed tumor cell metabolism and replication coincident with minimal carcass weight gain. Torosian et al[40] confirmed these observations and noted that nutritional repletion was synergistic with Adriamycin when treating rats with transplanted mammary adenocarcinomas.

Torosian's group elected to call the short interval of nutritional repletion prior to chemotherapy in their experiments "adjuvant, pulse total parenteral nutrition." Such pulsing of nutrients may explain experimental results Daly's group obtained when graded doses of methotrexate were given to rats with transplanted Walker-256 carcinosarcomas maintained on either IVH or allowed to drink the solution *ad libitum.*[41] Significant inhibition of tumor growth was found in both groups compared to saline-injected controls. Yet the intravenously fed animals also exhibited significant tumor growth inhibition when compared to animals that drank the 30% dextrose-5% amino acid solution *ad libitum.* Leucovoran rescue was used in all animals (Table 3). This result was repetitive but lacked explanation. Enterally fed animals did not drink the solution for 24 hr after methotrexate administration, whereas animals fed intravenously were nourished continuously. To resolve this issue, the experiment was repeated in all respects except animals fed enterally had catheters placed within their jejunum and the 30% dextrose-5% amino acid solution was infused continuously to avoid the failure of enteral nutritional intake for 24 hr after methotrexate administration. Under these circumstances, the response to methotrexate was the same for both intravenous and enteral groups and equal to the group fed intravenously in the previous experiment. In the experiment of Torosian et al[40] Adriamycin was more effective in those animals receiving adequate continuous nutritional intake. In Daly et al's experiment,[41] animals failing to maintain an adequate nutritional intake had a poorer response to methotrexate when compared to animals fed continuously by vein or by gut.

At the University of Florida, in the laboratory under the direction of Drs. Harry Sitren and Sam Mahaffey, the technique of total parenteral nutrition has been adapted to the mouse.[42,43] Unlike the rat, transplantable tumors in mice metastasize, thereby allowing study of a tumor system potentially more like that of human beings. Previously Buzby's group[44] demonstrated decreased tumor growth in parenterally fed rats bearing mammary adenocarcinomas when calories were provided as fat compared to dextrose. Our group wished to confirm these observations in a metastasizing mouse model.[45] Lewis lung carcinoma is an anaplastic, squamous cell carcinoma that metastasizes to the lungs with litte involvement of other organs and causes a pulmonary death. Swiss mice were implanted subcutaneously with fresh tumor and parenteral calories were provided by one of three diets: dextrose, fat or a dextrose-fat combination. Nitrogen, electrolytes, minerals, vitamins, calories, and volume were the same in all three groups. Tumor doubling time was slowest in the dextrose group; consequently, tumors in this group were significantly smaller at the conclusion of the experiment. Calories as fat, or as a combination of dextrose and fat, maintained tumor growth equal to the orally-fed, casein diet control animals. The results of Buzby's experiment were not duplicated. No doubt, the ability of any one calorie source to inhibit or maintain tumor growth depends on the animal species and the tumor models selected for study.

From these studies in mice, an interesting and yet to be explained result has been obtained (Mahaffey et al: Decreased lung metastasis and tumor growth in parenterally fed mice. J Surg Res (in press)). Pulmonary metastases as measured by surface pulmonary nodules were significantly fewer in the mice maintained on any one of the parenteral diets, regardless of caloric source, when compared with the mice that drank isocaloric amounts of the same diet or were fed a casein diet. In fact, fewer pulmonary metastases were observed when the mice were infused with a solution containing only the electrolytes and minerals of the parenteral solution and were maintained nutritionally by an oral casein diet. Possibly, a simple explanation exists for this repetitive observation, but presence of the catheter in the inferior vena cava, sepsis, or other more obvious answers do not appear to be operative.

Although acceleration of tumor growth in human beings has not been observed during short intervals of nutritional repletion, results from rodent experiments suggest that this possibility exists in the mammalian species, and that appropriate oncologic therapy should be instituted early during nutritional repletion. Data from rodents cannot be applied directly to malnourished cancer patients since the doubling times of cancers in human beings are measured in terms of weeks or months, and the cancer may not kill the patient for several years after the initial clone of malignant cells has developed. The doubling time of animal tumors can often be measured in hours or days, and this relatively rapid growth can result in death of animals within 5 to 7 weeks after initial tumor innoculation. Dietary protein depletion or repletion would be expected to have a more measurable and obvious effect on a tumor such as a Walker-256 carcinosarcoma or a transplanted Lewis lung carcinoma because of their rapid growth characteristics. As in rats, however, tumors in cachectic human beings have not been noted to be more responsive to cell-cycle specific chemotherapeutic agents during treatment with IVH; although such a possibility has yet to be subjected to a proper randomized-prospective clinical trial.

Unquestionably, Dr. Jonathan E. Rhoads was responsible for creating the environment in which my interest in nutritional metabolism developed. For the maturation process as a faculty member, I would like to thank Stanley Dudrick and my co-workers at The University of Texas Medical School at Houston between 1972 and 1982, especially John Daly, Bruce MacFadyen, and David Ota. Likewise, I owe a debt of gratitude to Renilda Hilkemeyer, Louise Cox, Mary Ann Rapp, and Sandra Norman, the nurses who participated in the development of the IVH program at the M. D. Anderson Hospital. For example, in 1981, Louise Cox and David Ota evaluated 57 cancer patients for ambulatory parenteral nutrition and discharged 28 patients to receive the nutrient solutions at home. In so doing, they developed the criteria for home parenteral nutrition in the cancer patient.[46]

I suspect the same is true today, as it was almost 10 yr ago when we wrote, "An enlightened approach to therapy of the malnourished cancer patient is to rehabilitate him nutritionally with IVH before, during and/or after all forms of therapy, whenever this highly desirable goal cannot be accomplished by enteral means."[47] Likewise, I have not changed my indications for the use of IVH in cancer patients since our initial publications. They are: (1) patients who satisfy the criteria for malnutrition and have a reasonable chance of responding to appropriate oncologic therapy; (2) patients who have been previously treated with oncologic therapy and are incapable of adequate enteral nutrition because of the malnutrition imposed by previous therapy; (3) nutritionally intact patients whose treatment plan necessitates multiple courses of chemotherapy, possibly combined with radiation therapy or surgery, when optimal nutritional status during treatment is a necessary goal.

REFERENCES

1. Dudrick SJ, Wilmore DW, Vars HM, Rhoads JE: Can intravenous feeding as the sole means of nutrition support growth in the child and restore weight loss in the adult? An affirmative answer. Ann Surg 1971;121:169–173.
2. Wilmore DW, Dudrick SJ: Safe long-term venous catheterization. Arch Surg 1969;98:256–258.
3. Copeland EM, MacFadyen BV Jr, McGown C, Dudrick SJ: The use of hyperalimentation in patients with potential sepsis. Surg Gynecol Obstet 1974;138:377–380.
4. Copeland EM, MacFadyen BV Jr, Dudrick SJ: Intravenous hyperalimentation in cancer patients. J Surg Res 1974;16:241–247.
5. Copeland EM, MacFadyen BV Jr, Lanzotti V, Dudrick SJ: Intravenous hyperalimentation as an adjunct to cancer chemotherapy. Am J Surg 1975;129:167–173.
6. Schwartz GF, Green HL, Bendon ML, et al: Combined parenteral hyperalimentation and chemotherapy in treatment of disseminated solid tumors. Am J Surg 1971;121:169–173.
7. Hermann VM, Garnick MB, Moore FD, Wilmore DW: Effect of cytotoxic agents on protein kinetics in patients with metastatic cancer. Surgery 1981;90:381–387.
8. Lanzotti VC, Copeland EM, George SL, et al: Cancer chemotherapeutic response and intravenous hyperalimentation. Cancer Chemother Rep 1975;59:437–439.
9. Copeland EM, Souchon EA, MacFadyen BV, et al: Intravenous hyperalimentation as adjunct to radiation therapy. Cancer 1977;39:609–616.
10. Souchon EA, Copeland EM, Watson P, Dudrick SJ: Intravenous hyperalimentation as an adjunct to cancer chemotherapy with 5-fluorouracil. J Surg Res 1975;18:451–454.
11. Issell BV, Valdivieso M, Zaren HA, et al: Protection against chemotherapy toxicity by IV hyperalimentation. Cancer Treat Rep 1978;62:1139–1143.
12. Jordan WM, Valdivieso M, Franman C, et al: Treatment of advanced adenocarcinoma of the lung with floraflur, doxorubicin, cyclophosphamide and cisplatin (FACP) with intensive hyperalimentation. Cancer Treat Rep 1981;65:197–206.
13. Valdivieso M, Bodey GP, Benjamin RS: Role of hyperalimentation as an adjunct to intensive chemotherapy for small cell bronchogenic carcinoma. Cancer Treat Rep 1981;65:145–151.
14. Clamon GH, Feld R, Evans WK, et al: Effect of adjuvant central IV hyperalimentation in survival and response to treatment of patients with small cell lung cancer: A randomized trial. Cancer Treat Rep 1985;69:167–177.
15. Popp MB, Fischer RJ, Wesley R, et al: A prospective randomized study of adjuvant parenteral nutrition in the treatment of advanced, diffuse lymphoma: Influence on survival. Surgery 1981;90:195–204.
16. Levine AS, Brennan MF, Ramo A: Controlled clinical trials of nutritional intervention as an adjunct to chemotherapy, with a comment on nutrition and drug resistance. Cancer Res 1982;42:744–781.
17. Shamberger RC, Brennan MF, Goodgame JT, et al: A prospective, randomized study of adjuvant parenteral nutrition in the treatment of sarcomas: Results of metabolic and survival studies. Surgery 1984;96:1–11.
18. Samuels ML, Selig DE, Ogden S, et al: IV hyperalimentation and chemotherapy for stage III testicular cancer: A randomized study. Cancer Treat Rep 1981;65:615–628.
19. Nixon DW, Moffitt S, Lawson DH, et al: Total parenteral nutrition as an adjunct to chemotherapy of metastatic colorectal cancer. Cancer Treat Rep 1981;65:121–128.
20. Copeland EM: Intravenous hyperalimentation and chemotherapy: An update. JPEN 1982;6:236–239.
21. Copeland EM, Dudrick SJ: Nutritional aspects of cancer. IN Current Problems in Cancer, Vol 1, No. 3, Hickey RC (ed). Year Book Medical Publishers, Inc, Chicago, 1976.
22. Yamada N, Koyama H, Hioki K, et al: Effect of postoperative total parenteral nutrition (TPN) as an adjunct to gastrectomy for advanced gastric carcinoma. Br J Surg 1983;70:267–274.
23. Mullen JM, Buzby GP, Matthews DC, et al: Reduction of operative morbidity and mortality by combined preoperative and postoperative nutritional support. Ann Surg 1980;192:604–613.
24. Dioniegi R, Guaglio R, Bonera A, et al: Clinical pharmacological aspects, application and effectiveness of total parenteral nutrition in surgical patients. Int J Clin Pharmacol Biopharm 1979;17:107–113.
25. Daly JM, Massar E, Giacco G, et al: Parenteral nutrition in esophageal cancer patients. Ann Surg 1982;196:203–208.

26. Copeland EM, MacFadyen BV Jr, MacComb WS, et al: Intravenous hyperalimentation in patients with head and neck cancer. Cancer 1975;35:606–611.
27. Muller JM, Dienst C, Brenner V, Pichimaier H: Preoperative parenteral feeding in patients with gastrointestinal carcinoma. Lancet 1982;1:68–71.
28. Senivkov MV, Khmeleviski IM, Zubov OG, et al: Parenteral feeding of patients with cancer of the larynx undergoing combination therapy. Vestn Otoinolaryngol 1978;2 68–72.
29. Heatley RV, Williams RHP, Lewis MH: Preoperative intravenous feeding-A controlled trial. Postgrad Med J 1979;55:541–545.
30. Holter AR, Fischer JE: The effects of perioperative hyperalimentation on complications in patients with carcinoma and weight loss. J Surg Res 1977;23:31–34.
31. Johnson LR, Lichtenberger LM, Copeland EM, et al: Action of gastrin on gastrointestinal structure and function. Gastroenterology 1975;68:1184–1192.
32. Johnson LR, Copeland EM, Dudrick SJ, et al: Structural and hormonal alterations in the gastrointestinal tract of parenterally fed rats. Gastroenterology 1975;68:1177–1183.
33. Castro GA, Copeland EM, Dudrick SJ, Johnson LR: Intestinal disaccharidase and peroxidase activity in parenterally nourished rats. J Nutr 1975;105:776–781.
34. Ryan GP, Dudrick SJ, Copeland EM, Johnson LR: Effects of various diets on colonic growth. Gastroenterology 1979;77:658–663.
35. Copeland EM, MacFadyen BV Jr, Dudrick SJ: Effect of intravenous hyperalimentation on established delayed hypersensitivity in the cancer patient. Ann Surg 1976;184:60–64.
36. Daly JM, Dudrick SJ, Copeland EM: Intravenous hyperalimentation: Effect on delayed cutaneous hypersensitivity in cancer patients. Ann Surg 1980;192:587–592.
37. Daly JM, Copeland EM, Dudrick SJ, Delaney JM: Nutritional repletion of malnourished tumor-bearing and non-tumor bearing rats: Effects on body weight, liver, muscle and tumor. J Surg Res 1980;28:507–518.
38. Nixon DW, Lawson DH, Kutner M, et al: Hyperalimentation of the cancer patient with protein-calorie under nutrition. Cancer Res 1981;41:2038–2045.
39. Daly JM, Reynolds HM, Rowlands BJ, et al: Tumor growth in experimental animals: Nutritional manipulation and chemotherapeutic response. Ann Surg 1980;191:316–322.
40. Torosian MH, Mullen JL, Miller E, et al: Adjuvant, pulse total parenteral nutrition and tumor response to cycle-specific and cycle-nonspecific chemotherapy. Surgery 1983;94:291–299.
41. Daly JM, Reynolds HM, Copeland EM, Dudrick SJ: Effects of enteral and parenteral nutrition on tumor responses to chemotherapy in experimental animals. J Surg Oncol 1981:16:79–86.
42. Sitren HS, Heller PA, Bailey LB, Cerda JJ: Total parenteral nutrition in the mouse: Development of a technique. JPEN 1983;7:582–586.
43. Mahaffey SM, Copeland EM, Talbert JL, et al: Further studies of a technique for total parenteral nutrition in the mouse. Nutr Res 1985;5:1121–1130.
44. Buzby GP, Mullen JL, Stein JP, et al: Host-tumor interaction and nutrient supply. Cancer 1980;45:2940–2948.
45. Mahaffey SM, Copeland EM, Economides E, et al: The effect of energy substrate manipulation in tumor growth and metastasis and intermediary metabolism in the parenterally fed mouse. J Pediatr Surg 1985;20:775–784.
46. Ota DM, Cox LC, Martin S, Copeland EM: Ambulatory home intravenous hyperalimentation. Cancer Bull 1982;34:218–220.
47. Copeland EM, Daly JM, Dudrick SJ: Nutrition as an adjunct to cancer treatment in the adult. Cancer Res 1977;37:2451–2456.

Discussion

Dr. Michael Torosian What is your endpoint in terms of clinical treatment of cancer patients? Do you look for weight changes, serum protein levels, nitrogen balance changes? What do you require in the preoperative period or before you administer chemotherapy?

Dr. Ted Copeland: Well, I have never done it very scientifically, and I suppose I basically use clinical judgement. The reason you are able to use clinical judgement is why the surgical training program has to be so long. When the male patients begin to shave or walk around the room or when the ladies put on lipstick, those kinds of things you can go by. You know as well as I do that you can use the tests, but, quite frankly, the patients that we have studied before chemotherapy or before surgery have been very malnourished patients. Common sense would tell you that they are malnourished. and common sense would frankly tell you when they would be able to withstand therapy. Sure, their transferins and all that other stuff go up, but we did not have those parameters to use early on simply because we were not able to measure those things, and serum albumin takes a long time to go up as you know. So, we used basic clinical judgement, and quite frankly, in the practice of medicine, that is what I usually still use. Yes, all those other things get measured, and yes, they do seem to correlate, but, by and large, I use a certain visceral feeling to tell me when the patient is ready to go.

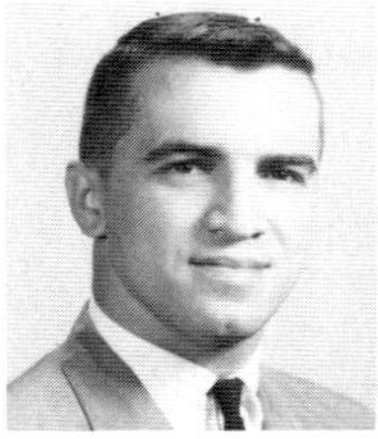

Introduction of Dr. Stan Dudrick

Dr. Clyde Barker: Our next speaker is Stan Dudrick. Stan graduated from the Hospital of the University of Pennsylvania residency in 1967. He had come to Penn Medical School from Franklin and Marshall, an institution on whose Board of Trustees he now serves. It was obvious even while Stan was a student and certainly when he was a resident that he was one of the most effective people on the scene. Although we did not realize it at the time, the fact that he was one of the most effective people in this group by definition meant that he was going to be a national leader in surgery, which he very soon became as he moved to the University of Texas at Houston as one of the youngest chairmen in the country. We all know of the many honors that have come to him since.

Much of the introduction that is appropriate for Stan I already gave before Ted's talk. I'll backtrack to show the title of this paper once more because it's so important in the development of the entire field of nutrition (Dudrick, S. J., Vars, H. M., Rawnsley, H. M., and Rhoads, J. E.: Total Intravenous Feeding and Growth in Puppies. *Fed Proc* 25:481, 1966). This short publication was really the beginning of the whole field of parenteral nutrition. It is considered by many to be one of the seminal pieces of work in all of medicine.

This 1968 abstract entitled "Reversal of Uremia and Body Wasting with Intravenous Essential Amino Acids" by Dudrick, S. J., Wilmore, D. W., Steiger, E., and Rhoads, J. E. (*Fed Proc* 28:808, 1968) described an early variation on the main theme of hyperalimentation in which Stan and his colleagues used the technique for purposes slightly different than nutrition per se. This interesting digression is appropriate as an introduction to Stan's intriguing topic of "Regression of Atherosclerosis by the Intravenous Infusion of Specific Biochemical Nutrient Substrates in Animals and Humans," which he will be speaking on today.

Dr. Dudrick's Introductory Remarks

Thank you very much Clyde and thank you all for being here. As Terry and I were flying to Philadelphia I asked her, "Is it okay for a guy my age to feel tingly all over and excited about going home and seeing my old buddies, my old professors, and Dr. Rhoads again?" She assured me that it was, and I must say that that is just the way I do feel looking out at this audience, however schmaltzy it might seem. I was trying to think of what made the group of people in this program so special. If I tried to put it in one word, I guess the word would be selfless. I don't know of any other group of people that mean anything to me who were so unselfish in helping each other to become educated, to be trained, and to take the best possible care of patients. We helped each other in our clinical responsibilities so that we would have time to go to the laboratory. We encouraged each other and lifted each other up when we were down about negative results or things that weren't looking so good. Although there were differences of opinion voiced periodically, the dominant theme was that everybody was still a friend; everybody could walk into anybody's office or operating room or look at anybody's patient. There was a great feeling of camaraderie. It thrills me to see that this still exists in this Department of Surgery. I think we get that from the top. Dr. Rhoads has always been that way and he ingrained us with that attitude. It's a wonderful tradition and heritage that we all owe to Dr. Rhoads.

I particularly enjoyed the wonderful turnout for Dr. Rhoads' birthday reception at the Union League last night. At the end of the evening I walked up to him and said, "Gee, Dr. Rhoads, this has been such a wonderful evening I can't wait for your ninetieth birthday." He said, "Well then you better start taking better care of yourself."

The one sadness for me today is that Harry Vars is not here to participate in this celebration. We owe so much to him. As Jim Thompson said in his talk, it was just wonderful to have had an opportunity to spend time with a walking encyclopedia, a kind, saintly man. I can't put it any better than Jim did in his eloquence. He meant a lot to all of us and through about 35 years in the Harrison Department of Surgical Research Harry Vars contributed greatly to all of us either directly or indirectly. My greatest regret today is that he doesn't have the joy of seeing some of the results that he spawned. But he was a wonderful man, a selfless man, who would allow me to work in the laboratory and do my thing while he went to the library to get books and do other things for me. Even before we started doing the work when I was up in Hazleton, Dutch Dyson would come down to Philadelphia in his Porsche even in the snow and load up on library books and bring them back to me so that I could read and do some of the basic ground work for the research work we were doing. Carter Nance would take off his fecal cytology gown and cover patients so we could get the lab work going. There are so many people—Harry Nelson, Bob Critchlow, Ed Kaplan, and others—who contributed greatly and it was nobody's particular turf. It wasn't Jerry Peskin's, Lenny Miller's, or Ted Copeland's turf. As you heard from Scott Jones, I don't know why Scott even put their names on the paper and himself as third. But these men all worked together throughout the residency program in a very unselfish way, the way Harry Vars and Dr. Rhoads always wanted us to do. I don't want to get too maudlin but I do want to pay tribute to Harry Vars, a man I know Dr. Rhoads would be particularly anxious to see given the appropriate tribute for what he did for all of us.

Dr. Rhoads, Happy Birthday and I surely do hope that, God willing, I'll still be around in ten years for your ninetieth.

Regression of Atherosclerosis by the Intravenous Infusion of Specific Biochemical Nutrient Substrates in Animals and Humans

STANLEY J. DUDRICK, M.D., F.A.C.S.

Preliminary studies in 400 New Zealand albino rabbits produced a reliable animal model of nutrient-induced atherosclerosis that stimulated that observed in humans. Atherosclerosis was then induced in an additional 1600 rabbits in sets of 40 animals each, maintaining plasma cholesterol concentrations between 1000 and 2000 mg/dL for 6–20 weeks. In each set, 10 control rabbits were killed to document baseline atherosclerosis, and the other 30 rabbits were assigned randomly to one of three groups of 10 rabbits. Groups of 10 rabbits were either continued on the atherogenic diet (group I), given standard laboratory rabbit pellets (group II), or infused continuously with specially formulated anticholesterol solutions *via* central venous catheters (group III) for 6 weeks. At autopsy, atherosclerotic lesions consistently involved 85–95% of the aorta in group I. In group II, atherosclerosis was comparable with the baseline control group with no regression. In group III, regression of atherosclerosis by 90–95% was consistently documented. Correlations between plasma amino acids and plasma cholesterol concentrations were established in four humans with severe atherosclerosis to maximize the cholesterol reduction capacity of the amino acid formulation. Infusion of the modified total parenteral nutrition solution induced prompt reduction in plasma cholesterol levels by 40–60% regardless of the initial level and was accompanied by evidence of regression of atherosclerosis after a 90-day infusion therapy period.

THE ROLE OF CHOLESTEROL in the etiology and pathogenesis of atherosclerosis has been debated by clinicians and investigators for many decades.[1] An elevated plasma cholesterol concentration is certainly not the only cause of, or contributing factor to, coronary heart disease. However, it appears that reducing elevated plasma cholesterol levels will decrease the risk, or is associated with a decreased risk, of myocardial infarction secondary to atherosclerotic coronary heart disease.[2,3]

During the past 20 years, as clinical applications of total parenteral nutrition (TPN) have been expanded, it has been documented that plasma cholesterol concentrations decline to low or low normal levels especially in puppies, infants, critically ill malnourished adults, and long-term home TPN patients. However, early attempts to correlate short-term TPN-induced hypocholesterolemia with regression of peripheral vascular disease by our team at the Hospital of the University of Pennsylvania in six patients studied for 1 month were unsuccessful. Subsequently, several patients in our series who had mesenteric infarction of the small bowel secondary to severe atherosclerosis required another abdominal operation after 3–5 years of nourishment entirely by vein. In four of these patients, the previously documented atherosclerosis in the major abdominal vessels had decreased dramatically or was undetectable at intraoperative evaluation. In six such patients in their fifth to eighth decades

From the Department of Surgery, The University of Texas Medical School at Houston, Hermann Hospital, Houston, Texas.

Presented at the 107th Annual Meeting of The American Surgical Association, Palm Beach, Florida, April 21–23, 1987.

Clinical Professor of Surgery, The University of Texas Medical School at Houston, Houston, Texas.

This article has been reproduced from *Annals of Surgery*, Vol. 206, No. 3, 1987.

TABLE 1. *Atherogenic Rabbit Diet Formulation**

Base formula
High fiber Purina Labchow 5326†
14.5% protein
1.7% fat
55 ppm cholesterol
42.4% nitrogen-free extract
8.9% ash
Water
22.5% crude fiber
40.9% neutral detergent fiber (cellulose, lignin, hemicellulose)
24.6% acid detergent fiber (cellulose, lignin)
Additives per kilogram of base formula
900 g fiber
80 g peanut oil
20 g crystalline cholesterol

* Teklad T.D. 82135, Teklad, Inc., Madison, WI.
† Purina Labchow 5326, Purina Mills, Inc., St. Louis, MO.

of life who died for reasons unrelated to their cardiovascular system after 3.5–15 years of home TPN, postmortem examination demonstrated minimal atherosclerosis or disease-free vessels.

Foremost among other workers who observed cholesterol lowering effects of fat-free TPN were Starzl et al.,[4,5] Folkman et al.,[6] and Yamashita et al.[7] who made novel clinical applications of this phenomenon to the management of patients with hyperlipoproteinemia, glycogen storage disease, and familial hypercholesterolemia.

The goals of this series of investigations were to: (1) strictly control nutrient substrate administration in rabbits and humans to determine the maximum dietary potential to reduce plasma cholesterol concentrations while maintaining adequate nutrition; (2) modify existing intravenous nutrient substrate mixtures to maximize their cholesterol reducing effects; (3) determine whether these diets, either directly or secondary to induced hypocholesterolemia, could arrest and/or induce regression of atherosclerosis; and (4) determine whether improved cardiovascular function and secondarily improved blood flow to vital tissues would thereby result.

Animal Studies

Preliminary laboratory investigations were done in 400 New Zealand albino rabbits to develop a reliable animal model of dietary-induced atherosclerosis. By systematically altering the fat, cholesterol, and fiber in the oral diet, a special formulation evolved that consistently induced atherosclerotic lesions comparable in composition, distribution, and gross and histologic appearance to those commonly occurring in humans. The atherogenic rabbit diet (Table 1) was subsequently fed to an additional 1600 animals in quantities sufficient to maintain plasma cholesterol levels at approximately 1000 mg/dL without untoward hepatobiliary or gastrointestinal complications. The severity of atherosclerosis in the major vasculature could be estimated by observing the appearance and extent of atheromatous deposits in the blood vessels of the iris. After 6–20 weeks of maintaining hypercholesterolemia, significant atherosclerosis was routinely demonstrated to affect 30–90% of the surface area of the great vessels, respectively; the lesions were histologically indistinguishable from those seen in humans (Figs. 1–3). By 6 months, some animals had myocardial infarctions, strokes, mesenteric vascular occlusions, and peripheral vascular occlusions secondary to severe atherosclerosis involving more than 95% of the surface of the great vessels and major tributaries.

A large series of experiments was done in sets of 40 rabbits in which plasma cholesterol levels were maintained at approximately 1000 mg/dL in all animals for 4.5 months. Ten animals in each group were killed to determine the gross and histologic extent and character of the atherosclerosis, and the remaining animals in each experiment were assigned randomly to one of three groups of 10 animals each. For the next 6 weeks, group I rabbits continued to be fed the atherogenic diet, group II rabbits were fed standard laboratory rabbit

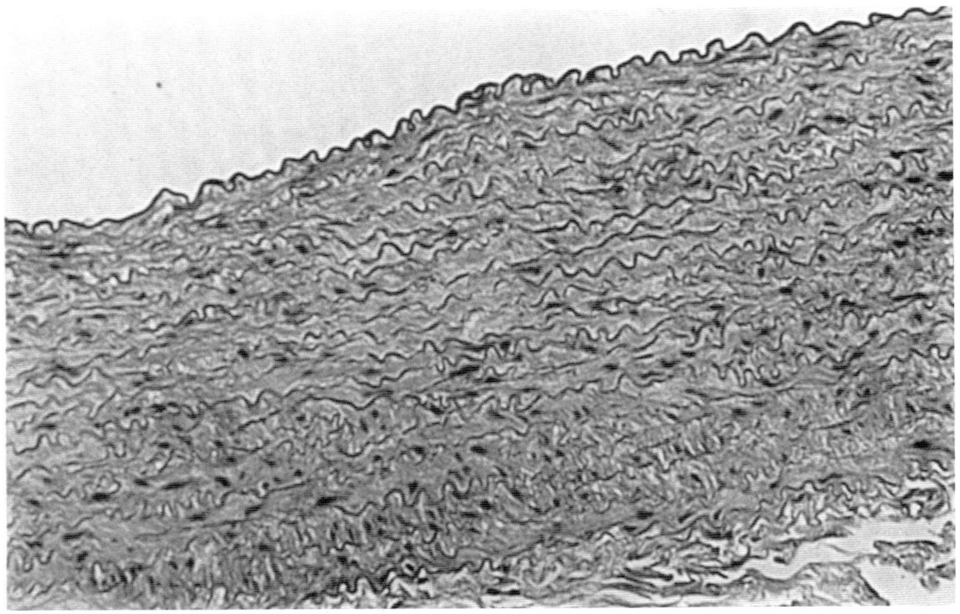

FIG. 1. Intermediate power full-thickness longitudinal section of a normal rabbit aorta. The thin darkly stained convoluted upper border of the specimen represents the entire thickness of the intima. The adventitia is visible in the lower right corner. The media, filled with elastin fibrils, extends between the intima and adventitia.

pellets, and group III rabbits were fed by continuous central venous infusions either with one of the six commercially available amino acid solutions listed in Table 2 or with specially formulated solutions designed to achieve a maximum plasma cholesterol lowering effect. All amino acid mixtures were administered continuously by pump over 24 hours together with all essential vitamins, minerals, and trace elements and all nonprotein caloric requirements as dextrose. All intravenous solutions were fat free. Blood samples were obtained weekly throughout the 6 months to monitor lipid profiles and standard biochemical and hematologic indices. Serum and urine amino acid profiles were obtained monthly, and all animals had autopsies at the end of the study.

In group I animals, complex atherosclerotic lesions consistently involved 85–95% of the great vessels. In group II animals, the atherosclerosis was comparable with that in the 4.5-month atherogenic control group with no evidence of significant progression or regression. In group III animals, significant regression of the atherosclerosis was consistently documented by 90–95% clearing of the surface area of the great vessels and major tributaries (Figs. 4–8).

In the first six sets of 40 rabbits, the group III animals received one of six commercially available amino acid solutions (Table 2). After the 6-week intravenous infusion period using these solutions, regression of atherosclerotic lesions varied from minimally detectable to 5–10% regression. By correlating plasma and urine amino acid concentrations with plasma cholesterol levels in these animals, changes in the percentages of the individual amino acids were made sequentially in the group III animals and all subsequent sets of rabbits. As a result of these manipulations, a 9.5% amino acid formulation evolved that induced 90–95% regression of the dietary-induced atherosclerosis within 6 weeks. The rabbit study was terminated at this point because the data obtained from this model indicated that the maximum atherosclerosis regression potential of the modified TPN solution had been achieved under the experimental conditions. No regression of atherosclerosis has been observed in long-term follow-up studies of 10 rabbits that were fed the atherogenic diet for 6 months and then fed the standard laboratory rabbit pellets for up to 2 years.

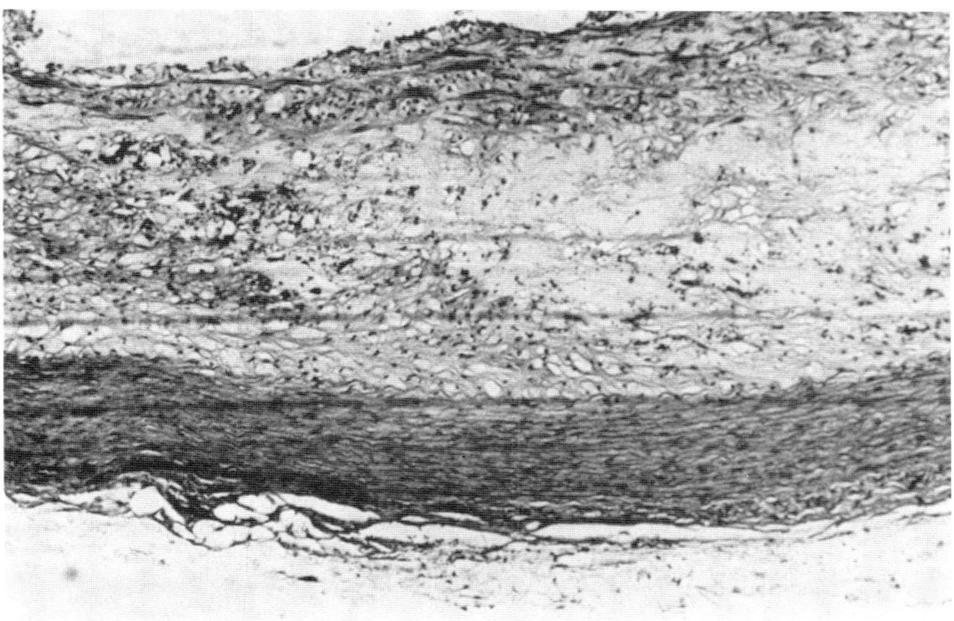

FIG. 2. Low power longitudinal section of the aorta from an animal fed a high-cholesterol diet for 4.5 months. The intima histologically fulfills the criteria of a complicated lesion with: (1) smooth muscle proliferation and expansion of the intima from 1 to 30 cells thick, (2) focal calcification is depicted by the darkly stained calcium deposits, (3) vacuolated appearance of foam cells, and (4) extracellular deposits of cholesterol as cholesterol clefts.

Patient Studies

Pilot Study: Case 1

A 40-year-old white man with Type IIB hyperlipidemia had an acute anterior myocardial infarction at age 32. After recovery, he was treated with clofibrate, Questran®, and Coumadin®. His plasma cholesterol levels ranged between 500 and 800 mg/dL and his serum triglyceride levels ranged from 800–1000 mg/dL. Dietary manipulation begun in 1977 maintained his plasma cholesterol to levels between 450 and 560 mg/dL. Cardiac catheterization in April 1984, showed 100% occlusion of his right coronary artery and diffuse atherosclerotic disease involving the left anterior descending and circumflex coronary arteries.

Due to the development of progressively increasing severity and frequency of angina pectoris, severe claudication after walking one block, daily dizziness and syncope, and episodic numbness in his extremities related to poor and/or absent pulses in his neck, arms, and legs, he agreed to undergo a 6-month period of intravenous anticholesterol therapy beginning in May 1985. A percutaneous subclavian central venous feeding catheter was inserted into the patient's superior vena cava, and a continuous infusion of the modified TPN solution that had ultimately evolved during the rabbit studies was begun after obtaining baseline biochemical and hematologic studies and instructing the patient in the basic principles and practices of ambulatory home TPN. The patient was allowed absolutely no food by mouth but could drink water *ad libitum.* The patient received no fat during the study, and all nonprotein caloric requirements were provided as dextrose. Since he was approximately eight pounds above his calculated ideal body weight, his formulation for the first few weeks was hypocaloric until he achieved his ideal body weight. Essential vitamins, minerals, and trace elements were provided in accordance with standard home TPN practices. Within 10 days of receiving the initial intravenous anticholesterol diet, his plasma cholesterol level dropped from his preinfusion baseline concentration of 508 mg/dL to 220 mg/dL, representing a greater than 50% reduction. During the 6 months that the patient received the anticholesterol therapy, he had no angina pectoris, dizziness or syncope; his

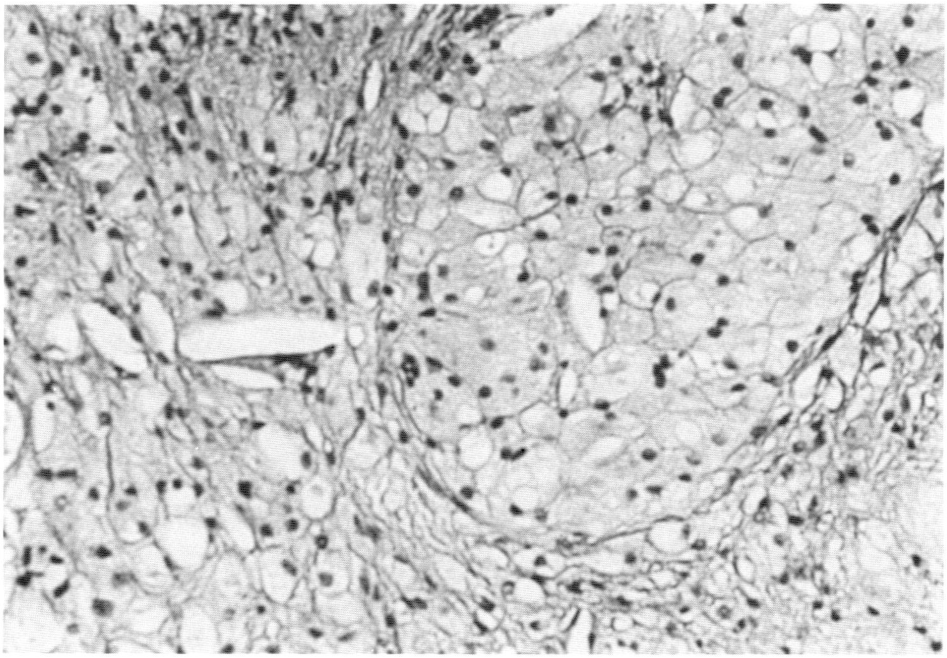

FIG. 3. This high power photomicrograph depicts the deposition of cholesterol and fats both intracellularly (foam cells) and extracellularly (cholesterol clefts).

peripheral pulses and perfusion improved greatly; the Doppler blood flow to his left leg increased 250% and to his right leg increased 300%; and the episodic numbness in his hands and feet disappeared completely.

After 4 weeks of therapy, the patient's general health, strength, and feeling of well being improved sufficiently, and he was begun on a graduated monitored treadmill exercise

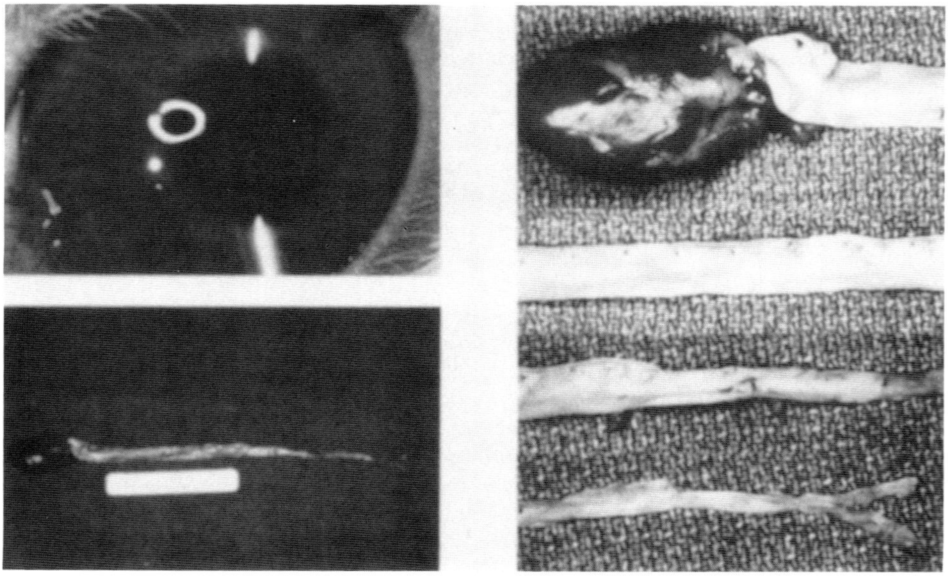

FIG. 4. Composite picture depicting a normal rabbit iris and intimal surface of the aorta with no evidence of atherosclerosis.

TABLE 2. *Percentage Composition of Intravenous Amino Acid Formulations*

Amino Acid	Travasol 8.5%*	FreAmine III 8.5%†	Aminosyn 10%‡	Travasol 10%*	FreAmine III 10%†	Novamine 11.4%§	Atheromine 10.3%*
Isoleucine	4.09	6.53	6.61	5.46	6.51	4.83	4.0–10.0
Leucine	5.30	8.53	8.64	6.65	8.59	6.70	5.0–10.0
Lysine	3.56	4.93	4.75	3.79	4.92	5.48	4.5–6.5
Methionine	4.36	4.38	3.23	3.20	4.40	4.25	3.5–5.5
Phenylalanine	4.19	4.21	3.20	4.03	4.18	5.30	4.5–7.5
Threonine	3.95	4.15	5.27	4.21	4.16	5.33	2.0–3.5
Tryptophane	0.98	0.92	0.88	1.05	0.91	1.03	1.0–2.5
Valine	4.39	6.94	8.22	5.90	6.97	6.92	4.0–9.0
Alanine	26.01	9.75	17.25	27.64	9.83	19.78	7.0–16.0
Arginine	5.51	5.57	5.59	5.94	5.57	5.90	9.0–18.0
Histidine	2.38	1.69	1.75	2.78	1.68	3.66	1.5–3.5
Proline	4.09	11.98	9.00	7.05	12.04	6.57	4.5–8.5
Serine	0.00	6.90	4.81	5.67	6.94	4.76	2.5–6.5
Tyrosine	0.27	0.00	0.32	0.29	0.00	0.20	0.0–1.0
Glycine	30.92	22.98	20.50	16.35	23.05	11.68	3.0–8.0
Glutamic acid	0.00	0.00	0.00	0.00	0.00	4.30	3.5–5.5
Aspartic acid	0.00	0.00	0.00	0.00	0.00	2.75	2.0–4.0
Cysteine	0.00	0.24	0.00	0.00	0.25	0.56	0.0–1.0
Total	100.00	99.71	100.00	100.00	100.00	100.00	100.00

* Baxter Healthcare Corp., Deerfield, IL.
† Kendall-McGaw Laboratories, Irvine, CA.
‡ Abbott Laboratories, North Chicago, IL.
§ Cutter Laboratories, Emeryville, CA.

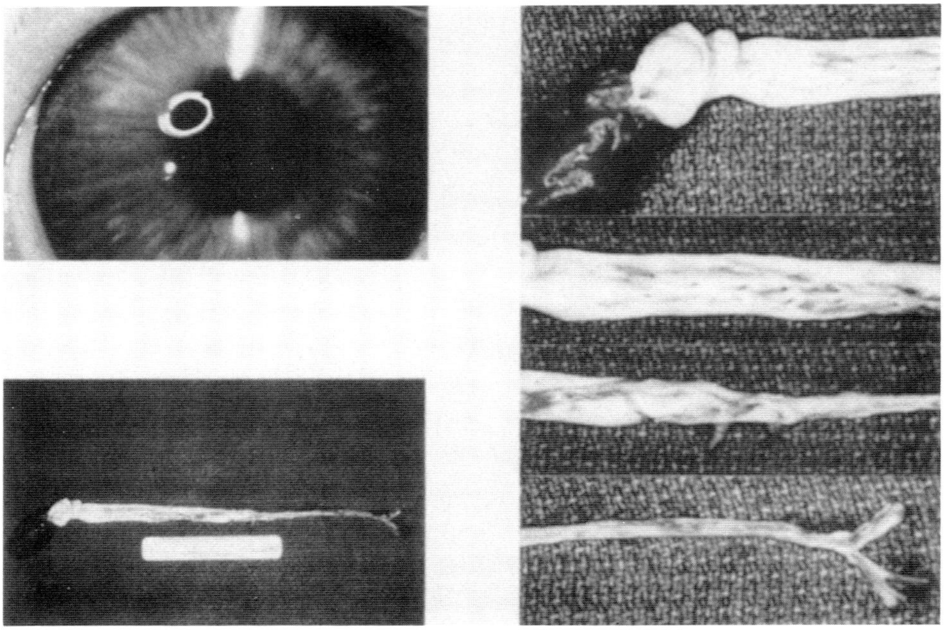

FIG. 5. Composite picture of the iris and aorta in a rabbit fed the high-cholesterol diet for 4.5 months. The lack of pigment in the iris allows direct visualization of the deposition of plaque in the vascular bed, which correlates positively with the atherosclerosis involving 90% of the aorta.

program. During the fifth week of his therapy, he walked 1 mile a day on the treadmill at 1 mile per hour and by the eighth week was walking 3.5–4 miles a day at 3.5 miles per hour without pain or claudication in his legs and with no angina pectoris. During the ninth week

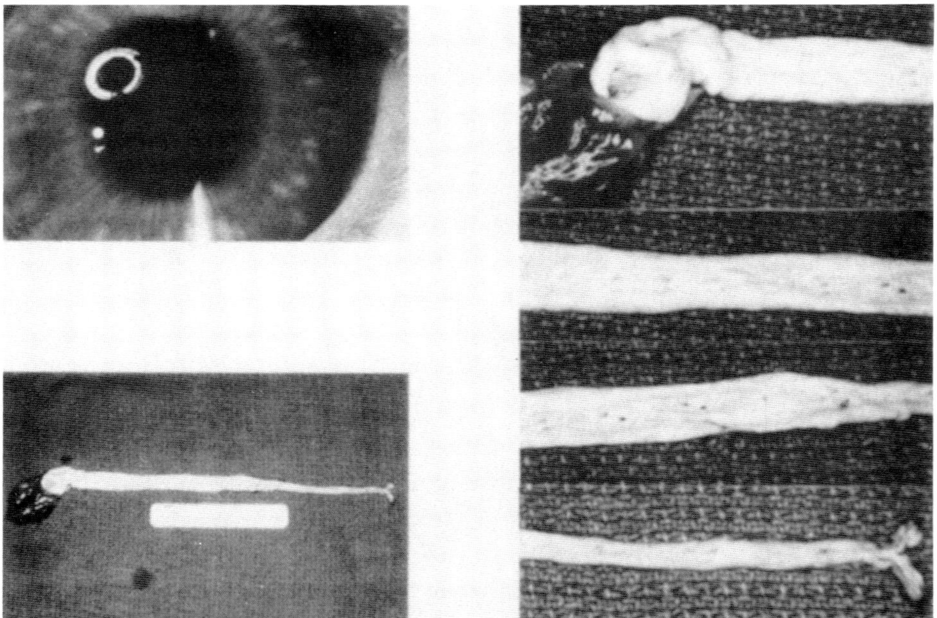

FIG. 6. Composite picture of the iris and aorta in a rabbit fed the high-cholesterol diet for 4.5 months and maintained on the high-cholesterol diet for an additional 6.5 weeks.

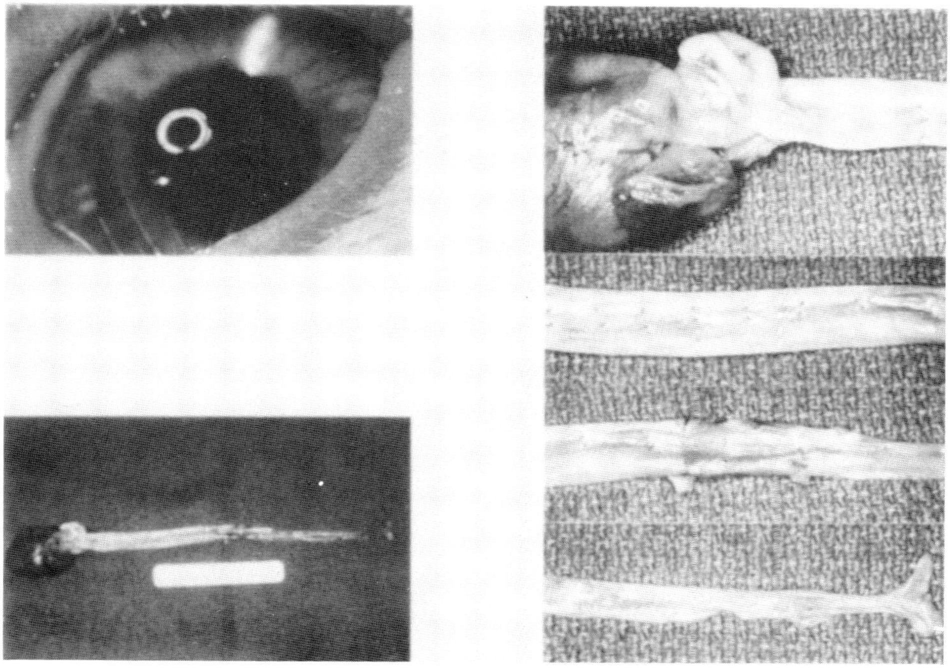

FIG. 7. Composite picture depicting the iris and aorta in a rabbit maintained on the high-cholesterol diet for 4.5 months before switching to low-cholesterol diet rabbit pellets for an additional 6 weeks.

of therapy he began to play 18 holes of golf several times a week scoring in the 70s, despite the handicap of having to wear the continuous intravenous infusion apparatus.

During the course of his therapy and study, frequent plasma and urine amino acid concentrations were determined and correlated with his plasma cholesterol level (Fig. 9). At point two, the branched chain amino acids, isoleucine, leucine, and valine, were increased in the formula. At point three, phenylalanine was increased and glycine was decreased in the formula. At point five, alanine was decreased, and glutamic acid and aspartic acid were increased. At point ten, proline and serine were decreased, and at point twelve, arginine was increased, whereas histidine was decreased.

On day 60 at point six, 500 mL of 10% soybean oil emulsion (10% Intralipid, KabiVitrum, Stockholm, Sweden) was infused into the patient over 6 hours, and the plasma cholesterol concentration rose promptly and dramatically more than 100 mg/dL to 365 mg/dL and remained above 300 mg/dL for 1 month. At that point 500 mL of 20% soybean oil emulsion (20% Intralipid, KabiVitrum) was infused over 6 hours, and the plasma cholesterol level again rose significantly but not as high nor as persistently as the initial infusion of the 10% soybean oil infusion. However, the persistent adverse effects on plasma cholesterol levels after infusions of such relatively small amounts of fat emulsion are obvious, dramatic, and disturbing.

Between days 140 and 150, the plasma concentration of arginine was approximately 100 μmol/L, and the urine concentration of arginine was approximately 40 μmol/L (Fig. 10). Because this represented the lower limit of normal for plasma arginine concentration, the dosage of arginine in the infusion mixture was doubled for the next 10 days. This resulted in a rise in the plasma amino acid concentration of arginine to approximately 200 μmol/L, the usual upper normal limit, whereas urine excretion of arginine increased. Concomitantly, the plasma cholesterol level dropped dramatically from 310 mg/dL to 230 mg/dL. At this point, the arginine dosage in the infusion mixture was tripled with essentially no change in plasma concentration of arginine, a dramatic increase in urinary excretion of arginine, and essentially no change in plasma cholesterol concentration. This sequence of events illustrates the manner in which the dosages of the various amino acids in the anticholesterol formulation

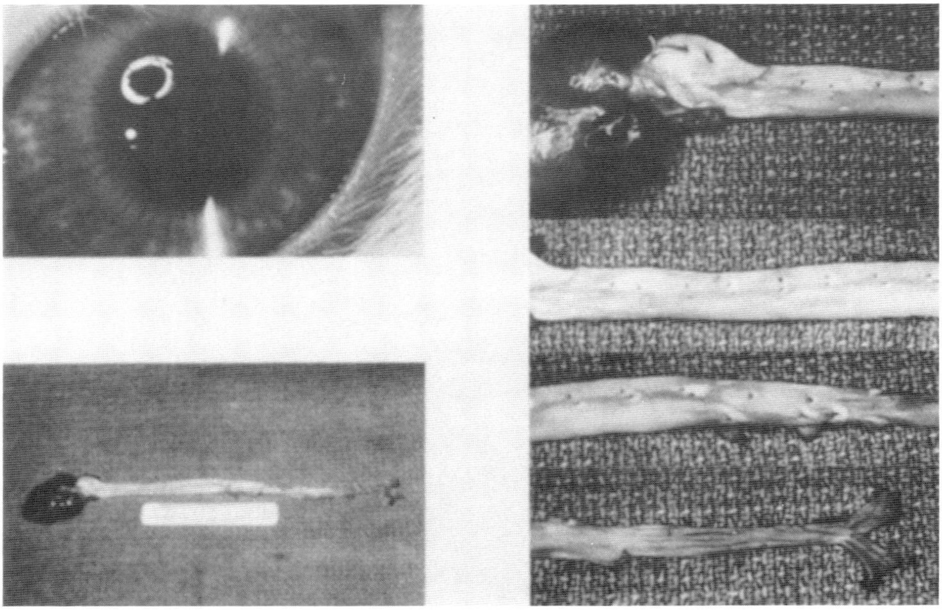

FIG. 8. Composite picture depicting the iris and aorta in a rabbit fed a high-cholesterol diet for 4.5 months and switched to a special mixture of nutrient substrates infused intravenously for an additional 6 weeks. The aortic surface is 95% free of atherosclerosis.

were derived. All other numbers in Figure 9 represent changes in dextrose calories in response to changes in the patient's body weight and activity.

The significant changes in plasma apolipoprotein B and triglyceride concentrations are illustrated in Figures 11 and 12.

Coronary angiography after the therapy indicated improved flow in the previously completely blocked right coronary artery and increased diameter and flow in the tributaries of the left coronary artery with the development of increased collateral coronary artery circulation, myocardial perfusion, and cardiac performance (Figs. 13 and 14). Coronary arteriographic analysis using computerized quantitative angiography[8] (Figs. 15 and 16) indicated

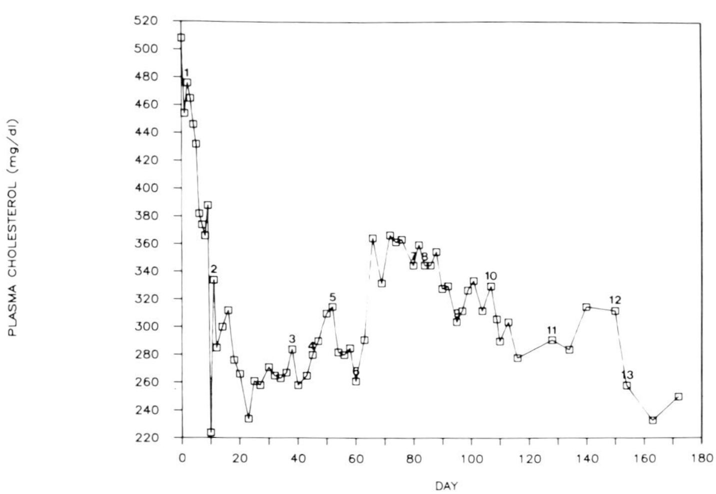

FIG. 9. Plasma cholesterol levels during 6 months of anticholesterol therapy. Numbered points denote significant changes in the components of the formula.

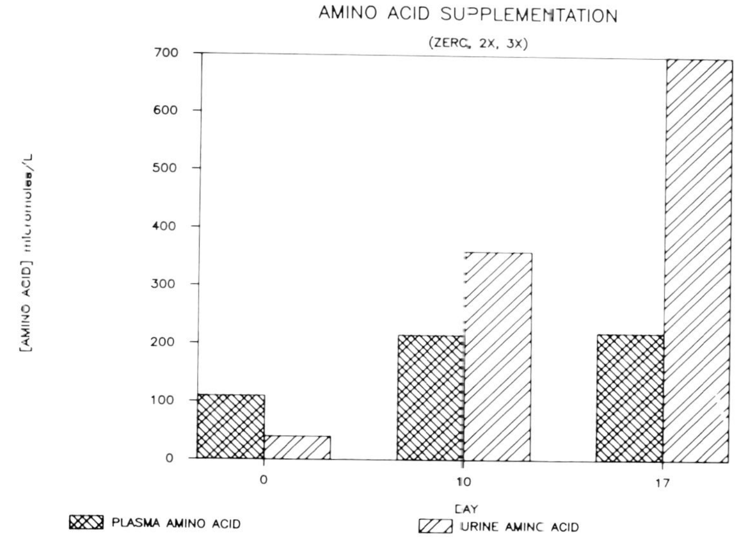

FIG. 10. Relative changes in plasma and urinary arginine levels with changes in the intravenous solution mixture.

regression of coronary atherosclerosis by an increase in the diameter in one of the branches of the left coronary artery from 1.19 mm before therapy to 1.30 mm after therapy and an increase in cross-sectional area from 1.12 mm^2 before therapy to 1.27 mm^2 after therapy. Coronary flow reserve increased from 3.6 to 4.2, consistent with the disappearance of his angina pectoris. These data assume even greater potential significance considering that the baseline angiography was performed more than 1 year before the initiation of the anticholesterol therapy and that the patient's continuing symptomatic deterioration during that interval indicated further progression of his coronary atherosclerosis during that year.

To date, the patient is 2 years post-initiation of his anticholesterol therapy and 18 months post-completion of his therapy. He has remained completely free of his initial presenting signs and symptoms, has returned to gainful employment as a Computer Systems Analyst,

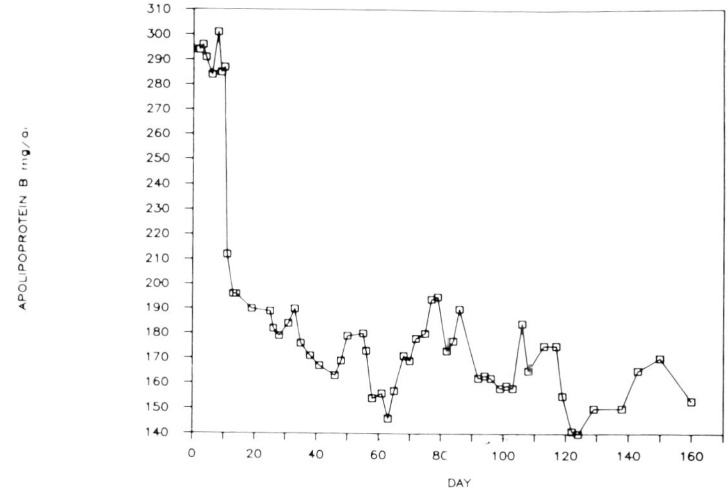

FIG. 11. Alteration of plasma apolipoprotein B levels during 6 months of anticholesterol therapy.

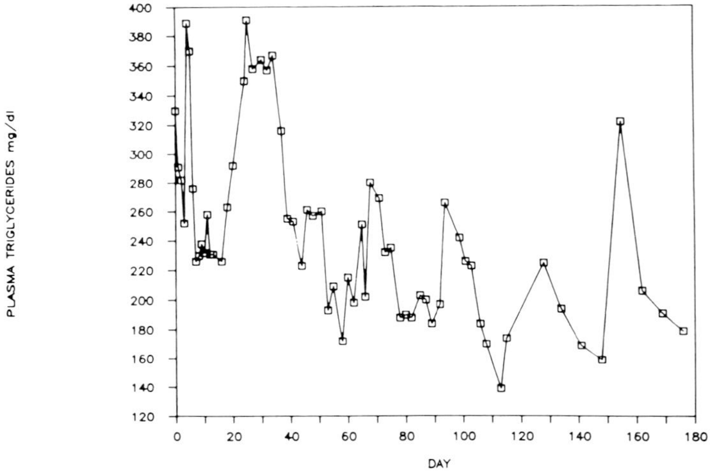

FIG. 12. Alteration of plasma triglyceride levels during 6 months of anticholesterol therapy.

engages in normal physical activity without limitations, plays golf regularly, and enjoys a feeling of good health and well being.

Home TPN Patients

To determine the extent of the increased effectiveness of the anticholesterol amino acid formulation (Atheromine, Baxter Healthcare Corp., Deerfield, IL) in lowering plasma cholesterol compared with the standard amino acid formulations used in home TPN, 30 patients with short bowel syndrome who had been receiving one of the six commercially available amino acid formulations for 4 months to 9 years were studied. The Atheromine solution that had evolved during the pilot patient study was substituted for the usual amino acid formula in each of the 30 patient volunteers for 7 days while monitoring plasma cholesterol levels daily. The upper and lower limits of the plasma cholesterol concentrations determined daily for these 30 patients are shown in Figure 17. Prompt reductions in plasma cholesterol concentrations by 40–60% occurred in all patients regardless of the initial baseline value or

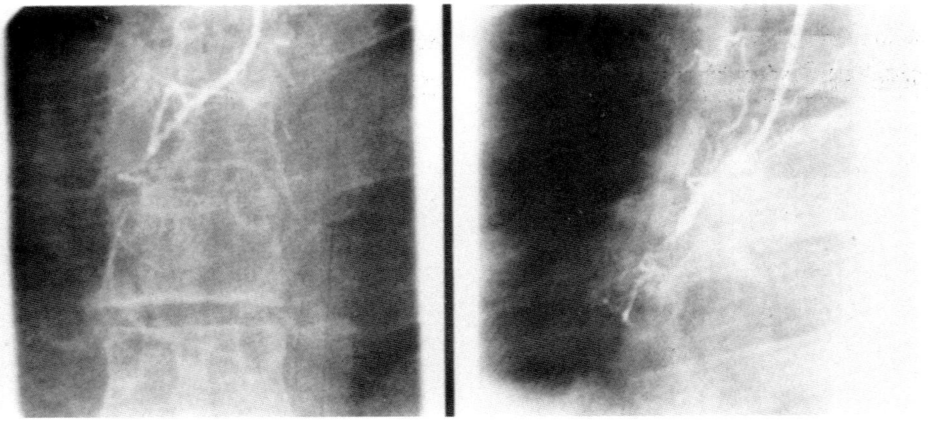

FIG. 13. Angiography shows complete blockage of the right coronary artery before treatment (*left*). Improved flow through the right coronary artery and greatly increased collateral blood flow occurred after therapy (*right*).

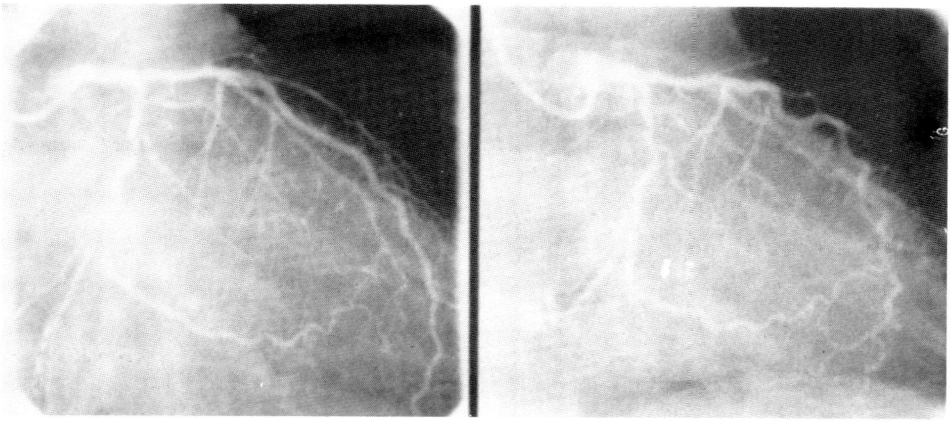

FIG. 14. Increased diameter and blood flow through the left anterior descending and circumflex coronary arteries occurred after therapy (*right*) compared with the pretreatment angiogram (*left*). Improved collateral circulation between the right and left coronary systems can be seen in the left lower quadrant of the right photograph.

the amino acid mixture that had been infused during their standard home TPN regimen. In one patient in whom the baseline cholesterol level was 168 mg/dL, a 58% drop in plasma cholesterol to 70 mg/dL occurred in 7 days. Even more dramatic and remarkable was a drop in plasma cholesterol from an already low value of 85 mg/dL by 65% to 30 mg/dL in 7 days.

Case 2

A 55-year-old man with severe coronary artery disease had a myocardial infarction in 1963 at the age of 31. A second myocardial infarction occurred in 1977 and required emergency coronary bypass to five vessels.

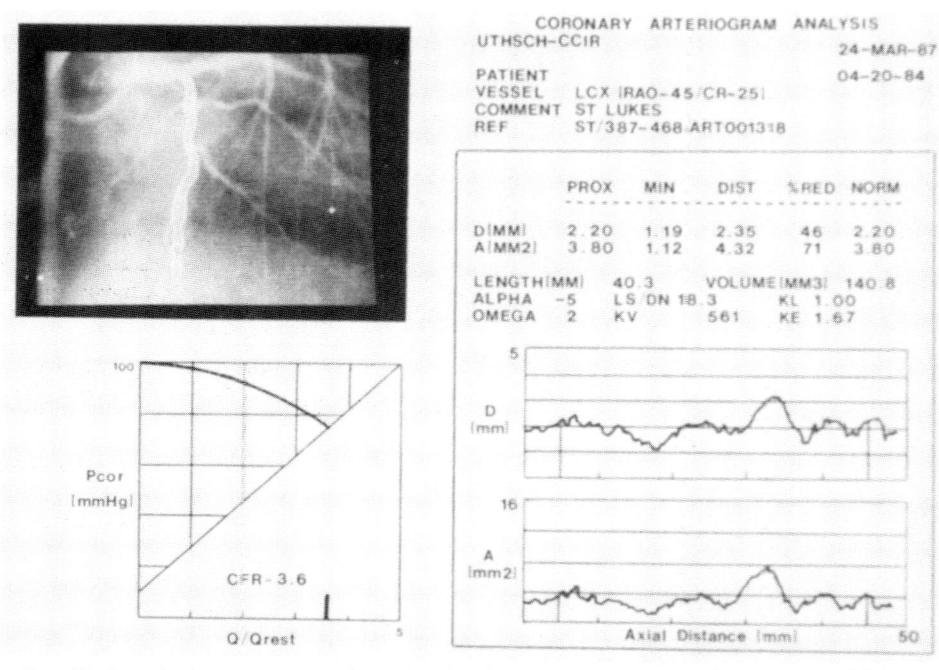

FIG. 15. Quantitative coronary angiography showing restricted coronary flow reserve of 3.6 before therapy.

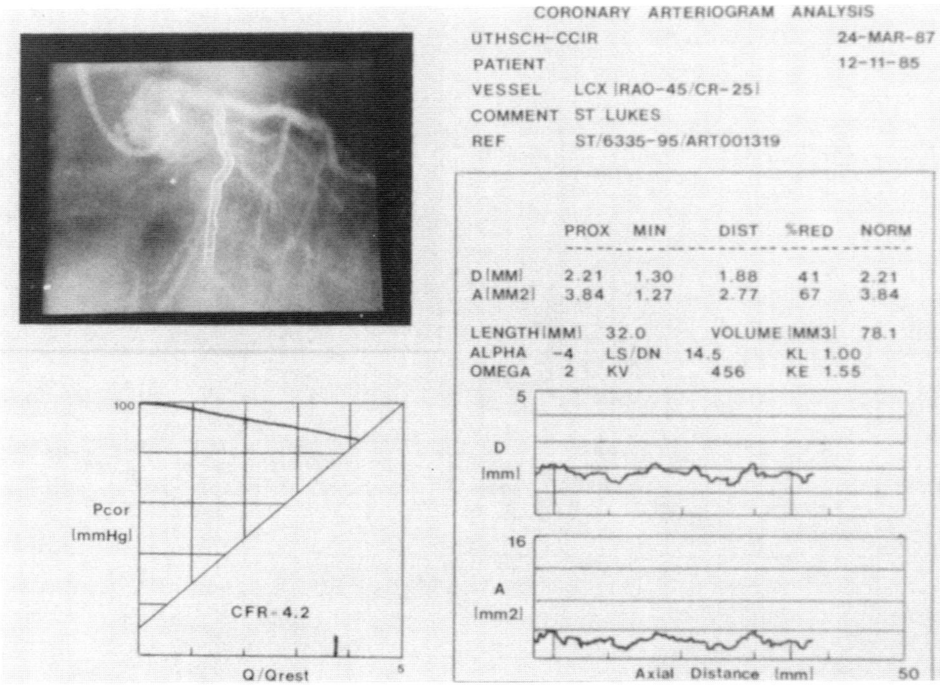

FIG. 16. Repeat quantitative coronary angiography showing 16% improved coronary flow reserve to 4.2 after therapy secondary to increased diameter and cross-sectional area of the artery.

Recurrent persistent angina pectoris developed in March 1985, and in December 1985, he had a third myocardial infarction. Before intravenous anticholesterol therapy, the patient had disabling crushing anterior chest pain 4–5 times per day, even at rest. Cardiac catheterization in 1985 showed three-vessel coronary artery disease with occlusion of the right coronary artery, extensive disease in the left anterior descending coronary artery, occlusion of a large marginal branch of the circumflex coronary artery, and occlusion of all of his

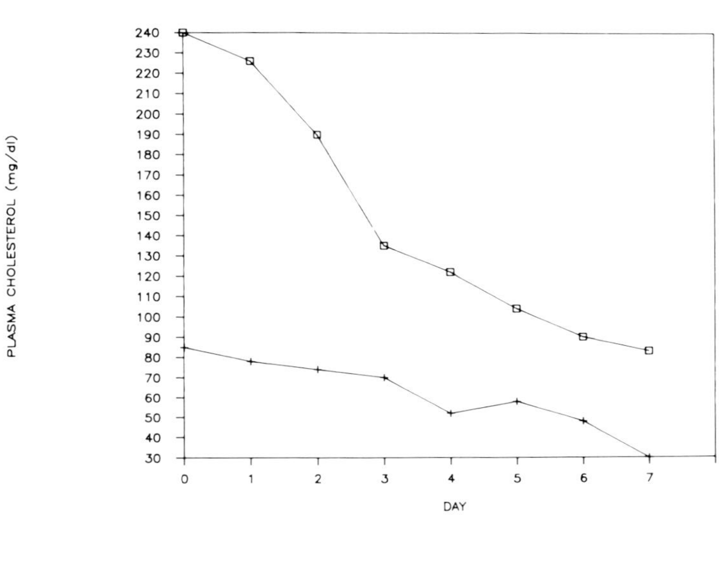

FIG. 17. Upper (□) and lower (+) levels of plasma cholesterol levels in home TPN patients (N = 30) during the first week of therapy.

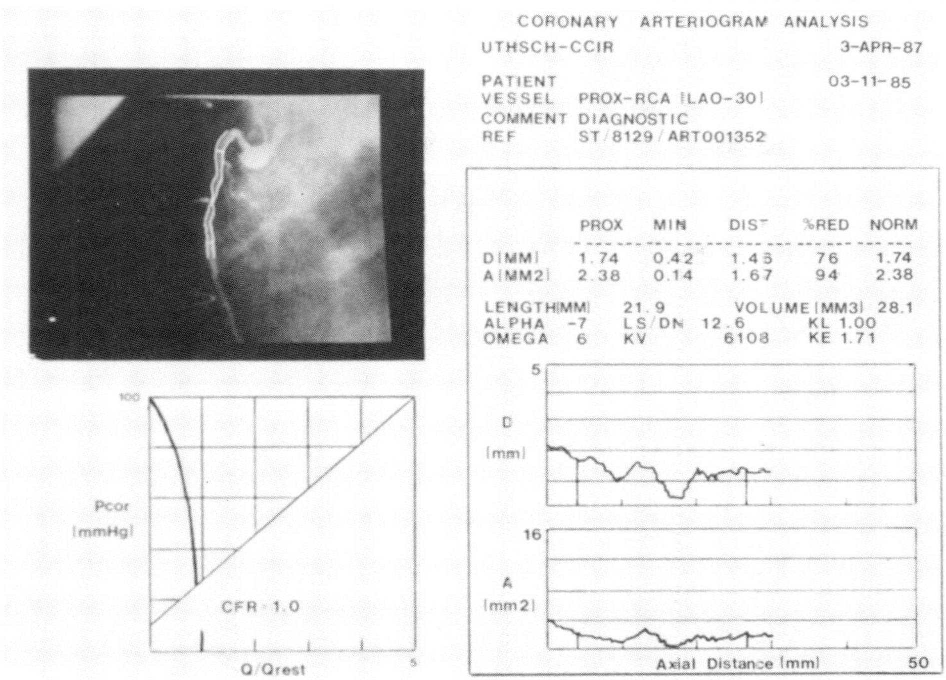

FIG. 18. Severely compromised coronary flow reserve before initiation of Atheromine therapy secondary to greatly decreased diameter and cross-sectional area of the right coronary artery.

bypass grafts with the exception of the left anterior descending graft, which was functioning poorly.

The patient denied angina pectoris after the first two days of anticholesterol therapy with the exception of one mild episode that occurred while riding a bicycle in 30-degree weather against a 45 mph wind for 2.5 miles, a great increase over his usual level of exertional activity.

His medications before anticholesterol therapy included Procardia®, Norpace®, Lanoxin®, Tenormin®, aspirin, nitroglycerin, and nitropaste. At the completion of 90 days of anticholesterol therapy, the patient's only cardiac medication was Lanoxin, and he denied chest pain despite a greatly increased level of physical activity. His initial plasma cholesterol level of 218 mg/dL declined by 39% to a low value during therapy of 123 mg/dL.

His follow-up evaluation included cardiac catheterization and quantitative coronary angiography, which documented an improvement in coronary flow reserve (CFR) from 1.0 to 2.3, an improvement of 130% (Figs. 18–20). Additionally, a pretherapy thallium treadmill test showed a perfusion defect involving the anterolateral, apical, and inferior segment of the left ventricle that did not show any evidence of reperfusion at rest. The post-therapy thallium treadmill test showed resolution of the perfusion defect in the anterolateral segment of the left ventricle. Stress defects and redistribution abnormalities in the apical posterior, lateral, and inferior segments of the left ventricle were not as severe as the pretreatment examination. There was definite evidence for improvement of perfusion of the left ventricle.

Case 3

A 45-year-old previously healthy white man had an inferior wall myocardial infarction that was complicated by ventricular fibrillation from which he was successfully resuscitated. Cardiac catheterization demonstrated a 50% narrowing of the midlateral anterior descending coronary artery, a 50% narrowing of the circumflex artery, and a normal right coronary artery. Despite treatment with an extremely low-fat, low-cholesterol diet and anticholesterol drugs, including nicotinic acid and cholestyramine, he was unable to decrease his plasma cholesterol level below 250 mg/dL.

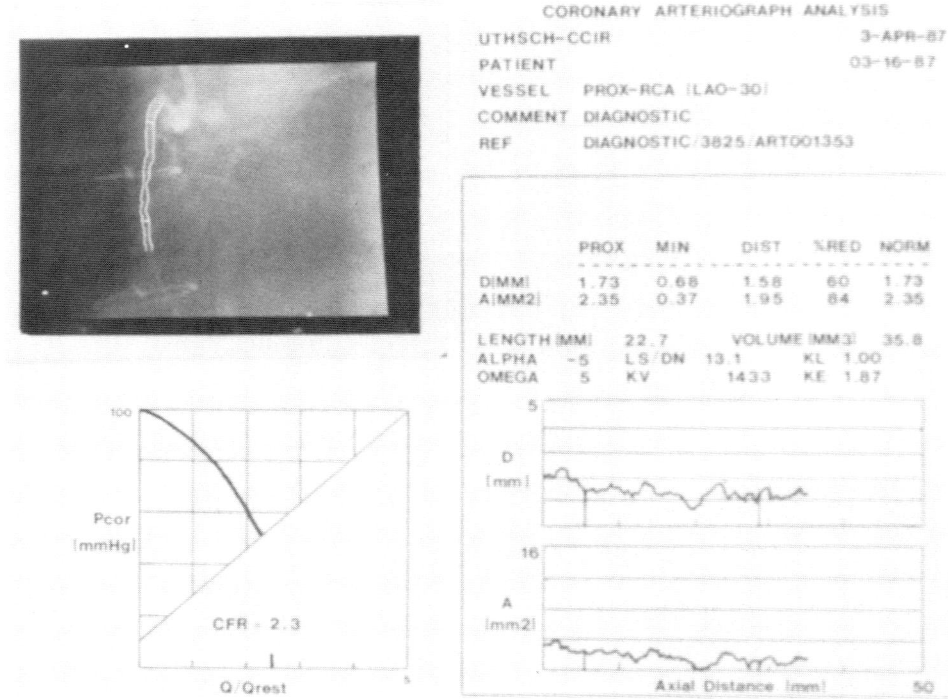

FIG. 19. Marked improvement in coronary flow reserve in right coronary artery after 3 months of Atheromine therapy with significantly increased diameter and cross-sectional area of the previously narrowed segment.

During 90 days of intravenous anticholesterol therapy, he lost approximately 1 pound and could be weaned from his cardiac medications (nifedipine and timolol). His plasma cholesterol declined 64% to a low level of 90 mg/dL.

Case 4

A 55-year-old white man with a history of recurrent coronary artery disease and several previous myocardial infarctions initially developed angina pectoris in 1971. Cardiac catheterization showed significant coronary artery disease for which he had an internal mammary coronary bypass (Weinberg procedure). In 1980, he had a myocardial infarction, and recurrent and persistent angina pectoris developed in 1981. At that time a second cardiac catheterization documented significant recurrent disease. He had saphenous vein aorta coronary bypass to three vessels with improvement for approximately 2 years until the development of recurrent chest pain primarily associated with exercise. He had cardiac catheterization again in 1983, which showed global hypokinesis with an ejection fraction of 26%, a totally obstructed left anterior descending and distal circumflex coronary artery, and significant disease of the distal right coronary artery.

His angina pectoris became progressively severe over the subsequent 3 years, and at the time of pretreatment evaluation he was having chest pain 4–5 times per day requiring nitroglycerin for relief. He could walk only 2 miles at a slow pace without the development of chest pain. His pretreatment medications included Procardia, Corgard®, and nitroglycerin.

After starting anticholesterol therapy, he had no further episodes of angina pectoris despite the development of a subclavian vein thrombosis necessitating placement of a second Hickman catheter and the development of a small bowel obstruction secondary to adhesions that required laparotomy. He lost 16 pounds during the 90-day treatment period and was able to reduce his cardiac medications by 50%.

His initial plasma cholesterol level of 252 mg/dL declined by 66.7% to a low of 84 mg/dL. His pretreatment positive thallium treadmill test remained positive post-treatment; how-

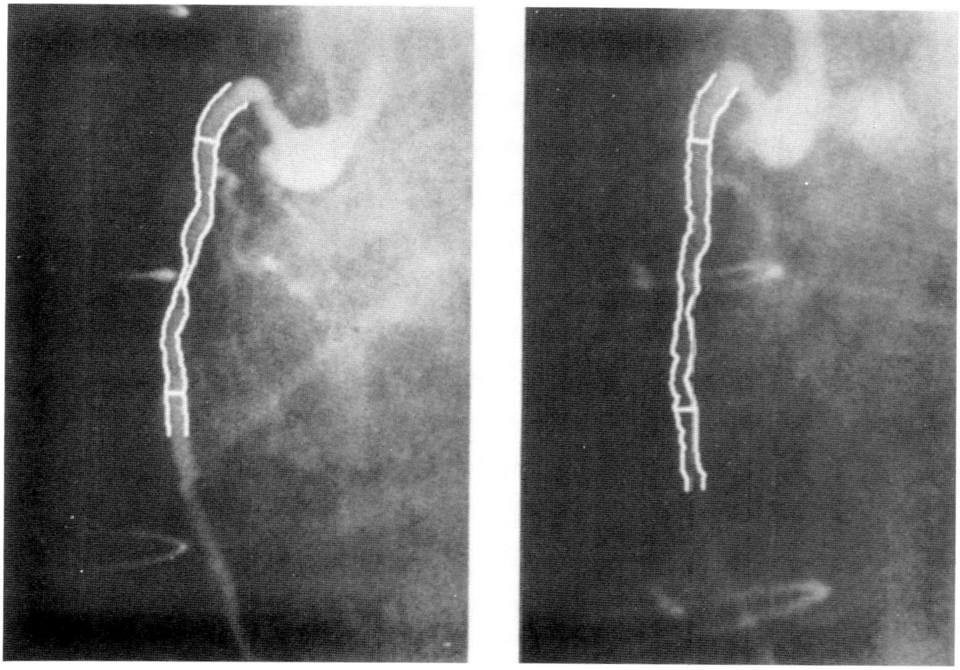

FIG. 20. Enlargement of right coronary angiograms before (*left*) and after (*right*) therapy demonstrating computer augmented vascular outlines.

ever, he was able to achieve a 25% higher heart rate during his post-treatment examination. Follow-up cardiac catheterization showed generalized severe coronary atherosclerosis with complete occlusion of the left anterior descending, circumflex, and right coronary artery and the development of an extensive collateral network with a patent but stenotic vein graft to the right coronary artery and an ineffective left internal mammary graft. His ejection fraction, however, on his post-treatment examination had increased to 55%, representing a 92% improvement.

During and since his therapy he has had no further angina pectoris despite a greatly increased level of activity.

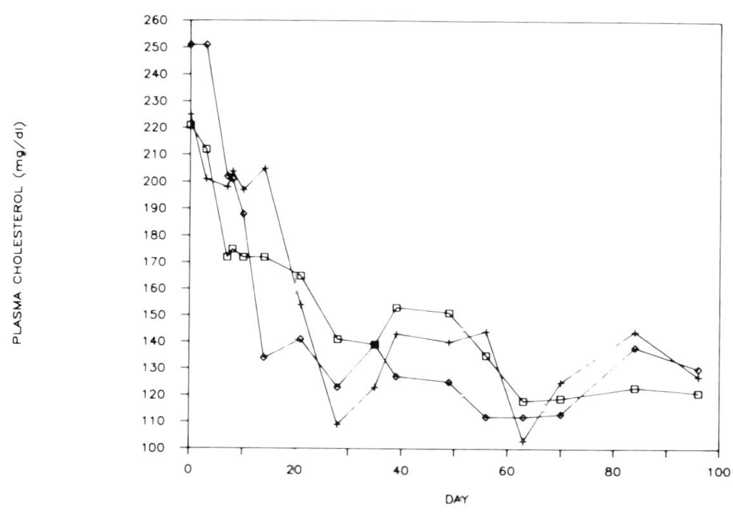

FIG. 21. Total plasma cholesterol levels of three patients during 90 days of Atheromine therapy.

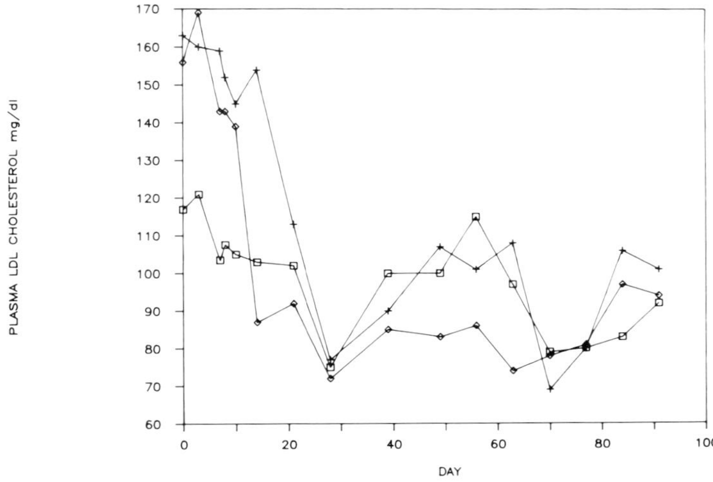

FIG. 22. Plasma VLDL cholesterol levels of three patients during 90 days of Atheromine therapy.

Figures 21–24 are graphic representations of the plasma concentrations of total cholesterol, LDL cholesterol, VLDL cholesterol, and HDL cholesterol during the 90-day period of the intravenous anticholesterol therapy in cases 2, 3, and 4.

Anticholesterol Solution Development

The anticholesterol therapy solution (Atheromine) consists of 18 L-amino acids formulated in quantities and ratios that are optimal for reducing plasma cholesterol concentrations in each patient. Starting with the base formula that evolved during the patient pilot study, modifications in the amino acid formulation are made depending on plasma and urine amino acid concentrations determined weekly until stable and then monthly thereafter. Figure 25 demonstrates the positive, negative, and neutral correlations between the individual plasma amino acids and plasma cholesterol concentrations derived from multiple determinations in three patients. Analyzing these data and plasma-to-urine ratios of the individual amino acids, the individual amino acids in the Atheromine can be adjusted to maximize its effectiveness in reducing plasma cholesterol concentrations.

Table 3 illustrates the average daily anticholesterol therapy solution that can be tailored to meet the nutritional needs of the patient while achieving maximum effectiveness in reducing plasma cholesterol concentration. Thus far, all patients have had the therapy on an ambu-

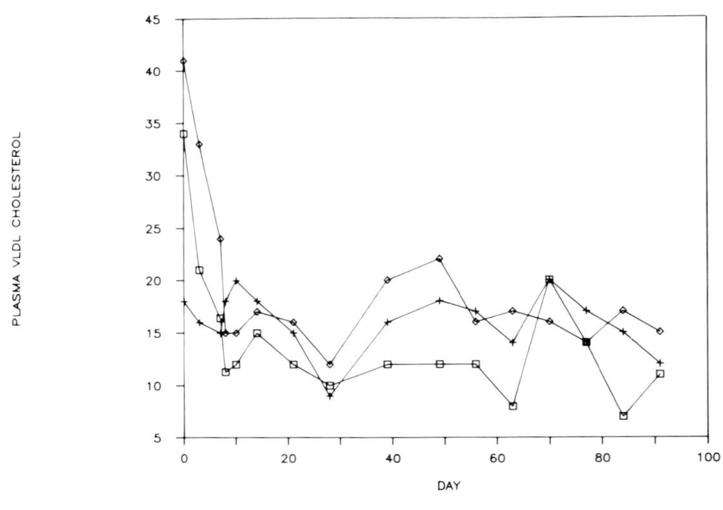

FIG. 23. Plasma LDL cholesterol levels of three patients during 90 days of Atheromine therapy.

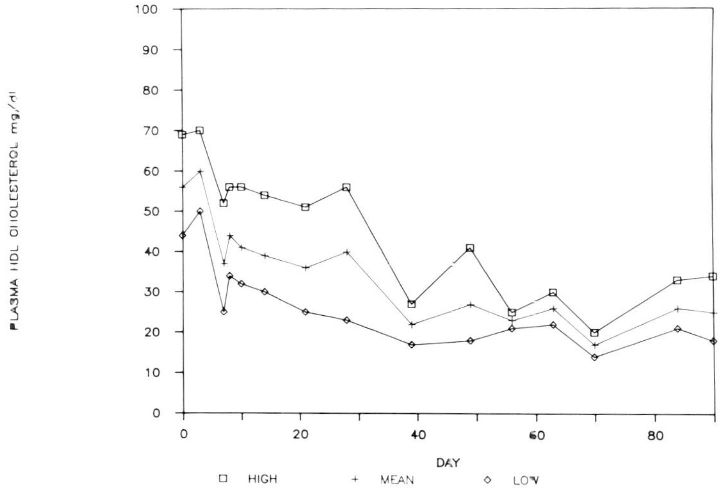

FIG. 24. Plasma HDL cholesterol levels of three patients during 90 days of Atheromine therapy.

latory basis using a lightweight, portable, computerized pump (Pancretec Inc., San Diego, CA) to guarantee desired infusion rates with maximum safety. No fat has been administered to the patients since the pilot study, and no evidence of biochemical or clinical fatty acid deficiency has been documented thus far. The cholesterol-reducing effects of the solution are greatly compromised by the oral intake of even minute amounts of lipid substrates and negated completely if the solution is infused by tube into the gastrointestinal tract in rabbits or in humans.

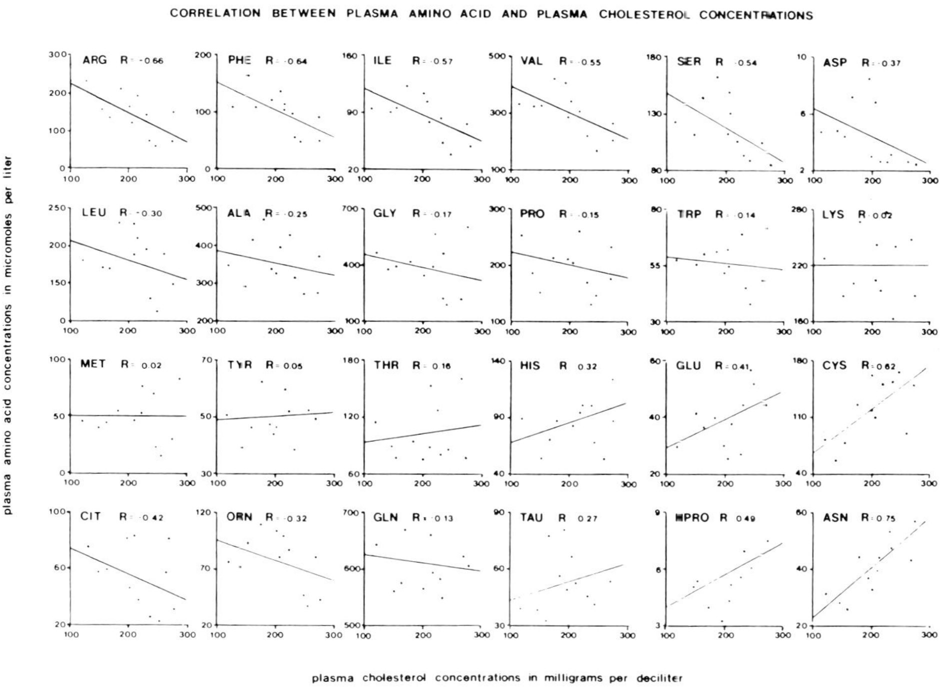

FIG. 25. Correlations between plasma amino acids and cholesterol levels in three patients during 90 days of Atheromine therapy. The first three rows represent the 18 amino acids in Atheromine and the bottom row represents metabolite amino acids.

TABLE 3. *Average Daily Anticholesterol Therapy Solution*

Amino acids 10.31%	1000 mL
Isoleucine	4.0–10.0%
Leucine	5.0–10.0%
Lysine	4.5–6.5%
Methionine	3.5–5.5%
Phenylalanine	4.5–7.5%
Threonine	2.0–3.5%
Tryptophane	1.0–2.5%
Valine	4.0–9.0%
Alanine	7.0–16.0%
Arginine	9.0–18.0%
Histidine	1.5–3.5%
Proline	4.5–8.5%
Serine	2.5–6.5%
Tyrosine	0.0–1.0%
Glycine	3.0–8.0%
Glutamic Acid	3.5–5.5%
Aspartic Acid	2.0–4.0%
Cysteine	0.0–1.0%
Dextrose 20–50%	1000 mL
Calcium gluconate	4.7–9.4 mEq
Magnesium sulfate	30–36 mEq
Potassium chloride	0–60 mEq*
Potassium acetate	0–60 mEq*
Potassium phosphate	20–40 mEq*
Sodium chloride	40–80 mEq†
Sodium acetate	0–40 mEq†
Trace elements (MTE-5)	4 mL
Zinc sulfate	4.0 mg
Copper sulfate	1.6 mg
Manganese sulfate	0.4 mg
Chromium chloride	16 μg
Selenium	80 μg
Multivitamins (MVC 9 + 3)	10 mL
Vitamin A	3300 I.U.
Vitamin D	200 I.U.
Vitamin E	10 mg
Vitamin B1	3 mg
Vitamin B2	3.6 mg
Vitamin B3	40 mg
Vitamin B5	15 mg
Vitamin B6	4 mg
Vitamin B12	5 mg
Vitamin C	100 mg
Biotin	60 μg
Folic Acid	0.4 mg
Total water volume	2200 mL
Optional additives as indicated	
Vitamin K (Aqua-Mephyton)	
Folic Acid (Folvite)	
Iron Dextran (Imferon)	
Cimetidine (Tagamet)	
Insulin (Humulin)	
Heparin	
Zinc sulfate	
Copper sulfate	

* Total daily potassium dose = 80 mEq.
† Total daily sodium dose = 80 mEq.

Discussion

Although atherosclerosis represents a spectrum of pathophysiology and clinical manifestations and although hypercholesterolemia represents only one of the causative or contributing factors to the development and progression of atherosclerosis, nonetheless a real and finite relationship between the two exists. Based on available epidemiologic studies, it is highly likely that the vast majority of atherosclerosis and its complications could be ameliorated, corrected, or avoided by strict adherence to an optimal diet providing only 100 mg of cholesterol, 20% of total calories as fat consisting of one-third saturated fat, one-third polyunsaturated fat, and one-third monounsaturated fat and a total caloric ration tailored to meet energy needs and maintenance of ideal body weight. However, it will be a major public health undertaking to convince Americans to make the radical changes in their current diets to achieve the optimal target diet outlined. Moreover, the changes in plasma cholesterol levels occur very slowly with oral dietary manipulation alone, and the hypercholesterolemic patient is usually discouraged within a few months of adhering to the diet because of the slow apparent progress. Moreover, it is difficult to achieve reductions of plasma cholesterol levels of greater than 8–10% by dietary manipulation alone.

The advantages of using a totally intravenous diet to stimulate reduction of plasma cholesterol levels are several: (1) the components of the diet can be finitely defined and precisely administered directly into the blood stream where they can immediately become involved in the appropriate biochemical reactions; (2) the cholesterol reduction effect of the optimal mixture of amino acids occurs rapidly to effect 40–60% reductions, which are unprecedented with any other single form of anticholesterol therapy; (3) the patient not only achieves prompt gratification and reward for the investment biochemically but also symptomatically as hyperlipidemia is reduced with corresponding decreased blood viscosity and increased microvascular perfusion; and (4) regression of atherosclerosis can be documented indirectly and/or directly by techniques that are currently rather crude but are destined to improve in simplicity, sophistication, and resolution.

This technique allows the application of clinical biochemistry directly to the management of a complex metabolic disorder with gratifying early biochemical and clinical results. The technique also allows a degree of control of the myriad biochemical processes of the body that is currently impossible to achieve with oral or enteral regimens. Thus the importance of any or all of the individual active components in the solution can be established finitely *via* direct intravenous infusion and without potentially detrimental modification by the digestive and absorptive processes of the alimentary tract. Eventually, however, the principles derived from the conscientious, meticulous study of the reactions and responses of patients with atherosclerosis to the intravenous nutrient mixtures herein described should allow the development of oral and enteral dietary formulations that will mimic or duplicate the biochemical milieu of the currently infused substrates after digestion, absorption, and assimilation. It is important that our efforts be directed toward achievement of these goals to allow the patient who has benefited from an intravenously induced hypocholesterolemia to maintain the accrued advantages after returning to a judicious oral diet after the intravenous therapy. The ultimate goal will be to prove the biochemical importance of maintaining much lower plasma cholesterol levels than we have accepted and tolerated as normal in the past not only to arrest and reverse atherosclerosis, but ultimately to prevent atherosclerosis. It is anticipated that this relatively pure biochemical approach to the management and control of the number one pathophysiologic process adversely affecting the health and longevity of our population will be rewarded with highly significant reductions in morbidity and mortality and greatly increase understanding of basic and clinical lipid and lipoprotein chemistry.

ACKNOWLEDGMENTS

The contributions of the following co-workers to this project are gratefully acknowledged: Phillip R. Adams, Elizabeth R. Blume, Pamela R. Dieffenbach, Richard W. Drummond, DeAnn M. Englert, Andrew S. Feste, Stanley J. Gerlich, Mary Lou Gilliam, John T. Gordy, Edward J. Guinn, Carolyn M. Henry, Rhona J. Huntsman, Phillip E. Locey, Jun Maeda, Hugh A. McAllister, Theron C. Mock, Jr., Carolyn E. Moore, Judy C. Negele, Joseph J. O'Donnell, Charles Peters, Jacqueline Ruiz, Sheila M. Theiler, Betty W. Trotter, and Christann M. Vasquez.

REFERENCES

1. Ross R. The pathogenesis of atherosclerosis: an update. N Engl J Med 1986;314:488–500.
2. Consensus Conference. Lowering blood cholesterol to prevent heart disease. JAMA 1985;253:2080–2086.

3. Stamler J, Wentworth D, Neaton JD. Is relationship between serum cholesterol and risk from premature death from coronary heart disease continuous and graded? JAMA 1986;256:2823–2828.
4. Starzl TE, Chase HP, Putnam CW, Porter KA. Portacaval shunt in hyperlipoproteinemia. Lancet 1973;II:940–944.
5. Starzl TE, Putnam CW, Porter KA, et al. Portal diversion for the treatment of glycogen storage disease in humans. Ann Surg 1973;178:525–539.
6. Folkman J, Philippart A, Crigler J. Portacaval shunt for glycogen storage disease: value of prolonged intravenous hyperalimenation before surgery. Surgery 1972;72:306–314.
7. Yamashita H, Okada A, Itakura T, et al. Total parenteral nutrition in familial hypercholesterolemia: importance of caloric control. Surgery 1986;99:327–335.
8. Gould KL. Quantification of coronary artery stenosis in vivo. Circ Res 1985;57:341–353.

Discussion

This discussion took place at the Rhoads Symposium.

Dr. Clyde Barker: Stan, when is it going to be that we can just use this formula instead of quinine water and not have to have the intravenous line but simply drink it with our cocktails in the afternoon?

Dr. Stan Dudrick: That is an excellent question Clyde and we are working on that now. We are doing some studies in patients giving amino acids in powder form and having our patients take some 40 to 80 capsules a day to see if we can duplicate, after they digest the capsule, the same thing we can accomplish by direct infusion into the bloodstream. But if you feed the rabbit the intravenous formula, the rabbit's digestive process destroys its effectiveness and it just does not work at all in either lowering cholesterol or regression of vascular lesions. So we are now going through a tedious process to try to come up with something that when digested and absorbed will mimic the results we create by intravenous injection. I think that arginine is probably the most important amino acid and the optimal profile of the amino acids is similar to that of vegetable or plant protein rather than animal protein. All of the other amino acids that we use are either egg or casein, which is milk protein, or combinations of egg and milk base and they're animal protein based. If you look at the correlation of hypercholesteronemia and atherosclerosis, the strongest correlation is not with high cholesterol per se or with high animal fat it's with animal protein intake and that's in epidemiological studies that started with Ansel Keys and that can still be reproduced today. So not only is total fat important, cholesterol is important and whether you eat it as animal protein or vegetable protein. What we might be able to do is let people eat some animal protein but give them a supplementary capsule of certain amino acids to help convert the animal protein while it's in the gut so that what's absorbed is a profile resembling plant protein. This might allow people to eat some of the things they enjoy without punishing them too badly and allowing them to live a little bit longer without dying of atherosclerosis or its complications.

Dr. Robert Reis: Stan, when you stop this intravenous feeding, how quickly does the atherogenesis process resume?

Dr. Stan Dudrick: The patient with the longest follow-up so far is 18 months from the end of therapy and two years from the beginning of therapy. He is symptom free. Although I have not felt justified in getting another arteriogram on him, his cholesterol level hovers around 300 (down from 508) on a diet that he tells us he's not following. He has the unfortunate attitude that I think a lot of patients are going to have: "When I get another angina attack or when I can't play 18 holes of golf, I'll come in and get washed out again." What we try to do is put patients on a 20-g fat diet of which about 7% is saturated fat, 7% monounsaturated, and 7% polyunsaturated and a 100-mg cholesterol maximum per day. With this we should be able to keep their cholesterol down to within about 20% of what the low was on the intravenous therapy. If you overcome the inertia intravenously you can knock the cholesterol down by 60% or so and then even if it goes back up by 20%, its still 40% below normal. That would get 90% or 95% of your patients down into the less than 180% mg per dc range where atherogenesis should stop.

Dr. Henry Moss: Stan, I certainly enjoyed your presentation. Merck and Company just recently announced a new product that is expected to be very effective in lowering cholesterol. Is there any common denominator between what they've done with their product and this form of therapy?

Dr. Stan Dudrick: What they are using is a blocking agent so if you are taking cholesterol precursors it will block their synthesis into cholesterol in the liver. That's also the mechanism by which nicotinic acid works to a lesser extent. There are also resins that bind the cholesterol and its precursors in the gut so that they're not absorbed. So there are several mechanisms by which cholesterol can be lowered. My concern for the moment is that their drug has already been around for about 7 years and they're still a little leery about releasing it because its predecessor did cause cataracts, so I think that when it comes out they may allow it to be used only in people over age 65. I think that their premise is that if it does accelerate cataracts you will at least have had 65 years of fairly good eyesight. I hope that these various methods will complement each other.

Dr. Clarence Dennis: Has this changed your view toward adding lipids to your total parenteral nutrition solutions?

Dr. Stan Dudrick: Yes it has. So far, Dr. Dennis, we haven't shown any fatty acid deficiency in our patients even though we've run them for 3 months and one man for 6 months (though he did have two units of intralipid) and he did not show fatty acid deficiency as manifested by either reversal of the ratio or measurements of individual fatty acids. We never were hyperenthusiasts for fat for calories. We always thought that you ought to give enough to promote normal essential fatty acid profiles, but believed that the people who advocated giving 40% to 60% of the total calories as intralipid were absolutely wrong. I think it has now been proven that there is another reason why they were wrong. I guess if patients have tremendous needs and could burn up all that fat, such as burn patients or some other hypermetabolic state, it might be okay. But I think that in a person who is not otherwise ill, you should feed him or her no more than 20% of their calories as fat and this probably ought to be pretty high on the unsaturated side. So it hasn't really changed our attitude because we've only given what is necessary for fatty acid normalcy in the first place. I think this will provide reinforcement that philosophy is better than pushing for 50% to 60% fat calories.

DISCUSSION

This discussion took place when this paper was presented at the American Surgical Association.

DR. EDWARD M. COPELAND, III (Gainesville, Florida): The work that Dr. Dudrick has presented represents a culmination of 7 years of effort. I was privileged to see this project begin when I was still in Houston and have had the chance to follow its progress by various visits to Dr. Dudrick's laboratory.

I have had access to the manuscript and you, the audience, have not. To be able to give the amount of data contained in this manuscript in 10 minutes is impossible. I implore you to read the manuscript when it becomes available. It is excellent and represents a Herculean effort for which Dr. Dudrick and his colleagues should be congratulated.

Many questions arose while reading the paper. The solution does not work if given by gut. Dr. Dudrick might comment as to why. Will it work in the "garden variety" atherosclerotic patient as opposed to someone who has hereditary hyperlipidemia? Obviously, there are more people with "garden variety" atherosclerosis than with the other types of hyperlipidemia diseases. Does it work possibly in those patients with atherosclerosis but no hypercholesterolemia?

The published formula, called "Atheromine," is a range of concentrations for the individual amino acids, rather than a specific concentration for each amino acid. The concentration range was derived from multiple formula changes in both rabbits and patients to get a solution that would lower cholesterol maximally.

A further question, therefore, is: those of us who will use the solution, will we have to measure the serum and urine amino acids, as well as plasma cholesterol and various other lipids, to manipulate the concentration of the substrates to produce the data that you have, or will there be a single solution that we will be able to use much like that which evolved for the treatment of renal failure and hepatic failure?

DR. HENRY BUCHWALD (Minneapolis, Minnesota): I thank Dr. Dudrick for the privilege of reviewing this manuscript beforehand. I start with a few historic remarks: the ability of intravenous hyperalimentation solutions to depress lipid levels was first noted by Dr. Judah Folkman in 1972 in his work with total parenteral nutrition (TPN) solutions for glycogen storage disease. This work was confirmed by Dr. Starzl, our Program Chairman, and associates in 1973, in the use of TPN solutions as a preoperative test of potential efficacy before consideration of a portacaval shunt in patients with familial homozygous hyperlipoproteinemia. Again, this effect of TPN solutions was confirmed by Torsuch and Lees (1975), Stein and Meiny, and associates (1975), Cywes et al. (1976), and Yamashita and co-workers (1986). Most important, all of these studies showed that once you stopped infusion of TPN solutions, the hypolipidemic effect disappeared and the lipid levels returned to baseline.

I next turn to some of the items in Dr. Dudrick's paper and comment on them. I am a little confused about the atherosclerosis in the rabbits used in these experiments. Traditionally, if you give rabbits enough oral cholesterol, or enough of a dietary stimulus, to raise their cholesterol concentration over 1000 mg/dL, and then continue to follow these rabbits, they get progressive atherosclerotic disease, and it is ever progressive disease until they die. Thus, I question the validity of the visual inspection used by Dr. Dudrick of these lesions. Could his means of assessment not have been refined by use of scanning electronic microscopy, Folch analysis of vessel lipid content, or even simple dye staining to obtain a more accurate assessment of progression and regression? Finally, with respect to the animal data, I do not understand how he gets his numbers of 85% and 95%.

In terms of the clinical data, I was privileged to read in Dr. Dudrick's manuscript about four case studies. Dr. Dudrick, you had preoperative and postoperative arteriograms in all four patients, but in only one patient, the one you cited in your presentation, did you conclude that there was actual evidence of atherosclerotic regression on the arteriogram. Your data showed increases in flow rate, changes in symptoms, and alterations in Dopplers, but only one case showed, as I read the manuscript, a decrease in atherosclerosis.

The TPN solution advocated by Dr. Dudrick has three features that distinguishes it from the standard TPN solutions. There is a decrease in glycogen, a decrease in alanine, and an increase in arginine. Most interestingly, if the same solution is given orally, as has been noted by Dr. Copeland, the effect is negated. I cannot understand why.

I conclude from the data presented that this is an interesting pilot study. The work needs to be repeated in a randomized controlled trial in humans and it should not precede a commercialization at this point of a product.

I ask Dr. Dudrick several questions: what is the significance of these changes in these three basic amino acids? Why are glycine, alanine, and arginine altered so differently from their concentrations in other TPN solutions? With Dr. Copeland, I would like to ask, must this formula be individualized per patient or can a standard formula be developed, or can the blending of the formula be codified so that other investigators can do the same thing?

Again, I repeat the question why doesn't your solution work orally? Amino acids are absorbed without change from the intestinal tract; thus, why would this solution not work when administered orally?

Finally, what do you postulate is the biochemical mechanism by which your solution, in an isocaloric state, works to lower the serum lipids?

DR. HAROLD URSCHEL, JR. (Dallas, Texas): That was a fascinating presentation, and it could potentially mobilize the large cardiovascular labor force from bench work to more creative pursuits.

Previous search for the ideal "Draino" included our experiments with intra-arterial hydrogen peroxide in the late 1960s and early 1970s. It was based on the fact that hyperbaric oxygen reduced blood lipids and in some cases reversed atherosclerosis.

We must be careful in extrapolating the efficacy of any antiatherosclerotic drugs solely on the base of animal atherosclerosis, particularly hyperlipidemic rabbit atherosclerosis. With intra-arterial hydrogen peroxide, these lesions could be reversed in virtually 100% of animals completely. Even the induced hyperlipidemic lesions in primates consistently disappeared with intra-arterial hydrogen peroxide.

We tried this in over 100 patients with significant atherosclerotic obstructive lesions, and the results varied dramatically from total reversal to minimal regression or no effect.

A 95% stenosis in a unilateral vertebral artery not amenable to surgery in a patient with severe basilar artery insufficiency disappeared with 19 treatments of intra-arterial peroxide. The patient became asymptomatic for 4 years and died of carcinoma.

These data were presented to the Society of Vascular Surgery in 1975. It was totally ineffective in occluded arteries and in severely calcified arteries. These are similar limitations to angioplasty (PTCA) today.

I ask Dr. Dudrick what are the limitations of his technique. One of the arteries that we saw treated was totally obstructed (the right coronary artery). The rapidity that Dr. Dudrick showed the angiograms reminded me of Ken Cooper's speed of showing them when he was trying to demonstrate the effect of exercise on reversal of atherosclerosis. When you flash those angiograms past that quickly, it is difficult to assess the results.

We used hydrogen peroxide for cardiac resuscitation and treatment of acute myocardial infarction by retroperfusion of the coronary sinus, but discontinued its use because of the effective dose response was so close to the toxic effect on the enzyme system. I would like to know about the toxic effects in your dose-response curves and any deleterious side effects.

I think this is exciting, but caution should be employed until the clinical results are carefully assessed.

DR. ANTHONY M. IMPARATO (New York, New York): Dr. Dudrick is to be complimented on the exhaustive laboratory investigations that he has done with rabbits and the follow-up attempts to duplicate the results in humans. Carotid bifurcation plaques as seen in the operating room in both symptomatic and asymptomatic ischemic stroke patients vary considerably from patient to patient sharing in common mainly their localization at the carotid bulb and their content of fibrous tissue. They may be and probably are the prototype arterial lesions that cause ischemia in other parts of the body as well. Their evolution can be deduced, probably accurately, from observations in humans in the operating room and subsequent microscopic study.

May I lay the groundwork for two questions that I would like to ask by showing some slides?

(Slide) A carotid plaque appears to start as fibro-intimal thickening (Slide) which can be reproduced in the experimental animal by specific alterations of blood flow without alteration of diet. These are some of the models and these are the lesions at 1 year.

In humans it can progress to fibro-intimal plaque with intraplaque hemorrhage totally contained within the fibrous covering. (Slide) That is an early hemorrhage contained. (Slide) Gradual transformation of the hemorrhage to atheromatous debris can occur (Slide) until the so-called cholesterol abscess results. At any stage in the evolution of this plaque, thrombosis of the vessel can occur or embolization of a portion of the arterial wall producing ischemic stroke.

(Slide) This shows the portion of the arterial wall that is missing having embolized.

Would Dr. Dudrick speculate as to how lowering serum cholesterol in the human might influence this complex process of plaques' evolution? By what mechanism might ischemia be improved or relieved by lowering cholesterol?

DR. HIRAM C. POLK, JR. (Louisville, Kentucky): Dr. Dudrick, in response to specific inquiry from Council, you said that you would present objective evidence in humans of regression of atherosclerosis as well as describe the nature of the solution used. Would you specifically respond on both those counts, taking an extra minute to do so in your closing discussion?

DR. JOHN H. SIEGEL (Baltimore, Maryland): I congratulate Dr. Dudrick on opening up a whole new era on nutritional therapy, but I have some questions. It seems that a good deal of the response he has shown is due to a hypocaloric-controlled starvation in which he specifically reduced gluconeogenic amino acids and, therefore, to some extent also reduced lipogenic precursors.

I wonder if he could address the following questions. In both the experimental model and in humans, was the total caloric input in excess of metabolic needs, or was the caloric input negative with respect to the actual metabolic rate that these animals had?

Secondly, what effects did this nutritional program have on insulin secretion relative to the hypercaloric atherosclerotic diet where insulin is increased, since elevated insulin output in the control hypercaloric phase might cause increased synthesis of fatty acids? Was there a specific negative insulin secretory effect of the TPN solution used during the hypocaloric therapeutic period? Did those levels change?

Thirdly, is there any evidence of alteration in free fatty acid re-esterification before or after the therapeutic TPN period, since we did notice that when he restarted lipids he raised triglyceride levels severely. Does the TPN antiatherosclerosis diet therapy alter the tendency for re-esterification of administered lipids?

DR. GEORGE H. A. CLOWES, JR. (Boston, Massachusetts): Dr. Dudrick, before you come up, I would like to ask one question also. It seems to me that what you have shown us is that substitution of certain amino acids, perhaps for caloric value or for synthetic value, have had what looks like a beneficial effect.

I ask whether you have any data as to actually how these amino acids are used, studies with a radioactive tracer, or some other system?

DR. STANLEY J. DUDRICK (Closing discussion): My sincere thanks to all of the discussants. I greatly appreciate the comments and questions; each one is valid and appropriate.

This vital area is one of complex biochemistry. I do not believe that we can describe, explain, manage, or treat every manifestation or complication of atherosclerosis in the same way. As Dr. Imparato showed, there are various stages in the development of complex atherosclerotic lesions. There are also various causes, contributing factors, initiating factors, classifications, distributions, complications, etc. One must do the best one can in preventing and treating the usual presenting problems, and what cannot be managed adequately biochemically will require operative management.

Dr. Clowes, there is an enormous amount of work in the basic science literature showing positive correlations between the dietary intake of various sources of food and mortality rates secondary to coronary heart disease. In men between the ages of 55 and 59, animal protein had the highest positive correlation of 0.78 with a p value of less than 0.05, followed by cholesterol (0.76), meat (0.70), total fat (0.68), eggs (0.67), sugar (0.64), total calories (0.63), and animal fat (0.63). No correlation is demonstrable at $p < 0.05$ for plant sterols, fish, vegetable fat, or vegetables, and a negative or beneficial correlation exists for starch or complex carbohydrate (−0.46) and vegetable protein (−0.40).

The formulation of this solution resulted from a series of tedious, obsessive-compulsive laboratory experiments and observations. The solutions that were most effective in the rabbits and most effective in humans resembled plant or vegetable protein in their amino acid composition. Having started with intravenous amino acid mixtures with profiles derived from animal protein, which includes all kinds of meat, cheese, eggs, milk, even skim milk, we arrived at a mixture of amino acids that is similar to that of plant protein. Therefore, it appears that we have documented the wisdom of ingesting a vegetarian diet, which has been well described in the basic literature, and we have done it under the precise, well-controlled nutritional and metabolic conditions that can only be achieved intravenously.

Dr. Clowes, we have demonstrated reproducible correlations between plasma amino acids and plasma cholesterol concentrations in a series of meticulous studies in several atherosclerosis patients. Of the 18 component amino acids in the intravenous mixture, very strong inverse correlation between the plasma amino acid and the plasma cholesterol level was demonstrated for arginine, phenylalanine, isoleucine, valine, serine, aspartic acid, and leucine in decreasing order of importance and significance. The inverse correlations are not as significant for alanine, glycine, proline, or tryptophan. No correlation could be demonstrated between plasma cholesterol and plasma lysine levels, and there have been several published reports indicating that high arginine to lysine ratio has a positive correlation with lowering plasma cholesterol in animals.

Plasma methionine, tyrosine, and threonine show little or no correlation with plasma cholesterol levels, whereas histidine, glutamic acid, and cysteine show direct correlations between their plasma levels and plasma cholesterol level in increasing order of significance. Metabolite amino acids that are not in the mixture but appear in the plasma in significant amounts include citrulline, ornithine, glutamine, taurine, hydroxyproline, and asparagine. Strong inverse relationships exist for citrulline and ornithine, which are derivatives of arginine, the most important amino acid in the mixture. The inverse relationship for glutamine and cholesterol is less impressive, and the relationships between taurine, hydroxyproline, and asparagine are direct in increasing order of significance.

Dr. Buchwald, evidence for regression of atherosclerosis has been demonstrated clearly in three patients reported in this paper. There was not sufficient time in this 10-minute presentation to show all of the data included in the 25 figures in the paper.

Dr. Polk, the formula is presented with upper and lower limits for each component amino acid and compared with the currently available clinical intravenous amino acid mixtures. Starting at the median value for each amino acid, the mixture is individually formulated optimally for each patient based on plasma and urine amino acid and cholesterol levels. To date, this is the only manner in which the formula can be used clinically, but we are currently working toward an FDA approved formula suitable for mass production and distribution. The components of the mixture and the principles for their safe and effective formulation and use in patients are outlined in the paper. Your second question has been answered in my response to Dr. Buchwald's query.

Dr. Copeland, when the amino acid mixture is administered *via* the alimentary tract in either rabbits or patients, the digestive processes destroy the effectiveness of the active ingredients in reducing plasma cholesterol or inducing regression of atherosclerosis. Therefore, we are currently engaged in studies to produce amino acid mixtures that when digested and absorbed, will mimic the milieu that we induce by direct central venous infusion.

I regret that there is insufficient time to discuss or answer the other comments and questions.

Introduction of Dr. Cleon Goodwin

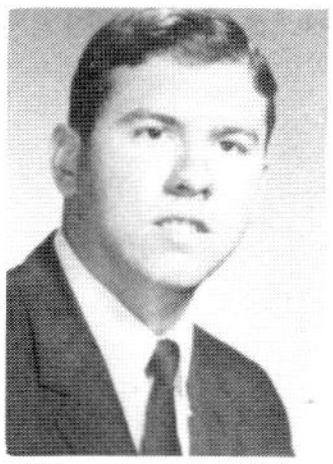

Dr. Clyde Barker: It is evident that Cleon Goodwin has become much more famous since he left Penn. This slide is his yearbook picture and as you can see from the caption they had Cleon mixed up with someone else. While Cleon was in the residency at HUP he worked with Bob Forster and Len Miller on oxygen delivery and had the good fortune to also spend some time with Basil Pruitt in San Antonio where Bill Curreri and Doug Wilmore were also working—sort of a Harrison Department annex as Cleon has said. After finishing his residency in 1976 he returned to Dr. Pruitt's burn unit where he worked until 1983, when he moved to Cornell where he is now in charge of the Burn Unit. He will speak today on his paper entitled "Colloid Increases Lung Water After Massive Fluid Resuscitation."

Dr. Goodwin's Introductory Remarks

Happy Birthday Dr. Rhoads and thank you Dr. Barker for the invitation. I consulted Gary Hart about changing my name before I came, so that is why there was a mix-up. I would like to talk about my introduction to surgical research under Dr. Rhoads' tutelage and Dr. Leonard Miller's. It all began when I was completing my second year of residency. I came home one day and my wife said that she had gotten a call from Dr. Rhoads who told her that I had been elected to do research for two years in colonoscopy and colon physiology. Since this was not my favorite topic, I realized that I was having the first political crisis of my surgical career. Sort of like the intern Dr. Kaplan referred to, I chose the scrambled eggs instead of the vanilla coke. I began discussing my interest in metabolism and particularly oxygen transport in tissue with Dr. Miller. He and Dr. Rhoads then secured a place for me in Dr. Robert Forster's laboratory in the Department of Physiology. Dr. Forster's major interest was oxygen supply to tissues and its regulation, and this was an excellent foundation for my fledgling research career.

I had just come off a clinical rotation on Dr. Johnson's service and when Dr. Forster told me I was to do nothing but read for about 3 to 4 months, I found I could only stand to do that for so long. So I began to wander around the Richards Building, which was a particularly fertile area at that time. There were researchers everywhere doing projects on a variety of topics in physiology and biochemistry and all within walking distance of the Harrison Department. Up on the sixth floor Dick Park had a laboratory where he was looking at the effects of chronic hypoxia with physiological models. Being an interested surgical resident who had tired of reading after a few hours, I went up to his lab and learned to do this procedure with Dick. We did a fair number of dogs using the model to examine a variety of physiological events and especially to evaluate the effects of hypoxia.

Colloid Increases Lung Water After Massive Fluid Resuscitation

CLEON W. GOODWIN, M.D.

THERMAL INJURY of sufficient duration and intensity causes coagulation necrosis and cell death in the affected tissue. Loss of capillary integrity leads to loss of isotonic fluid from the intravascular space into the tissue surrounding the injury, and in burns exceeding 25% of the total body surface, additional plasma volume may be lost into the unburned tissue.[1] Massive edema may form in burned tissue, and its severity depends on both the extent and depth of injury and on the volume of infusate. With the loss of intravascular volume, cardiac output, blood pressure, and urinary output fall; if the intravascular volume deficits of sufficient magnitude are not replaced, acidosis and hypovolemic shock ensue. The loss of plasma volume is too rapid and too massive in patients with extensive burns to allow effective restoration of the intravascular volume deficit by the translocation of fluid from the interstitial and intracellular compartments.

With adequate fluid resuscitation, the fall in plasma volume and total body blood flow can be limited. Although cardiac output is restored usually to near normal levels during the latter half of the first 24 hours postburn, plasma volume is not restored to normal levels until the end of the second postburn day.[2] While the net plasma volume deficit is dependent on the amount of infused resuscitation fluid, the rate of plasma volume loss into the surrounding tissue is not affected by fluid restoration during the first 18 to 24 hours after injury. Subsequently, capillary integrity returns to normal, fluid infusion effectively restores intravascular volume, and cardiac output begins to rise to supranormal levels typical of the early postinjury hypermetabolic response.[3] The rate of fluid infusion is dictated by the patient's physiologic response to resuscitation. Animal studies of organ blood flow distribution indicate that the kidney is the most poorly perfused organ after thermal injury.[4] By implication, when renal function is adequate, other vital organs usually are being perfused satisfactorily, and urinary output is the most reliable and readily accessible index of effective resuscitation.

Before the realization that severe thermal injury was associated with massive loss of isotonic fluid into the injured tissues, a syndrome of "burn shock" was described in which thermally injured patients failed to respond to the then customarily administered quantities of fluid.[5] Subsequently, the effectiveness of massive quantities of balanced electrolyte solutions in replacing not only the intravascular volume deficit but also that of the entire functional extracellular space was demonstrated,[6] and the use of such volume replacement has virtually eliminated renal failure and cardiovascular collapse as a cause of early postburn death. The failure of cardiac output to return rapidly to normal after infusion of fluid volumes estimated to be necessary for adequate resuscitation has been ascribed to the presence of a circulating myocardial depressant factor.[6,7] Myocardial depression also has been postulated to explain the inability of fluid infusions to reestablish organ perfusion in certain categories of burned patients, especially those at either age extreme.[8] However, the existence of such a myocardial depressant factor has been proposed on the basis of decreased cardiac output, and this hemodynamic variable does not directly indicate myocardial performance.

The lung participates in the pathophysiologic alterations associated with large plasma volume losses and administration of massive resuscitation volumes after thermal injury. In the absence of inhalation injury, successful resuscitation commonly restores systemic and pulmonary hemodynamic indices to normal, with no subsequent pulmonary complications. Inhalation injury accentuates fluid requirements during resuscitation and predisposes a

From the New York Hospital–Cornell Medical Center, New York, New York.

TABLE 1. *Serial Changes in Lung Water and Cardiac Output as a Function of Fluid Composition: Lung Water is Normalized to the Patients' Measured Lung Volumes*

Treatment		Postburn day							
		0.5	1.0	1.5	2.0	2.5	3.0	5.0	7.0
Coloid	LW	0.130	0.125	0.120	0.123	0.141	0.144	0.167	0.173
	CO	4.30	5.28	4.51	4.65	5.30	6.74	7.70	10.20
Crystalloid	LW	0.130	0.122	0.124	0.137	0.138	0.139	0.149	0.137
	CO	4.07	4.55	4.29	4.89	5.45	6.83	8.28	9.19

LW: lung water, ml/ml alveolar volume; CO: cardiac output, l/min.

patient to the development of acute pulmonary edema during the first postburn week.[9] Early pulmonary edema may also occur in patients with no coexisting inhalation injury or preexisting cardiovascular disease when edema in the burn wound is being rapidly mobilized during the fourth to the eighth postburn days.

The formulas commonly used to estimate the resuscitation fluid needs of burned patients vary widely in terms of both the volume and composition of the fluids recommended. The majority of patients show a satisfactory clinical response to resuscitation no matter what established formula is used to predict fluid requirements. This observation is a reflection of the physiologic tolerance of the patients treated, since volume and salt dosage of the various formulas for the first 24 hours postburn alone differ by more than twofold. Although virtually all formulas provide for administration of colloid-containing fluids in the second 24 hours postburn, the recommended colloid-containing fluid for the initial 24 hours postburn ranges from a volume equal to that of electrolyte-containing fluid administered to no colloid-containing fluid at all. As in the case of resuscitation of other trauma patients, controversy exists over whether colloid-containing fluids are necessary, desirable, or even deleterious. Proponents of colloid-containing fluid as a part of initial postburn resuscitation have claimed that inclusion of such solutions reduces the volume of fluid required for resuscitation, maintains urinary output at a higher level than with an equal volume of crystalloid fluid, better supports cardiac output, and minimizes loss of fluid into the pulmonary interstitium and other tissues. Conversely, many think that the immediate postburn increase in capillary permeability permits leakage of blood-borne colloid, and that colloid-containing fluid is retained within the circulation to no greater an extent than an equal volume of non-colloid electrolyte solution in the immediate postburn period.[10] That school also believes that colloid-containing fluid has no specific beneficial effect in terms of changes in lung water volume and, in fact, may be deleterious when given in large amounts.[11]

To compare the effect of resuscitation solution composition on lung water after thermal injury, we studied 50 patients who were randomized to receive crystalloid or colloid-containing resuscitation solutions. Our results indicate that the addition of colloid to crystalloid solutions produces no important hemodynamic benefits and is associated with increased accumulation of lung water after the immediate resuscitation.

Material and Methods

Patient Sample

Fifty thermally injured patients were studied serially after informed consent was obtained from them for participation in research protocols approved by institutional review. Control of resuscitation was obtained within 4 hours of injury, and all patients were admitted within 12 hours of injury. Patients were assigned by a random numbers table to receive either crystalloid or colloid resuscitation. Patients in the crystalloid arm were given lactated Ringer's solution and those in the colloid arm were given 2.5% albumin-lactated Ringer's solution. During the first 24 hours, fluid was administered at a rate sufficient to stabilize vital signs and to produce a urinary output of 30 to 50 ml/h. Resuscitation requirements for each treatment group are indicated in Table 1. Plasma volume was replaced on the second postburn day by colloid equivalent to plasma in a dosage of 0.3 to 0.5 ml/kg body weight/% body surface burn. After the initial 24-hour resuscitation phase, 5% dextrose in water was administered at a rate that allowed each patient's weight to return to preburn levels by postburn day 7 to 10, and which maintained serum sodium and osmolal concentrations in the normal range. No patients had evidence of inhalation injury or other pulmonary disease based on clinical evaluation and on normal fiberoptic bronchoscopy, ^{133}xenon ventilation-perfusion lung scan, chest roentgenogram, and arterial blood gases.[13] None of the patients demonstrated microbiologic or clinical evidence of pulmonary infection during the 7 days of the studies.

Lung Water Protocol

Lung water and cardiac output were measured every 12 hours (6:00 AM and 6:00 PM) for the first 3 postburn days and once daily (6:00 AM) on postburn days 5 and 7. Extravascular lung water and cardiac output were determined by a standard rebreathing method, using two gases of differing solubility. Lung tissue volume measured by this method has been shown to reflect with high reliability changes in lung water content in both animals and humans with normal and edematous lungs.[14–19] After several minutes of quiet breathing to become accustomed to the mouthpiece and noseclip, the patient exhaled to residual volume and began breathing into a reservoir bag containing 1.5% dimethyl ether (soluble gas), 7% helium (insoluble gas), 30% oxygen, and balance nitrogen. Six to eight maximal rebreathing maneuvers were carried out for 15 to 20 seconds. The concentrations of each test gas were measured by a time of flight medical mass spectrometer (MGA 1100A, Perkin Elmer Corp., Pomona, CA). Changes in reservoir bag volume were measured with a previously calibrated data acquisition dry spirometer (Model 843, Ohio Instrument Company, Houston, TX). A fiberoptic photographic recorder (Model 1858, Honeywell, Inc.) with a frequency response of 5000 Hz recorded the electrical output of the helium, dimethyl ether, and bag volume signals. The signals tracings and calibration standards were digitized off-line from the photographic paper by a microcomputer that corrected the raw data for the time of passage of gases through the sampling system, for gas consumption by the mass spectrometer (60 ml/min), and for anatomic and apparatus dead space in the first end expiratory volume cycle. The disappearance of the soluble gas was plotted on semilogarithmic paper so that its slope (pulmonary capillary blood flow) and time zero intercept (tissue volume) could be calculated. To detect tracer gas recirculation, indicated by a decrease in the logarithmic washout slope, serial least squares lines were calculated through at least three of the first six rebreathing points and the zero intercept. The line yielding the best squared correlation coefficient was chosen for subsequent calculations. All measurements were made in duplicate, and intervals of at least 5 minutes between each study were observed to allow exhalation of any soluble gas that may have accumulated in the body. To compare measurements among individuals of different sizes, lung water is expressed as ml/ml alveolar volume for each patient. The normal range in this laboratory is 0.110 to 0.120 ml/ml alveolar volume. In the absence of significant pulmonary shunting, pulmonary capillary blood flow is identical to cardiac output. Thermodilution cardiac outputs were measured in conjunction with the rebreathing measurements in selected patients.

Statistical Analyses

Data describing patient characteristics are reported as mean ± standard deviation (SD), while experimentally derived data are reported as mean ± standard error of mean (SEM). A one-way analysis of variance was used to examine serial changes of physiologic indices within each treatment group with time. A two-way analysis of variance was used to detect treatment differences between the crystalloid and colloid groups. When physiologic indices of the treatment groups were compared with the reported values for the normal subjects, statistical difference was assessed with a one-tailed test using the t distribution.[12] Statistical differences with $P < 0.05$ were accepted as significant.

Results

Fifty patients were randomized consecutively into two treatment groups of 25 patients each to receive either colloid or crystalloid fluid for resuscitation. The mean patient age was 29 ± 8 years in the colloid groups and 27 ± 9 years in the crystalloid groups, while their burn sizes were 50 ± 20% and 43 ± 12% of the body surface, respectively. Neither characteristic is significantly different between treatment groups. The crystalloid-treated patients received significantly more fluid (3.74 ± 1.28 ml/kg body weight/% burn) than the colloid-treated patients did (2.89 ± 1.27 ml/kg body weight/% burn; $P < 0.01$). By the end of the 7-day study, five patients in the colloid-treated group demonstrated roentgenographic evidence of pulmonary edema, as did one patient in the crystalloid-treated group. Eleven patients receiving colloid resuscitation died later during their hospital courses, while three patients treated with crystalloid resuscitation eventually died.

The serial changes in lung water and cardiac index over the 7-day study period are outlined in Table 1. Lung water in the colloid-treated patients increased significantly during the first postburn week ($P < 0.0001$). In contrast, lung water in the crystalloid-treated patients did not change significantly during the 7-day study ($P > 0.10$). Measured lung water levels in each treatment group were statistically different from each other ($P < 0.001$). The effect of resuscitation fluid composition is demonstrated further when lung water is evaluated as a linear function of time postburn by the following regression equations: LW(Coll) = 0.116 + 0.009 PBD, $r^2 = 0.87$, and LW(Crys) = 0.128 + 0.003 PBD, $r^2 = 0.43$ (PBD = postburn day). Cardiac indices increased significantly during the 7-day period of study ($P < 0.01$). At no point during this study were significant differences in cardiac index found between treatment groups.

Discussion

All of the patients reported in these studies were in the young adult age group, and none had clinical evidence or a history of heart disease. Coexisting inhalation injury was excluded on the basis of diagnostic criteria having an accuracy of 96%.[13] In this protocol, resuscitation fluid for the first 24 hours consisted of either lactated Ringer's solution or lactated Ringer's solution containing 2.5% albumin (2.5 g/dl). Volume requirements were estimated as 2 ml/kg body weight/% burn and the actual infusion rate was adjusted to maintain urinary output at 30 to 50 ml/h. The colloid-treated and crystalloid-treated patients had burns of similar extent, but the former group required significantly less fluid to achieve clinically adequate resuscitation. Hourly urinary output was adequate in both groups. Cardiac output was higher in the colloid-treated group at both 12 and 24 hours postburn, but this difference was statistically insignificant. Cardiac output in the two groups was statistically indifferent to resuscitation fluid composition across the entire duration of the study.

Using a noninvasive rebreathing technique, measured lung water was found to be influenced by composition of resuscitation solutions. While lung water content in colloid-treated patients increased significantly during the 7-day study, lung water in patients receiving only crystalloid fluids remained unchanged during that study interval. The differential effect of treatment on each group was statistically significant. Both groups displayed qualitatively similar responses in lung water after thermal injury. During the initial 36 hours after injury, lung water in both groups tended to decrease. Subsequently, lung water in the crystalloid-treated group returned to levels found immediately after injury. Patients receiving colloid-containing fluids demonstrated a progressive rise in lung water, beginning at the end of the second postburn day and continuing until the end of the study, greatly exceeding the original admission values. This temporal sequence corresponds clinically to the reabsorption of burn wound edema that occurs after resuscitation.

The validity of the rebreathing method for estimating lung water requires a brief examination. The volume in which the soluble tracer gas distributes during rebreathing measures lung tissue volume, not water volume. However, since water comprises more than 80% of the lung tissue volume, the tissue volume measurements reflect primarily lung water content. Moreover, the solid structures of the lung can be reasonably assumed to remain constant during the time of this study, and any change in lung tissue volume represents a change in lung water content. Since lung size is variable even in patients of the same height and weight, measured lung water was normalized by each patient's simultaneously measured alveolar volume. If anything, this approach may lead to underestimation of lung water, especially in those patients in whom clinically significant pulmonary edema develops, since the tracer gas will not enter nonventilating portions of the edematous lung. We attempted to avoid patients in whom pulmonary edema was likely to develop during the first postburn week, but radiologic evidence of interstitial edema did develop in a few patients. Since this complication occurred primarily in colloid-treated patients, their progressive increase in lung water may be underestimated.

The goals of fluid resuscitation are the restoration of vital organ function and the establishment of hemodynamic stability at the least physiologic cost. In thermal injury, as in most situations of severe nonhemorrhagic fluid depletion, major deficits of the interstitial and intracellular compartments coexist with more clinically obvious intravascular volume depletion.[20] While colloid solutions primarily replace intravascular deficits, crystalloid solutions will rapidly and more completely replenish all compartments. Early studies of burn injury demonstrated that colloid-containing solutions administered to animal models more rapidly restored cardiac output to normal than did crystalloid solutions when administered on an equal volume basis.[21] However, both types of solutions produced identical effects on vital signs, pulmonary and systemic vascular resistance, arterial blood gases, plasma lactate, and lung histology. When indices of adequate intravascular fluid volume, such as venous filling pressures or urinary output, serve as guidelines for fluid administration, colloid and crystalloid solutions appear to be equally affective in restoring cardiac output and hemodynamic stability.[22,23] To achieve comparable hemodynamic effects, larger volumes of crystalloid solution must be administered, usually two to four times the equivalent volume of colloid solutions. As a result, patients resuscitated with crystalloid solutions gain more weight, develop more peripheral edema, and have a lower plasma oncotic pressure than similar patients resuscitated with colloid-containing solutions.

In an animal model, Moylan *et al.* found that sodium and fluid volume doses do exert independent effects on the early postburn restoration of cardiac output, with 1 mEq of sodium exerting the same hemodynamic effect as approximately 13 ml of salt-free fluid volume.[10] In that study, restoration of cardiac output was influenced little by inclusion of colloid in the resuscitation regimen. In our patients, colloid solutions failed to demonstrate any clinical advantage over crystalloid solutions when resuscitation was guided by standard clinical indices, such as blood pressure, pulse rate, and hourly urinary output. Pulmonary capillary wedge pressure in our patients was characteristically below 5 mmHg during resuscitation and stayed below 10 to 12 mmHg for the remainder of the postburn week. Any attempt to guide fluid infusion rate during resuscitation by elevating pulmonary capillary wedge pressure or cardiac output into the normal range, particularly with crystalloid patients, caused marked increase in urinary output and did not further improve other vital signs. Weight gain and peripheral edema did not indicate overexpansion of the intravascular volume or compromise of organ function.

Thermal injury is associated with significant alterations in pulmonary microvascular dynamics.[24,25] In both clinical and laboratory studies, elevation of pulmonary artery pressure and pulmonary vascular resistance have been measured within the first 12 hours postburn.[21] Some investigators have related these changes in patients to the effect of fluid resuscitation and have considered pulmonary systolic arterial pressure to correlate with interstitial pulmonary fluid.[26] Others have considered the changes to reflect acute lung injury, particularly inhalation injury. In our study patients, neither resuscitation regimen was associated with elevated pulmonary artery pressure above the normal range, suggesting that neither regimen produced pulmonary edema during resuscitation and that screening for inhalation injury in these patients was effective. The measurements of lung water in the first 2 days postburn confirm, in both treatment groups, the absence of pulmonary edema.

The relationship between changes in pulmonary artery pressure and vascular resistance and changes in lung water appears to be dependent on the primary site of flow resistance. If the increase is precapillary, as would be consistent with the measurements of cardiac output and pulmonary capillary wedge pressure in our studies and those of others, one would not anticipate an increase in lung water. If the site of the increased resistance is at the capillary or postcapillary level, as would occur with left ventricular failure or direct capillary injury, one would expect an increase in lung water. The rarity of pulmonary edema in burn patients during resuscitation suggests that the increase in pulmonary vascular resistance resides at a precapillary site. The similarity in lung water changes during the first 48 postburn hours in the two treatment groups reflects the similarity of changes of pulmonary hemodynamic indices in both groups, and speaks against a specific effect of colloid on transcapillary movement of fluid in the lung immediately after cutaneous thermal injury. Since protein sieving by the pulmonary microvasculature appears to remain normal during postburn resuscitation, the infusion of colloid at this time appears to protect intravascular volume and to inhibit fluid loss into the pulmonary interstitium. This hypothesis is supported by the slight fall in measured lung water in both treatment groups during the first 36 hours after burn injury.

The fall of plasma oncotic pressure in burn patients after massive crystalloid resuscitation is not associated with an increase in pulmonary extravascular lung water.[27,28] In animal models of other hypovolemic states, infusion of colloid-containing fluid has been associated with a greater increase in lung water than occurred with infusion of crystalloid fluid.[29,30] Albumin is distributed widely throughout the body, with two-thirds located in extravascular sites. Injected albumin is distributed across the capillary membrane according to biphasic kinetics, characterized by a fast exchange rate and by a much slower exchange rate.[31,32] Thus, albumin infused during resuscitation will equilibrate across the pulmonary capillary, even if protein sieving is unaffected by burn injury. The extracellular albumin present in the lung after resuscitation will promote subsequent fluid retention within the lung interstitium. Since this occurs at the time of rapid mobilization of burn wound edema fluid, the albumin may exert a subtracting effect on the intravascular fluid volume.[11] This hypothesis is supported by the significantly greater lung water measured in the colloid-treated group at 7 days. Clinical observations are consistent with this concept (five of the colloid-treated patients showed roentgenographic changes consistent with early pulmonary edema by the seventh postburn day, while only one crystalloid-treated patient demonstrated this complication).

We used colloid solutions containing 2.5% albumin, and the average patient in the colloid treatment group received 300 to 350 g of albumin during the first 24 hours after burn injury. This colloid concentration is similar to the albumin concentration recommended in the Evans formula.[33] In studies assessing the effect of varying doses of colloid on resuscitation and survival after hypovolemic shock, 2 g/kg body weight of albumin produced the optimal beneficial effect.[34] Colloid solutions of 6% were no more effective than 3.5% solutions. Patients in our colloid group received approximately 4 g/kg body weight of albumin during resuscitation. Since this dosage was more than two times that of previously demonstrated effective levels, we did not evaluate resuscitation solutions with even higher concentrations of colloid. Based on our current findings, it is entirely possible that the use of higher concentrations of albumin may lead to even more pronounced changes in lung water. Although the numbers of patients in each treatment group are insufficient for statistical analysis at this time, the raw mortality data suggest that the addition of colloid to crystalloid resuscitation solutions may have later deleterious effects. When used according to the above described resuscitation guidelines, crystalloid solutions appear to be the preferred fluid for the treatment of acutely burned patients.

REFERENCES

1. Arturson G. Pathophysiological aspects of the burn patient syndrome. Acta Chir Scand 1961;271:135.
2. Pruitt BA Jr, Mason AD Jr, Moncrief JA. Hemodynamic change in the early postburn patient: The influence of fluid administration and of a vasodilator (Hydralazine). J Trauma 1971;11:36–46.
3. Pruitt BA Jr. Advances in fluid therapy and the early care of the burn patient. World J Surg 1978;2:139–150.
4. Asch MJ, Mason AD Jr, Pruitt BA Jr. Regional blood flow in the burned unanesthetized dog. Surg Forum 1971;22:55–56.
5. Blalock A. Experimental shock: VIII. The importance of the local loss of fluid in the production of the low blood pressure after burn. Arch Surg 1931;22:610–616.
6. Baxter CR, Shires T. Physiological response to crystalloid resuscitation of severe burns. Ann NY Acad Sci 1968;150:874–894.
7. Baxter CR. Fluid volume and electrolyte changes of the early postburn period. Clin Plast Surg 1974;1:693–709.
8. Shoemaker WC, Vladeck BC, Bassin R *et al.* Burn pathophysiology in man: I. Sequential hemodynamic alterations. J Surg Res 1973;14:64–73.
9. Morgan A, Knight D, O'Connor N. Lung water changes after thermal burns. Ann Surg 1978;187:289–293.
10. Moylan JA, Mason AD Jr, Rogers PW, Walter HL. Postburn shock: A critical evaluation of resuscitation. J Trauma 1973;13:354–358.
11. Goodwin CW, Long JW, Mason AD, Pruitt BA. Paradoxical effect of hyperoncotic albumin in acute burned children. J Trauma 1981;21:63–65.

12. Rosner B. Fundamentals of Biostatistics. Boston: Duxbury Press, 1982;175–183.
13. Agee RN, Long JM III, Hund JL *et al.* Use of ^{133}xenon in early diagnosis of inhalation injury. J Trauma 1976;16:218–224.
14. Petrini MF, Peterson BT, Hyde RW. Lung tissue volume and blood flow by rebreathing: theory. J Appl Physiol 1978;44:795–802.
15. Peterson BT, Petrini MF, Hyde RW, Schreiner BF. Pulmonary tissue volume in dogs during pulmonary edema. J Appl Physiol 1978;44:782–795.
16. Overland ES, Ravinder NG, Huchon GJ, Murray JF. Measurement of pulmonary tissue volume and blood flow in persons with normal and edematous lungs. J Appl Physiol 1981;51:1375–1383.
17. Friedman M, Kaufman SH, Wilkins SA. Analysis of rebreathing measurements of pulmonary tissue volume in pulmonary edema. J Appl Physiol 1980;48:66–71.
18. Farney RJ, Morris AH, Gardner RM, Armstrong JD Jr. Rebreathing pulmonary capillary and tissue volume in normals after saline infusion. J Appl Physiol 1977;43:246–253.
19. Cander L, Forster RE. Determination of pulmonary parenchymal tissue volume and pulmonary capillary blood flow in man. J Appl Physiol 1959;14:541–551.
20. Shires T, Colin D, Carrico J, Lightfoot S. Fluid therapy in hemorrhagic shock. Arch Surg 1964;88:688–693.
21. Asch MJ, Feldman RJ, Walker HL *et al.* Systemic and pulmonary hemodynamic changes accompanying thermal injury. Ann Surg 1973;178:218–221.
22. Siegel DC, Cochin A, Geocaris T, Moss GS. Effects of saline and colloid resuscitation on renal function. Ann Surg 1972;177:51–57.
23. Virgilio RW, Rice CL, Smith DE *et al.* Crystalloid vs colloid resuscitation: Is one better? Surgery 1979;85:129–139.
24. Demling RH, Will JA, Belzer FO. Effect of major thermal injury on the pulmonary microcirculation. Surgery 1978;83:746–751.
25. Harms BA, Bodai BI, Kramer GC, Demling RH. Microvascular fluid and protein flux in pulmonary and systemiccirculations after thermal injury. Microvasc Res 1982;23:77–86.
26. Martyn JAJ, Snider MT, Szyfelbein SK, Burke JF. Right ventricular dysfunction in acute thermal injury. Ann Surg 1980;191:330–335.
27. Tranbaugh RF, Lewis FR, Christensin JM, Elings VB. Lung water changes after thermal injury: The effects of crystalloid resuscitation and sepsis. Ann Surg 1980;192:479–488.
28. Lam V, Goodwin CW Jr, Treat RC, Martin DL, Mason AD Jr, Pruitt BA Jr. Does pulmonary extravascular water vary with colloid oncotic pressure after burn injury. Am Rev Respir Dis 1979;119:139.
29. Schloerb PR, Hunt PT, Plummer JA, Cage GK. Pulmonary edema after replacement of blood loss by electrolyte solutions. Surg Gynecol Obstet 1972;135:893–896.
30. Holcroft JW, Trunkey DB. Extravascular lung water following hemorrhagic shock in the baboon: Comparison between resuscitation with Ringer's lactate and plasmanate. Ann Surg 1974;180:408–417.
31. Berson SA, Yalow RS, Schreiber SS, Post J. Tracer experiments with I^{131} labeled human serum albumin: Distribution and degradation studies. J Clin Invest 1953;32:746–768.
32. Rothschild MA, Bauman A, Yalow RS, Berson SA. Tissue distribution of I^{131} labeled human serum albumin following intravenous administration. J Clin Invest 1955;34:1354–1358.
33. Evans EI, Purnell OJ, Robinett PW *et al.* Fluid and electrolyte requirements in severe burns. Ann Surg 1952;135:804–817.
34. Dawidson I, Eriksson B, Gelin L-E, Soderberg R. Oxygen consumption and recovery from surgical shock in rats: A comparison of the efficact of different plasma substitutes. Crit Care Med 1979;7:460–465.

Dr. Goodwin's Closing Remarks

In closing, I would like to explain my relationship with Dr. Rhoads, beginning when I was a resident. In all honesty, as a resident I did not see Dr. Rhoads very much. My one rotation on the Rhoads' service was partly consumed by my vacation. However, immediately after I finished my residency I began to see Dr. Rhoads more frequently. The very first paper that I presented after finishing my residency was at a British meeting in 1977. As most of you know, the British can be particularly caustic critics and after I suffered through some of this trauma a very nice question came from the back. In this small town in England it was from Dr. Rhoads who was sitting at the back of the audience. Having heard Dr. Thompson describe his contacts with Dr. Rhoads at meetings around the world I have concluded that this sort of experience is more the rule than the exception and that it's just one more way in which Dr. Rhoads supports his trainees. However, my wife, bless her heart, had this alternative explanation. She said that Dr. Rhoads was probably there because he knew some people needed more help than others. Whether that is true or not Dr. Rhoads, I certainly do appreciate all of your help.

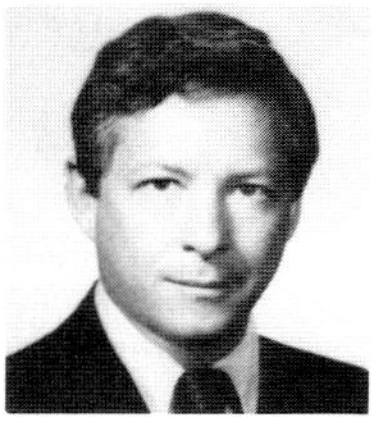

Introduction of Dr. Harvey Sugerman

Dr. Clyde Barker: The next paper will be given by Harvey Sugerman. I failed to find a photograph of Harvey in our files except for a xerox copy of one that was so faded I couldn't use it, but he looks exactly the same now as he did then. During his residency, Harvey worked with Leonard Miller on shock, and I clearly remember one experience I shared with him at that time about 15 years ago. I had just done my first liver transplant, and the patient really needed the help of someone who was an expert on shock. Harvey put in one of the first Swan-Ganz catheters used at HUP and provided that help. Unfortunately, it wasn't enough. Following his residency, Harvey fulfilled his military requirement with the Army in Germany and then spent several years in community practice before returning (as those of us who knew him predicted he would) to the mainstream of academic surgery. As a faculty member at the Medical College of Virginia, where he is now Professor of Surgery, he has been a very productive investigator in the field of metabolism. As Dr. Rhoads told us last night, he has just been elected to membership in the American Surgical Association. Harvey will speak today on his article entitled "Oxygen Delivery."

Dr. Sugerman's Introductory Remarks

Thank you, Clyde. I would like first of all to tell you how I came to be in the surgical residency program at Penn which many of us entered by serendipitous routes. I happened to be a medical intern at HUP. Perhaps that's one of the reasons there was not a picture in my folder. I would come back to the medical ward from a very boring morning in medical clinic taking care of patients with hypertension and diabetes only to discover that Drs. Dudrick and Copeland had made rounds on Ward D and whisked all my interesting patients off to the surgical suite. So, I figured the only way I could continue in the management of these sick patients was to switch over to Surgery, and I was delighted to be accepted into Dr. Rhoads' program.

I must also say that I also owe staying in the program to the kindness and compassion of Dr. Rhoads. When I had finished my two years in the laboratory and had come back onto the clinical rotations, a log jam occurred and about seven of us landed in the same year. We got together, and for some reason or another, I was the one elected to meet with Dr. Rhoads to suggest that perhaps not all should finish at HUP in the same year but that instead maybe a few of us should be farmed out to other hospitals for this final year, as was the custom in those days. When I went into his office, I wasn't worried about my being one of those to be farmed out. However, Dr. Rhoads said to me, "Well Harvey," and after about 10 minutes, it wasn't so clear exactly what we were talking about, but I was hoping that I was correct in thinking I would still be in the program after our conversation. I have been grateful to Dr. Rhoads ever since that he decided to allow me to continue at HUP after I had set up that politically unwise meeting.

My interest in oxygen delivery began during my two years in the Shock and Trauma Unit. As you heard, there was a lot of shock and very little trauma, but the tradition under Drs. Rhoads and Ravdin of employing principles of basic physiology and biochemistry to improve the care of surgical patients made a major impact on many of us.

Oxygen Delivery

HARVEY J. SUGERMAN, M.D.

IN 1969 the issue of oxygen delivery was a hot topic in the clinical Shock and Trauma Research Unit at the Hospital of the University of Pennsylvania (HUP). Oxygen–hemoglobin equilibrium curves and fuzzy looking chest radiographs were the subject of daily discussion. These may not sound like exciting topics for those interested in advancing the cutting edge of surgery, but the philosophy at HUP at that time was to apply biochemistry and physiology to the optimal care of our seriously ill surgical patients. This approach was in the Penn tradition as a result of Dr. Jonathan Rhoads' and Dr. Isadore Ravdin's commitment to the basic sciences and is emphasized by the Ravdin Lecture in Basic Sciences at the annual meeting of the American College of Surgery.

In 1969, I had the opportunity of working with Drs. Leonard Miller and Frank Oski to study the effects of alterations in 2,3-diphosphoglycerate (2,3-DPG) on the oxygen–hemoglobin equilibrium curve. We noted precipitous decreases in 2,3-DPG after massive transfusions with old blood stored in acid–citrate–dextrose (ACD)[1] or total parenteral nutrition (TPN) without phosphate supplementation.[2] Hemodynamic study of one patient with a markedly left shifted oxygen–hemoglobin equilibrium curve documented a severe impairment in oxygen delivery (Fig. 1).

The clinical importance of 2,3-DPG was validated in the study of two children, one with a hexokinase (HK) deficiency, who could not produce 2,3-DPG as a result of decreased erythrocyte glycolysis, and another with pyruvate-kinase (PK) deficiency, who had markedly increased levels of 2,3-DPG due to the block at the end of glycolysis.[3] Both children had similar degrees of anemia. The HK child was extremely weak, excused from physical education and, when studied, had difficulty with oxygen delivery during exercise which was totally dependent on cardiac output and the development of a metabolic acidosis which shifted the curve to the right helping to unload oxygen. The PK child was an active basketball player and had an almost unlimited oxygen reserve due to his markedly right-shifted oxygen–hemoglobin equilibrium curve.

Since these studies, it has become established that phosphate is a critical element in the nutritional cocktail of TPN patients. It is obvious that high-energy phosphate bonds in 2,3-DPG, ATP, and creatine-phosphate (PO_4) are vital to cellular function of erythrocytes, leukocytes, and neurologic tissue, as well as all other organs in the body. It is now unforgivable for patients to become hypophosphatemic. Furthermore, partially as a result of studies initiated in our laboratories,[4] erythrocyte storage has doubled, from 21 to 42 days with the use of citrate–phosphate–adenine (Adsol) to preserve *in vitro* erythrocyte ATP and 2,3-DPG production.

In 1969, the Adult Respiratory Distress Syndrome (ARDS) exploded on the scene as a major determinant of the morbidity and mortality of surgical patients. The relationship of acute respiratory failure to critically ill surgical patients was first appreciated in the Second World War, where it was known as the "Traumatic Wet Lung syndrome." It became more apparent during the Korean conflict and, especially, during the Vietnamese War where it was known as "shock lung" or "DaNang lung." Surgeons were interested in the problem because of its relationship to multiple transfusions, long bone fractures (pulmonary fat embolism syndrome), necrotizing pancreatitis, pulmonary contusion, burn inhalation injury, and septicemia. In fact, more than 75% of ARDS patients are on a surgical service. The topic was the subject of a major symposium published in 1968.[5]

From the Department of Surgery, Medical College of Virginia, Virginia Commonwealth University, Richmond, Virginia.

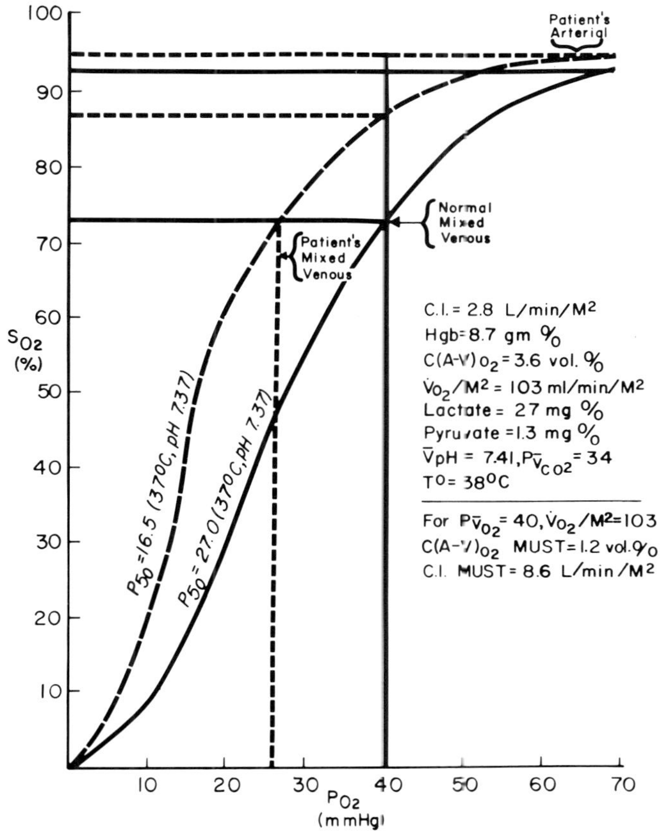

FIG. 1. Normal oxygen hemoglobin equilibrium curve, P_{50} = 27.0 (solid line), and markedly left shifted curve, P_{50} = 16.5 (dashed line), in patient with TPN-induced hypophosphatemia. This patient had a low cardiac index associated with her anemia (Hgb 8.7 g%) and very low PvO_2 (27 torr). To maintain a normal PvO_2 of 40 torr, her cardiac index would have to rise markedly to 8.6 l/minute/M^2.

In 1969 Ashbaugh and co-workers published their famous study[6] on the use of positive end-expiratory pressure (PEEP) for the treatment of the ARDS, which was the first time that this phrase was used. The use of PEEP had been condemned by Cournand *et al.*[7] in 1947 when it was noted that it could decrease cardiac output; however, this study involved volunteers who had normal pulmonary function and compliant lungs. Ashbaugh and co-workers were unaware of this study and, in their initial report, did not study the effect of PEEP on cardiac output.

When we first applied PEEP to our patients with septic-induced ARDS at HUP, it was suggested that PEEP would markedly decrease cardiac output and oxygen delivery and that we would be killing our patients. However, since they were dying anyway due to the need to progressively increase the level of inspired oxygen and there was no other solution, we believed that PEEP warranted further study. Safe and rapid bedside right heart catheterization had recently been developed by Swan and Ganz, permitting the study of cardiac output, oxygen delivery and consumption in critically ill patients. Our study demonstrated that levels of PEEP between 5 and 15 cm water (H_2O) were unassociated with a significant decrease in cardiac output and that this appeared to be due to the decrease in pulmonary compliance in ARDS patients and the failure to transmit the PEEP pressures to the pulmonary capillary bed[8] (Fig. 2). Furthermore, the worse the arterial blood gas, the stiffer the lung, the more PEEP that is needed, the more PEEP that can be used without decreasing cardiac output. A level of PEEP, however, can be reached in any patient that will decrease cardiac output.[9,10]

The use of the term ARDS probably was unfortunate as the problem can be seen in infants and adolescents. It has been taught that the syndrome is due to an increased pulmonary capillary permeability with the leak of protein-rich fluid into the pulmonary interstitium and, subsequently, the alveolus, leading to alveolar collapse, the perfusion of unventilated alveoli or ventilation–perfusion (V/Q) mismatch, and hypoxemia refractory to an increased

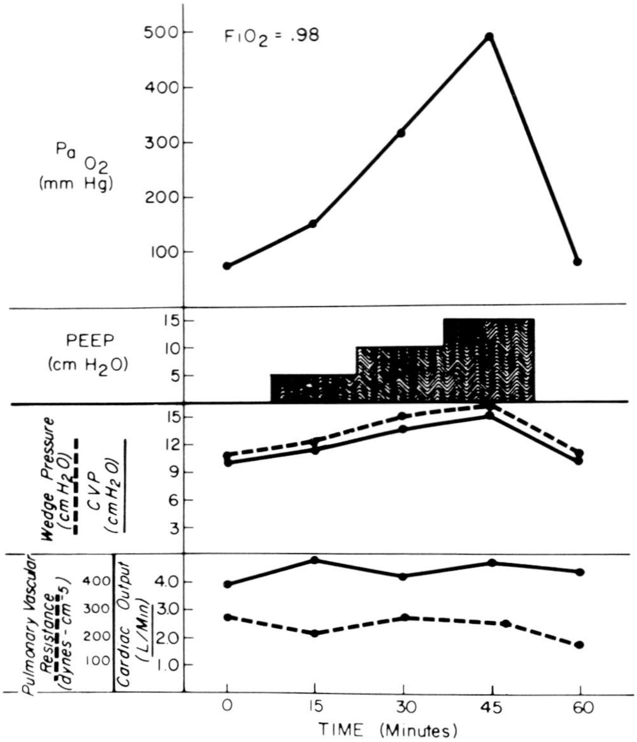

FIG. 2. Effect of 0, 5, 10, 15 and 0 cm H_2O PEEP, for 15-minute intervals each, on PaO_2, wedge pressure, central venous pressure (CVP), cardiac output, and pulmonary vascular resistance in patient with septic-induced ARDS. Notice absence of fall in cardiac output with PEEP and attenuation of PEEP pressure transmission on wedge pressure. (Reprinted with permission from Sugerman HJ *et al.* Continuous positive end-expiratory pressure ventilation (PEEP) for the treatment of diffuse interstitial pulmonary edema. J Trauma 12:263–274, © by Williams & Wilkins, 1972.)

inspiratory oxygen concentration.[11] Thus, it has been suggested that the process be called "permeability pulmonary edema" to contrast it to "cardiogenic pulmonary edema" as seen in congestive heart failure. However, there is recent evidence that the process also may include a significant element of bronchospasm with a decreased airflow into the alveoli, also leading to alveolar collapse and a V/Q mismatch.[12]

In our 1972 study, we noted a marked improvement in the chest radiograph 12 hours after the application of PEEP and presumed that PEEP was driving interstitial fluid and protein out of the lung.[9] Subsequent studies, using a technique to measure pulmonary albumin flux, have failed to confirm this hypothesis[13] (Fig. 3). Furthermore, application of PEEP was associated with an immediate improvement in the chest radiograph secondary to a sudden increase in pulmonary air volume, documented by the increase in functional residual capacity[13] (Figs. 4A–4D). It is important to appreciate this fact when viewing chest radiographs in critically ill surgical patients being mechanically ventilated with PEEP.

Over the years between completing the surgical residency and my return to academic surgery, I had continued to mull over a way to measure the apparent primary pathophysiologic process in ARDS, namely the leak of a protein-rich fluid into the pulmonary interstitium and alveoli. During the time spent in the Shock and Trauma Unit at HUP, I had the opportunity of working with Dr. Bryan Marshall in the Department of Anesthesiology who was also interested in ARDS. At that time, the technique of measuring alterations in extravascular lung water (EVLW) was based on the double isotopic dilution method of Chinard and Enns.[14] Volunteers underwent insertion of radial artery and right heart catheters. The EVLW was measured by the double isotopic dilution technique in the sitting and supine positions, and supine exercising with a bicycle ergometer, producing marked changes in cardiac output. The greater the cardiac output, the more EVLW was measured, documenting the dependence of this technique on flow and pulmonary vascular recruitment (Fig. 5).[15] Since critically ill surgical patients have marked fluctuations in cardiac output, this technique would be of no value for the clinical measurement of EVLW. Since that time, the technique of EVLW measurement has been developed using Evans blue (cardiogreen) dye as the intravascular marker and heat as the water marker.[16] Heat is a very rapidly diffusing

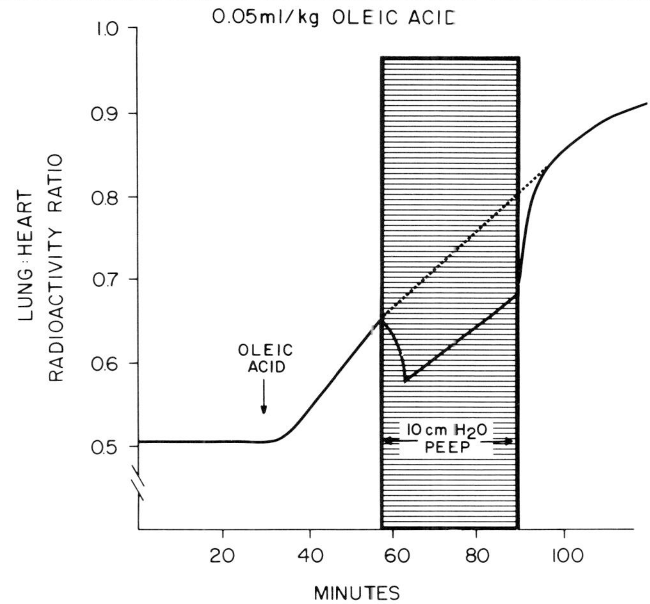

FIG. 3. Lung:heart radioactivity ratio of dog after 20 mCi ^{99m}TC-HSA; 0.05 ml/kg oleic acid given IV at 30 minutes and 10 cm H_2O PEEP from 60 to 90 minutes after radiopharmaceutical. Significant decrease ($P < 0.001$) in ratio was seen within 2 minutes of application of PEEP. Upon release of PEEP, ratio rose to level predicted (dotted line) had PEEP had not been used. "Slope of injury" during PEEP paralleled slope predicted without PEEP. (Reprinted with permission from Sugerman HJ *et al.* Scintigraphy and radiography in oleic acid pulmonary microvascular injury: Effects of positive end-expiratory pressure (PEEP). J Trauma 22:179–185, © by Williams & Wilkins, 1982.).

indicator, so that the thermal-cardiogreen method is minimally affected by cardiac output in most clinical situations. It is, however, quite invasive requiring the insertion of both a right heart catheter (usually required for clinical reasons) and a 5-French femoral artery catheter.

Measurement of the accumulation of EVLW is a static technique requiring multiple points over time to determine if water is accumulating or decreasing. The measurement of increased pulmonary albumin flux is a dynamic method. With the support of Dr. Lazar Greenfield at the Medical College of Virginia, we began investigations into the use of the gamma camera to detect increased pulmonary albumin flux. In the first study, we noted that intravenously administered technetium 99m (^{99m}TC)-tagged human serum albumin (TC-HSA) could be seen accumulating in the lung (Fig. 7) from its initial location in the heart (Fig. 6).[17] However, measurement of albumin flux required a computerized gamma camera, where lung–heart radioactivity ratio curves could be constructed. In the normal lung, the lung–heart radioactivity ratio remained constant until an increased capillary permeability occurs, as with the intravenous administration of oleic acid, when a rapid increase in the ratio, which we have called the slope index (SI), is seen (Fig. 8).[17] In further studies, the SI was noted to be proportional to the dose of oleic acid[18] and much greater with TC-HSA than TC-tagged erythrocytes.[19] Because of the previously mentioned effects of alterations in pulmonary vascular recruitment on the measurement of EVLW,[15] pulmonary vascular recruitment was increased by inflating a left atrial balloon or opening a large aortocaval shunt. In this study, we noted a marked change in the lung:heart (L:H) radioactivity ratio with an acute alteration in pulmonary vascular recruitment, but this stabilized within 5 minutes after equilibration, when the ratio again became constant.[20] Thus, for the measurement to be valid, it is important that the patients' cardiovascular hemodynamics be stable for the 45 minutes required for measurement of SI.

As previously mentioned, the technique was used to study the effects of PEEP on pulmonary albumin flux and refuted our previous theory that PEEP decreased the leak of albumin in ARDS.[13] In this study, after the initial change in L:H ratio with the application of PEEP, the SI was parallel to the slope had PEEP not been used (Fig. 3). Thus, the improved chest radiograph with PEEP is not due to a decreased amount of EVLW or protein, but due to a decreased density as a result of the increased pulmonary air volume (Figs. 4A–4D). Clinical studies[21] have shown that patients with elevated SI have a significantly lower $(a/A)O_2$ ratio while being ventilated with a significantly higher amount of PEEP (Fig. 9).

Having developed a technique for measuring increased albumin flux, it became our goal to determine if pharmacologic intervention could reduce the leak of protein with the hope of

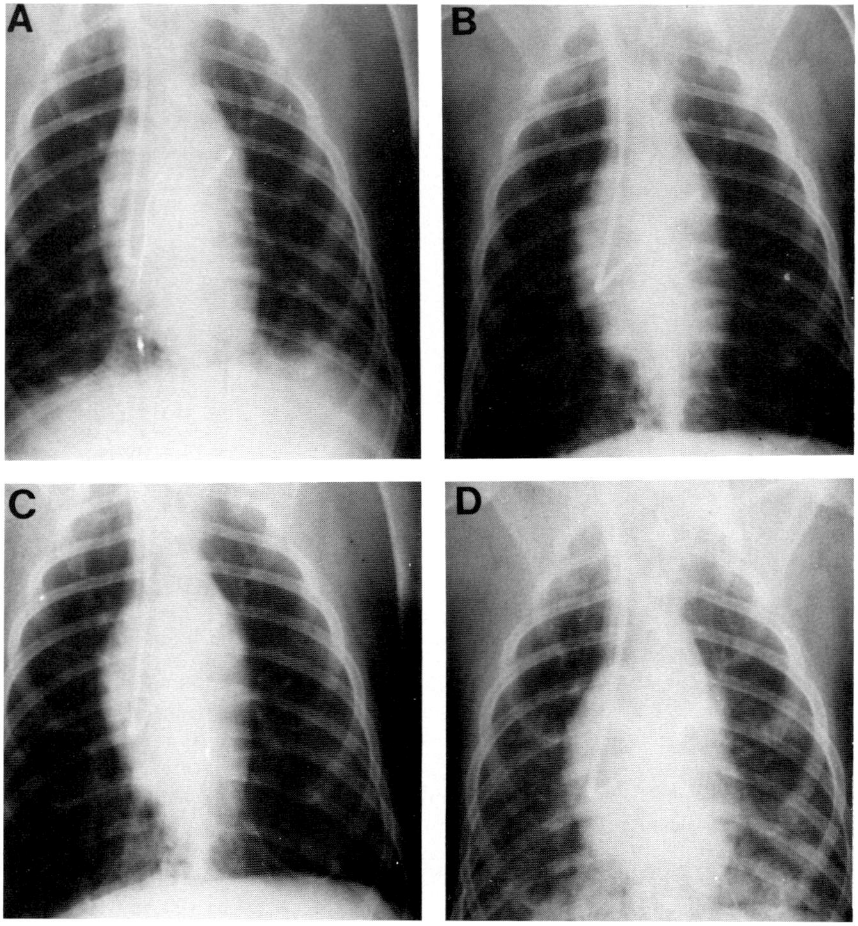

FIGS. 4A–4D. Chest radiograph in a dog showing (A, top left) a subtle infiltrate 30 minutes after the administration of 0.3 ml/kg oleic acid (B, top right) which appeared to resolve within 2 minutes after the application of 10 cm H_2O PEEP. (C, bottom left) The infiltrate was again apparent after 30 minutes of PEEP but (D, bottom right) became very prominent 2 minutes after PEEP was removed. (Reprinted with permission from Sugerman HJ *et al.* Scintigraphy and radiography in oleic acid pulmonary microvascular injury: Effects of positive end-expiratory pressure (PEEP). J Trauma 22:179–185, © by Williams & Wilkins, 1982.)

decreasing the duration of mechanical ventilation, intensive care unit stay and death. It is estimated that there are at least 150,000 cases of ARDS per year in the United States and that the mortality continues to hover around 50% to 65%.[22,23] Our initial studies were unable to find a pharmacological agent which would alter the increased albumin flux after oleic acid, the presumed culprit in pulmonary fat embolism syndrome after long bone trauma,[24] or acid aspiration,[25] both presumably secondary to a direct injury to the pulmonary capillary membrane and unlikely to be relieved with drug therapy. Septic induced ARDS, however, is likely to be an indirectly mediated injury and more likely responsive to drug treatment. In this regard, we have found that ibuprofen, the blocker of cyclo-oxygenase activity and prostaglandin production, caused a decrease in pulmonary artery pressure (PAP) and prevented the fall in PaO_2 after intravenous *Pseudomonas,* but did not alter the increased pulmonary capillary permeability determined by both thermal-cardiogreen EVLW and computerized gamma scintigraphic measurement of albumin flux.[12] Methylprednisolone[26] or the serotonin blocker, ketanserin,[27] also failed to prevent *Pseudomonas*-induced increased permeability.

Presumably, septic-induced ARDS is secondary to the release of multiple mediators of inflammation and treatment will probably require polypharmacy. To this end, a combina-

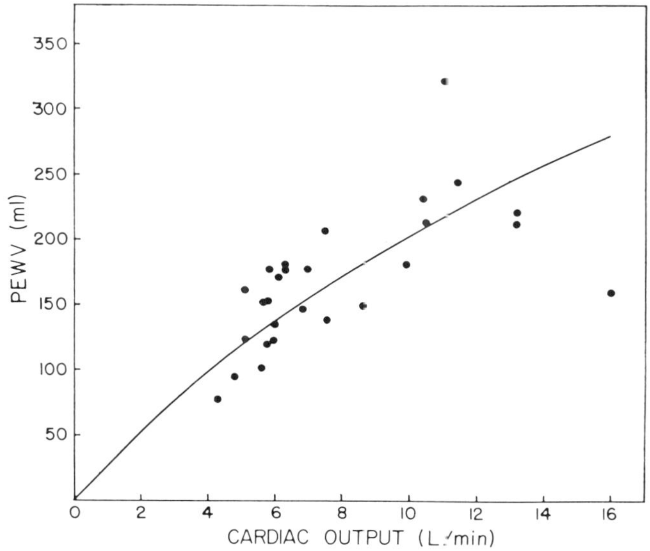

FIG. 5. Effects of changing cardiac output on pulmonary extravascular water volume (PEWV) measured by double isotopic dilution technique. Increasing cardiac output increased the amount of water measured, making the technique perfusion dependent. (Reprinted with permission from Marshall *et al.* Effects of posture and exercise on the pulmonary extravascular water volume in man. J Appl Physiol 1971;31:375–379.)

tion of five agents, Poly 5, was studied in the porcine pseudomonas model and included the nonspecific inflammatory blocker, methylprednisolone (30 mg/kg), the serotonin blocker, ketanserin (0.2 mg/kg), the prostaglandin blocker, ibuprofen (12.5 mg/kg), the H_1 blocker, diphenhydramine (3 mg/kg), and the H_2 blocker, cimetidine (150 mg) given intravenously (IV) 20 minutes and 120 minutes after the onset of the pseudomonas infusion. This combination lowered the early marked rise in PAP to control levels (Fig. 10), prevented the fall in PaO_2 (Fig. 11), cardiac output and systemic artery pressure and prevented the increased permeability as measured by EVLW and scintigraphic albumin flux (Fig. 12). Subsequent studies have shown that deletion of both methylprednisolone and ketanserin was associated with a fall in cardiac output, but the remaining combination (CID) of prostaglandin blockade

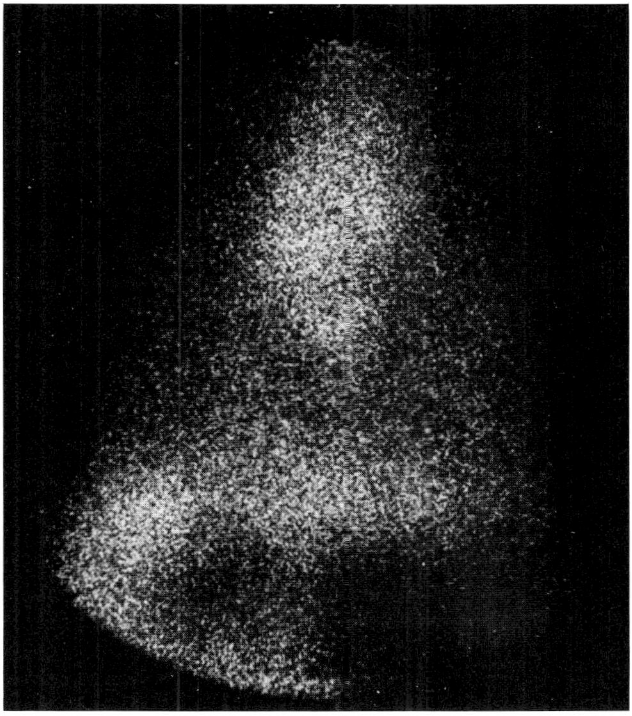

FIG. 6. Gamma camera scintiscan of the heart and lungs of a normal dog 2.5 hours after the administration of 5 mCi ^{99m}TC-HSA before the administration of 0.3 ml/kg oleic acid, showing concentration of radioactivity in the cardiac region. (Reprinted with permission from Sugerman HJ *et al.* Preliminary report: Gamma camera detection of oleic acid alveolar–capillary albumin leak. J Surg Res 1980;29:93–99.)

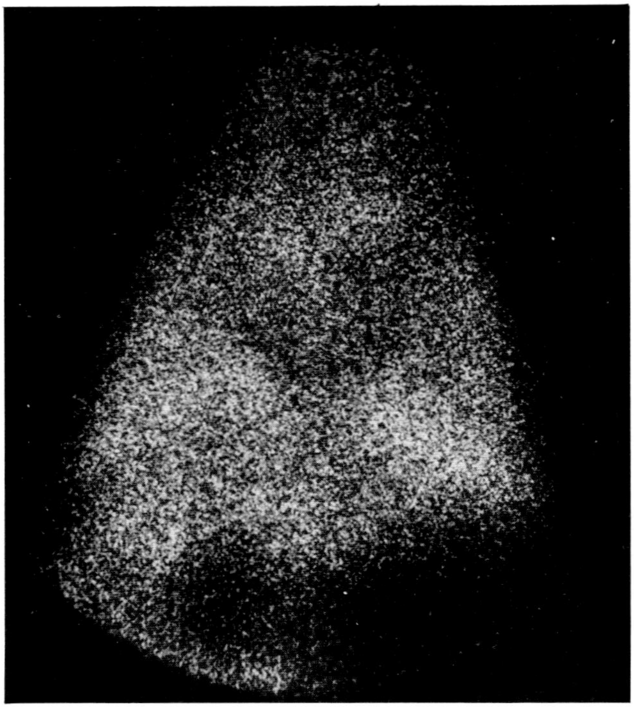

FIG. 7. Gamma camera scintiscan of the heart and lungs of dog shown in Figure 6, 45 minutes after the administration of 0.3 ml/kg oleic acid, showing redistribution of radioactive albumin into the pulmonary regions. (Reprinted with permission from Sugerman HJ *et al.* Preliminary report: Gamma camera detection of oleic acid alveolar–capillary albumin leak. J Surg Res 1980;29:93–99.)

with ibuprofen and histamine blockade with both the H_1-receptor blocker, diphenhydramine, and the H_2-receptor blocker, cimetidine, prevented the increased pulmonary capillary permeability (Fig. 12) after *Pseudomonas* as well as improved PAP (Fig. 10), PaO_2 (Fig. 11), and systemic pressure.[29] Deletion of any one of these three agents caused a marked deterio-

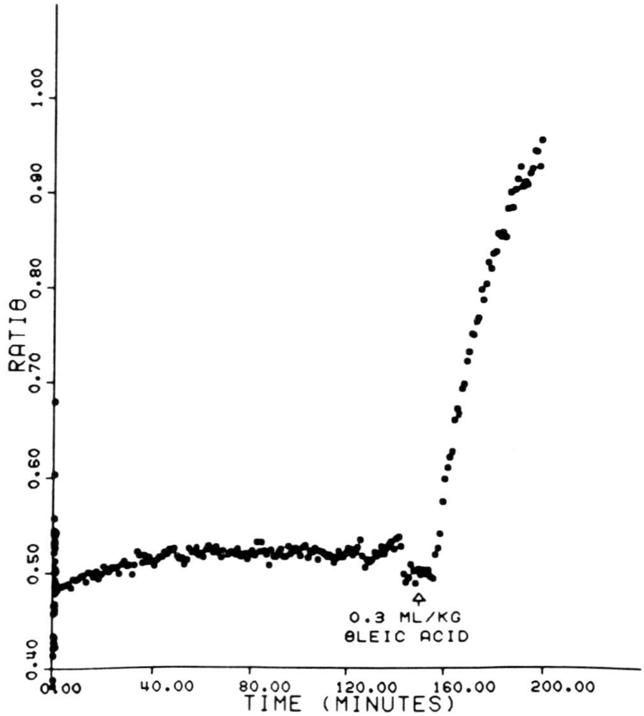

FIG. 8. Computer constructed lung:heart radioactivity ratio curve following 5 mCi ^{99m}TC-HSA in dog given 0.3 ml/kg oleic acid. The increase in lung:heart radioactivity became statistically significant within 7 minutes ($P < 0.05$) and within 9 minutes ($P < 0.001$) after the administration of oleic acid. (Reprinted with permission from Sugerman HJ *et al.* Preliminary report: Gamma camera detection of oleic acid alveolar–capillary albumin leak. J Surg Res 1980;29:93–99.)

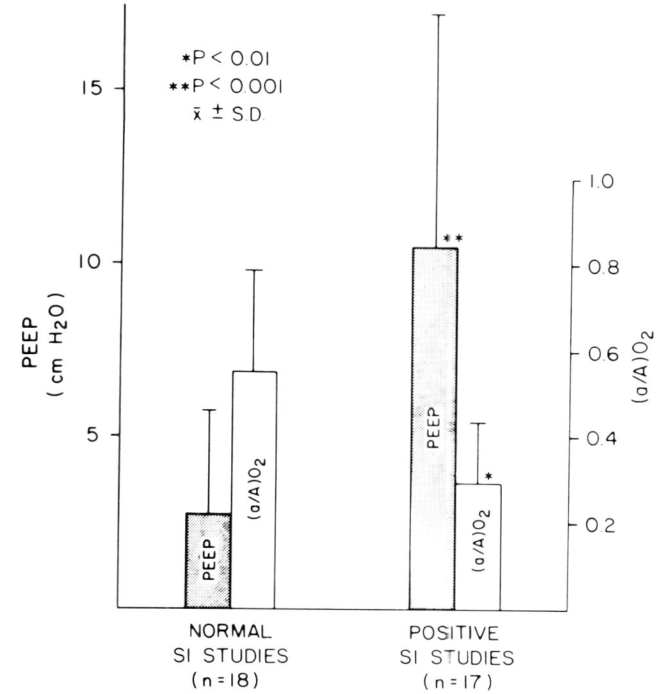

FIG. 9. Patients with positive SI had a significantly lower mean $(a/A)O_2$ ratio while receiving a significantly higher level of PEEP than those with a normal SI. (Reprinted with permission from Sugerman HJ *et al.* Gamma scintigraphic analysis of albumin flux in patients with acute respiratory distress syndrome. Surgery 1984;95:674–682.)

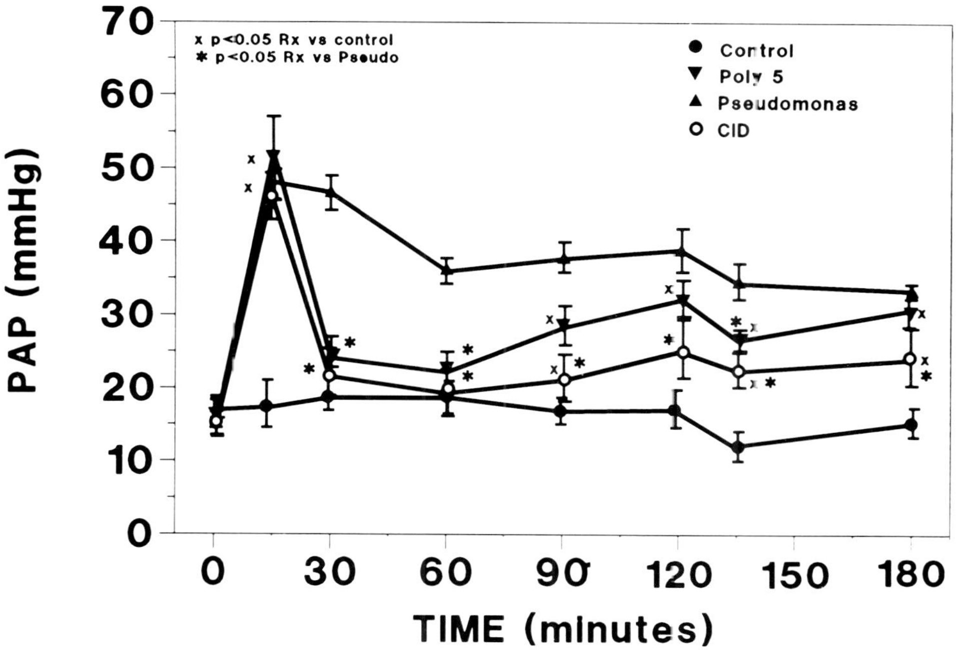

FIG. 10. Mean pulmonary arterial pressure: Treatment with a combination of cimetidine, ibuprofen, and diphenhydramine (CID) resulted in a significant reduction in pulmonary arterial pressure (PAP) compared to *Pseudomonas* alone. Treatment with Poly 5 (including CID + methylprednisolone and ketanserin) produced a more transient amelioration. (Reprinted with permission from Sielaff TD *et al.* Successful treatment of ARDS by histamine and prostaglandin blockade in a porcine Pseudomonas model. Surgery 1987;102:350–357.)

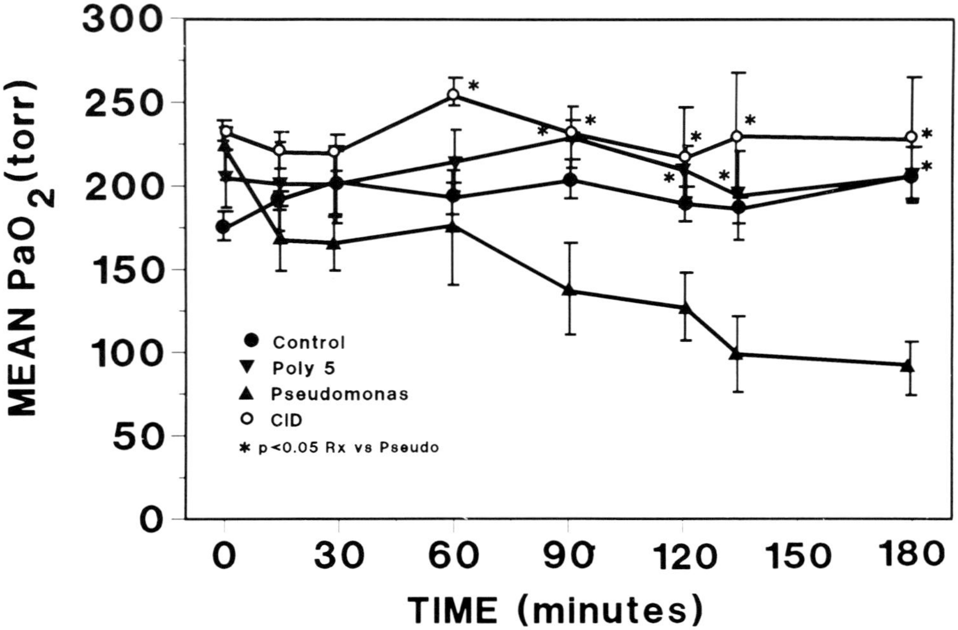

FIG. 11. Maintenance of arterial oxygen tension (PaO_2) at control levels with CID or Poly 5 after a continuous infusion of *Pseudomonas* in the pig which, untreated, caused a marked fall in PaO_2. (Reprinted with permission from Sielaff TD *et al.* Successful treatment of ARDS by histamine and prostaglandin blockade in a porcine Pseudomonas model. Surgery 1987;102:350–357.)

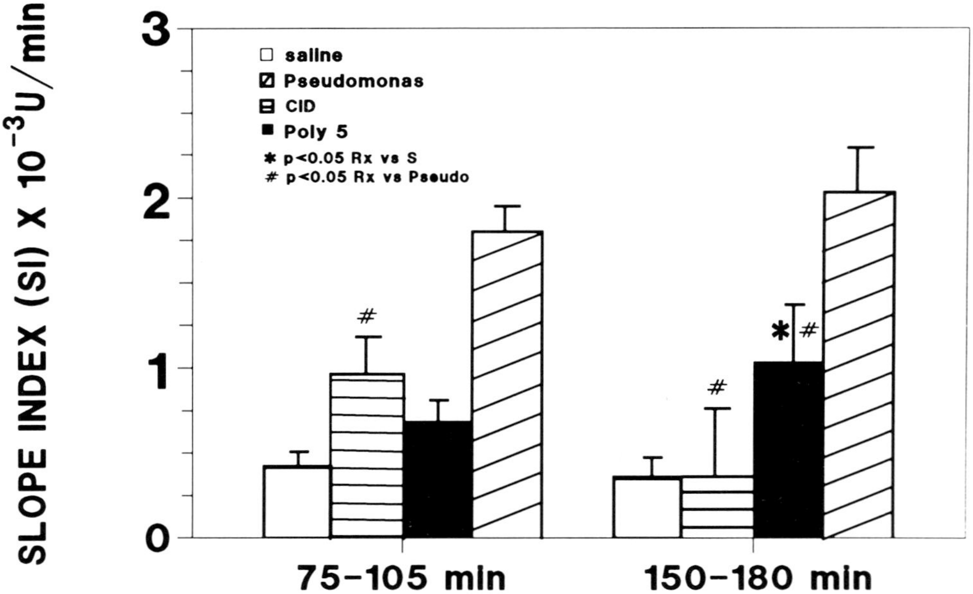

FIG. 12. Albumin flux (gamma scintigraphic measurement): Treatment with CID prevented a significant increase in slope index (SI) seen with *Pseudomonas* alone as compared to control animals. Treatment with Poly 5 resulted in a significant increase in SI 150-180 above control. (Reprinted with permission from Sielaff TD *et al.* Successful treatment of ARDS by histamine and prostaglandin blockade in a porcine Pseudomonas model. Surgery 1987;102:350–357.)

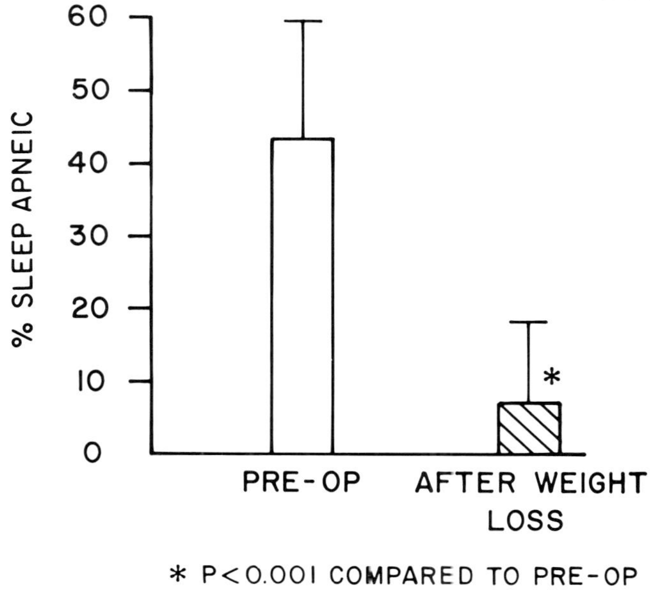

FIG. 13. Reduction in percent of sleep apneic (mean ± SD) in 22 patients with obstructive sleep apnea syndrome after weight loss induced by gastric surgery. (Reprinted with permission from Sugerman HJ *et al.* Gastric surgery for respiratory insufficiency of obesity. Chest 1986;89:81–86.)

ration in this model. Perhaps this combination therapy will be of value in the treatment, or prevention of septic-induced ARDS as well as multisystem organ failure associated with sepsis and septic shock. A clinical study now is being planned.

My interest in oxygen delivery, begun as a resident at HUP, has continued to influence me and was a major motivation to study the morbidly obese patient with respiratory insufficiency after gastric surgery for weight reduction. These unfortunate individuals may suffer from the obstructive sleep apnea syndrome (SAS), the obesity hypoventilation syndrome (OHS), or both as in the Pickwickian syndrome. This term was coined to describe a 52-

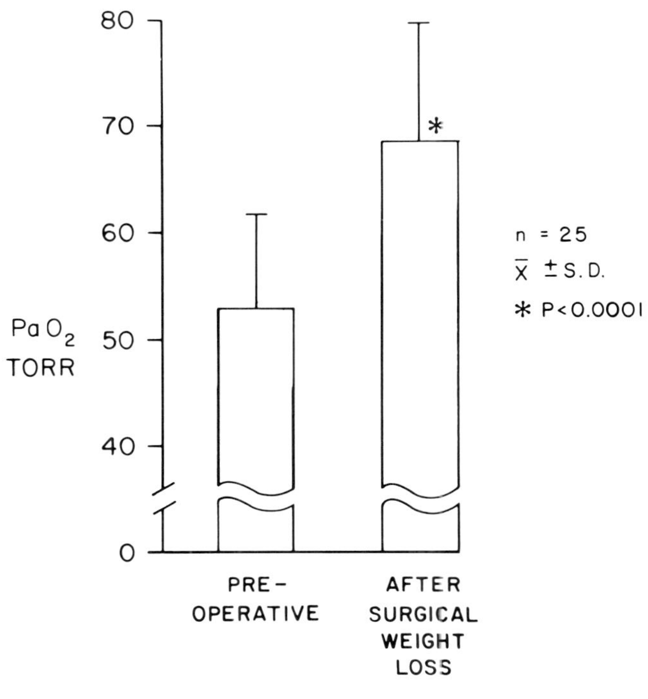

FIG. 14. Increase in PaO_2 in patients with obesity hypoventilation syndrome after surgically induced weight loss. (Reprinted with permission from Sugerman HJ *et al.* Gastric surgery for respiratory insufficiency of obesity. Chest 1986;89:81–86.)

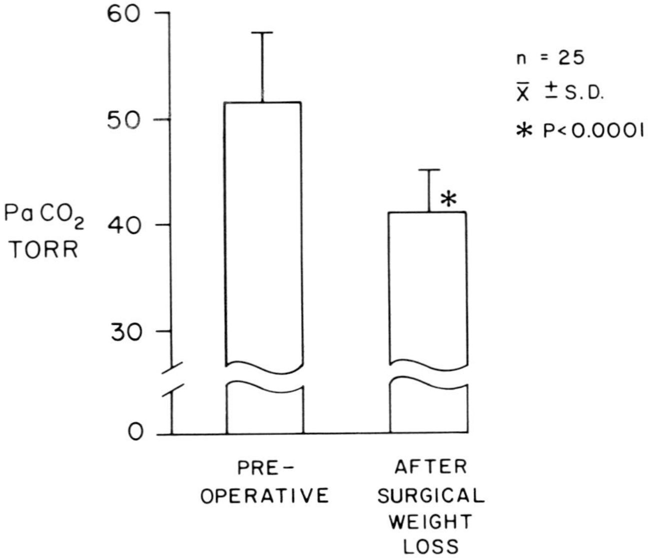

FIG. 15. Decrease in $PaCO_2$ in patients with obesity hypoventilation syndrome after surgically induced weight loss. (Reprinted with permission from Sugerman HJ *et al.* Gastric surgery for respiratory insufficiency of obesity. Chest 1986;89:81–86.)

year-old man who fell asleep in a poker game with a winning hand containing three aces and two kings, known as a full house.[30] Gastric surgery-induced weight loss will produce a marked decrease in sleep apnea (Fig. 13), significant improvements in PaO_2 (Fig. 14), $PaCO_2$ (Fig. 15), and lung volumes (Fig. 16).[31,32]

In conclusion, I am indebted to the philosophy instilled in me as a HUP surgical resident. This philosophy is exemplified by the career of Dr. Jonathan Rhoads who has supported studies in the basic sciences as the fundamental underpinning for advancements in surgery. This tradition dates from the beginning of surgery at the University of Pennsylvania and continues now under the baton of Dr. Clyde Barker. It is obviously vital to cut well and sew well; but the provision of adequate fuel to support the patients' metabolic machinery and

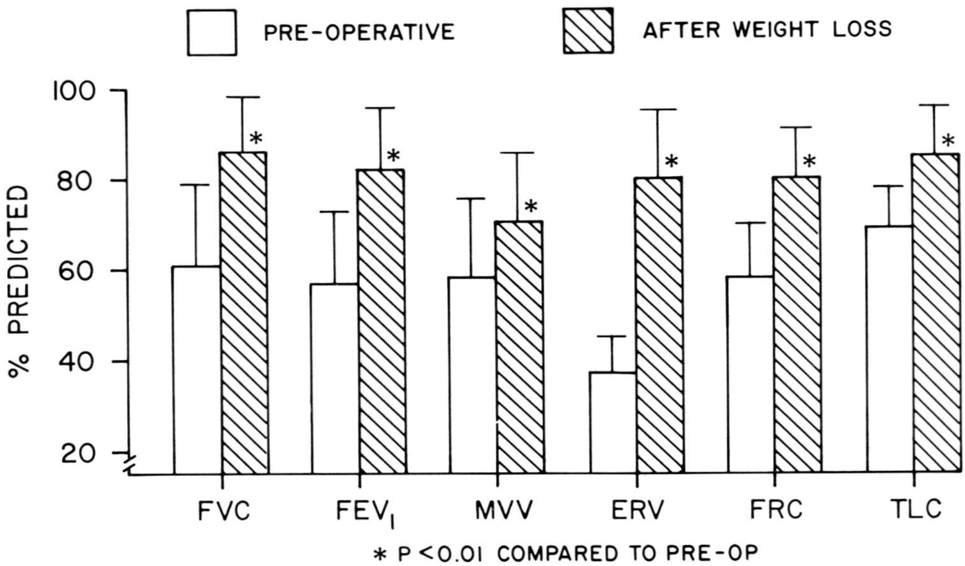

FIG. 16. Improved pulmonary function (mean ± SD) in 26 patients with obesity hypoventilation syndrome after weight loss after gastric surgery. (Reprinted with permission from Sugerman HJ *et al.* Gastric surgery for respiratory insufficiency of obesity. Chest 1986;89:81–86.)

efforts to correct or prevent multisystem organ failure are equally important for our patients to get well.

REFERENCES

1. Sugerman HJ, Davidson DT, Vibul S, Delivoria-Papadopoulos M, Miller LD, Oski FA. The basis of defective oxygen delivery from stored blood. Surg Gynecol Obstet 1970;131:733–741.
2. Travis SF, Sugerman HJ, Ruberg RL *et al.* Alterations of red-cell glycolytic intermediates and oxygen transport as a consequence of hypophosphatemia in patients receiving intravenous hyperalimentation. N Engl J Med 1971;285:763–768.
3. Oski FA, Marshall BE, Cohen PJ, Sugerman HJ, Miller LD. The role of the left-shifted or right-shifted oxygen–hemoglobin equilibrium curve. Ann Intern Med 1971;74:44–46.
4. Oski FA, Sugerman HJ, Miller LD. Experimentally induced alterations in the affinity of hemoglobin for oxygen: I. *In vitro* restoration of erythrocyte 2,3-diphosphoglycerate and its relationship to erythrocyte purine nucleoside phosphorylase activity in a variety of species. Blood 1972;39:522–524.
5. Eiseman B, Ashbaugh DG. Pulmonary effects of nonthoracic trauma: Proceedings of a conference conducted by the committee on trauma, Division of Medical Sciences, National Academy of Sciences–National Research Council. J Trauma 1968;8:621–756.
6. Ashbaugh DG, Bigelow DB, Petty TL, Levine BE. Acute respiratory distress in adults. Lancet 1967;2:319–323.
7. Cournand A, Motley HL, Werko L, Richards DW. Physiological studies of the effects of intermittent positive pressure breathing on cardiac output in man. Am J Physiol 1948;152 162–174.
8. Sugerman HJ, Olofsson KB, Pollock TW, Agnew RF, Rogers RM, Miller LD. Continuous positive end-expiratory pressure ventilation (PEEP) for the treatment of diffuse interstitial pulmonary edema. J Trauma 1972;12:263–274.
9. Monaco V, Burdge R, Newell J *et al.* Pulmonary venous admixture in injured patients. J Trauma 1972;12:15–23.
10. Falke KJ, Pontoppidan H, Kumar A, Leith DE, Geffin B, Laver MB. Ventilation with end-expiratory pressure in acute lung disease. J Clin Invest 1972;51:2315–2323.
11. Robin ED, Carey LC, Grenvik A *et al.* Capillary leak syndrome with pulmonary edema. Arch Intern Med 1972;130:66–71.
12. Lee CC, Sugerman HJ, Tatum JL, Wright TP, Hirsh PD, Hirsch JI. Effects of ibuprofen on a pig Pseudomonas ARDS model. J Surg Res 1986;40:438–444.
13. Sugerman HJ, Strash AM, Hirsch JI *et al.* Scintigraphy and radiography in oleic acid pulmonary microvascular injury: Effects of positive end-expiratory pressure (PEEP). J Trauma 1982;22:179–185.
14. Chinard FP, Enns T. Transcapillary pulmonary exchange of water in the dog. Am J Physiol 1954;178:197–202.
15. Marshall BE, Teichner RL, Kallos T, Sugerman HJ, Wyche MQ Jr, Tantum KR. Effects of posture and exercise on the pulmonary extravascular water volume in man. J Appl Physiol 1971;31:375–379.
16. Oppenheimer L, Elings V, Lewis FR. Thermal dye lung water measurements: Effects of edema and embolization. J Surg Res 1979;26:504–509.
17. Sugerman HJ, Hirsch JI, Strash AM *et al.* Preliminary report: Gamma camera detection of oleic acid alveolar–capillary albumin leak. J Surg Res 1980;29:93–99.
18. Sugerman HJ, Strash AM, Hirsch JI *et al.* Sensitivity of scintigraphy for detection of pulmonary capillary albumin leak in canine oleic acid ARDS. J Trauma 1981;21:520–527.
19. Sugerman HJ, Hirsch JI, Tatum JL, Strash AM, Sharp DE, Greenfield L. Comparative scintigraphy in oleic acid pulmonary microvascular injury. Crit Care Med 1982;10:31–33.
20. Sugerman HJ, Tatum JL, Strash AM, Hirsch JI, Greenfield LJ. Effect of pulmonary vascular recruitment on gamma scintigraphy and pulmonary capillary protein leak. Surgery 1981;90:388–395.
21. Sugerman HJ, Tatum JL, Burke TS, Strash AM, Glauser FL. Gamma scintigraphic analysis of albumin flux in patients with acute respiratory distress syndrome. Surgery 1984;95:674–682.
22. Fein AM, Lippman M, Holtzman H, Eliraz A, Goldberg SK. The risk factors, incidence, and prognosis of ARDS following septicemia. Chest 1983;83:40–42.
23. Fowler AA, Hamman RF, Good JT *et al.* Adult respiratory distress syndrome Risk with common predispositions. Ann Intern Med 1983;98:593–597.
24. Sugerman HJ, Blocher CR, Hirsch JI, Strash AM, Tatum JL. Failure of various agents to decrease oleic acid pulmonary albumin leak. J Surg Res 1983;34:456–462.
25. Buchman SR, Sugerman HJ, Tatum JL, Wright TP, Blocher CR, Hirsch JI. HCl-induced pulmonary albumin leak in dogs. Surgery 1984;96:163–170.
26. Harvey CF, Sugerman HJ, Tatum JL, Sielaff TD, Blocher CR. Ibuprofen and methylprednisolone in a pig Pseudomonas ARDS model. Circ Shock 1987;21:175–183.
27. Sielaff TD, Kellum JM, Sugerman HJ, Kuemmerle JF, Tatum JL. Serotonin receptor blockade improves cardiac output and hypoxia in porcine ARDS. J Surg Res 1987;43:118–127.
28. Sielaff TD, Sugerman HJ, Tatum JL, Kellum JM, Blocher CS. Treatment of porcine Pseudomonas ARDS with combination drug therapy. J Trauma 1987;27:1313–1322.
29. Sielaff TD, Sugerman HJ, Tatum JL. Successful treatment of ARDS by histamine and prostaglandin blockade in a porcine Pseudomonas model. Surgery 1987;102:350–357.

30. Burwell CS, Robin ED, Whaley RD, Bickelmann AG. Extreme obesity associated with alveolar hypoventilation: A Pickwickian syndrome. Am J Med 1956;21:811–818.
31. Sugerman HJ, Fairman RP, Lindeman AK, Mathers JA, Greenfield LJ. Gastroplasty for respiratory insufficiency of obesity. Ann Surg 1981;193:677–685.

Discussion

The following is a discussion of Dr. Goodwin's and Dr. Sugerman's papers.

Dr. Henry Moss: The first paper I ever wrote was with Dr. Ravdin on wound healing, and in this paper we concluded that there was no substance that would enhance the rate of wound healing beyond normal. I know that Dr. Ravdin strongly felt that there were factors that could retard wound healing, but that there were none that could accelerate or enhance it. I'd like to ask Cleon if that has changed in any way. Will hyperoxygenation or any other factors accelerate wound healing?

Dr. Cleon Goodwin: We started out thinking that if we made animals hypoxic this would have an influence, but we quickly disabused ourselves of this. But, I don't know of a substance that accelerates wound healing. The usual things, such as adequate nutrition, specific vitamins, etc., are influential but like hyperbaric oxygen will not accelerate wound healing beyond normal.

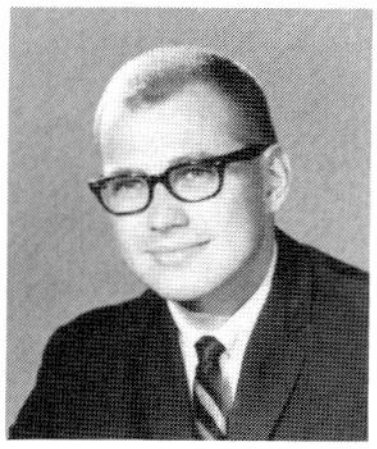

Introduction of Dr. Douglas Wilmore

Dr. Clyde Barker: Our next speaker, Doug Wilmore, was Dr. Rhoads' chief resident in 1971 and is clearly one of the star graduates of our program. As Stan Dudrick acknowledged earlier today, while Doug was still a resident at HUP he had an important role in the early development of parenteral nutrition. His work in San Antonio with Basil Pruitt after leaving our program has also been mentioned. Since then Doug has risen rapidly in the surgical world to become President of the Society of University Surgeons, and recently he was called to take over Francis Moore's famous laboratory at Harvard. He has become the acknowledged expert on sophisticated and innovative metabolic studies such as he will describe today as he presents his paper entitled "Positive Nitrogen Balance With Human Growth Hormone and Hypocaloric Intravenous Feeding."

Dr. Doug Wilmore's Introductory Remarks

Dr. Rhoads, there is no greater joy or pleasure for any of us as students than being called to recite before our teacher. I join all others today in saying what a great pleasure it is to be here enjoying such an opportunity. Dr. Rhoads, thanks so much for your influence on my career.

Positive Nitrogen Balance With Human Growth Hormone and Hypocaloric Intravenous Feeding

J. McK. MANSON, F.R.C.S. AND D. W. WILMORE, M.D.

Nitrogen equilibrium cannot be achieved in surgical patients without adequate nitrogen and calorie intake, frequently requiring central venous feedings. To investigate the hormonal environment under which nitrogen retention might be achieved during hypocaloric feedings, we administered peripheral vein nutrition with growth hormone (GH) to four healthy male patients. The intravenous diets provided 50% of estimated energy requirements (mean 566 kcal/m^2/day) and adequate nitrogen (6 gm/m^2/day). Each subject was studied for two 7-day periods; 10 mg of GH was given daily during one period and placebo during the other. Administration of GH decreased weight loss, caused retention of nitrogen, potassium, and phosphorus in amounts closely matching their proportions in skeletal muscle, and stimulated insulin production. GH also raised serum levels of free fatty acids and glycerol, increased urinary excretion of ketones, and favored fat oxidation in the postabsorptive state. Hyperinsulinemia and increased lipolysis and ketogenesis may augment the primary effects of GH. Further studies at adequate and approximately 30% of adequate calorie intake confirmed these findings. Maintenance of body protein with GH may allow improved nutritional care of catabolic patients that was previously unrecognized.

LOSS OF BODY PROTEIN is a characteristic response after critical illness such as injury or infection. This negative nitrogen balance can be attenuated or reversed by providing calories, nitrogen, and other essential nutrients. When enteral feeding is impossible or inadequate, central venous infusion of hypertonic nutrient solutions is usually necessary to meet the increased energy requirements associated with these hypermetabolic states.

Growth hormone (GH) is a potent anabolic agent that stimulates protein synthesis and cell growth. GH has been administered to hypercatabolic burn patients in an effort to improve nitrogen balance.[1,2] These studies suggested that GH can reduce nitrogen loss when administered with adequate quantities of protein and energy. In early studies with bovine GH and reduced calorie intakes, the anabolic effects of GH were negligible.[3] Other studies demonstrated that GH administration to fasting obese subjects also failed to promote nitrogen retention, a response associated with heightened ketoacidosis.[4]

Human GH, extracted from cadaver pituitary glands, has always been in short supply. However, GH is now synthesized by recombinant DNA techniques, and the ready availability of the hormone has stimulated renewed interest in the possible role for this anabolic agent in hospitalized patients. In this pilot study we administered GH to normal volunteers to determine the effects of both GH and caloric intake on protein, fat, carbohydrate, and mineral metabolism. All nutrients were administered by the intravenous route.

From the Department of Surgery, Brigham and Women's Hospital and the Harvard Medical School, Boston, Massachusetts.

Presented at the Forty-seventh Annual Meeting of the Society of University Surgeons, Richmond, Va., Feb. 13–15, 1986.

Supported in part by a National Institutes of Health Trauma Center grant P50 G.M. 29327-05 and Clinical Research Center grants 29-9299, AM 15191 and A1 15614.

This article has been reproduced with permission from *Surgery*, Vol. 100, No. 2, August 1986.

TABLE 1. *Characteristics of Subjects and Calorie Intakes Received*

Subject	Age (yr)	Weight (kg)	Height (cm)	Body surface area (m^2)	Total calorie intake ($kcal/m^2/day$)* Adequate calories	50% of Adequate	30% of Adequate
01	25	76.3	178	1.94	1166	583†	—
02	38	78.2	185	2.01	1144	572†	403
03	31	63.4	175	1.76	—	560	396
04	29	70.2	183	1.85	—	551	—

* These values reflect the energy provided by both the protein (6 gm nitrogen/m^2/day or ~150 kcal/m^2/day) and nonprotein caloric components of the diets.

† GH is given as human GH; in other studies recombinant methionyl-GH was used.

Materials and Methods

Subjects

Eight paired studies were performed in four healthy male subjects (Table 1). Medical history and examination were normal in each subject, as were screening blood tests, a glucose tolerance test, chest roentgenogram, and electrocardiogram.

Study Design

The study protocol was reviewed and approved by the Committee for the Protection of Human Subjects from Research Risks, Brigham and Women's Hospital, Boston, Mass.

Each study consisted of two 7-day periods. The periods were separated by at least 2 weeks and were identical except that during one the subjects received GH, 10 mg (20 IU), at 8:30 AM subcutaneously each day and during the other a similar volume of saline solution was injected. The subjects were unaware which treatment they were receiving. GH was given during the first period in half the studies and during the second period in the other half; the order was determined by random design. In two studies human GH (Aselacrin, provided by Serono Pharmaceuticals Ltd., Randolph, Mass.) was used, and in the other six recombinant methionyl-GH (Protropin, provided by Genentech Inc., South San Francisco, Calif.) was administered.

The basal metabolic requirements were calculated for each subject from standard tables based on sex, age, height, and weight.[5] An additional 25% was added to the basal requirement to allow for minimal activity in the hospital setting, and this quantity (basal +25%) was determined as the subjects' energy requirement. In two studies this quantity of energy was provided; this level of support will be referred to as "adequate." In four studies only one half of this quantity of energy was administered; this diet will be referred to as "50% of energy requirements." In two further studies the fat emulsion was removed from the energy component of the '50%' diet and only carbohydrate was infused as the nonprotein calorie source; this diet will be referred to as "30% of energy requirements." At all levels of calorie intake the nitrogen provided was constant at 6 gm/m^2/day (approximately 1 gm of protein/kg/body wt/day) and satisfied maintenance requirements. The caloric value of the amino acids was subtracted from the total caloric content of the diet, and the remaining calories were supplied as carbohydrate and fat in a ratio of 60:40, except the '30%' diet in which fat was omitted entirely. Nutrient solutions were prepared in the manufacturing pharmacy from commercially available amino acids (10% Travasol, Travenol Laboratories Inc., Deerfield, Ill.), 50% glucose, minerals, and vitamins on the day before each 7-day study with an Automix High Speed Compounder (Travenol Laboratories Inc.).

Parenteral nutrition was administered via an infusion pump from a 3 L bag that held the required nutrients for a 24-hour period (6:00 AM to 6:00 AM). Fat emulsion (10% Intralipid, Cutter Laboratories, Berkeley, Calif.) was administered via a side arm in the intravenous line at a rate of 100 ml/hr starting at 1:00 PM. Mineral and vitamin infusion was constant in all studies, and the volume of fluid infused was also the same in all studies (3 L/day).

Parenteral diets adequate in calories required central vein infusion and a central line was passed under fluoroscopic control via the antecubital fossa; dressings at the catheter entrance site were changed every third day. All other infusions were administered via a peripheral venous catheter placed in the forearm and the infusion site was changed every 2 days.

Subjects were given distilled water to drink ad libitum, but no other oral intake was allowed. They were allowed to walk in their rooms and on the ward and watch television.

At 6:00 AM on the seventh day of the study, the intravenous infusion was discontinued and the infusion catheter removed. The appropriate injection (saline solution or GH) was given at 8:30 AM. After a 5-hour fast, gas exchange analysis was performed and blood samples were obtained.

Measurements

The subjects were weighed at 6:00 AM each day. Throughout the study daily blood pressure and 4-hourly pulse and oral temperature were recorded. At 7:00 AM each day oxygen consumption and carbon dioxide production were measured with a Metabolic Measurement Cart (Beckman Instruments Inc., Fullerton, Calif.). The volume of distilled water taken each day was recorded.

Peripheral venous blood samples were obtained each morning at 8:00 AM, except the first and last mornings when blood was drawn at 6:00 AM (before infusion of the first bag of intravenous solution was started and before the last bag was discontinued), for blood urea nitrogen, glucose, sodium, and potassium. On days 1, 4, and 7, blood was drawn for serum insulin, β-hydroxybutyrate and acetoacetate, free fatty acids, glycerol, inorganic phosphate, albumin, total protein, bilirubin, and hepatic transaminases. Hematocrit and white cell count were determined on day 4. On days 1, 4, and 6, blood was also drawn at 12:30 PM for GH estimation and later in the study for free fatty acids and glycerol determination.

Urine was collected throughout the study during 24-hour periods coinciding with the duration of infusion of one bag of nutrient solution (6:00 AM to 6:00 AM). Urine was analyzed for total nitrogen, urea, ammonia, creatinine, acetoacetate and β-hydroxybutyrate, C-peptide, potassium, sodium, inorganic phosphorus, and calcium. Subjects passed stool only once per 7-day study, on the second or third day. This output was attributed to oral intake before commencement of the study and was discarded. Samples of intravenous solution from each infusion period were analyzed for glucose, nitrogen, sodium, and potassium content.

At 11:00 AM on the seventh day of the study, after a 5-hour fast, gas exchange measurements were performed and peripheral blood samples of insulin, free fatty acids, glycerol, and ketones were obtained.

All metabolite determinations in blood, plasma, or urine used standard analytic techniques previously described.[6] Radioimmunoassay techniques were used for the determination of insulin,[7] GH,[7] and C-peptide.[6] Nitrogen concentration in urine and parenteral nutrient solutions were determined by the macro-Kjeldahl technique.

Calculations

The daily weights obtained during each study period were plotted against time and the best fit linear regression was determined. The slope of each line was used to calculate the weight change during the 6-day period of parenteral nutrition. This method used all seven weight measurements and thus did not rely solely on the measurements taken on the first and last days of each study.

Daily balances were calculated as the difference between intake (amount in nutrient fluid) and urine output. Insensible loss of sodium was estimated at 6 mEq/day and of potassium at 4 mEq/day,[8] and these values were added to the urinary losses for calculation of the sodium and potassium balance. Average daily balance was calculated for each subject but the first 24-hour period was not included and was regarded as a "lead-in period." Thus the mean balance for a substance represents the average for days 2 through 6. The mean values for all subjects in a group were then averaged. The nitrogen, sodium, and potassium content of the intravenous solution was determined for each study; the values obtained for the electrolytes were consistently within 2% of the prescribed concentrations, and electrolyte intake as prescribed was used in the balance calculation. The nitrogen content of the solutions was determined at the same time that urinary nitrogen measurements were made. Measured intake values were used for the nitrogen balance calculations.

Metabolic rate, fat oxidation, and carbohydrate oxidation were calculated from oxygen consumption, carbon dioxide production, and urinary nitrogen excretion according to the equations of de Weir.[5] Metabolic rate for each day was derived from gas exchange measurements taken at the beginning and the end of the 24-hour period and nitrogen excretion during the same period. The values for each day were averaged to derive the mean for the 6-day period, and the mean value for each level of calorie intake was calculated from these values. Energy content of the nutrient solution was calculated from manufacturers specifications per unit volume and the quantity of nutrient administered.

Statistical Analysis

Statistical analysis was performed with a VAX 11/780 computer (Digital Equipment Corporation, Maynard, Mass.) and a standard software package (Minitab 82.1, Penn State University) to apply linear regression methods and paired *t* testing. A similar response was observed after administration of human and recombinant GH, and hence all the GH treatment data have been combined.* Results are expressed as mean ± SEM. Differences in means were accepted as significant when $p < 0.05$. In the analysis of metabolic rate data, the value from each study day was used to determine differences between control and GH periods by analysis of variance.

Results

The studies were well tolerated by the subjects. Three of the four subjects reported that during the GH phase of the hypocaloric diets they "felt better" than during the comparable control period and experienced fewer symptoms of inadequate nutrient intake such as mild fatigue and weakness. There were no complications associated with the intravenous infusions or catheters.

There were no significant differences in blood pressure and daily mean or maximum oral temperature during control and GH periods. GH administration was related to a rise in mean pulse rate from 71 ± 2 bpm to 76 ± 2 ($p < 0.01$).

The change in body weight that occurred during the 6 days of parenteral nutrition was significantly different between control and GH periods. This alteration also depended on the quantity of energy infused (Fig. 1). The weight changes in the subjects who received adequate diets were −0.4 ± 0.2 kg./m^2/6 days during the control period and +0.3 ± 0.1 during GH, in the subjects who received 50% of energy requirement they were −1.3 ± 0.2 kg/m^2/6 days during the control period and −0.4 ± 0.2 during GH ($p < 0.001$), and in the subjects who received 30% of energy requirements they were −1.4 ± 0.4 kg/m^2/6 days during the control period and −0.6 ± 0.5 during GH.

All basal preinfusion blood values were within normal limits at the start of the studies, and there were no major differences in these values between GH and control periods (Table 2). With administration of parenteral nutrients, glucose, insulin, and phosphate levels rose slightly. With GH therapy the increase in glucose and insulin was more prominent; insulin concentration more than doubled, a disproportionate increase when compared with a rise in glucose of only 5% to 15%. Blood urea nitrogen values fell with GH treatment. Early morning concentrations of the lipid substrates were not altered. However, plasma concentrations of glycerol and free fatty acids determined from plasma samples obtained at 12:30 PM, 4 hours after GH injection at the apparent height of lipolytic activity, were elevated at this time when compared with control values.

There was no significant difference in serum sodium, albumin, total protein, or liver transminases between day 1 and the periods of parenteral nutrition with or without GH.

Urine volume appeared less during GH treatment than during the control period (Table 3). Since intravenous intake was constant and there was no difference in oral intake (50% calories, control 458 ± 110 ml/m^2/day, GH 421 ± 57; all studies, control 437 ± 57, GH 440 ± 48), this reflected an alteration in fluid balance, probably indicating that water retention

* The data from all studies are public record and on file with the Food and Drug Administration, Rockville, MD.

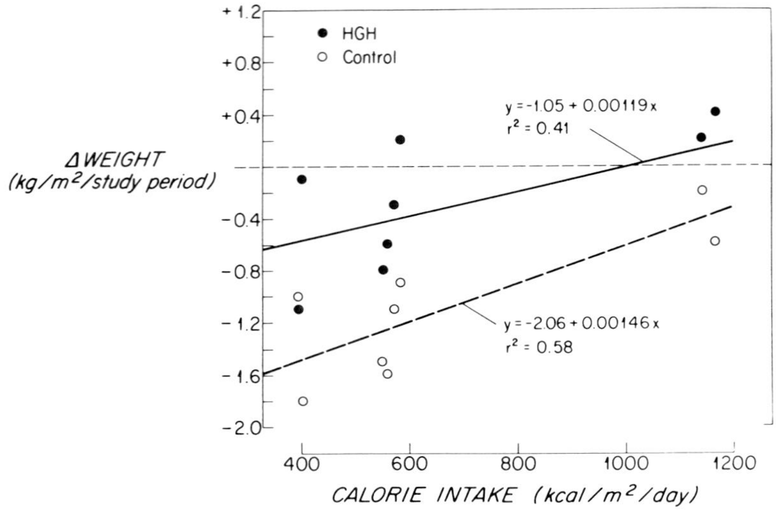

FIG. 1. Increase in caloric intake decreased weight loss during control and GH study periods. At all levels of caloric intake GH treatment was associated with a decrease in weight loss compared with control.

occurred with GH. However, insensible water losses were not measured and may have been altered because of changes in heat production associated with GH treatment.

With GH treatment there was a decreased excretion of nitrogen and urea and an increased excretion of C-peptide and ketones.

During the control periods there was negative balance of nitrogen, potassium, and phosphorus; losses of these substances were generally greater as calorie intake decreased (Table 4). With administration of GH, positive balance of these substances occurred (Fig. 2) at all levels of calorie intake (Fig. 3). Increased urinary excretion of calcium occurred during GH treatment.

Metabolic rate was greater during GH treatment than during the control period. At the 30% calorie intake level, metabolic rate was 892 ± 46 kcal/m^2/day compared with 845 ± 14 during control ($p < 0.02$) and during the adequate level of calorie intake 856 ± 10 kcal/m^2/day with 716 ± 28 during control ($p < 0.01$). Metabolic rate was not significantly different at the 50% calorie intake level (754 ± 69 kcal/m^2/day during GH compared with 795 ± 66 during control).

Five hours after the discontinuation of the intravenous infusion on the seventh day of study, oxygen consumption and carbon dioxide production tended to be higher with GH treatment (Table 5). Calculation of fuel oxidation demonstrated increased fat oxidation after GH treatment when compared with control periods. Respiratory quotient tended to be lower during GH treatment (0.78 ± 0.02) compared with control periods (0.79 ± 0.02; not significant). Simultaneous serum determinations demonstrated increased concentrations of free fatty acids and glycerol during GH study periods, despite elevated insulin concentrations.

Discussion

For more than 30 years investigators have evaluated the effects of GH in human subjects. These past studies have demonstrated the unique properties of GH in improving nitrogen balance. Because of the short supply of GH before 1985, clinical studies were limited and much of the knowledge of the metabolic actions of GH came from animal investigations or studies that used bovine growth hormone, a substance that is now known to have unpredictable anabolic activity in humans. After such investigations it was proposed that the protein anabolic effect of GH occurred only when adequate nutrient intake was provided; during inadequate nutrient intake GH failed to stimulate protein retention.[3] From these data investigators formulated the 'critical level' hypothesis that proposed that adequate calories and nitrogen were necessary for GH to express its' anabolic effects. This hypothesis was

TABLE 2. *Blood or Serum Values (mean ± SEM)*

	Basal values (AM studies)		Infusion values*: 50% of adequate calories		Infusion values*: All studies	
	Control	GH	Control	GH	Control	GH
Glucose (mg/dl)	85 ± 3	84 ± 3	91 ± 6	96 ± 5†	94 ± 4	108 ± 7
Insulin (μU/ml)	11 ± 1	9 ± 1	12 ± 3	25 ± 6†	16 ± 4	37 ± 14
GH (ng/ml)	—	—	4.2 ± 2.9	33 ± 10†	2.7 ± 1.5	42 ± 8§
Sodium (mEq/L)	142 ± 1	142 ± 1	141 ± 1	140 ± 1	142 ± 1	140 ± 1†
Potassium (mEq/L)	4.2 ± 0.1	4.2 ± 0.1	4.4 ± 0.1	4.5 ± 0.1	4.5 ± 0.1	4.5 ± 0.1
Phosphate (mg/dl)	3.9 ± 0.2	3.9 ± 0.2	4.3 ± 0.2	4.4 ± 0.2	4.4 ± 0.1	4.5 ± 0.2
Blood urea nitrogen (mg/dl)	15 ± 1	15 ± 1	15 ± 1	9 ± 1‡	14 ± 1	9 ± 1§
β-Hydroxybutyrate (mmol/L)	0.08 ± 0.02	0.05 ± 0.01	0.05 ± 0.01	0.02 ± 0.01	0.05 ± 0.01	0.02 ± 0.01
Acetoacetate (mmol/L)	0.05 ± 0.01	0.03 ± 0.01†	0.03 ± 0.01	0.02 ± 0.01	0.03 ± 0.01	0.02 ± 0.01
Glycerol (mg/dl) AM	1.28 ± 0.12	1.39 ± 0.07	1.52 ± 0.19	1.39 ± 0.13	1.45 ± 0.10	1.46 ± 0.08
12:30 PM	—	—	—	—	1.41 ± 0.09	2.00 ± 0.11§ (n = 5)
Free fatty acids (μEq/L) AM	629 ± 65	826 ± 71	716 ± 74	946 ± 152	730 ± 52	896 ± 80
12:30 PM	—	—	—	—	850 ± 66	1265 ± 188§ (n = 5)

* Glucose, potassium, and blood urea nitrogen are mean of daily samples (days 2–7); all other values are mean of day 4 and day 6 or 7 determinations.

† $p < 0.05$, when compared with control by paired t test.

‡ $p < 0.01$.

§ $p < 0.001$.

supported by studies in fasting obese volunteers; nitrogen excretion was not reduced with GH administration. However, in these studies marked ketoacidosis accompanied GH administration and this perturbation caused increased ammonia excretion and altered nitrogen metabolism.[4] The critical level hypothesis was not supported by our observations with human or m-GH in normal human subjects: GH administration with hypocaloric parenteral diets containing some carbohydrate and adequate quantities of amino acids resulted in prompt and significant nitrogen retention.

The GH-induced retention of nitrogen was accompanied by positive balance of both potassium and phosphorus, intracellular constituents that are essential components of lean body mass. The retention of each gram of nitrogen was accompanied by approximately 5 mEq of potassium and 67 mg of phosphorus (these figures are calculated as the difference in the balances of these substances during control and GH studies). Previous investigators suggest that for every gram of nitrogen retained as skeletal muscle, approximately 3 mEq of potassium is retained, although greater quantities of potassium may be retained under certain circumstances.[9] For every gram of nitrogen retained in skeletal muscle, approximately 66 mg of phosphorus is retained.[8] Because the quantitative relationships between these elements is so similar to their relative proportions in skeletal muscle, these data support the thesis that the nitrogen retained during GH treatment was primarily in the form of skeletal muscle.

The alterations in body weight that occurred during control and GH periods support, in part, these balance data. For example, the subjects who received 50% of adequate calories lost approximately 0.9 kg./m^2/6 days more weight during the control periods when compared with GH treatment. The difference in cumulative nitrogen balance between these two periods was approximately 14 gm N/m^2/6 days. This amount of nitrogen would account for 85 to 90 gm of protein and 350 to 400 gm of hydrated tissue. While the gain in lean tissue can in part explain the differences in weight loss, other factors such as fluid retention also account for differences in weight change. The subjects excreted 200 ml/m^2/day less urine during GH treatment than during control periods. Assuming that insensible loss was constant during study period (an assumption that may be inappropriate because of the alterations in metabolic rate that occurred with GH treatment), this 200 ml of fluid retention represents 1.2 kg during the 6-day study period. This fluid weight in addition to the 350 gm of lean tissue is within the error term of the weight difference observed. However, this retained fluid was not accompanied by signs of peripheral edema or significant sodium retention, suggesting that the water may have been retained as intracellular fluid. Glycogen storage could also account for some fluid retention and facilitate intracellular potassium deposition. Further studies are required to confirm this speculation.

Some of the metabolic alterations observed, including fluid retention, may reflect short-term changes that are altered with time. The increased excretion of calcium with GH treatment has been previously observed,[10] but calcium loss returns to normal with time.[11] Long-term studies coupled with more detailed analysis of body composition are required to assess the impact of this treatment on body tissues and fluid compartments.

While GH has direct tissue effects that can be demonstrated in vitro, it is thought that many of the protein anabolic properties of the hormone are mediated by a second substance, which is synthesized primarily in the liver in response to GH.[12] This substance, called insulin-like growth factor (IGF I), is thought to directly stimulate protein synthesis in skeletal muscle and other tissues. The nitrogen-retaining properties of GH may in large part depend on IGF I synthesis, and the production of this substance may be altered in various disease states, including malnutrition and liver dysfunction.[13,14] IGF I levels were determined on the last day of five of the total of eight paired studies, and these data revealed a threefold increase in IGF I during GH treatment when compared with controls.

In addition to the increased elaboration of IGF I, GH administration stimulated insulin production as characterized by hyperinsulinemia and increased C-peptide excretion, both of which increased twofold, while blood glucose values rose only 5% to 15%. Because insulin is a potent anabolic agent, this hormone may have augmented net nitrogen retention. However, during this state of hyperinsulinemia, increased fat was mobilized and oxidized (Tables 4 and 5). This response was uncharacteristic of usual hormonal control; elevated insulin concentrations inhibit lipolysis and suppress ketogenesis. Because ketones are thought to

TABLE 3. *Urinary Excretion (mean of days 2 through 6 ± SEM, all expressed/m²/day)*

	50% Adequate calories		All studies	
	Control	GH	Control	GH
Urine volume (ml)	1583 ± 47	1360 ± 111	1483 ± 60	1285 ± 70*
Nitrogen (gm)	7.5 ± 0.2	5.1 ± 0.4†	7.3 ± 0.3	5.0 ± 0.2‡
Urea nitrogen (gm)	6.6 ± 0.1	4.3 ± 0.4†	6.3 ± 0.3	4.1 ± 0.3‡
Ammonia (gm)	0.28 ± 0.03	0.28 ± 0.02	0.27 ± 0.02	0.29 ± 0.02
Creatinine (gm)	0.90 ± 0.02	0.91 ± 0.01	0.91 ± 0.01	0.89 ± 0.02
C-Peptide (nmol)	6.2 ± 0.7	11.8 ± 1.5†	7.2 ± 0.6	17.4 ± 2.9†
β-Hydroxybutyrate (mmol)	0.23 ± 0.03	0.76 ± 0.12*	0.23 ± 0.02	0.66 ± 0.10‡
Acetoacetate (mmol)	0.28 ± 0.04	1.52 ± 0.03*	0.26 ± 0.02	1.14 ± 0.03*

* $p < 0.05$, when compared with controls by paired t test.
† $p < 0.01$.
‡ $p < 0.001$.

TABLE 4. *Nitrogen and Mineral Intake, Excretion, and Balance (mean of days 2 through 6 ± SEM, all expressed/m²/day)*

	50% of adequate calories					All studies				
		Excretion		Balance			Excretion		Balance	
	Intake	Control	GH	Control	GH	Intake	Control	GH	Control	GH
Nitrogen (gm)	6.0 ± 0.1	7.5 ± 0.2	5.1 ± 0.4*	−1.4 ± 0.2	+0.9 ± 0.4*	6.0 ± 0.1	7.3 ± 0.3	5.0 ± 0.2†	−1.2 ± 0.3	+1.0 ± 0.3†
Sodium (mEq)	54	54 ± 2	52 ± 12	−2.8 ± 2.2	+0.4 ± 1.9	53	53 ± 1	50 ± 2	−2.9 ± 1.8	+0.6 ± 1.1
Potassium (mEq)	54	57 ± 1	48 ± 4	−4.6 ± 2.5	+4.1 ± 3.0	53	57 ± 2	46 ± 3*	−5.6 ± 1.9	+5.7 ± 2.2*
Calcium (mg)	212	130 ± 7	175 ± 8*	+82 ± 10	+37 ± 9*	209	129 ± 5	185 ± 10†	+81 ± 4	+25 ± 10†
Inorganic phosphorus (mg)	246	335 ± 17	180 ± 18*	−89 ± 10	+67 ± 20*	243	364 ± 22	216 ± 19†	−120 ± 21	+2.8 ± 19†

* $p < 0.01$, when compared with controls by paired t test.
† $p < 0.001$.

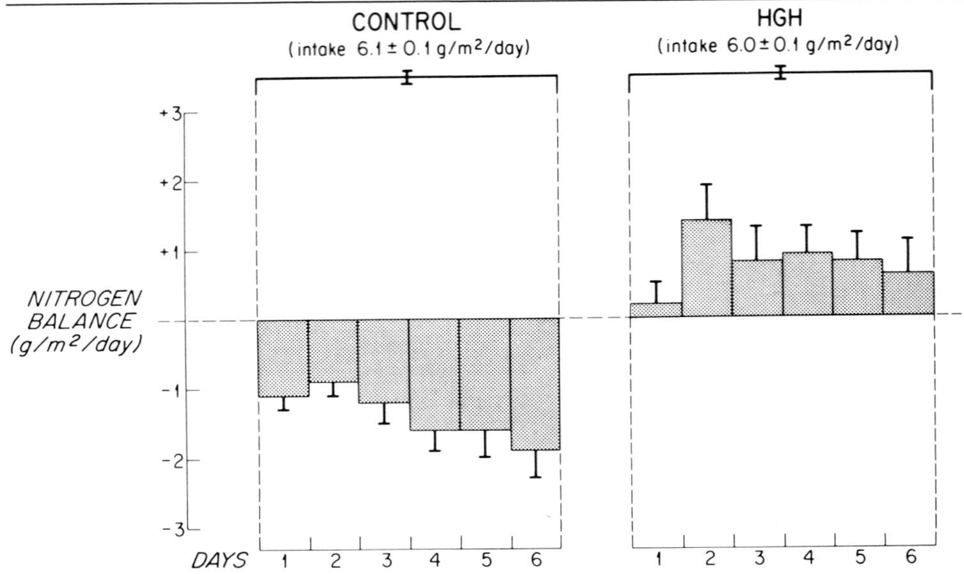

FIG. 2. Mean daily nitrogen balance during control and GH study periods at 50% adequate intake. During control periods the nitrogen balance was persistently negative. With GH treatment the nitrogen balance was positive.

diminish net skeletal muscle protein breakdown[15] and may augment the protein sparing effect of insulin,[16] this environment of hyperinsulinemia and increased ketone production may be an additional mechanism to explain the nitrogen-sparing action of GH.

Under normal circumstances, when adequate protein is present in the diet, hypocaloric intake is associated with loss of body protein for at least several weeks. At this time, mechanisms associated with adaptation to more prolonged periods of inadequate food intake and protein wasting are initiated, and protein equilibrium may then occur. This study demonstrates that positive nitrogen balance can be achieved by administering as little as 140 gm of carbohydrate and an adequate quantity of amino acids along with GH. Body fat was utilized as the additional fuel and the resulting hormonal-substrate environment favored the

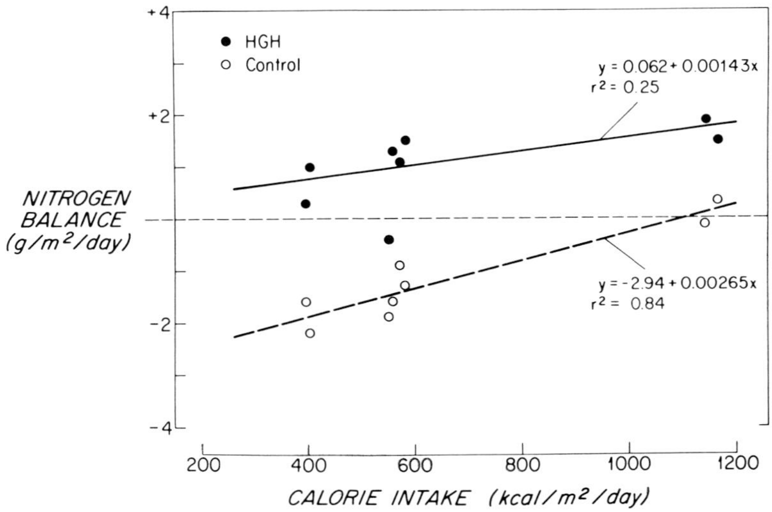

FIG. 3. Nitrogen balance during constant nitrogen intake varied with calorie provision. In the control studies nitrogen equilibrium was achieved with adequate calories. With GH administration nitrogen balance was positive at all levels of intake.

TABLE 5. *Gas Exchange Data and Serum Levels at 11:00 AM on Day 7 After a 5-hour Fast (all studies, mean ± SEM)*

	Control	GH
$\dot{V}_{O_2}$ (L/m^2/day)	170 ± 9	187 ± 9
$\dot{V}_{CO_2}$ (L/m^2/day)	135 ± 9	145 ± 10
Metabolic rate (kcal/m^2/day)	778 ± 43	860 ± 46
Fat oxidation (gm/m^2/day)	43 ± 5	59 ± 4*
Carbohydrate oxidation (gm/m^2/day)	46 ± 12	44 ± 15
Insulin (μU/ml)	6.8 ± 1.0	17.9 ± 3.4†
Serum free fatty acids FFA (μEq/L)	924 ± 41	1[illegible]16 ± 90*
Serum glycerol (mg/dl)	1.28 ± 0.14	1.71 ± 0.06*

* $p < 0.05$, when compared with controls by paired t test.
† $p < 0.01$.

net synthesis of lean body mass. It is not known what responses would occur if the dose of GH was varied; further studies are required to evaluate the dose response effects and determine long-term consequences of such therapy. However, this pilot study suggests that GH and possibly other growth factors that will become available as a result of recombinant DNA technology may allow improved nutritional care for catabolic patients that was here before unrecognized.

ACKNOWLEDGMENTS

We acknowledge the technical support of Michael Colpoys, Lourdes Holejko, Ramona Faris, and Elaine Brown. We also thank Sheila Driscoll, Rita O'Donnell, and the staff of the Clinical Research Center of the Brigham and Women's Hospital for their care of the subjects and Kathleen Benfell and Barbara Lapidas-Brown of the hospital pharmacy for their work in preparing the intravenous solutions.

REFERENCES

1. Liljadahl S-O, Gemzell C-A, Plantin L-O, Birke G. Effect of human growth hormone in patients with severe burns. Acta Chir Scand 1961;122:1–14.
2. Wilmore DW, Moylan JA Jr, Bristow BF, Mason AD Jr, Pruitt BA Jr. Anabolic effects of growth hormone and high caloric feedings following thermal injury. Surg Gynecol Obstet 1974;138:875–884.
3. Prudden JF, Pearson E, Soroff HS. Studies on growth hormone-II. The effect of growth hormone on the nitrogen metabolism of severely burned patients. Surg Gynecol Obstet 1956;102:695–701.
4. Felig P, Marliss EB, Cahill GF Jr. Metabolic response to growth hormone during prolonged starvation. J Clin Invest 1971;50:411–421.
5. Wilmore DW. The metabolic management of the critically ill. New York, 1977, Plenum Publishing Corp.
6. Bessey PQ, Watters JM, Aoki TM, Wilmore DW. Combined hormonal infusion simulates the metabolic response to injury. Ann Surg 1984;200:264–281.
7. Juan C, AvRuskin TW. A combined immunoassay of human growth hormone and insulin. J Clin Endocrinol 1971;33:150–152.
8. Consolazio CF, Johnson RE, Pecora LJ. Physiological measurements of metabolic functions in man. New York, 1963, McGraw-Hill Inc.
9. Randall HT. Water, electrolytes and acid base balance. *In* Goodhart RS, Shils ME, editors: Modern nutrition in health and disease, ed 6. Philadelphia, 1980, Lea & Febiger, p 377
10. Henneman PH, Forbes AP, Moldawer M, Dempsey EF, Carrol EF Effects of human growth hormone in man. J Clin Invest 1960;39:1223–1238.
11. Gertner JM, Horst RL, Broadus AE, Rasmussen H, Genel M. Parathyroid function and vitamin D metabolism during human growth hormone replacement. J Clin Endocrinol Metab 1979;49:185–188.
12. Schwander JC, Hauri C, Zapf J, Froesch ER. Synthesis and secretion of insulin-like growth factor and its binding protein by the perfused rat liver: dependence on growth hormone status. Endocrinology 1983;113:297–305.
13. Smith HF, Latham MC, Azubuike JA, Butler WR, Phillips LS, Pond WG, Enwonwu CO. Blood plasma levels of cortisol, insulin, growth hormone and somatomedin in children with marasmus, kwashiorkor, and intermediate forms of protein–energy malnutrition. Proc Soc Exp Biol Med 1981;167:607–611.
14. Wu A, Grant DB, Hambley J, Levi AJ. Reduced serum somatomedin activity in patients with chronic liver disease. Clin Sci Mol Med 1974;47:359–366.
15. Sherwin RS, Hendler RG, Felig P. Effect of ketone infusions on amino acid and nitrogen metabolism in man. J Clin Invest 1975;55:1382–1390.

16. Johnson DJ, Pressler VM, Colpoys MF, Smith RJ, Wilmore DW. Insulin-ketone interaction: a possible mechanism for post injury branched chain amino acid anticatabolic properties. Surg Forum 1985;36:54–56.

DISCUSSION

This discussion took place at the Society of University Surgeons.

DR. MURRAY BRENNAN (New York, N.Y.): I am always hesitant about questioning anything that Dr. Wilmore has thought through, but the question I have is how can it be true? If the nitrogen balance is as stated and does differ from zero, the only explanation I could think of was that either it is a transient phenomenon and when you stop all nitrogen retained would be lost because they were normal volunteers not previously depleted, receiving hypocaloric feeding, or you have created a situation of pubertal acromegaly with never-ending retention of nitrogen! Would you explain that?

DR. GEORGE BLACKBURN (Boston, Mass.): Would you share with us the values of serum ketoacids, acetoacetate, and β-hydroxy-butrate and particularly point out that in the face of an increased C-peptide and serum insulin, one would expect a decrease in the rates of ketogenesis. While you have shown us a small excretion and an unusual ratio, oxidative ketone body acetoacetate being greater than reduce form β-hydroxy-butrate. Do you have any other evidence to the influence of growth hormone on the rates of ketogenesis compared with control?

DR. R. A. FORSE (Montreal, Quebec): You have indicated that the study was done for a 7-day period. Was this a crossover study design or did you do one study followed by another? As well, did you arrange for the volunteers to have a period of time between studies to allow them to normalize? Finally, do you have any data on the resting energy expenditure during the studies?

DR. JOSEF FISCHER (Cincinnati, Ohio): Could you tell us what the serum glucose level and the glucose excretion were? Since you have made a reasonable argument for perhaps an indirect effect through insulin, I suppose the question as to a possible role for insulin is, is it direct or is it secondary to hyperglycemia?

DR. JOHN BORDER (Buffalo, N.Y.): You have extrapolated this in your concluding remark to sick men. You have studied normal men with up and down regulation and anabolic regulation of metabolism. I would submit that it is a bit premature to extrapolate it to sick men.

DR. MICHAEL CALDWELL (Providence, R.I.): A number of years ago we showed that somatomedin will inhibit glucagon-stimulated gluconeogenesis from alanine. This effect was in an isolated, perfused rodent liver preparation in the absence of insulin. Therefore, have you considered direct effects of growth hormone or its messengers to decrease gluconeogenesis in your studies?

DR. MANSON (closing): Dr. Brennan asked whether the nitrogen retention might be a transient phenomenon. Of course the study lasted only 7 days and we cannot say that the effect would have continued for 14 or 21 days. Such studies as have been done in which growth hormone was given for longer periods include the work of Henneman and coworkers in 1960, not on normal subjects but on patients with pituitary disease. They showed similar effects to ours, lasting for 3 to 4 weeks. Such studies have not been done on normal volunteers as yet, and this data are not available at this time. Our nitrogen and mineral data suggest strongly that the nitrogen retained was in the form of skeletal muscle tissue.

Dr. Blackburn asked about serum ketones. We did measure serum ketones and were unable to show a significant difference between control and growth hormone periods. This was rather surprising in the face of marked ketonuria; however, in this study we did note that timing of determinations was critical. Blood for ketone determination was taken early in the morning before growth hormone injections, and this may explain the lack of a growth hormone-mediated rise. Samples of free fatty acids and glycerol taken at the same time also revealed no rise during growth hormone treatment, but samples taken 4 hours after an injection revealed a significant rise in both these lipid substrates (see Table 2).

Dr. Forse asked about study design. Control and growth hormone studies on any particular subject were separated by at least 2 weeks. Order was determined by "random design," that is, if in the first paired study the control period was first, in the next pair the growth hormone period would be first, and so on.

Growth hormone administration was associated with a rise in early morning metabolic rate, although this finding was not consistent at all levels of caloric intake. The slight increase in pulse rate most probably reflects this slight degree of hypermetabolism.

Dr. Fischer, when all studies were taken together, there was a small but insignificant rise in serum glucose levels. On the final day we examined the response under control and growth hormone conditions, to a 100 gm oral glucose load (data not reported here), and did reveal significant peripheral glucose resistance during growth hormone treatment.

Dr. Caldwell asked about a direct effect of somatomedin on blocking hepatic gluconeogenesis. This may well be. In five of our eight paired studies, serum levels of somatomedin C were determined, and highly significant rises were noted during growth hormone treatment.

Dr. Border asked about extrapolating these data derived from normal volunteers to sick patients, and indeed this requires caution. However, as I am sure you are all aware, it is not normally possible to observe positive nitrogen balance in normal volunteers under usual hospital ward conditions. To observe this effect during hypocaloric feedings is a unique finding. Studies that have been done in burn patients suggest that growth hormone may have effects similar to those we have demonstrated in volunteers.

The availability of growth hormone and other polypeptide growth factors, thanks to recombinant DNA technology, holds great promise for the improved nutritional care of critically ill surgical patients.

Discussion

This discussion took place at the Rhoads Symposium.

UNIDENTIFIED DISCUSSANT: In the treated animals, the wet weight of the bowel was increased. Could this have been due to edema or is it real growth?

DR. DOUG WILMORE: There was normal histology and the DNA content was also increased, so it was increased cellularity and not edema. If you think about the length of the gastrointestinal tract, it's comprised of billions of cells so very dramatic changes are possible.

DR. MARSHALL ORLOFF: Doug, any comments about other growth factors such as epidermal growth factor?

DR. DOUG WILMORE: Well, I think all of them are exceedingly important, particularly for the gastrointestinal tract. Epidermal growth factor may be a key player, although the studies are not quite as clear in that regard. But the gastrointestinal tract has receptors for insulin like growth factor I and insulin like growth factor II and epidermal growth factor. Insulin like growth factor I is available in recombinant form, although it is made when you give growth hormone so you sort of get two for one. We are using those sorts of things in models of bowel resection and in animals in which we have taken out 90% of the small bowel we can grow them up again. So, I really wonder whether this is not a better answer than bowel transplantation. The answer to bowel loss may be to use growth factors to stimulate and grow the population of cells needed.

UNIDENTIFIED DISCUSSANT: Have you studied enteroglucogan or any similar hormones because there are also receptors for those and they also have the property increasing tissue.

DR. DOUG WILMORE: We have not, although we have talked with Professor Bloom about it and should discuss it further. It may well be that glutamine, in addition to having a direct trophic effect, may stimulate enteroglucogan, which may be a very important influence.

DR. JOHN HOWARD: Do you think that growth factors influence stress ulcers?

DR. DOUG WILMORE: People have reported that. I have not studied it but others have suggested it.

DR. ED KAPLAN: As I understand it, growth hormone is being used by the weight-lifting athletes and I know it has been used in thoroughbred racing. The insidious aspect is that it can be used in ways that cannot be detected because the half-life is about three minutes. It disappears very rapidly through the intestines where it's present.

Doug, you have purposely kept the nutrition about half normal and have given growth hormone. If you gave the amount of protein that you normally would and gave growth hormone, would it enhance growth rate?

DR. DOUG WILMORE: We have done only a few studies where we have looked at that very important question. If only half of the nutritional component is given you use your own body fat. That is the major benefit of that approach. We have had patients on half the normal calories for over a month and then they do, in fact, gain weight. What they are doing is losing their body fat while gaining muscle mass, and since muscle is hydrated and fat is not the exchange works out well. These people should be cautious, although this is antecedal, but several of these people have gotten up and out of bed and have started walking around and doing things like that. We have the nuclear magnetic resonance guys poised to study muscle size and muscle adenosine triphosphate. Basil, you may remember the young man we had on growth hormone back in the 1970s who started chasing the nurses. We could break the code on the blind study because of the interest that the treated patients started to have in other things besides their injuries. So, there clearly is an associated euphoria and feeling of well being. If you think about discharging patients from the hospital earlier and wanting them to eat and repair and get well, this is a tremendous concept.

DR. BASIL PRUITT: Doug, in your earlier study with the extracted growth hormone it was your feeling that the effect depended on a patient receiving his or her estimated calorie needs. I found it interesting that in these studies you get an effect with less than estimated colony needs. Is that just a dose effect since you had a fixed dose with your earlier study?

DR. DOUG WILMORE: These clearly were not hypermetabolic patients but were patients in a resting state. They may have had infection in association with their wounds or fistulae but these were now drained. In the burned patients that I have studied I have never really reduced calorie intake. We have also studied several people who were paralyzed and on ventilators and still see the same kind of positive effect suggesting that we can make skeletal muscle even in paralyzed people, which is a dramatic effect.

DR. TED COPELAND: It almost sounds too good. What is the downside risk? I mean, it does not make a lot of sense for you to lie in bed and make skeletal muscle just throughout the skeletal muscular system. We always make muscle in response to a need and I guess one of the things I worry about is not skeletal muscle but cardiac muscle. Is the cardiac muscle getting bigger in these people? No biological system gives you something for free. So, what is the downside risk of this one?

DR. DOUG WILMORE: Well, it is hard to know Ted. I think one of my big concerns is whether it stimulates tumor growth. I mean, we are talking about real growth stimulation, so I think if we start treating patients with tumors we have to be very concerned about those kinds of effects. The other side of that is if we are ready for it we might well be able to stimulate tumor growth and put the right blocking drugs in that system. So, this may be another way to manipulate the system in the future. In general, for the short periods of time that we have studied so far, we see very little on the downside. You know it may well be that all of the short kids in the country will someday be getting growth hormone and will be growing up to be Bill Walton's size, and it may well be that in 20 years or so the Japanese will win the Olympics in basketball.

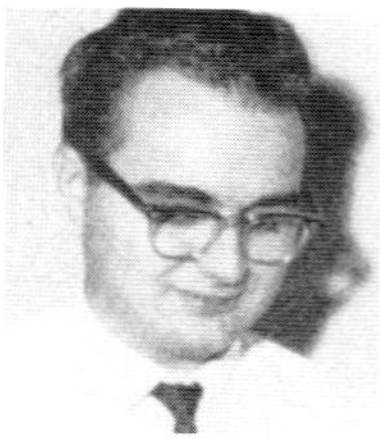

Introduction of Dr. P. William Curreri

Dr. Clyde F. Barker: Bill Curreri was a very good HUP resident who finished in 1968. He was productive in research while in the residency, working with Ben Miller. We've heard something about his continued contributions to the study of burns with Basil Pruitt and then with Tom Shires as he followed him from Dallas to Seattle to Cornell, where Bill headed the burn unit. Along the way, he became President of the University Surgeons. He is now Professor and Chairman of Surgery at the University of South Alabama College of Medicine. Today, he is going to present his article entitled "Microvascular Filtration in Burned and Non-Burned Tissue After Thermal Injury."

I was able to find a number of papers in Dr. Rhoads' bibliography which indicate that he has been interested in burns at least since 1941 when this one was published: Rhoads, J. E., Wolff, W. A., and Lee, W. E.: The Use of Adrenal Cortical Extract in the Treatment of Traumatic Shock of Burns. *Ann of Surg* 113:955–968, 1941.

Dr. Curreri's Introductory Remarks

Thank you, Clyde, and Dr. Rhoads. When I was a resident here, Dr. Ravdin had a large map of the United States in his office, and on that map were a number of pins, each one representing the location of a resident who had finished the program. It got to the point where there were different colors for pins, because there was more than one resident in some cities. I remember walking into his office one time while he was studying this map. I asked him what he found to be of such great interest. He said to me something I have never forgotten. He said a surgeon could perform several thousand operations in his lifetime, and that although these would benefit a number of people, he felt a much larger meaning was given to his life by the opportunity he had to pass on surgical principles to a large number of young people who would then not only practice surgery but also train their own residents.

I cannot help thinking how much pride Dr. Rhoads must have in the attendance today of all the professors and all of the chairmen he trained who are not only passing on the surgical principles he taught but also passing on the principles of education and research that he considers so important. This applies not only to the present generation but to several generations of surgeons to come, all of whom in a sense will have enjoyed the benefit of his wise council.

Two things I remember about Dr. Rhoads particularly stand out in my mind. One pertains to the operating room, which was the place I think his wry humor was most apparent. I clearly remember one night when he had a patient sent to him from St. Elsewhere General Hospital at about 2:00 AM. The patient had been operated on multiple times at the other hospital for regional enteritis and presented now with a wound that was breaking down, a number of GI fistulae, and septic shock. This was in the days before CAT scans, but I was fairly certain the patient had not only fistulae but intra-abdominal abscesses and was going to die if we didn't operate on him. I called Dr. Rhoads and he agreed. He came into the Hospital about 3:00 AM, and at just about that time, I got called away to see another sick patient. Dr. Rhoads went with the patient up to the operating room, and by the time I got there, he was already scrubbed and gowned. I scrubbed rapidly, and as I came into the operating room, Dr. Rhoads had already draped the patient. I was rushing around trying to catch up with him, and he said to me, "Do you mind if I start?" I said "Of course, I don't mind." By the time I got my gloves on and turned around, he had already opened the wound with his hands and scooped out a lot of necrotic debris. I asked, "Dr. Rhoads what have you found?" He looked at me and said, "Bill, I think I've just done a right colectomy." It was the only 30-second right colectomy I've ever seen in my life. I've heard more of his former residents say this about Dr. Rhoads than any other thing. The thing for which they most remember him is his uncanny ability to get in the damnedest complicated messes (usually created by other surgeons) and be able to figure an original way out. Many, many times when I've been operating and found something totally unexpected or something I've not ever seen in my previous experience, I have asked myself how Dr. Rhoads would handle this and I usually came up with a solution that was satisfactory. I think that many of the residents would say that.

Another thing I remember about Dr. Rhoads is that he was extraordinarily stimulating in terms of impressing all of us with the need to do basic research, and I believe this was one of the most important things in ensuring our future careers. The residents from this program have certainly more than held their own in terms of the excellence of their research programs and in maintaining NIH support. I think that's largely because of the encouragement that Dr. Rhoads gave us to work with basic scientists. I thought I would present today some work that has come out of our laboratory in the last two to three months that illustrates how young surgeons can still do basic research. Because of Dr. Rhoads' inspiration, a second generation of residents are now being stimulated to do this.

Microvascular Filtration in Burned and Nonburned Tissue After Thermal Injury

ROGER M. PITT, M.D., JAMES C. PARKER, PH.D., AUBREY E. TAYLOR, PH.D., AND P. WILLIAM CURRERI, M.D.

THERMAL INJURY increases microvascular permeability, resulting in rapid edema formation in burned skin. Increased permeability also has been reported to develop in nonburned skin when injury exceeds 40% of the body surface area.[1-3] Burn wound edema is thought to be the result of direct heat damage or vasoactive mediators released from damaged tissue whereas edema in nonburned tissue is thought to be the result of mediators or the hypoproteinemia which occurs with fluid resuscitation after large burns.[1]

Previous experimental models of thermal injury have evaluated edema formation by measurement of weight or volume changes,[4] extravasation of dyes or labeled proteins,[3,5] or measurement of lymph flow and lymph to plasma protein concentration ratios.[6] Although these experimental approaches to the study of edema formation after thermal injury have yielded important information, the pathophysiology of postburn edema formation and the role of mediators in this process remains unclear.

Since thermal injury is known to disrupt the integrity of the microvascular membrane,[7] the rate of transvascular fluid flux is a major factor influencing the rate of edema formation. The rate of transvascular fluid flux (Jv) is determined by the balance of Starling forces which act at the capillary membrane as seen in the Starling equation:

$$Jv = Kf[(P_c - P_I) - \sigma(\pi_c - \pi_I)]$$

These forces are capillary hydrostatic pressure (P_c), capillary interstitial pressure (P_I), capillary oncotic pressure (π_c), and interstitial oncotic pressure (π_I). The rate of fluid flux also is determined by the permeability characteristics of the membrane which are described by the reflection coefficient (σ) and the filtration coefficient (Kf). The reflection coefficient is a surface area independent coefficient which describes the permeability of the membrane to macromolecules whereas the filtration coefficient is a surface area dependent coefficient which describes the water conductance of the membrane. Since all of these factors are potentially altered after thermal injury and will affect the rate of microvascular filtration, we have developed a model of thermal injury which allows us to perform a Starling force analysis of microvascular filtration in burned and nonburned tissue after thermal injury.

Methods

Burns were performed in mechanically ventilated mongrel dogs under sodium pentobarbital anesthesia (30 mg/kg, intravenously [IV]). In Group I (N = 4), 3 l of 100°C water were poured over the shaved flank, back, and side resulting in an approximately 40% body surface area burn. Animals were resuscitated with lactated Ringer's solution at a rate of 2 ml/kg/% burn over the first 6 hours postburn. Animals in Group II (N = 5) received a 100°C scald burn to the left paw. In both groups, cannulas were placed in the jugular vein, carotid artery, femoral artery, and a branch of the lateral saphenous vein just above the left ankle. The arterial and saphenous vein catheters were connected to calibrated pressure transducers (Statham Model P 23) and pressures were recorded (Grass Model 7D polygraph). A cannula was placed in a prenodal lymphatic just above the ankle and lymph flow (Q_L) was measured using calibrated micropipets. Lymph and venous blood were collected in

From the Departments of Surgery and Physiology, College of Medicine, University of South Alabama, Mobile, Alabama.

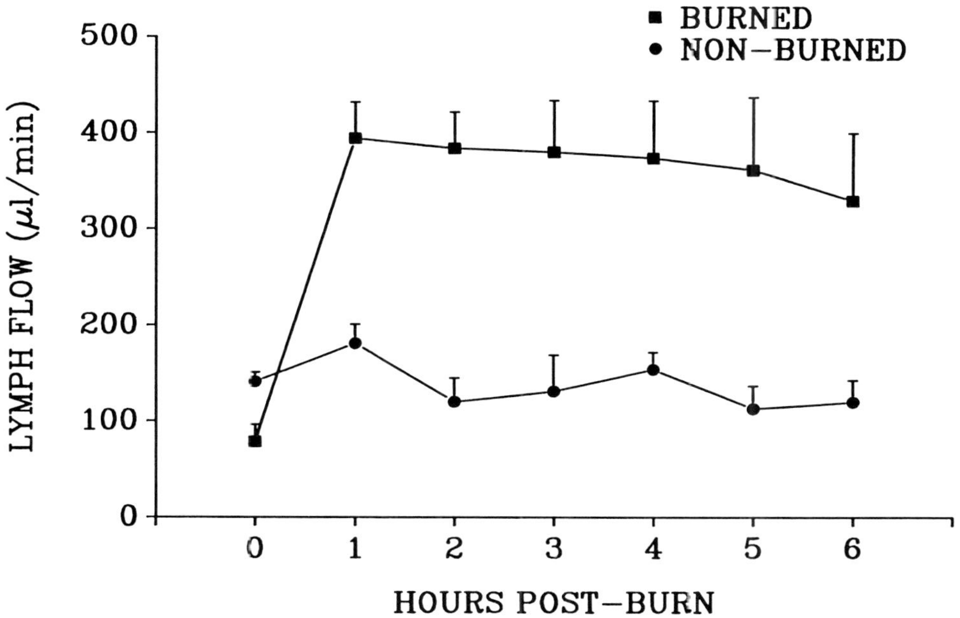

FIG. 1. Lymph flow in burned and nonburned tissue after thermal injury.

heparinized tubes and lymph (C_L) and plasma (C_p) total protein concentrations were measured using a calibrated protein refractometer (American Optical).

The paw was mechanically flexed 60 times a minute to maintain constant lymph flow and lymph was collected until Q_L and C_L reached steady state levels. Venous pressure was then elevated by tightening a tourniquet placed around the thigh underneath the femoral artery and vein. The Q_L and C_L were measured every 30 minutes until the minimal C_L/C_P was obtained. The burn was then performed and Q_L and C_L were measured at 30 minutes and 1 hour postburn and then hourly until 6 hours postburn.

Capillary pressure (P_C) was measured by the venous occlusion technique.[8] The ratio of pre-to-post capillary resistance (R_A/R_V) was calculated as follows:

$$R_A/R_V = P_A - P_C/P_C - P_V$$

where P_A is femoral artery pressure, P_C is capillary pressure, and P_V is saphenous vein pressure.

Data in the text and figures are presented as means ± SE. Comparisons between preburn and postburn data were performed by ANOVA and the Neuman-Keuls test. *P* values of less than 0.05 were accepted as statistically significant.

Starling Force Analysis

The reflection coefficient was calculated from the minimal C_L/C_P ratios[9] using the formula, $\sigma = 1 - C_L/C_P$. The filtration coefficient was calculated as, $Kf = Q_L/P_C - \sigma(\pi_P - \pi_L)$ where Q_L is lymph flow, P_L is capillary pressure, σ is the reflection coefficient and π_P and π_L are the plasma and lymph protein oncotic pressures. This calculation assumes that lymph flow is equal to the rate of microvascular filtration, lymph oncotic pressure is equal to interstitial oncotic pressure and plasma oncotic pressure is equal to capillary oncotic pressure. The calculation ignores the effect of interstitial hydrostatic pressure. Both π_L and π_P were calculated from the total protein concentrations in lymph and plasma using the Navar equation.[10]

Results

Figure 1 shows the effect of thermal injury on lymph flow in burned and nonburned skin. Lymph flow in burned skin increased from 78.3 ± 18.0 μl/minute to 394.1 ± 38.4 μl/minute

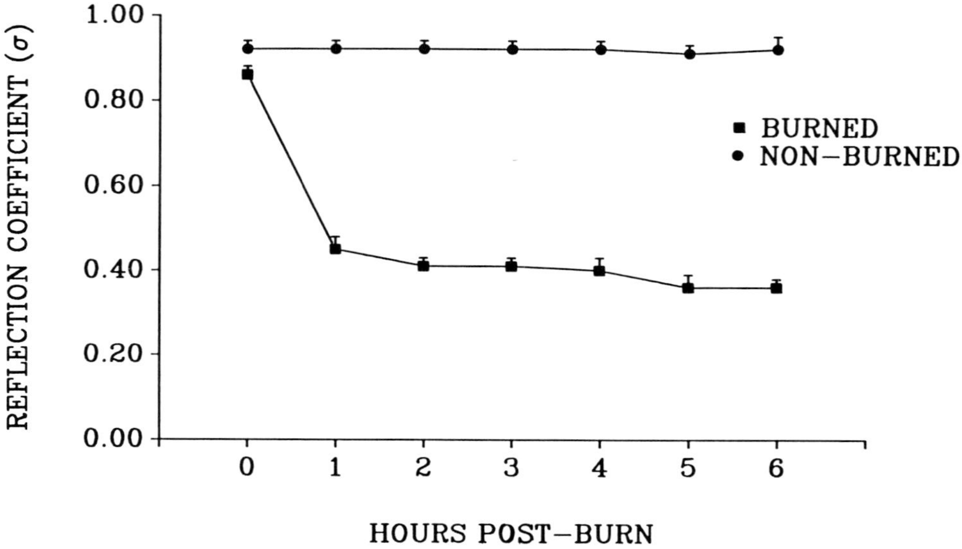

FIG. 2. Reflection coefficient in burned and nonburned tissue after thermal injury.

($P < 0.05$) at 1 hour postburn and remained significantly greater than control for the 6-hour study period. In contrast, lymph flow in nonburned skin was unchanged after thermal injury. The reflection coefficient in burned skin decreased from 0.86 ± 0.01 to 0.45 ± 0.03 ($P < 0.05$) at 1 hour postburn and was 0.36 ± 0.02 ($P < 0.05$) at 6 hours (Fig. 2). The reflection coefficient was unchanged in nonburned skin. The finding of increased lymph flow and a decreased reflection coefficient in burned skin indicates a marked increase in permeability compared to nonburned skin where there was no evidence of increased permeability.

Figure 3 shows that the plasma to interstitium oncotic pressure gradient decreased in both burned and nonburned skin. The gradient in burned tissue decreased because of the leakage

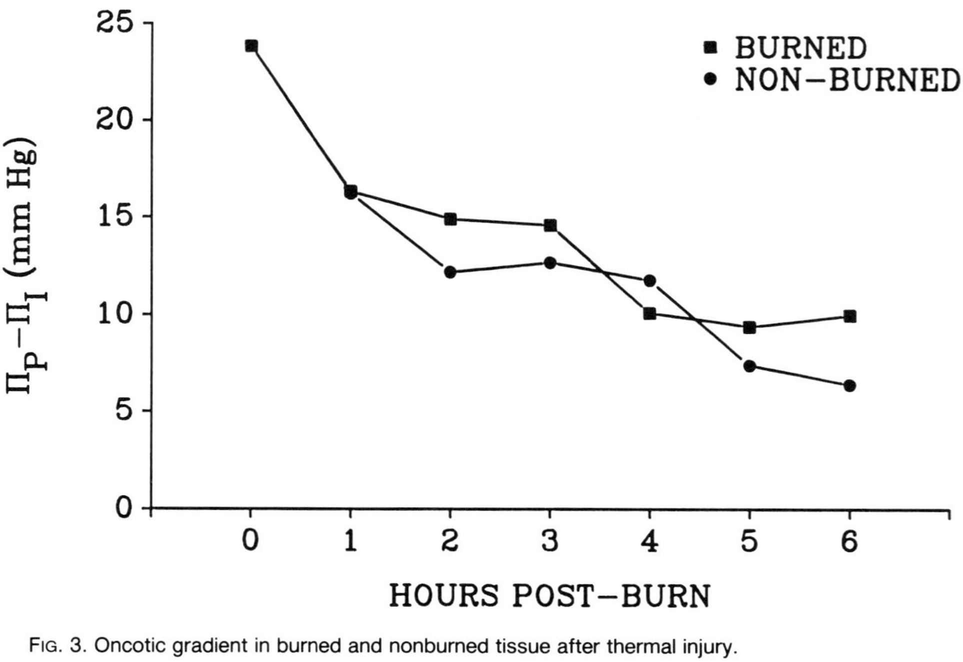

FIG. 3. Oncotic gradient in burned and nonburned tissue after thermal injury.

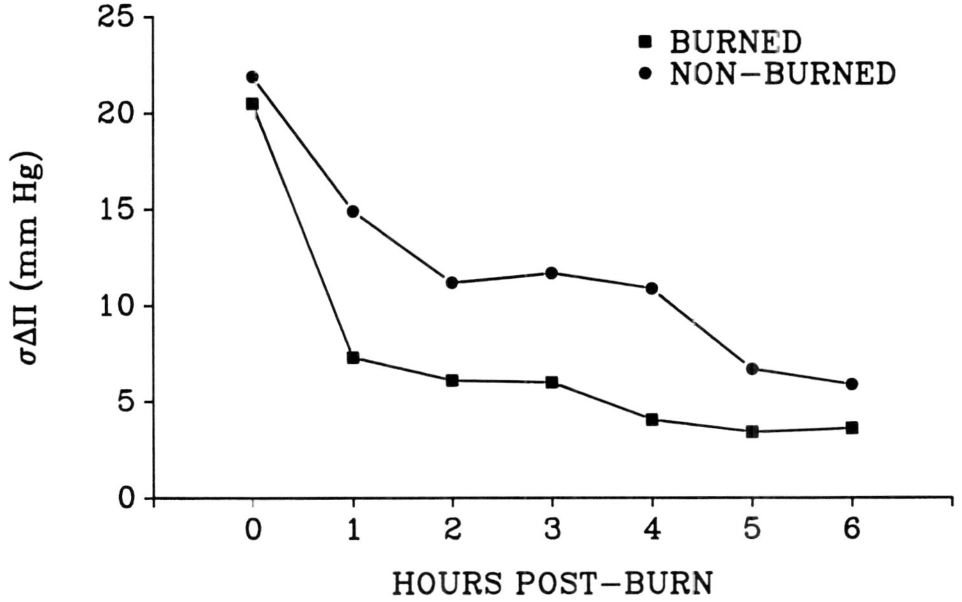

FIG. 4. Effective oncotic gradient ($\sigma\Delta\pi$) in burned and nonburned tissue after thermal injury.

of plasma proteins through the damaged microvasculature and into the interstitium whereas the gradient in nonburned tissue decreased because of the development of hypoproteinemia which occurred with resuscitation. In contrast, the effective oncotic pressure gradient ($\sigma\Delta\pi$) decreased more in burned skin (Fig. 4). Because the reflection coefficient decreased in burned tissue, the effective oncotic gradient was 3.7 ± 0.7 mmHg at 6 hours postburn in burned skin whereas it was 12.0 ± 4.3 mmHg ($P < 0.05$) in nonburned skin. The fall in the oncotic pressure gradient (control minus 6-hour gradient) was 16.9 mmHg in burned skin and 10.0 mmHg in nonburned skin.

Capillary pressure increased from 47.8 ± 8.3 mmHg to a maximum of 80.5 ± 13.2 mmHg ($P < 0.05$) in burned skin and remained significantly elevated at three hours postburn (Fig. 5). Capillary pressure was unchanged in nonburned skin. Increased capillary pressure was accompanied by a fall in the ratio of pre-to-post capillary resistance in burned tissue (Fig. 6). We previously have observed that the fall in pre-to-post capillary resistance is caused entirely by a decline in precapillary resistance since postcapillary resistance is unchanged.[11] The ratio of pre-to-post capillary resistance was unchanged in nonburned skin.

Although the fall in the effective oncotic pressure gradient of 10.0 mmHg in nonburned skin favors increased microvascular filtration and thus lymph flow, we observed no change in lymph flow. The filtration coefficient (calculated from the fourth equation) decreased from 0.048 ± 0.001 ml/minute/mmHg/100 g to 0.0036 ± 0.001 ml/minute/mmHg/100 g ($P < 0.05$) at 6 hours postburn in nonburned skin (Fig. 7). Since the filtration coefficient is a surface area dependent variable, this finding implies a decrease in microvascular surface area available for fluid flux in nonburned soft tissue. In contrast, Kf increased from 0.0029 ± 0.001 ml/minute/mmHg/100 g to a maximum of 0.0951 ± 0.0025 ml/minute/mmHg/100 g ($P < 0.05$) in burned tissue.

Discussion

Edema in Burned Tissue

The results of these experiments demonstrate that by applying a Starling force analysis to microvascular filtration in burned tissue, four factors are present which favor increased microvascular filtration: (1) increased permeability to macromolecules, (2) increased water conductance of the microvascular membrane, (3) decreased effective plasma to interstitium oncotic pressure gradient, and (4) increased capillary pressure. Whereas increased capillary

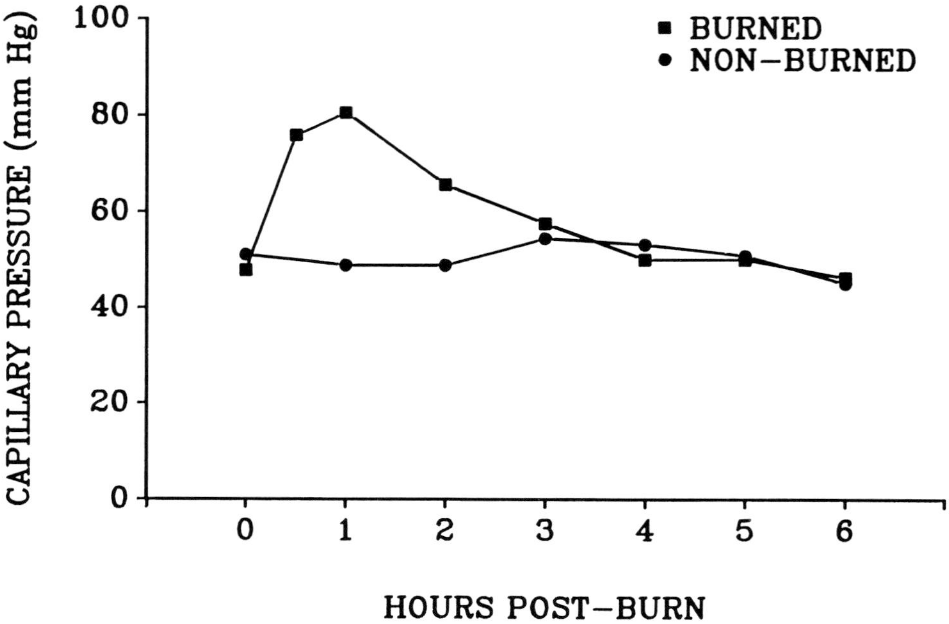

FIG. 5. Capillary pressure in burned and nonburned tissue after thermal injury.

pressure is transient, it accounts for 59% of the increase in filtration at 30 minutes postburn and 67% at 1 hour (Fig. 8). Over the first 3 hours postburn, increased capillary pressure accounts for greater than 50% of the total increase in filtration. The effect of increased capillary pressure in the first 3 hours postburn is amplified by the increase in the filtration coefficient since the effect on filtration of any given capillary pressure will be greater the larger the Kf. Thus, whereas one can analytically separate pressure from permeability effects, they act together to increase microvascular filtration in burned tissue.

The observation that increased capillary pressures have a significant role in causing

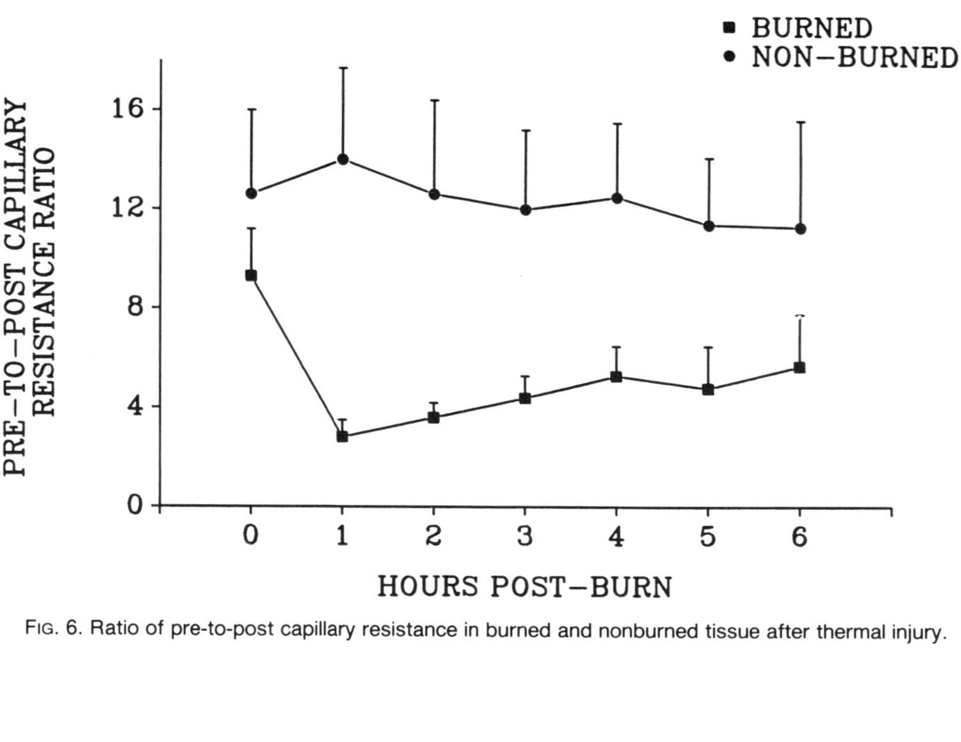

FIG. 6. Ratio of pre-to-post capillary resistance in burned and nonburned tissue after thermal injury.

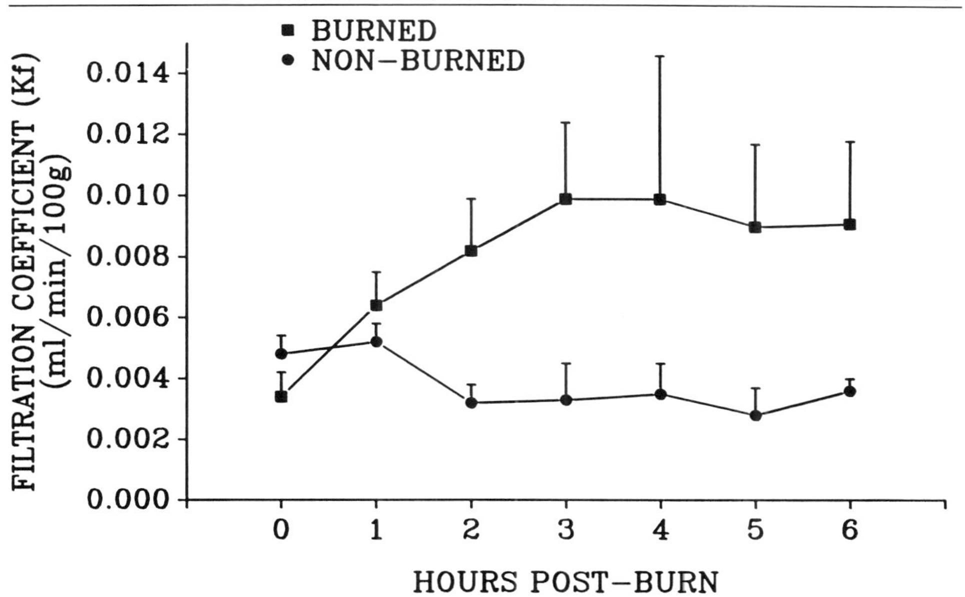

FIG. 7. Filtration coefficient in burned and nonburned tissue after thermal injury.

increased microvascular filtration has important implications for the study of experimental burns. Thermal injury may be considered as a type of severe inflammatory response. Studies have demonstrated the presence of histamine,[12] prostaglandins,[13] kinins,[14] and substance P[15] in burn wound fluid or lymph draining burned tissue. Other studies have implicated oxygen-free radicals as a cause of microvascular injury in burned tissue.[16] Despite the demonstration of vasoactive substances in the burn wound, attempts to attenuate burn wound edema by blocking their effects usually have been met with limited success.[1] How-

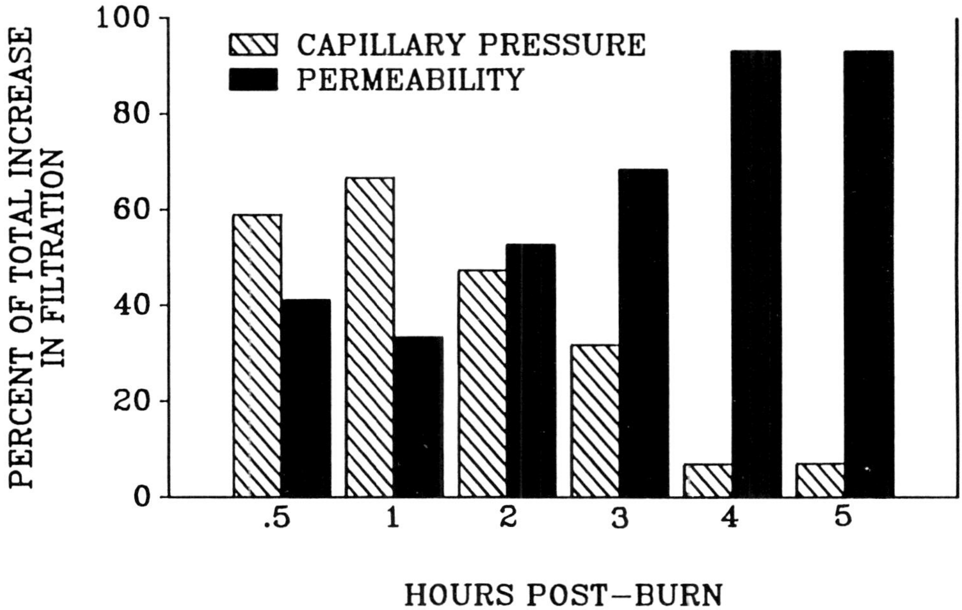

FIG. 8. Relative contributions of increased capillary pressure and permeability to increased filtration in burned tissue. The contribution of increased capillary pressure was calculated as $Kf(P_c \text{ observed} - P_c \text{ control})$.[11]

ever, a few studies have demonstrated that pharmacologic interventions can significantly reduce the amount of edema formation in the early postburn period. Szabo *et al.* demonstrated that terbutaline prevents edema formation in rabbits in the first 2 hours after thermal injury.[17] However, terbutaline failed to prevent edema at 4 hours. Horakova and Beavan have shown that depletion of histamine stores reduces edema by 50% at 1 hour postburn in rat paws.[12] Saria has shown that a substance P antagonist decreases Evans blue dye extravasation in burned rat paws at 5 minutes postburn; however, edema at 2 hours was no different from untreated controls.[18] Bjoerk and Arturson demonstrated that pretreatment with catalase or superoxide dismutase results in a small but statistically significant decrease in paw volume at 3 hours postburn.[16] However, the greatest effect was seen with cimetidine pretreatment which caused systemic hypotension. In none of these studies were capillary pressures measured. It is therefore impossible to determine whether these interventions decreased edema formation because of effects on capillary pressure or permeability.

Although prevention of pre-capillary vasodilitation may have a significant effect on edema formation in the early postburn period, and our data suggests that it would, it is not clear that such an effect would significantly decrease long-term edema formation. It also is possible that prevention of precapillary vasodilation could adversely affect wound healing since capsaicin pretreatment, which depletes substance P stores, adversely affects experimental skin flap survival.[19]

Although it has not been demonstrated, it is likely that only by preventing the increase in microvascular permeability as well as the increase in capillary pressure, will the prolonged phase of burn wound edema and plasma volume loss be significantly altered.

Edema in Nonburned Tissue

Although there is clearly edema formation in burned tissue after thermal injury, the development of edema in nonburned soft tissue is less clearly established. Leape demonstrated no increase in the water or albumin content of nonburned skin 4 hours after a 50% burn in rhesus monkeys.[5] However, Harms *et al.* found a transient increase in lymph flow in nonburned skin after a 30% burn in sheep.[6] This was accompanied by no change in the lymph to plasma protein concentration ratio. These findings were interpreted as demonstrating a transient increase in permeability in nonburned soft tissue. In contrast to Leape, Carvajal *et al.* observed a transient increase in water content and extravasation of labelled albumin in the nonburned skin of rats.[3]

We observed no increase in permeability in nonburned soft tissue after thermal injury. Of the measured or calculated Starling forces, only the decrease in the effective plasma to interstitium oncotic pressure gradient favored increased microvascular filtration. Despite the fall in the effective oncotic gradient, we observed no increase in lymph flow indicating that there was no increase in microvascular filtration. Thermal injury has been demonstrated to result in vasoconstriction in nonburned tissue.[20] This would explain the observed increase in postburn peripheral vascular resistance which is seen after large burns.[21,22] Vasoconstriction in nonburned soft tissue would decrease the surface area available for microvascular fluid exchange and tend to decrease the filtration coefficient, thus opposing the tendency for increased filtration caused by the fall in the oncotic gradient. That hypoproteinemia plays a significant role in increased microvascular filtration in nonburned tissue has been demonstrated by Demling *et al.*[23] They were able to eliminate the increase in nonburned lymph flow by restoring plasma protein concentrations to preburn levels. Our findings suggest that microvascular filtration in nonburned tissue depends primarily upon the extent of hypoproteinemia and the microvascular surface area in nonburned tissue. Whereas nonburned tissue edema may be minimal compared to burn wound edema, the cummulative effect may be significant in terms of plasma volume loss.

Conclusion

In summary, we observed no change in the reflection coefficient in nonburned skin. While there was a 10 mmHg fall in the effective oncotic gradient, we observed no change in lymph flow indicating that there was no net change in microvascular filtration. The calculated filtration coefficient decreased suggesting that the fall in the oncotic gradient was offset by a decrease in the microvascular surface area available for fluid exchange. Burned tissue was characterized by a marked decrease in the reflection coefficient and an increase in the filtration coefficient, indicating a marked increase in microvascular permeability. Filtration was further favored by a 16.9-mmHg fall in the effective oncotic gradient. Finally, capillary pressures were significantly increased for the first 3 hours postburn and accounted for greater than 50% of the total increase in filtration. The value of the experimental model presented here is that it allows us to separate the various factors affecting microvascular filtration. Specifically, we can separate pressure from permeability effects and thus more completely evaluate the role of mediators in postburn edema formation.

REFERENCES

1. Demling RH, Burns. In: Staub NC, Taylor AE, eds. Edema. New York: Raven Press, 1984;579.
2. Arturson G. Microvascular permeability to macromolecules in thermal injury. Acta Physiol Scand 1979;463:111.
3. Carvajal HF, Linares HA, Brouhard BH. Relationship of burn size to vascular permeability changes in rats. Surg Gynecol Obstet 1979;149:193.
4. Arturson G, Jakobsson OP. Oedema measurements in a standard burn model. Burns 1985;12:1.
5. Leape LL. Initial changes in burns: Tissue changes in burned and unburned skin of Rhesus monkeys. J Trauma 1970;15:969.
6. Harms BA, Bodai BI, Kramer GC, Demling RH. Microvascular fluid and protein flux in pulmonary and systemic circulations after thermal injury. Microvasc Res 1982;23:776.
7. Cotran RS. The delayed and prolonged vascular leakage in inflammation: II. An electron microscope study of the vascular response after thermal injury. Am J Pathol 1965;46 589.
8. Konthuis RJ, Granger DN, Taylor AE. A new method for estimating capillary pressure. Am J Physiol 1985;246:H880.
9. Granger DN, Taylor AE. Exchange of macromolecules across the microcirculation. In: Renkin EM, Michel CC, eds. Handbook of Physiology, sect. 2: The Cardiovasculary System, Vol. 4, part 1. Bethesda, MD: American Physiology Society, 1984;467.
10. Navar PD, Navar LG. Relationship between colloid osnotic pressure and plasma protein concentration in the dog. Am J Physiol 1977;233:H295.
11. Pitt RM, Parker JC, Jurkovich GJ, Taylor AE, Curreri PW. Analysis of altered capillary pressure and permeability after thermal injury. J Surg Res (in press).
12. Horakova Z, Beavan MA. Time course of histamine release and edema formation in the rat paw after thermal injury. Eur J Pharmacol 1974;27:305.
13. Harms BA, Bodai BI, Smith N, Gunther R, Flynn J, Demling RH. Prostaglandin release and altered microvascular integrity after burn injury. J Surg Res 1981;31:274.
14. Arturson G. Prostaglandins in human burn wound secretion. Burns 1977;3:112.
15. Jonsson DE, Brodin E, Dalsgaard CJ, Haegenstrand A. Release of substance-P-like immunoreactivity in dog paw lymph after scalding injury. Acta Physiol Scand 1986;126:21.
16. Bjoerk J, Arturson G. Effect of cimetidine and hydrocortisone, superoxide dismutase and catalase on the development of oedema after thermal injury. Burns 1983;9:249.
17. Szabo G, Magyar Z, Posch E. Effect of terbulatine on peripheral lymph flow, protein concentration and transport, and edema formation after thermal injury in rabbits. Lymphology 1985;18:76.
18. Saria A. Substance P in sensory nerve fibres contributes to the development of oedema in the rat hind paw after thermal injury. Br J Pharmacol 1984;82:217.
19. Kjartansson J, Dalsgaard CJ, Jonsson CE. Decreased survival of experimental critical flaps in rats after sensory denervation with capsaicin. Plast Reconstr Surg 1987;79:218.
20. Jelenko C, Jennings WD, O'Kelly WR, Byrd HC. Threshold burning effects on distant microcirculation. Arch Surg 1973;106:317.
21. Asch MJ, Feldman RJ, Walker HL *et al.* Systemic and pulmonary hemodynamic changes accompanying thermal injury. Ann Surg 1973;175:218.
22. Hilton JG, McPherson MB, Manullo DS. The relationship between post-burn increases in peripheral resistance and vasopression. Burns 1986;12:410.
23. Demling RH, Kramer G, Harms B. Role of thermal injury-induced hypoproteinemia on fluid flux and protein permeability in burned and non-burned tissue. Surgery 1984;90:136.

DISCUSSION

DR. HARVEY SUGERMAN: Just one question, Bill. Weren't you surprised that you didn't see any increase in permeability in non-burned tissues if increased permeability is due to release of mediators that are floating around? Do you think these mediators are cleared?

DR. WILLIAM CURRERI: No, I am not surprised at all. The unburned area is so large that although there may be very small changes, these have little significance. You must also remember that the effect of mediators on different types of capillary membranes may be influenced by injury itself. First of all, some of the mediators are present in high concentration in the wound. Secondly, there is no question that there is some damage to capillaries by any injury, and this may set them up to be highly effected by mediators while normal capillaries may not be. Clearly, we could not show any capillary permeability change. There is edema formation, but edema formation that would occur with small amounts of non-injured tissue appears to be clearly related to filtration rather than to permeability changes and filtration changes are going to be somewhat dependent on the degree to which we resuscitate the animal and the drug the animal is receiving. If you under-resuscitate, you will have increased peripheral resistance but decreased surface area and decreased filtration. If you over-resuscitate or give them vasodilators or beta blockers, you are likely to see different effects simply because you change surface area somehow.

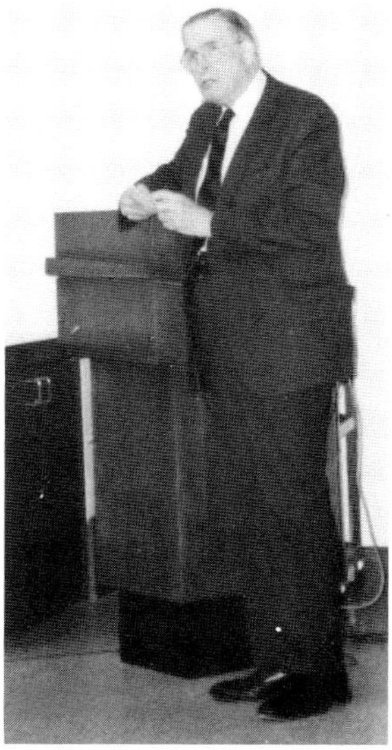

Closing Remarks of Dr. Jonathan E. Rhoads

Ladies and gentlemen, I really appreciate this, and I am very grateful to Clyde and Dode Barker who conceived it and made it a reality with the special help of Jack Mackie, John Daly, and Gordon Buzby, as well as the tireless efforts of Frances Ramirez. I had no idea we'd get such a wonderful turnout of former residents and old friends I perceive three elements in what has been said today. First, there was a lot of really good science. Secondly, there have been some very flowery compliments which remind me of Dr. Libby Rose's comment about flowers, "You should send them while people can still smell them." The third element was some rather scurrilous stories. I'll deal with the third element first. My dissecting partner in medical school was a man, who was for a good while on Bill Longmire's faculty, David Sprong. One of his favorite shibboleths was this, although I am sure it wasn't original, "I deny the allegations and I defy the alligators."

I have no thought of attempting any sort of summarization of today's scientific program. These papers all stand on their own. However, I would like to acknowledge the fact that all science does not originate here. I'm afraid that some of the speakers, by implying that it does, may have created a rather unfortunate impression on some of my friends from other institutions. I would particularly like to express appreciation to Basil Pruitt for having accepted a number of our residents into his program and giving them a postgraduate course in physiology and pathophysiology that they probably could not have gotten anywhere else.

I think we are all conscious of the fact that in an economic sense we as surgeons collect for operations that depend for their validity and effectiveness on the contributions of others. There is no way we can repay these investigators on whose shoulders we so clearly stand. I think of Ravdin, Wangensteen, and Blalock, and, in an earlier group, perhaps Coller and Graham and many others all of you can think of. Perhaps the best we can do is to accept the obligation of contributing, in our turn, new elements in the discipline of Surgery. We've certainly heard today from people who have done that, and there are many others in the group who have done it too. One of the recent Nobel Prize winners in economics (who like most economists quarrelled with his colleagues a great deal) said when he received the Nobel Prize that success was not so much in the plaudits of one's contemporaries as in the degree to which one's ideas and concepts became imbedded in one's discipline. I think a great deal of what we heard today is or will be imbedded in the discipline of Surgery.

I will spare you the rest of the cards I prepared. All I really want to say now is that it has been a tremendous satisfaction to me to hear this program, and I hope that the forthcoming volume (which I believe the speakers are committed to preparing) will come to fruition, since I think many of you will want to study portions of it, and I look forward to studying all of it. Thank you very, very much.

List of May 8th Birthday Reception Attendees

Ms. Diane Adler
Dr. and Mrs. Francis H. Adler
Mr. and Mrs. Gustave G. Amsterdam
Dr. and Mrs. Arthur Asbury
Dr. and Mrs. Robert Austrian
Mr. and Mrs. Samuel Ballam, Jr
Mr. Lester Balsham and Ms. Marjorie Balsham
Dr. and Mrs. William J. Bank
Mr. and Mrs. Richard P. Bansen
Dr. Donna Barbot and Dr. William McGowan
Dr. and Mrs. Clyde F. Barker
Dr. and Mrs. Harold Barker
The Reverend and Mrs. Sidney E. Barnes
Dr. and Mrs. Stanley Baum
Dr. Joseph Bavaria
Dr. William Beck
Dr. and Mrs. Herman Beerman
Dr. Whitfield J. Bell
Mr. and Mrs. Donald C. Bergus
Miss Elizabeth C. Berrang
Dr. Richard Best
Mr. Ray Bickert
Mr. and Mrs. Raymond Bissey
Dr. Nadia Blanchet
Dr. and Mrs. Lewis W. Bluemle
Dr. and Mrs. Michael Born
Dr. Herbert Bowles
Mrs. Francis Boyer
Dr. Kenneth Brayman
Dr. and Mrs. Charles Bridges
Dr. and Mrs. Carl T. Brighton
Dr. and Mrs. John R. Brobeck
Mr. E. W. Brown, Jr
Mr. and Mrs. Francis G. Brown
Mr. and Mrs. George Brown
Mr. Richard Brown
Dr. and Mrs. John W. Bryfogle
Mr. and Mrs. Howard Butcher, III
Dr. and Mrs. Michael Caldwell
Mr. and Mrs. Samuel D. Caldwell
Dr. and Mrs. Thomas H. Cannard
Miss Marian Carbone
Mr. and Mrs. H. Robert Cathcart and Theresa
Dr. and Mrs. C. Gene Cayten
Mr. Henry M. Chance, II
Dr. Anna Marie Chirico
Dr. Winston Chu
Dr. and Mrs. Robert Clancy
Mr. and Mrs. George R. Clark
Mr. and Mrs. Norris Claytor
Dr. and Mrs. Maurice C. Clifford
Mrs. Thomas Cooch
Dr. and Mrs. Lewis L. Coriell
Dr. and Mrs. David Cornfield
Dr. and Mrs. Malcolm Cox
Mr. and Mrs. Harold Cramer
Dr. Paul Creary
Dr. Robert Crichlow
Mr. and Mrs. Victor Crown
Dr. William Curreri
Dr. and Mrs. Don Dafoe
Dr. and Mrs. Gordon Danielson
Dr. and Mrs. Robert Darrow
Dr. and Mrs. Richard A. Davis
Mr. and Mrs. Roger Decker
Dr. and Mrs. James M. Delaplane
Dr. and Mrs. Robert DeLong
Dr. and Mrs. Clarence Dennis
Dr. and Mrs. Curtis Dohan
Mrs. Sally Donohue
Mr. and Mrs. C. Morris Dorrance, Jr
Dr. and Mrs. Stanley Dudrick
Mr. and Mrs. John W. Eckman
Dr. Stanley Edeiken
Dr. and Mrs. Richard N. Edie
Mr. and Mrs. David Engler
Dr. Clair and Samuel Fagin
Mr. Charles Farrell
Mrs. Harry Fields
Dr. Steven Fishman and Guest
Mr. and Mrs. Otto Folin
Dr. and Mrs. Robert E. Forster
Dr. and Mrs. Thomas G. Frazier
Dr. and Mrs. Sidney Friedman
Dr. and Mrs. Roland M. Frye
Dr. and Mrs. John Gatti
Mr. and Mrs. Kenneth W. Gemmill
Dr. and Mrs. Steve Glorsky
Dr. and Mrs. David R. Goddard
Dr. and Mrs. Robert L. Goodman
Dr. and Mrs. Louis Green
Mr. and Mrs. William Gross, IV
Dr. and Mrs. Frazier Gurd
Dr. and Mrs. Joseph Hafkenschiel
Dr. and Mrs. C. William Hanson, Jr

Dr. James Hardy
Mr. and Mrs. John Harkins
Mr. and Mrs. Britton Harris
Dr. and Mrs. Jonathan K. Hetzel
Mr. and Mrs. Theodore Hetzel
Dr. and Mrs. Charles L. Hobbs
Miss Elizabeth H. Hoffer
Mrs. Jo Arena Holt
Mr. and Mrs. Harold Horton
Mrs. Abram Hottel
Dr. Charles Huggins
Mrs. William Y. Inouye
Dr. Danny O. Jacobs
Dean William and Mrs. Jeffers, Jr
The Reverend and Mrs. Stanley R. Johnson
Dr. Edwin Kaplan
Dr. and Mrs. Norman S. Kato
Mr. and Mrs. Thomas C. Kaesmeyer
Dr. and Mrs. Calvin F. Kay
Dr. Jeff and Dr. Roseanne Kappa
Professor and Mrs. Adam Kendon
Mr. Benjamin S. Kendon
Dr. Lawrence Kerr
Dr. and Mrs. Alfred G. Knudson, Jr
Dr. and Mrs. Jacob Kolff
Dr. and Mrs. Irving B. Kravis
Dr. and Mrs. Scott Kripke
Dr. and Mrs. Joseph F. Kusiak
Dr. and Mrs. G. Clayton Kyle
Dr. and Mrs. Christian J. Lambersten
Dr. Gerald S. Lazarus
Dr. and Mrs. Paul R. Leberman
Miss Jean Lee
Dr. Kant Lin
Mr. and Mrs. John D. Lohmeyer
Dr. William Longmire
Dr. John Looby
Dr. Julius Mackie
Dr. Ellen Mahony and Guest
Dr. and Mrs. Terrance R. Malloy
Dr. and Mrs. Philip A. Marden
Dr. and Mrs. E. Wayne Marshall, Jr
Dr. Donald B. Martin
Mr. and Mrs. James McCabe
Ms. Marty McCartney
Dr. Peter and Dr. Elaine McCombs
Mrs. Noreen McHugh
Mrs. Lorraine Meehan
Mr. and Mrs. John Meyers
Dr. and Mrs. John J. Mikuta
Dr. Elizabeth E. Miller
Mr. and Mrs. John A. Miller
Dr. and Mrs. Wallace T. Miller
Ms. Maureen Milligan
Dr. Donald Moyer and Guest
Dr. and Mrs. Henry Moss
Mr. and Mrs. Stanton Moyer
Ms. Donna Muldoon
Dr. and Mrs. Morton G. Murdock
Dr. and Mrs. Frederick Murtagh, Jr
Mr. and Mrs. Christopher Nicholson
Dr. and Mrs. Jesse T. Nicholson
Dr. and Mrs. Robert F. Norris
Dr. and Mrs. Moreye Nusbaum
Dr. Helen and George O'Bannon
Mr. and Mrs. Peter Obbard
Mrs. Ginny Parkinson
Dr. David L. Paskin
Mr. and Mrs. Edward T. Pennock
Mr. and Mrs. Art Piper
Dr. and Mrs. Leldon P. Pitt
Dr. and Mrs. Robert S. Pressman
Mr. and Mrs. James B. Pritchard
Dr. Edward C. Raffensperger
Ms. Fran Ramirez
Dr. and Mrs. Robert R. Rascoe, Jr
Mr. and Mrs. R. Stewart Rauch, Jr
Mrs. Carolyn Ravdin
Mrs. Robert G. Ravdin and Family
Mr. and Mrs. William Ravdin
Miss Caroline P. Rhoads
Mr. Charles J. Rhoads
Drs. David and Elizabeth Rhoads
Dr. Donald Rhoads
Mr. Edward O. F. Rhoads
Dr. and Mrs. Jonathan E. Rhoads, Jr and Family
Dr. and Mrs. John M. Rhoads
Mrs. John Rhoads
Mr. and Mrs. Philip G. Rhoads
Mr. and Mrs. Philip Rhoads and Family
Mr. P. Garrett Rhoads, Jr
Mr. and Mrs. Richard H. Rhoads
Mr. and Mrs. William Rhoads
Mrs. Edgar P. Richardson
Mr. and Mrs. Wallace Ritchie
Dr. Elizabeth Rose
Dr. James Roseman
Dr. and Mrs. Robert Rout
Dr. and Mrs. George E. Ruff
Dr. and Mrs. Edward Savage
Dr. and Mrs. John J. Sayen
Dr. and Mrs. George Schumate
Dr. and Mrs. Luis Schut
Mr. C. Edward Schwartz
Dr. and Mrs. Alfred M. Sellers
Dr. and Mrs. Kenneth Seton
Mr. Donald T. Sheehan
Dr. and Mrs. Donald Silberberg
Dr. Linda Skinner and Guest
Dr. and Mrs. Barry Slaven
Dr. and Mrs. Henry A. Sloviter
Dr. and Mrs. Brian Smale
Miss Elizabeth C. Smith
Dr. and Mrs. James B. Snow, Jr
Mrs. Arnold Snyder

Dr. Andrew P. Somlyo
Dr. and Mrs. George L. Spaeth
Dr. and Mrs. Thorne Sparkman, Jr
Dr. Russell Stahl and Dr. Debbie DeMarco
Dr. and Mrs. William C. Stainback
Dr. and Mrs. Robert Stein
Dr. and Mrs. Edward J. Stemmler
Dr. and Mrs. Robert B. Stevens
Dr. and Mrs. David Stokes
Mr. and Mrs. S. Emlen Stokes
Mr. and Mrs. F. Joseph Stokes
Dr. Harvey Sugerman
Dr. and Mrs. Elliot Sussman
Dr. and Mrs. Leslie N. Sutton
Mrs. Horace Swain
Dr. and Mrs. Timothy R. Talbot
Miss Julia T. Talmadge
Mr. and Mrs. Robert E. Tatnall
Dr. and Mrs. John W. Thomas
Dr. James Thomas
Mr. John Togne
Dr. and Mrs. Joseph C. Touchstone
Mr. and Mrs. Robert L. Trescher
Mr. Edwin E. Tuttle
Mr. and Mrs. Sylvain Van Gobes
Dr. and Mrs. Frederick Wagner
Dr. and Mrs. Aaron Wahrman
Dr. Marc Wallach
Dr. and Mrs. S. Reid Warren
Dr. and Mrs. George L. Weinstein
Mr. and Mrs. Edward Weiss
Dr. Claude Welch
Dr. and Mrs. Robert Welty
Dr. Arthur F. Whereat
Dr. Doug Wilmore
Mrs. Nancy Wink and Husband
Dr. and Mrs. J. Edwin Wood
Dr. and Mrs. Myron Yanoff
Dr. Jack Yu
Dr. and Mrs. Felix Zandman

May 8th Birthday Reception

About 450 of Dr. Rhoads' friends and colleagues attended this reception, which was held in the Lincoln Hall of the Union League of Philadelphia.

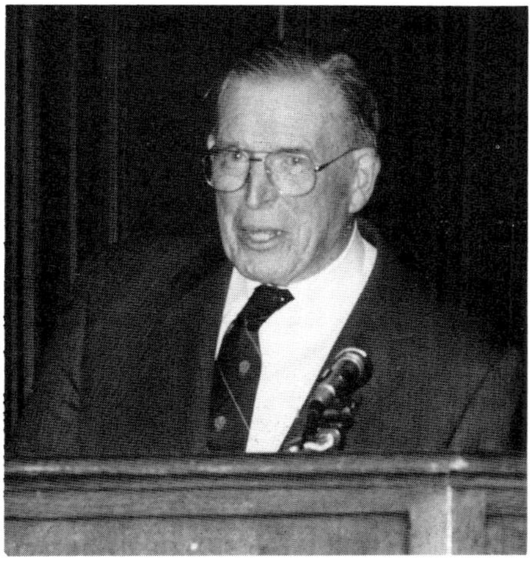

Dr. Rhoads addresses guests at the May 8th Birthday Reception at the Union League.

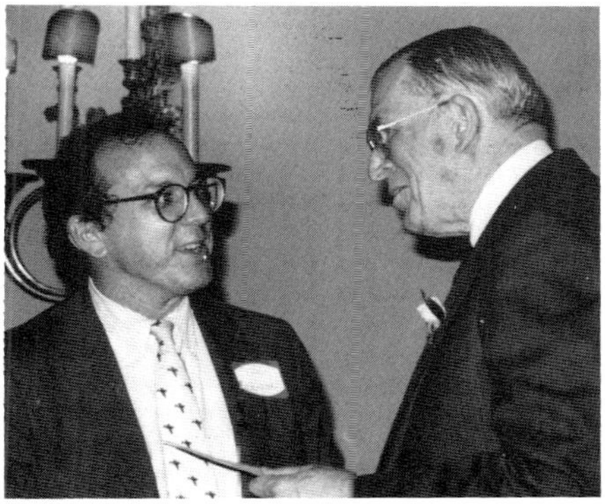

Thomas Frazier—HUP chief resident 1974–75 and President of the Ravdin-Rhoads Society, presents Dr. Rhoads with a $10,000.00 contribution from the Society for his research fund.

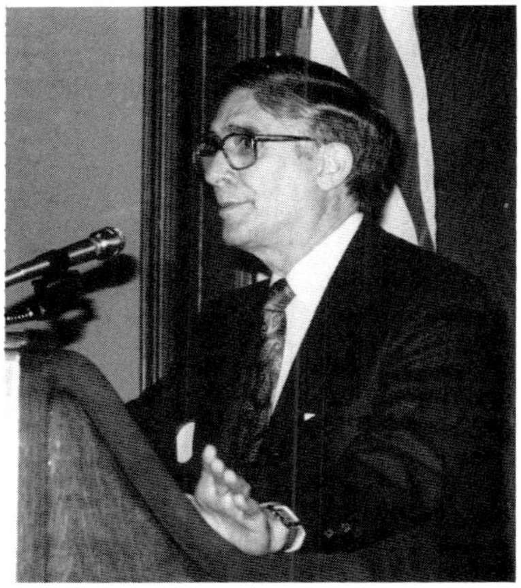

Edward Stemmler, Dean of the School of Medicine, University of Pennsylvania and Medical Center Executive Vice President addresses guests at the May 8th reception.

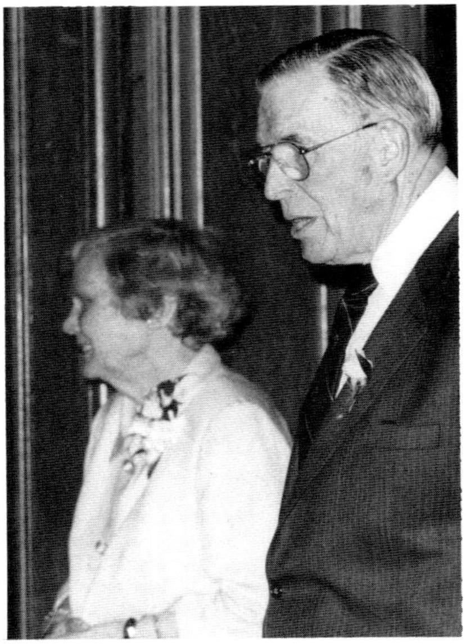

Dr. and Mrs. Rhoads at the reception on May 8th at the Union League.

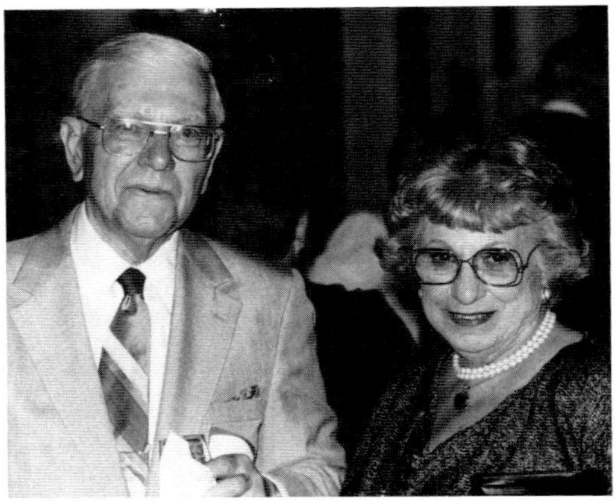

Mr. Robert Dunlop, University of Pennsylvania Trustee and Director of the Glenn Meade Trust, and Mrs. Charlotte Snyder.

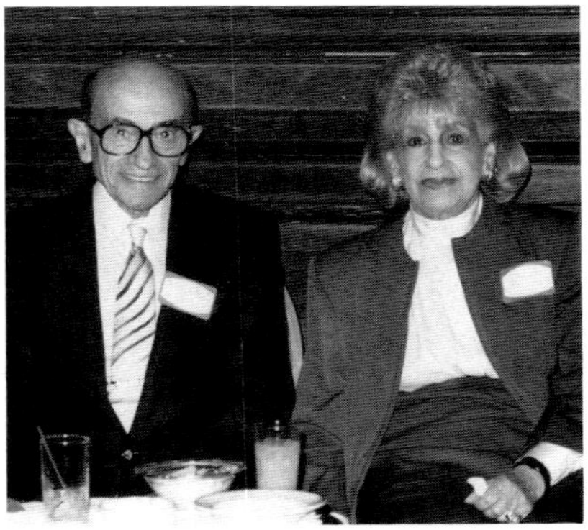

Hilda and Arthur Cohn, benefactors of the Humanitarian Award of the Kain Mosas Group for Cancer Research (Philadelphia Division of the American Cancer Society) which Dr. Rhoads received in 1963.

List of May 9th Symposium Banquet Attendees

Dr. and Mrs. Clyde Barker
Dr. and Mrs. Harold Barker
Dr. Anne Barnes and Husband
Dr. and Mrs. Scott Bartlett
Dr. William Beck
Dr. Whitfield Bell and Jane M. Oppenheimer
Dr. Gordon Buzby
Dr. Michael Caldwell
Dr. and Mrs. Gene Cayten
Dr. Winston Chu
Dr. and Mrs. Robert Coffey
Dr. and Mrs. Isidore Cohn
Dr. Edward Copeland
Dr. Robert Crichlow
Dr. William Currieri
Dr. and Mrs. Donald Dafoe
Dr. and Mrs. Gordon Danielson
Dr. and Mrs. Robert Darrow
Dr. and Mrs. Daniel Dempsey
Dr. and Mrs. William DeMuth
Dr. and Mrs. Clarence Dennis
Dr. Karen Deveney
Dr. and Mrs. Stanley Dudrick
Dr. and Mrs. William Dyson
Dr. and Mrs. L. Henry Edmunds
Dr. and Mrs. James Finnegan
Dr. Ira Fox
Dr. and Mrs. Jerrald Friedman
Dr. and Mrs. William Glenn
Dr. and Mrs. Herman Goldstein
Dr. Cleon Goodwin
Mr. and Mrs. Crawford Greenwalt
Dr. and Mrs. Ward Griffin
Dr. and Mrs. Frazer Gurd
Dr. and Mrs. Ralph Hamilton
Dr. and Mrs. Victor Hanson
Dr. and Mrs. William Hardesty
Dr. James Hardy
Dr. Charles E. Hartford
Dr. and Mrs. Clark Hargrove
Dr. George Hartzell
Dr. Hazel Holst and Friend
Dr. and Mrs. John Howard
Dr. Charles Huggins
Dr. Danny Jacobs
Mrs. Julian Johnson
Dr. Scott Jones
Dr. Edward Kaplan
Professor and Mrs. Margaret Rhoads Kendon and their daughter Gudrun
Dr. and Mrs. James Knecht
Dr. and Mrs. Thomas Langfitt
Dr. and Mrs. Don LaRossa
Dr. Lasalle Leffall
Dr. Stan Levenson
Dr. and Mrs. Harry Light
Dr. William Longmire
Dr. Barbara Lundy
Dr. Dennis Lynch
Dr. and Mrs. Julius Mackie
Dr. Len Miller
Dr. Francis Moore
Dr. and Mrs. James Muller
Dr. and Mrs. Harry Muller
Dr. and Mrs. Fred Murtagh
Dr. and Mrs. Richard Myers
Dr. Simon Myint
Dr. and Mrs. Ali Naji
Dr. Carter Nance
Dr. and Mrs. Harry Nelson
Dr. and Mrs. Paul Nemir
Dr. and Mrs. Raymond Noble
Dr. and Mrs. Barry Noone
Dr. and Mrs. Lloyd Nyhus
Dr. and Mrs. James O'Neill
Dr. and Mrs. Marshall Orloff
Dr. Jack Orr and his son Jonathan
Dr. and Mrs. C. Dick Park
Dr. and Mrs. Lewis Patterson
Dr. and Mrs. Leonard Perloff
Mrs. Thomas Pollock
Dr. and Mrs. Basil Pruitt
Dr. and Mrs. Peter Randall
Dr. and Mrs. Mark Ravitch
Dr. and Mrs. Robert Reis and their son Ronald
Ms. Caroline Rhoads
Mr. Charles Rhoads
Mr. Edward Rhoads
Mr. and Mrs. George Rhoads and their children Thomas and James
Dr. and Mrs. Jonathan Rhoads, Jr and their children Mary Teresa and Ruth Anne
Dr. and Mrs. Jonathan E. Rhoads
Mr. and Mrs. Philip Rhoads and their children Philip Jr., Deborah, and Joanna

Dr. and Mrs. Brooke Roberts
Dr. and Mrs. Ernest Rosato
Dr. and Mrs. Frank Rosato
Dr. James Roseman
Dr. Henry Royster and Daughter
Dr. and Mrs. Harry Schumacher
Dr. and Mrs. C. William Schwab
Dr. and Mrs. Clete Schwegman
Dr. Howard Silberman
Dr. David Skinner and daughter Kristen
Mrs. Gardner Smith
Dr. and Mrs. Pat Spagna
Dr. and Mrs. Frank Spencer
Dr. George Stephenson
Mrs. Larry Stephenson
Dr. Harvey Sugerman
Dr. James Thomas
Dr. James Thompson
Dr. Hillary Timmis
Dr. and Mrs. Michael Torosian
Dr. and Mrs. Santi Vibul
Dr. and Mrs. John Waldhausen
Dr. Marc Wallach
Dr. and Mrs. Alan Wein
Dr. Leonard Weiner
Dr. Claude Welch
Dr. and Mrs. Robert Welty
Dr. and Mrs. Linton Whitaker
Dr. and Mrs. Doug Wilmore
Dr. Robert Witmer
Dr. and Mrs. Francis Wood

May 9th Symposium Banquet at Philosophical Hall

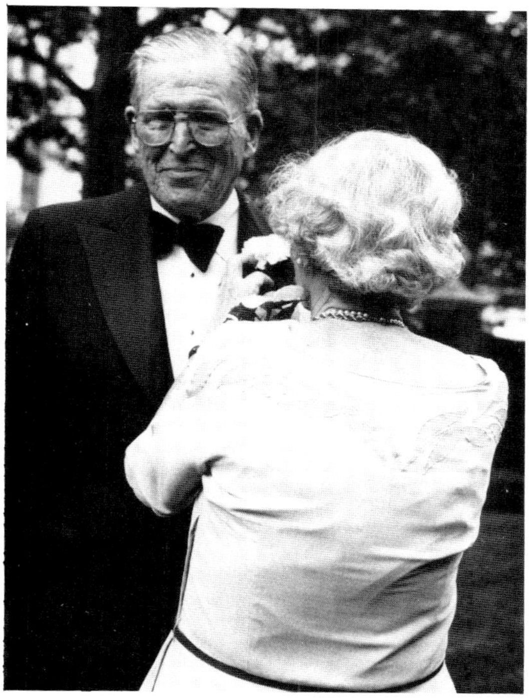

Mrs. Rhoads assists Dr. Rhoads in preparing for reception.

Reception in the Jefferson Garden, May 9, 1987.

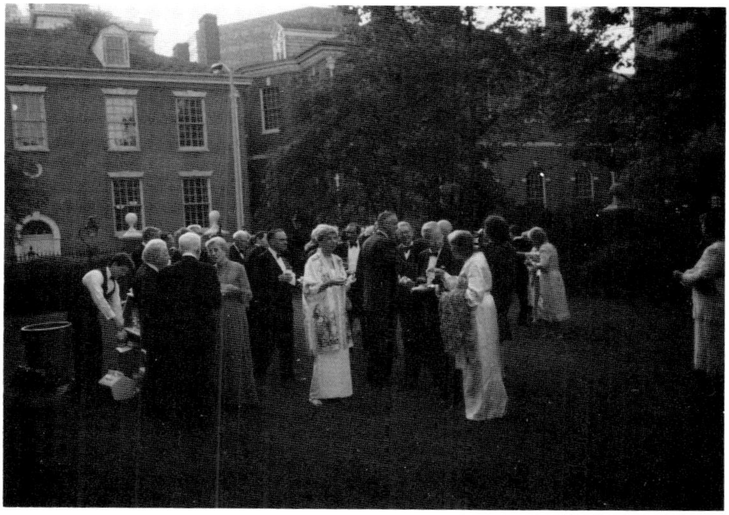

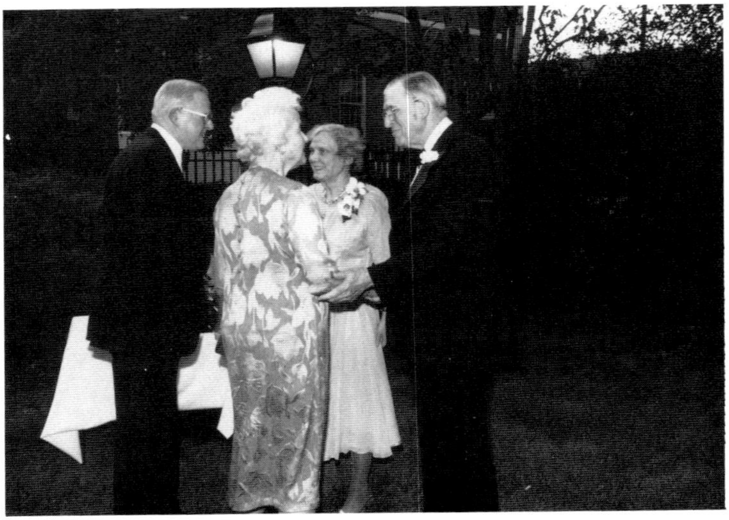

Dr. and Mrs. Rhoads greet Dr. and Mrs. Frazier Gurd. Dr. Gurd was Harrison Department of Surgical Research Fellow, 1946–47, and is Emeritus Professor of Surgery, McGill University.

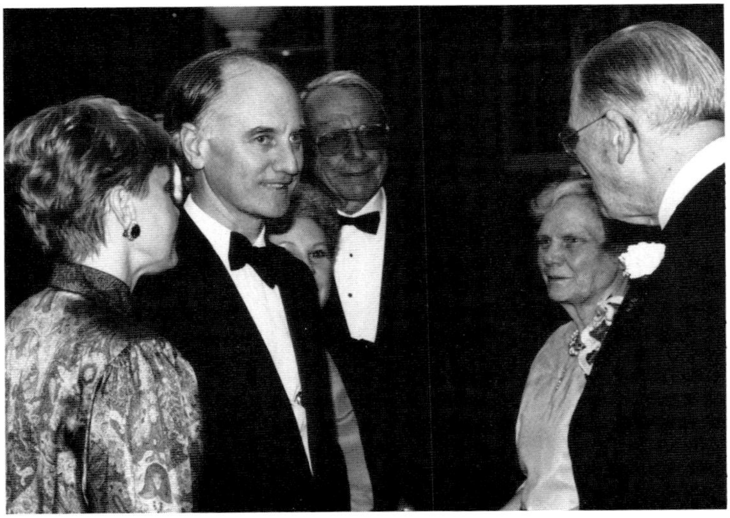

Dr. and Mrs. Linton Whitaker, Dr. William Dyson, and Dr. and Mrs. Rhoads.

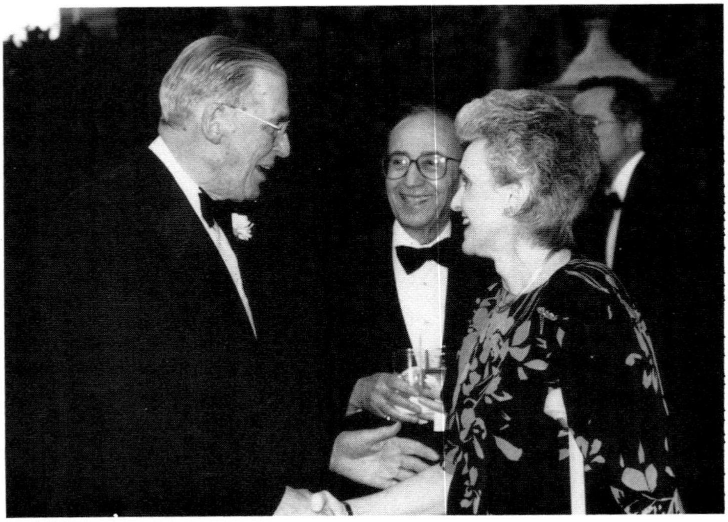

Dr. Rhoads with Dr. and Mrs. Herman Goldstine. Dr. Goldstine is Executive Officer of the American Philosophical Society.

Dr. Rhoads greets Mrs. Harold Barker.

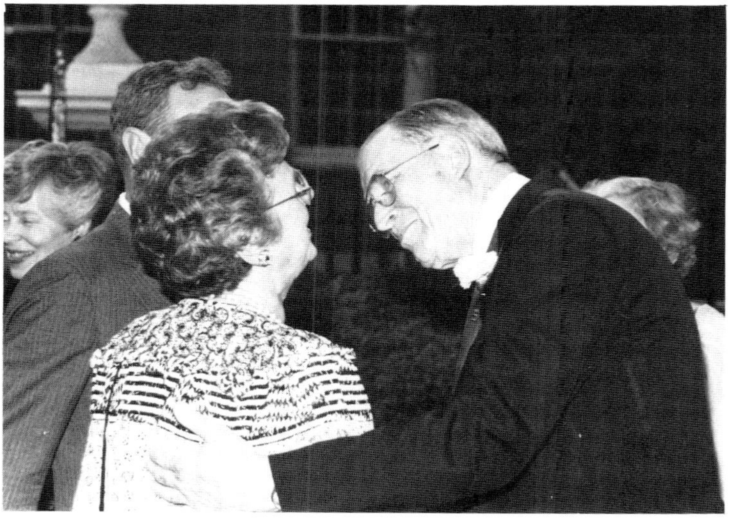

Dr. Rhoads and Dr. and Mrs. William H. Muller, Jr. Dr. Muller is former Chief of Surgery, Vice President of Health Affairs, University of Virginia.

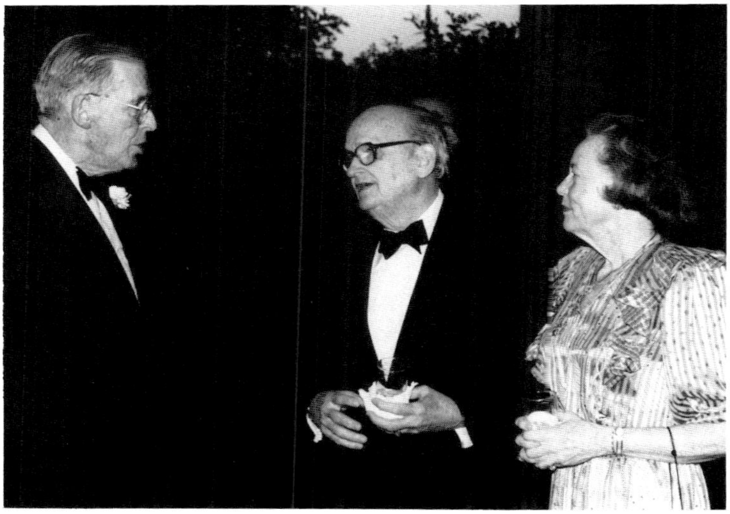

Dr. Rhoads greets Dr. and Mrs. Frank Rosato. Dr. Rosato was HUP Chief Resident, 1965–66, and is Chairman of Surgery, Thomas Jefferson University Hospital. In the background, Dr. Lloyd Nyhus, Chairman of Surgery, University of Illinois.

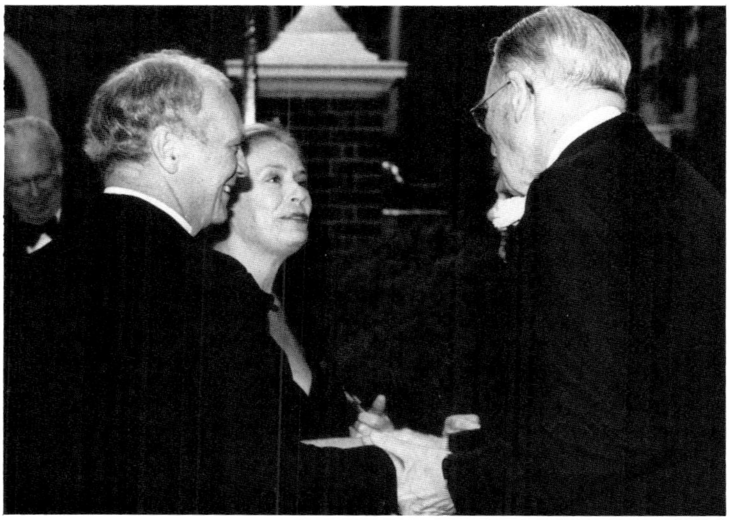

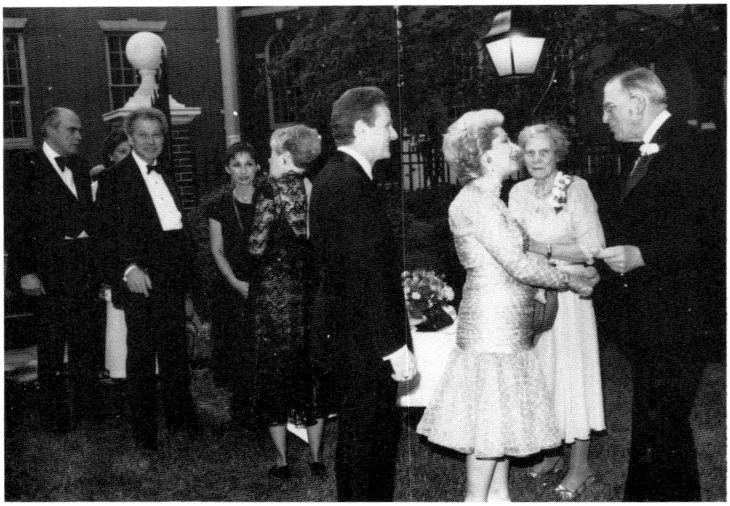

Dr. and Mrs. Rhoads greet Dr. and Mrs. Isadore Cohen. Dr. Cohen is Chairman of Surgery, Louisiana State University. Also shown are Dr. C. Dick Park, HUP Chief Resident, 1968–69, Dr. and Mrs. Douglas Wilmore, and Mrs. Clyde Barker.

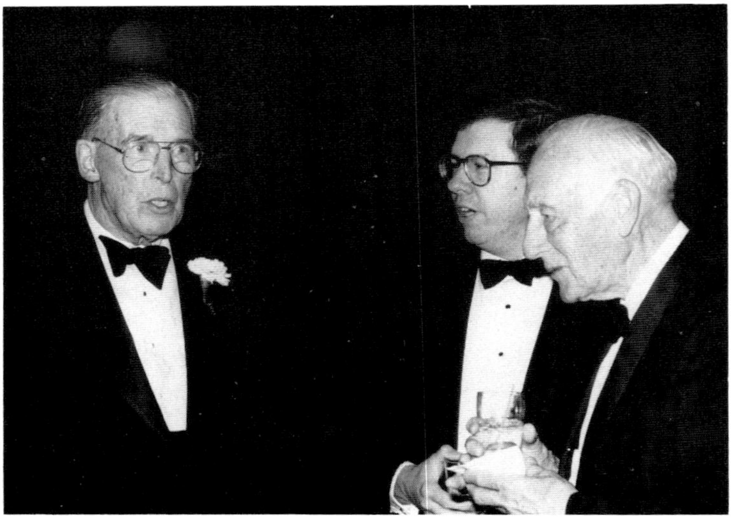

Dr. Rhoads and symposium speaker Dr. Cleon Goodwin, Chief Resident at HUP in 1976–77 and Associate Professor of Surgery at Cornell University. Also shown is Dr. Claude Welch, Massachusetts General Hospital.

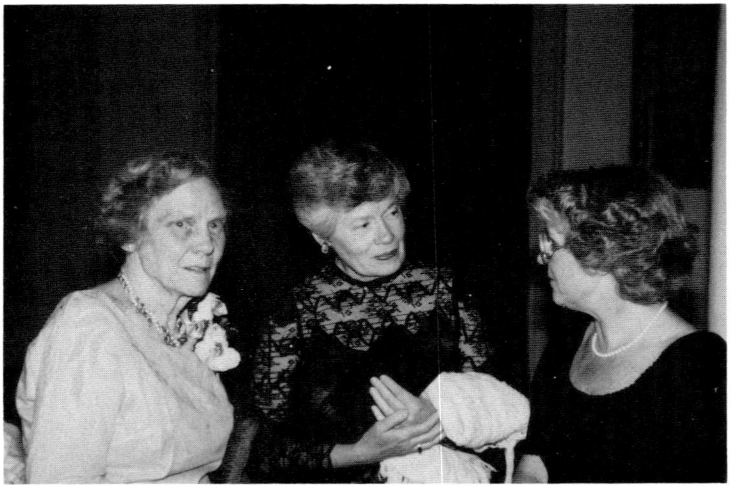

Mrs. Rhoads, Mrs. C. Barker, and Mrs. Dudrick.

Symposium speaker, Basil Pruitt, Director of US Army Institute of Surgical Research, San Antonio, Texas; symposium speaker Douglas Wilmore, HUP Chief Resident, 1970–71, and Professor of Surgery, Harvard Medical School; and after dinner speaker William Longmire, Professor and former Chairman of Surgery, UCLA.

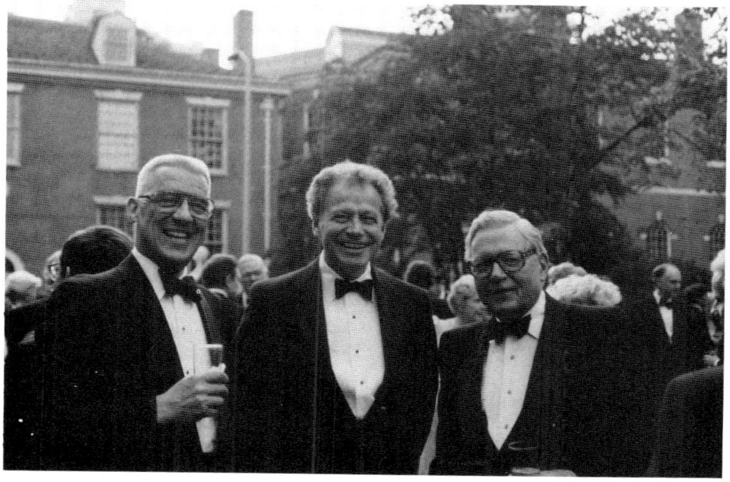

Dr. and Mrs. Richard Myers, Chairman Emeritus Bowman Grey Medical School, and symposium speaker Dr. James Thompson, HUP Chief Resident, 1958–59, and Chairman of Surgery, University of Texas Medical Branch, Galviston.

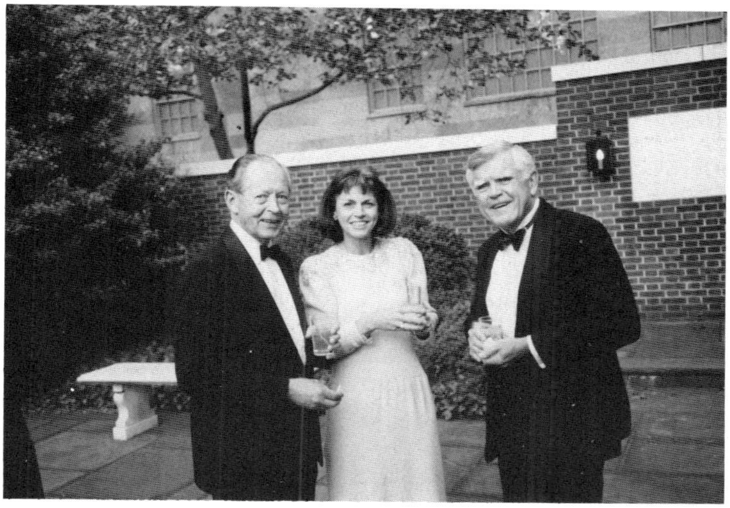

Dr. William Glenn, Professor of Surgery, Yale University, and Dr. Rhoads.

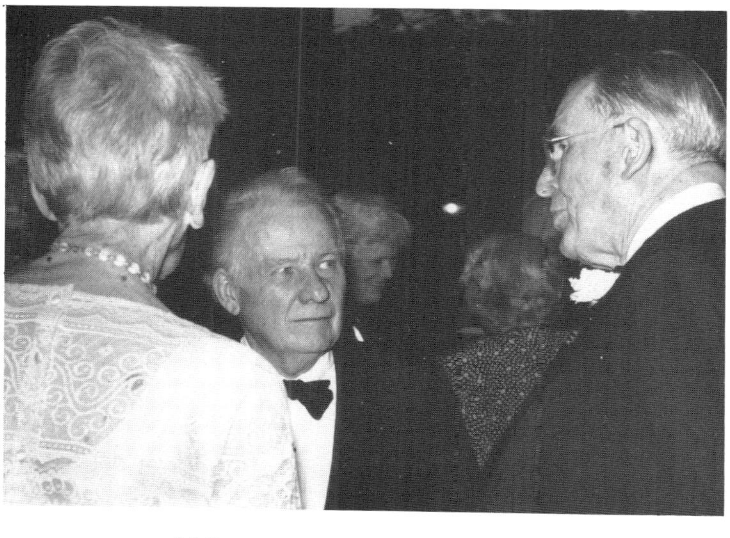

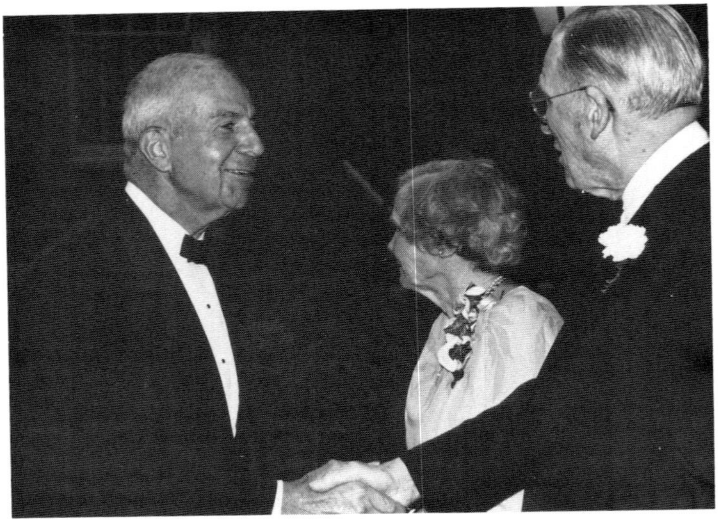

Dr. and Mrs. Rhoads with Dr. Paul Nemir, HUP Chief Resident, 1950–51, and Chairman Emeritus Department of Surgery, Graduate Hospital, Emilie Roland T. de Hellebranth Emeritus Professor of Surgery.

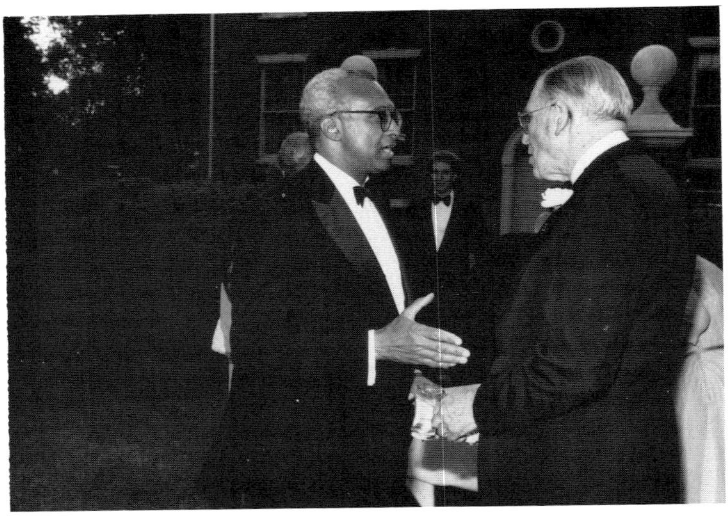

Dr. Rhoads and Dr. LaSalle Leffall, Chairman of Surgery, Howard University. In the background is Marc Wallack, HUP Chief Resident, 1976–77, and Chief of Surgery, Cedars Sinai Hospital, Miami.

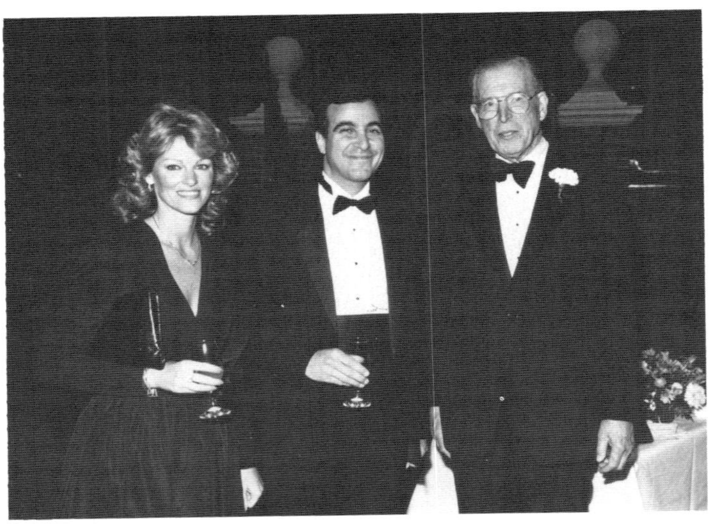

Dr. Rhoads with Dr. and Mrs. Michael Torosian. Mrs. Torosian is Acting Director of Nursing at HUP. Dr. Torosian, HUP Chief Resident from 1984–85, is Assistant Professor of Surgery at HUP.

Mrs. Jonathan Rhoads, Jr. (Julia) with her daughters Mary Teresa and Ruth Anne.

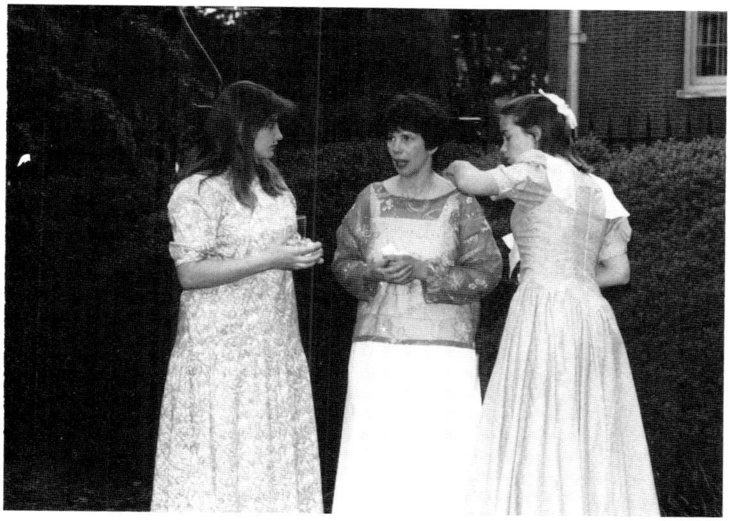

Shown from left to right: Dr. William Demuth, Chief Resident HUP, 1952–53, and Professor of Surgery, Penn State University; Bob Witmer, Chief Resident HUP, 1950–51; Dr. and Mrs. Robert Welty, Chief Resident CHOP, 1946; Dr. Hazel Holst; and after dinner speaker Dr. William Longmire.

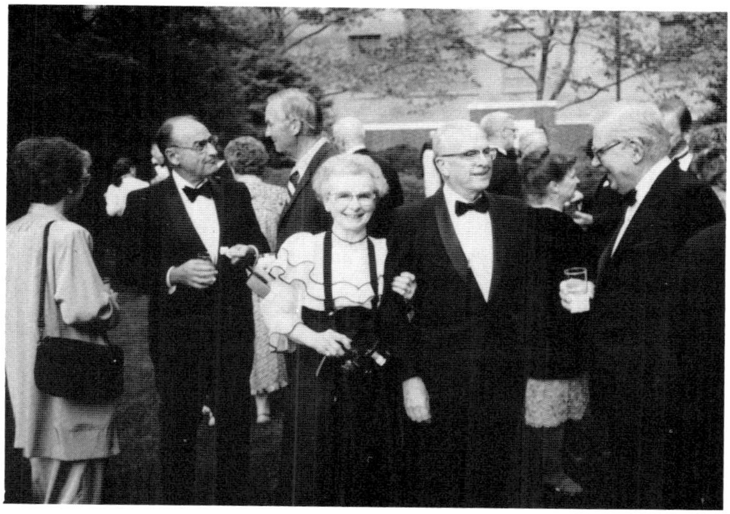

Dr. Brooke Roberts, HUP Chief Resident, 1950–51, Professor Emeritus of Surgery, University of Pennsylvania, and Acting Chairman of the Department of Surgery, 1981–83, with symposium speaker Dr. James Thompson.

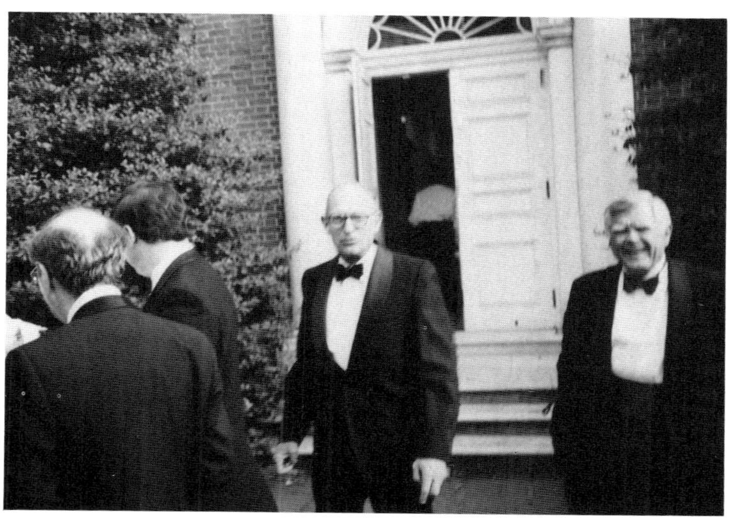

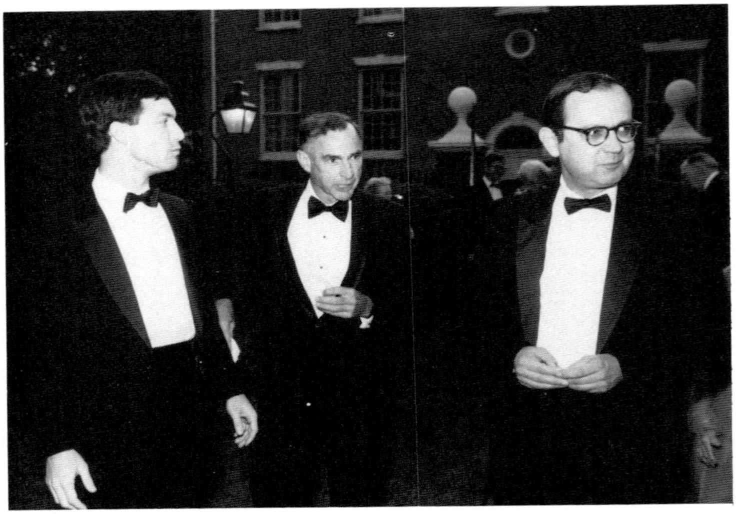

Dr. Jack Orr, HUP Chief Resident, 1958–59 with his son and Dr. Leonard Miller, Professor and former Chairman of Surgery, University of Pennsylvania.

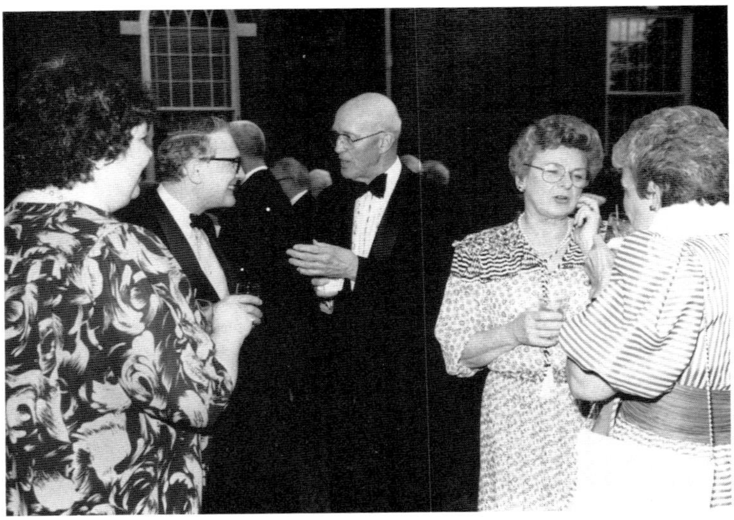

Former University of Pennsylvania Chiefs of Plastic Surgery, Dr. Peter Randall and Dr. Henry Royster. Mrs. Harold Barker and Mrs. Harry Shoemaker.

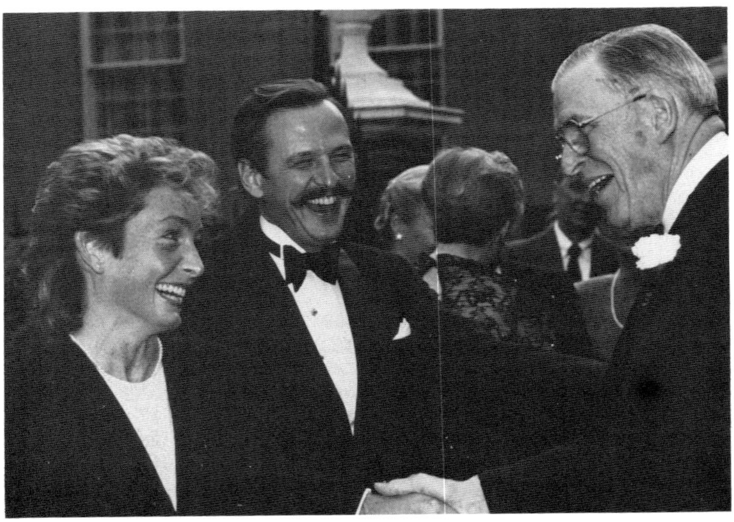

Dr. Rhoads greets Drs. Clark and Ellen Hargrove. Dr. Ellen Hargrove is a HUP surgical resident. Dr. Clark Hargrove, HUP Chief Resident, 1978–79, is Assistant Professor of Surgery at HUP.

Dr. and Mrs. Daniel Dempsey, HUP Chief Resident, 1985–86, and Assistant Professor of Surgery, Temple University. In the background are Dr. Hilary Timmis, HUP Chief Resident, 1961–62, and Dr. Lloyd Nyhus, Chief of Surgery, University of Illinois.

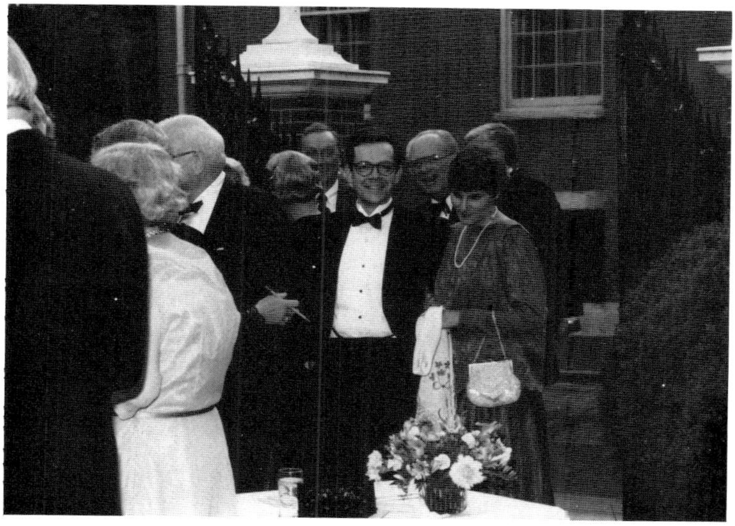

Dr. Rhoads' son, Edward, and Dr. Danny Jacobs, HUP Chief Resident, 1985–86, and Assistant Professor of Surgery, Harvard University.

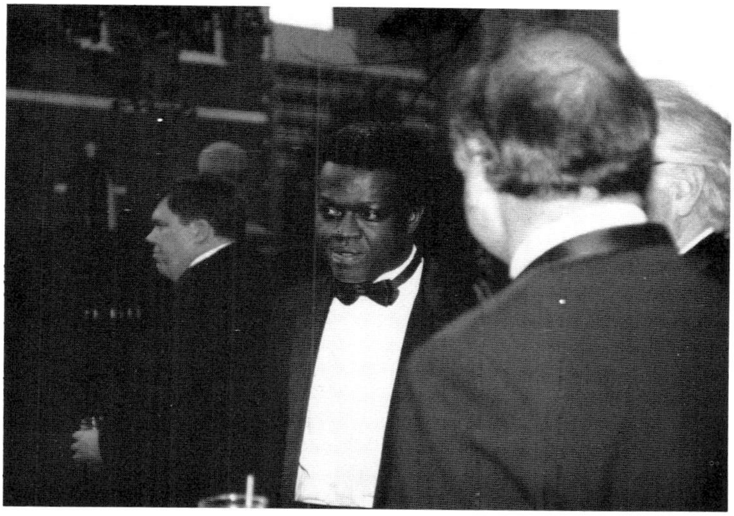

Dr. Danny Jacobs and Dr. Gordon Buxby, HUP Chief Resident, 1980–81, Assistant Professor of Surgery at HUP, and Co-Chairman of Rhoads Birthday Symposium.

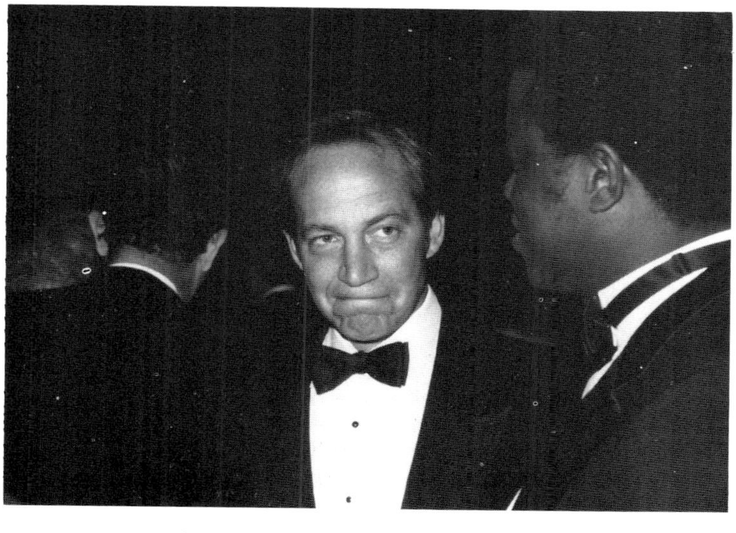

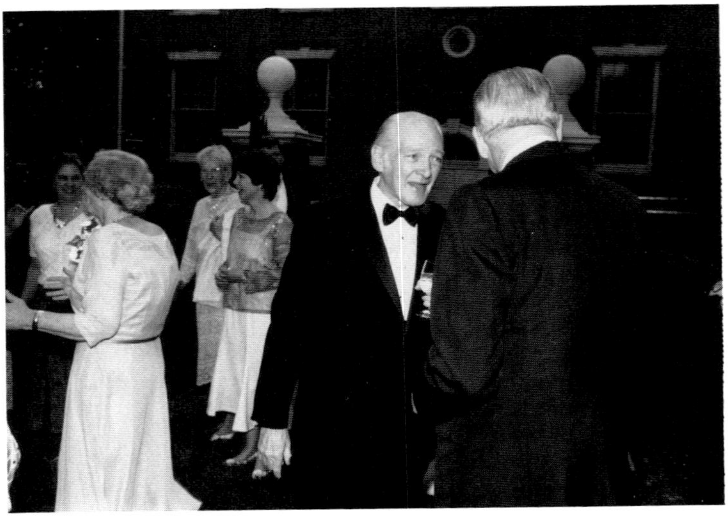

Shown from left to right: Margaret Kendon, Dr. Rhoads' daughter; Mrs. Jonathan Rhoads; Mrs. Rhoads' sister, Caroline; Mrs. Jonathan Rhoads, Jr. (Julia); Dr. Cletus Schwegman; and Dr. Rhoads.

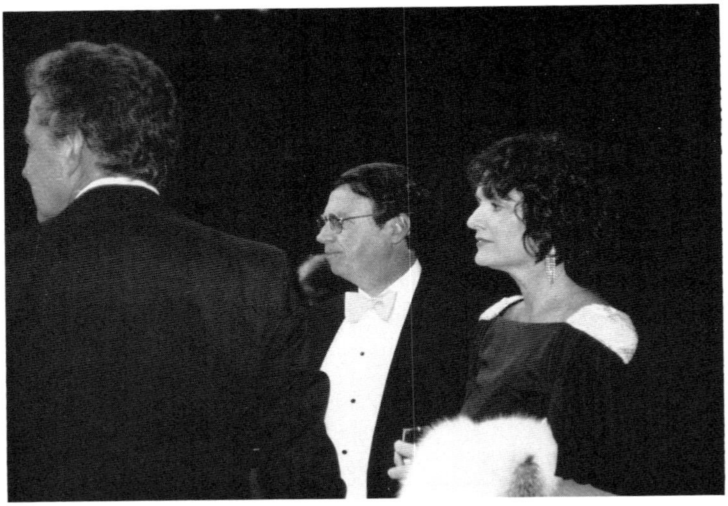

Dr. Douglas Wilmore and Dr. and Mrs. Ernest Rosato, Chief Resident HUP, 1967–68, and Professor of Surgery, University of Pennsylvania.

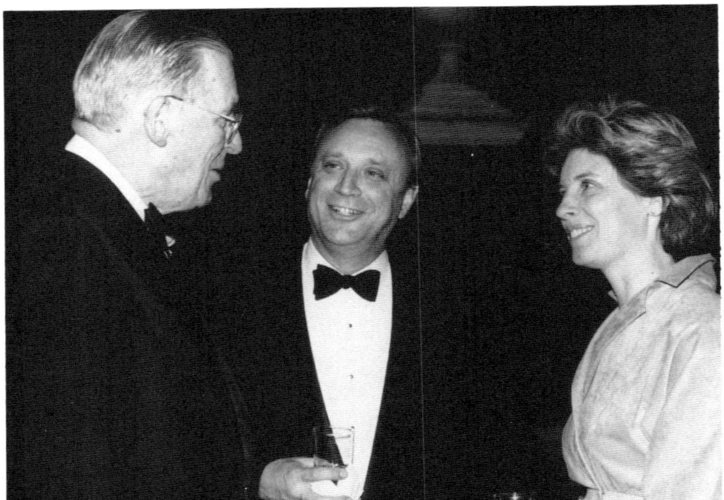

Dr. Rhoads with Dr. and Mrs. Don LaRossa. Dr. LaRossa is Associate Professor of Plastic Surgery at HUP.

Symposium speaker Dr. Scott Jones, Mrs. Thomas Langfitt, symposium speaker Dr. Thompson, and Dr. Thomas Langfitt, former Chief of Neurosurgery and Vice President for Health Affairs, University of Pennsylvania.

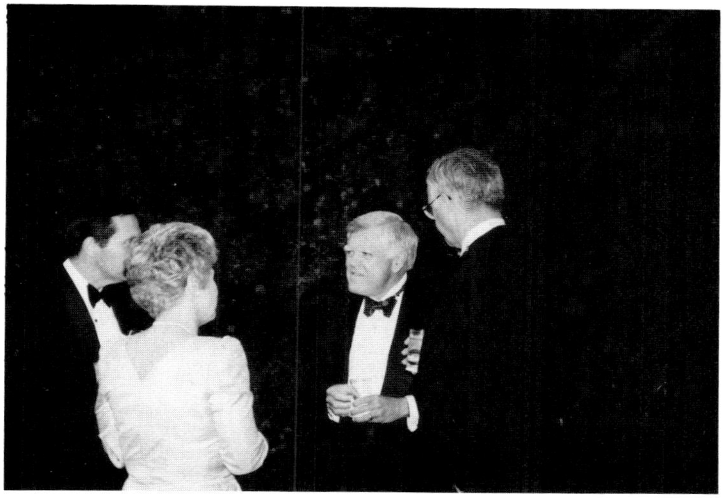

Dr. and Mrs. Rhoads with Dr. Howard Silberman, HUP Chief Resident, 1971–72, and Professor of Surgery at the University of Southern California.

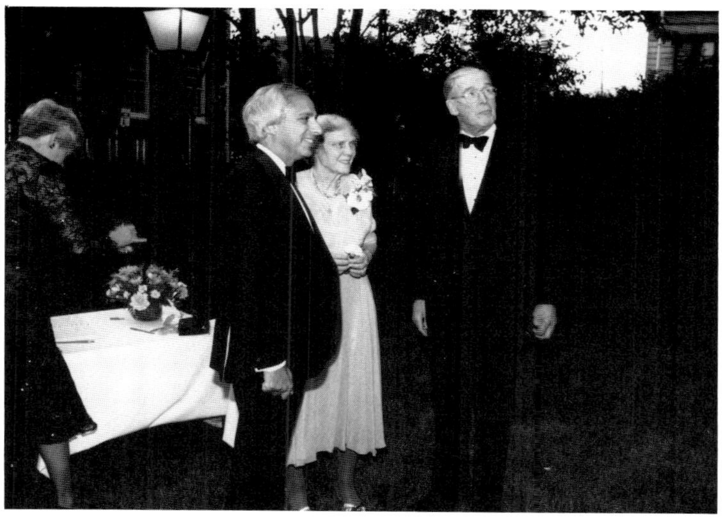

Shown from left to right: Mrs. Stanley Dudrick; Mrs. Ward O. Griffin; Dr. Claude Welch; Dr. Ward Griffin, Secretary of American Board of Surgery; Dr. Leonard Miller, Professor of Surgery, University of Pennsylvania; and symposium speaker Dr. John Waldhausen, Chairman of Surgery, Pennsylvania State University.

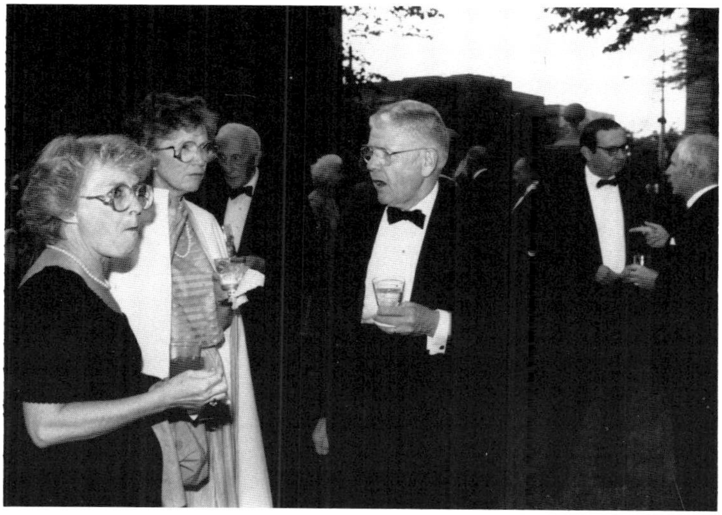

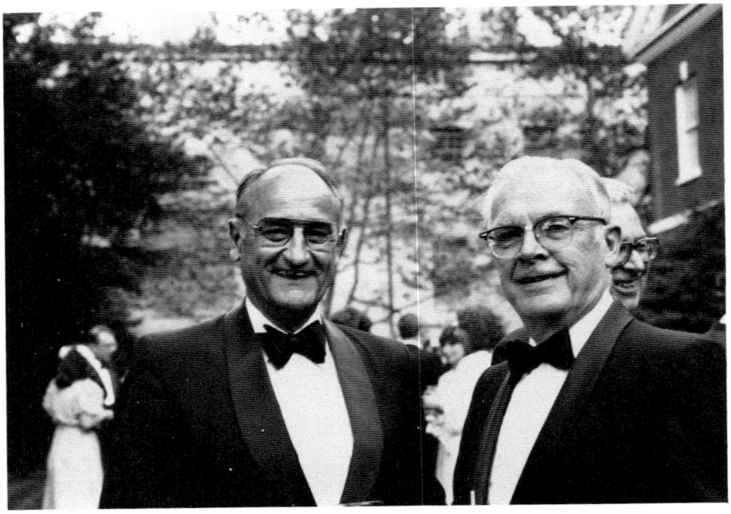

Dr. William DeMuth, HUP Chief Resident, 1952–53, and Emeritus Professor of Surgery, Penn State; Dr. Robert Welty, Chief Resident CHOP 1946; and Dr. Harold Barker, Chief Resident HUP, 1951–52, and Emeritus Professor of Surgery, Columbia University.

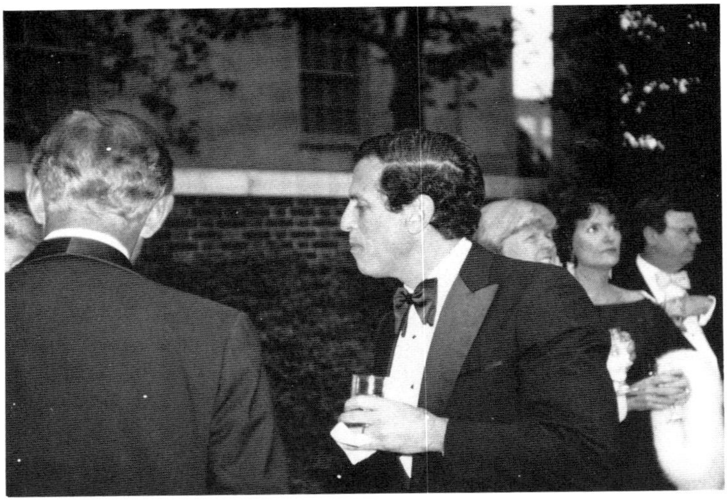

Symposium speaker Dr. Edwin Kaplan, HUP Chief Resident, 1966–67, and Professor of Surgery, University of Chicago. Also Mrs. Paul Nemir, and Dr. and Mrs. Ernest Rosato.

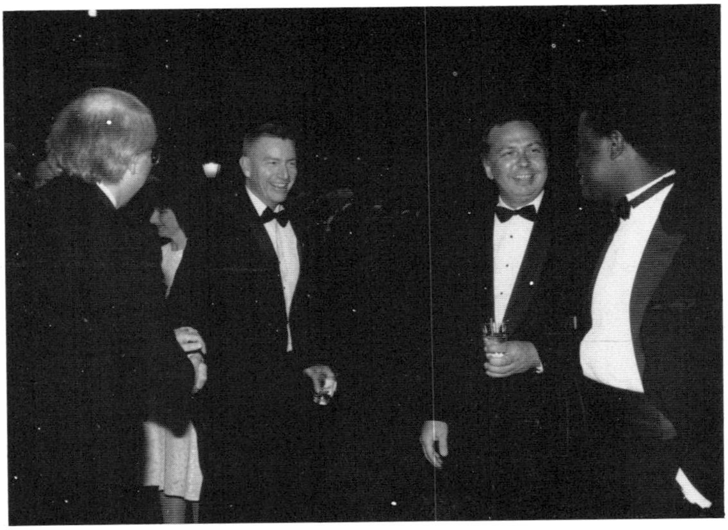

Mrs. Thomas Pollock, wife of HUP Chief Resident, 1977–78 with Dr. Clyde Barker, Dr. James Mullen, and Dr. Danny Jacobs.

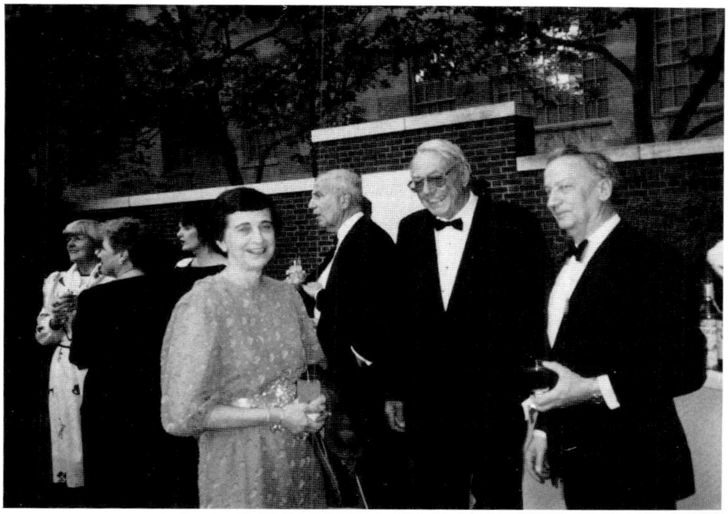

Shown from left to right: Mrs. Louis Patterson, Dr. Paul Nemir, Dr. William Dyson, and Dr. Louis Patterson.

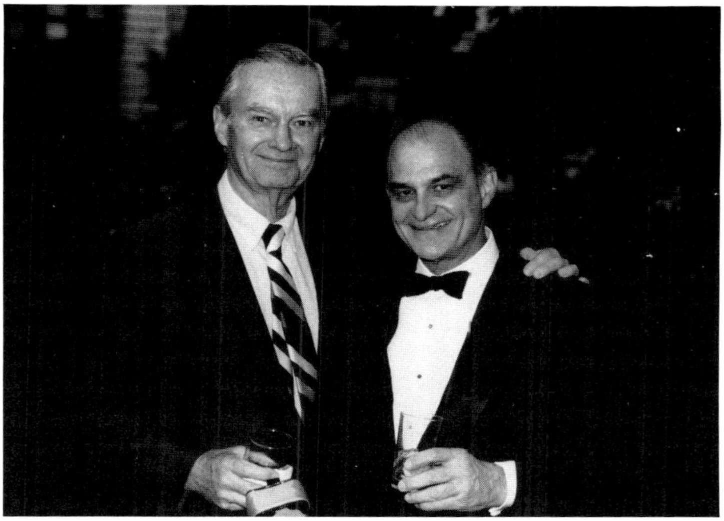

Dr. Robert Witmer, HUP Chief Resident, 1950–51, and Dr. Harry Light, HUP Chief Resident, 1960–61.

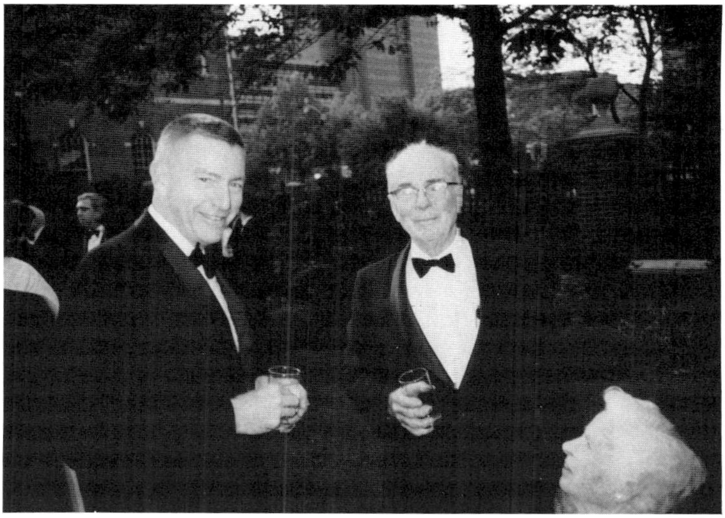

Dr. Clyde F. Barker and Dr. and Mrs. Francis C. Wood, Chairman Emeritus of Medicine, University of Pennsylvania.

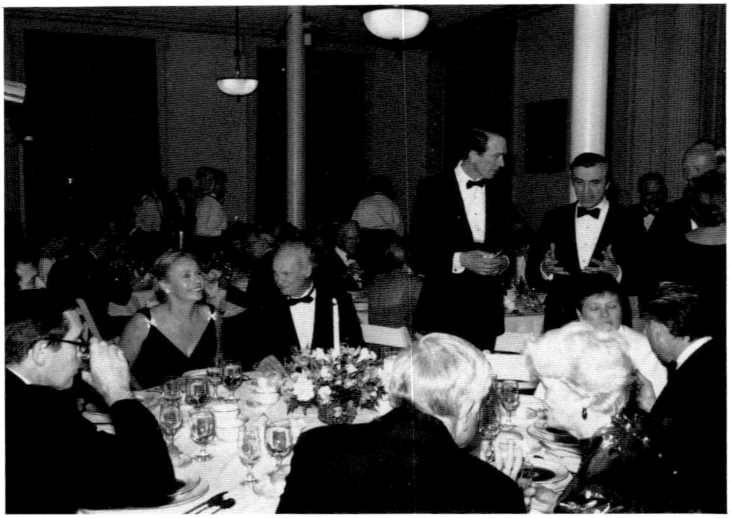

Dr. Scott Jones, Dr. and Mrs. Frances Rosato, Dr. Gordon Danielson, and Dr. Stan Dudrick.

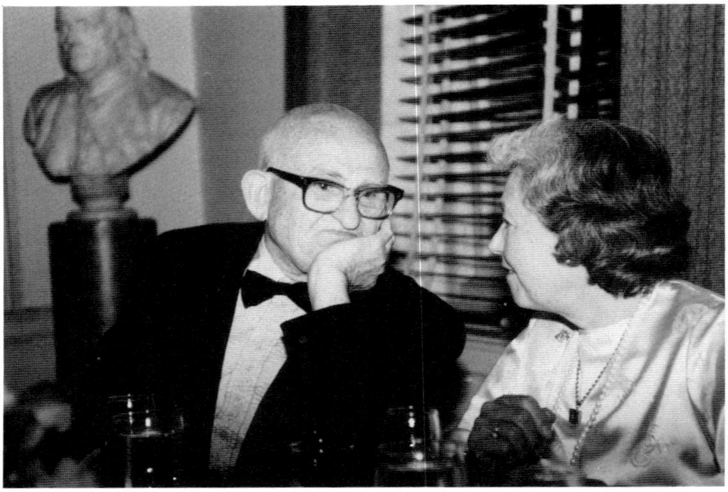

Symposium speaker Dr. and Mrs. John Howard. Dr. Howard was HUP Chief Resident, 1949–50, and is Professor of Surgery, University of Ohio (Toledo).

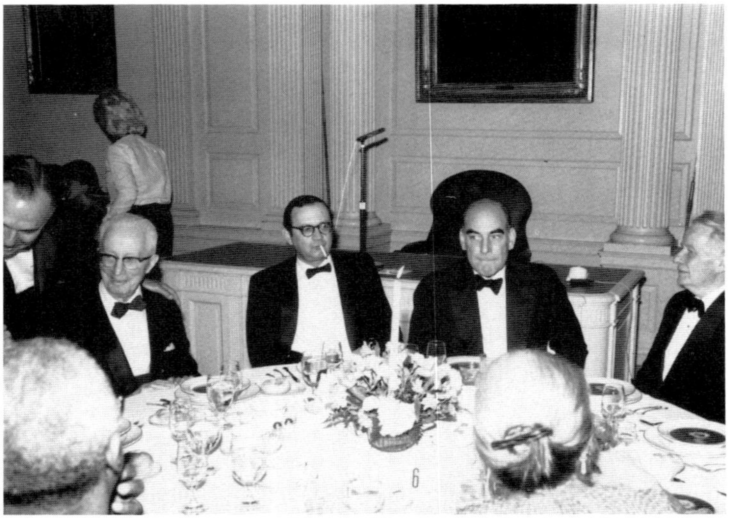

Dr. Frank Spencer; Dr. George Stephenson; Dr. Leonard Miller; Dr. Robert Crichlow, HUP Chief Resident, 1962–63, and Chairman of Surgery, Dartmouth; and Dr. William Glenn.

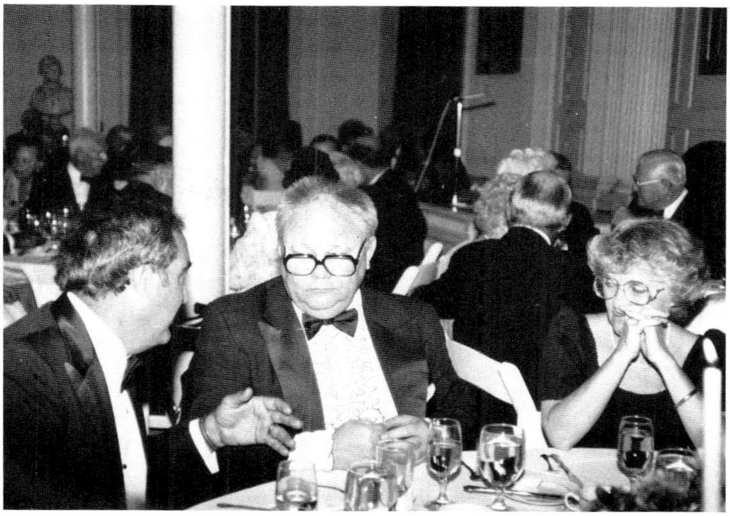

Symposium speaker Dr. William Curreri, Chief Resident HUP, 1967–68, and Chairman of Surgery, University of South Alabama; Symposium speaker Dr. Carter Nance, Chief Resident HUP, 1965–66, and Chairman of Surgery, St. Barnabas Medical Center; and Mrs. Dudrick.

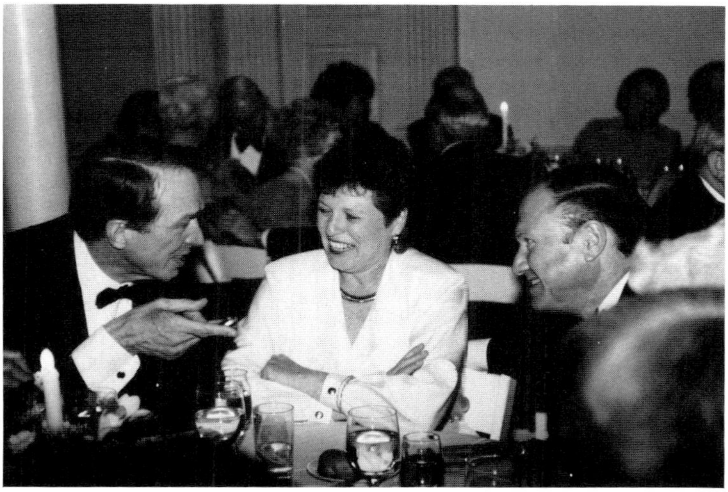

Symposium speaker Dr. Gordon Danielson, HUP Chief Resident, 1961–62, and Professor of Surgery, Mayo Medical School; Mrs. Danielson; and Dr. Marshall Orloff, Chief Resident HUP, 1957–58, and Professor and former Chairman of Surgery, University of California, San Diego.

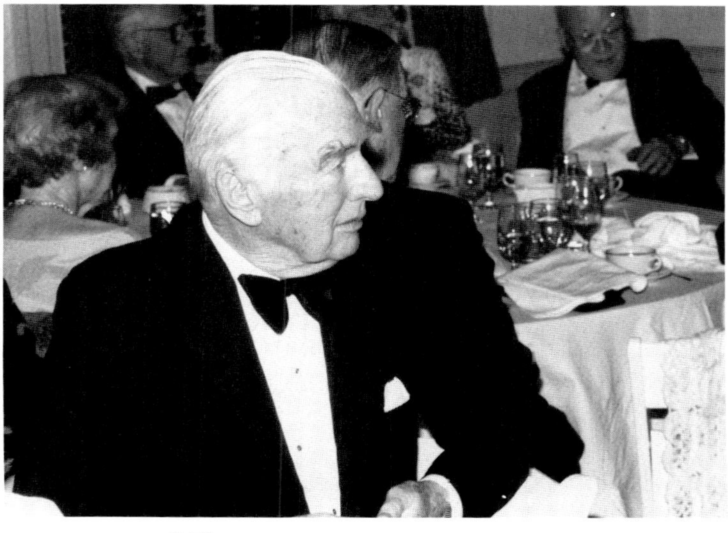

Crawford Greenwalt, Past President of the American Philosophical Society, Mrs. Rhoads, and Francis Moore, with Whitfield Bell in the background.

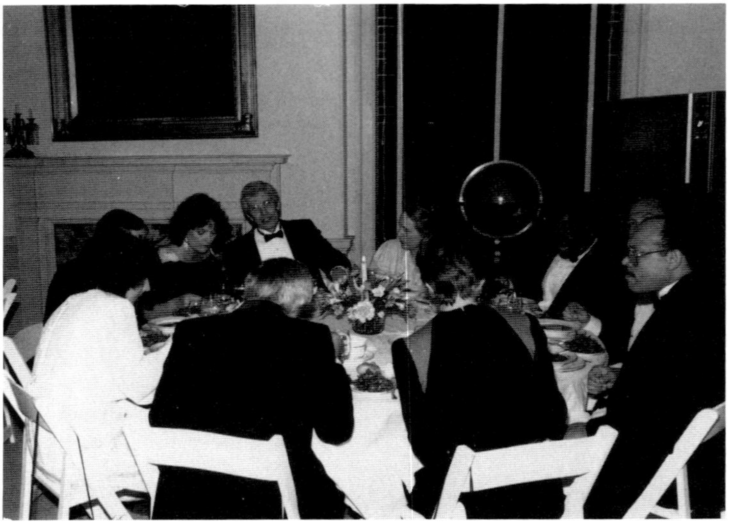

Mrs. Ernest Rosato; Dr. and Mrs. Leonard Perloff, HUP Chief Resident, 1970–71, and Associate Professor of Surgery, University of Pennsylvania; Dr. Danny Jacobs; and Dr. James Thomas, HUP Chief Resident, 1973–74, and Associate Professor of Surgery, University of Kansas.

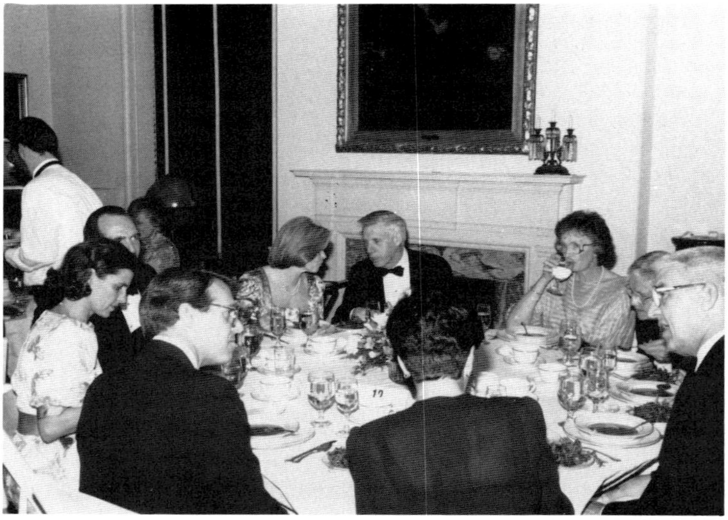

Mrs. Henry Edmunds; Dr. William Schwab, Professor of Surgery, HUP; Mrs. Gardner Smith; Dr. Henry Edmunds, Professor of Surgery, University of Pennsylvania; Dr. and Mrs. Ward Griffin; and Dr. Basil Pruitt

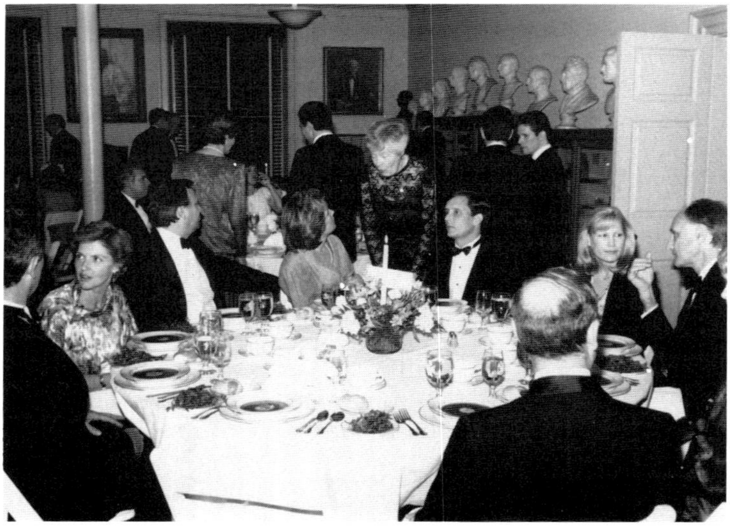

Shown from left to right: Mrs. Henry Edmunds; Dr. and Mrs. Don LaRossa; Mrs. Clyde Barker; Dr. and Mrs. Scott Bartlett; Dr. Donald Dafoe, HUP Chief Resident, 1980–81, and Associate Professor of Surgery, University of Pennsylvania; and Dr. and Mrs. Linton Whitaker. Dr. Whitaker is Professor of Surgery and Chief of Plastic Surgery at the University of Pennsylvania.

Dr. Pat Spagna, HUP Chief Resident, 1964–65, and Professor of Surgery, Medical College of Pennsylvania; Dr. Michael Caldwell, HUP Chief Resident 1981–82, and Associate Professor of Surgery, Brown University; Mrs. Spagna; Dr. Harry Light, HUP Chief Resident, 1960–61; Mrs. Light; and Dr. Harry Nelson, HUP Chief Resident, 1962–63.

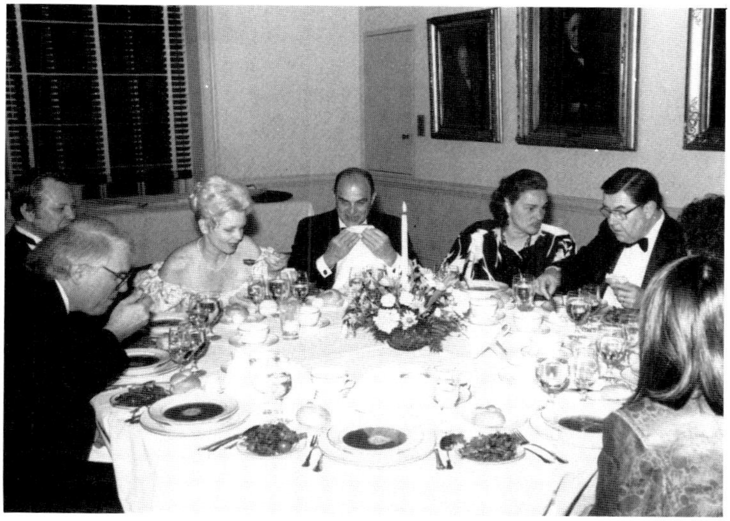

Dr. Michael Caldwell with Dr. and Mrs. Pat Spagna.

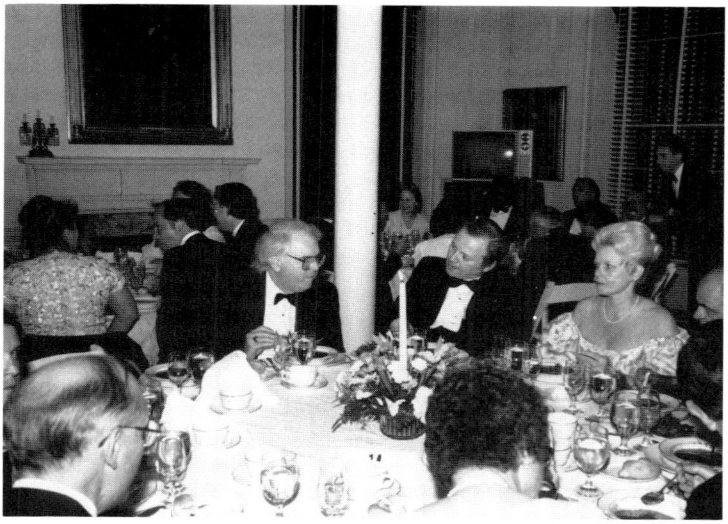

Dr. Alan Wein, Mrs. Larry Stephenson, Drs. Ellen and Clark Hargrove, and Dr. Marc Wallack.

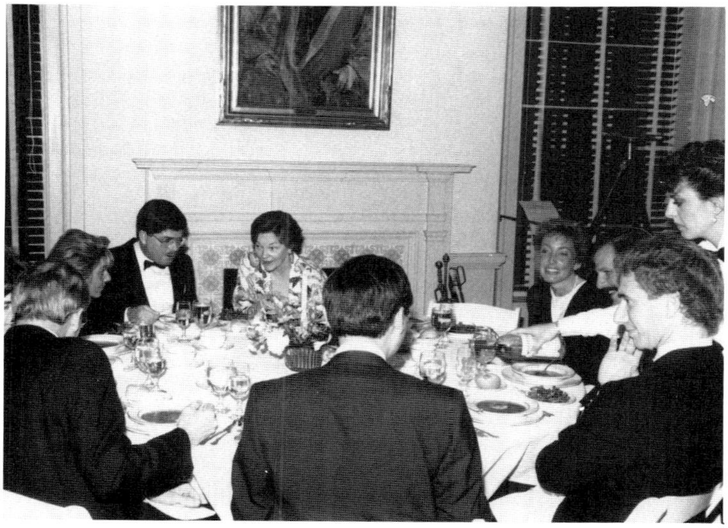

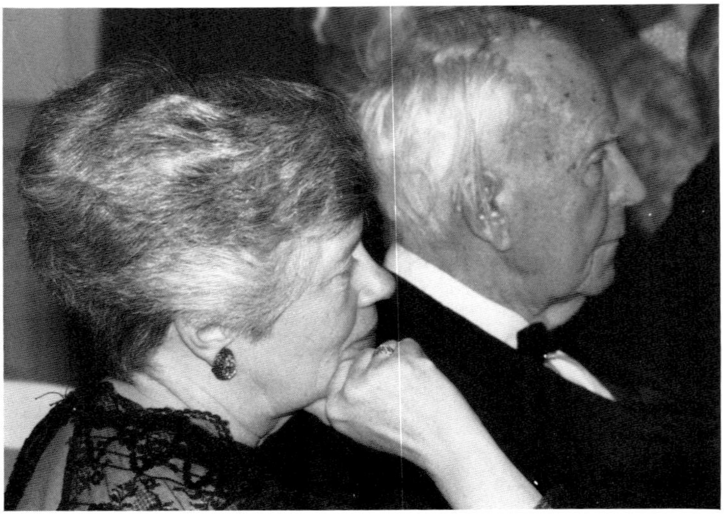

Mrs. Clyde Barker and Charles Huggins, Nobel Laureate, listen to Dr. Rhoads' after dinner remarks.

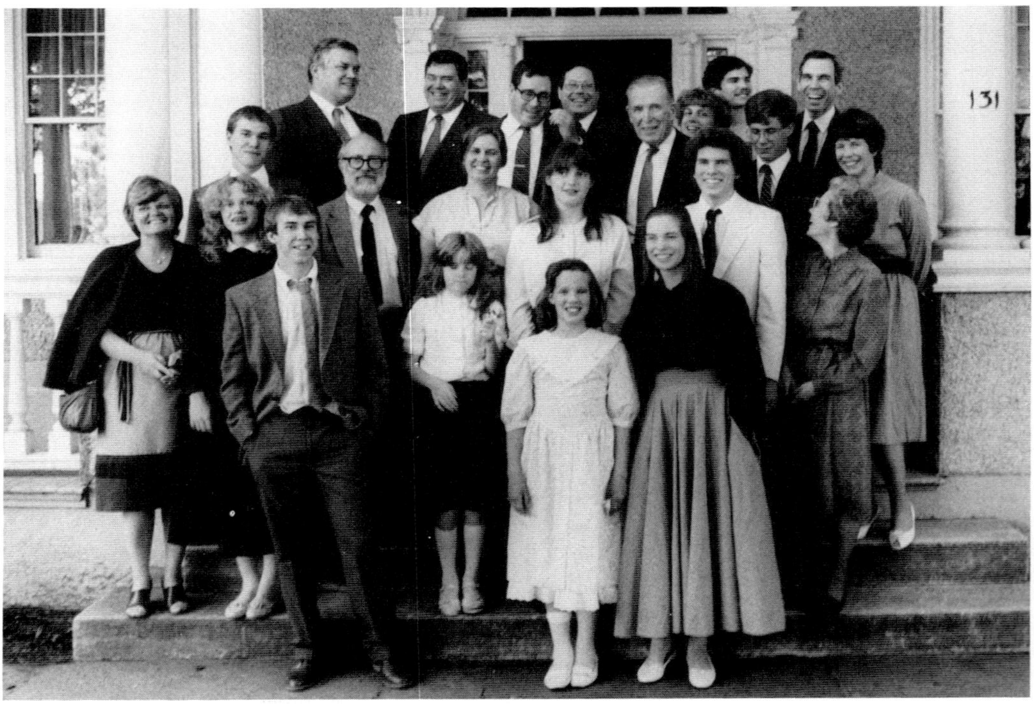

Dr. Jonathan E. Rhoads with his family, May 1987. Front row (left to right): *Barbara Rhoads, Mrs. Philip Rhoads, her daughter Deborah, Benjamin Kendon, Joanna (Philip and Barbara's daughter), and Margaret and Mary Teresa (Jonathan Jr. and Julia's daughters).* Middle row (left to right): *Angus Kendon (Adam and Margaret's son), Adam Kendon (Margaret's husband), Margaret (Dr. Rhoad's daughter), Ruth Anne Rhoads, James Rhoads, and Frances Rhoads.* Back row (left to right): *Dr. Rhoads' sons, Jonathan E. Rhoads, Jr., Edward Rhoads, Charles Rhoads, and Philip Rhoads; Dr. Rhoads; Margaret's daughter, Gudrun; George's son, Thomas; Philip's son, Philip; Dr. Rhoads' son, George; and Jonathan E, Rhoads, Jr.'s wife, Julia.*

Sketches of Dr. Rhoads by Friends

These sketches were presented after the banquet held at Philosophical Hall on May 9, 1987.

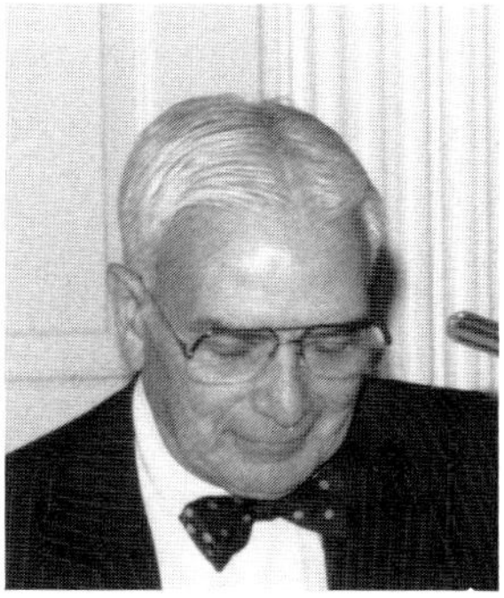

Harris B. Shumacker Jr., M.D.

MAY I OFFER a toast to the "Birthday Boy," Jonathan Rhoads. I do this, not because he and Terry and I have known one another since we entered a medical school down the road in Baltimore, one year minus sixty, and not because we graduated together. Not because we have been the closest of friends for nearly sixty years, but because he really is a great surgeon and because this occasion reminds me of another birthday that Jonathan had. Now I won't tell you exactly when it was, but it was a few decades ago. I believe that he and my wife Myrtie disagree by about one decade, but I think Myrtie is right. Nevertheless, on that occasion, Mealy Gibbon knew of a new drug. I can't remember whether it had been approved by the FDA or not, nor whether the FDA existed in those days, but it was supposed to give one a new hold on life, to give him vigor, vitality, and longevity. And since that time my wife has conducted a controlled, double-blind study of long duration and has come out with a slightly different interpretation. And so we thought that it was an important enough occasion that it couldn't be written in prose. I can't write poetry and so my wife has written this very brief toast, to which I ask you all to drink.

When you were young and sixty and Geritol was new,
Mealy thought it was neaty and gave a draught to you.
But now the years are kinder, there's naught you need to take.
Instead you need a halter and heavy duty brake.

Harris B. Shumacker, Jr., M.D.

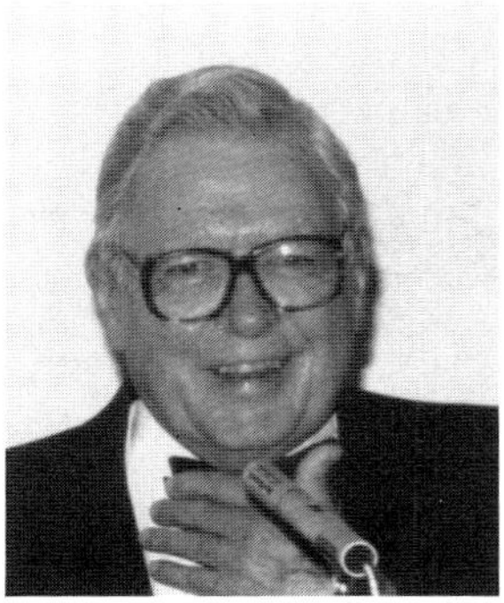

William Longmire M.D.

THANK YOU VERY much, Dr. Barker, Dr. and Mrs. Rhoads, former residents of this wonderful surgical service, and ladies and gentlemen. First, I would just like to express to all of you my appreciation for being invited to come across the continent to participate in this auspicious occasion. I know we've had a wonderful day. Some beautiful papers have been presented, and there are other speakers to follow me this evening, so I thought that I might open by quoting a little saying from Henry VIII as he spoke to each of his six wives, "I won't keep you long." Harry Shumacker has already referred to the fact that Jonathan and he attended one of those unnamed medical schools down the coast a bit. Unfortunately, since I came along a few years later, I missed knowing Jonathan during his medical school days at Johns Hopkins by a couple of years. It wasn't until the great Depression had ended and we were well into those somewhat "heady" post World War II years of the 1950s that Jonathan and I first became acquainted as members of an NIH study section.

I wonder if I might have that first of a few slides that I have of a very personal nature. I don't know whether any of you will be able to identify Dr. Rhoads or not, but in case you can't, he is the gentleman here in the lower right hand corner. ("Hasn't changed a bit," Harry Muller just said). Some of the other people you can see in the background are: Harry Shumacker, Edgar Poth, Richard Warren, Roy Cohen, Simione, and a number of other people in that group. This was taken at the Bohemian Club in San Francisco at a meeting of the Society of University Surgeons in 1949, so there have been a few changes in the faces since that period.

I think our real friendship started when I was appointed as a very junior member of the Surgery Study Section of the NIH. Being very much impressed with this appointment and the recognition that I thought it entailed, when I was given a grant to review, I spent a good deal of time preparing, editing, and typing my remarks, giving them just the right degree of witty, pithy, sarcasm to indicate to my colleagues that I had reviewed the grant very carefully. Well, after the first meeting or so I was very much surprised to look across the table and see Jonathan, who was one of the senior members of that group at that time, presenting his grant reviews from some handwritten notes on the back of a used envelope. As a matter of fact, the slide that you now see was made a few years later and I don't think he was preparing a grant review but more likely his presidential address to the American Surgical Association or the American College of Surgeons. But I quickly learned to appreciate something that I have witnessed over and over again during our thirty years' association, both at work and at play. Those apparently casually scribbled handwritten notes very succinctly distilled the essential components of the pros and cons I had struggled to analyze with such verbose prose. His comments presented a judgment based on such clearly stated logic that there could be little question regarding his recommendations. Some years later, before the Board of Regents of the American College of Surgeons, I would witness some particularly difficult and divisive issue that would be debated to a draw with, at times, heated and emotional arguments. Finally, after all had had their say but the question remained unresolved, and those on both sides of the issue were anxiously searching for a mutually acceptable solution, it would be Jonathan, head bowed, eyes wrinkled, who would slowly summarize the arguments presented and end his discussion with a conclusion so logical, so just, and so straightforward, that all sides rejoiced to have the problem so clearly outlined and so wisely resolved. As I look back on that time, I think we had some successes and we had some failures. I guess one of the great successes, Jonathan, was when we were able to recruit Rollo Hanlon to be the Director of the American College of Surgeons. And I suppose that one of the not so great successes was the time when our financial advisors put a fair amount of the endowment funds in Penn Central.

Well, of course, Jonathan is fond of quoting, I think it was Boswell, when he says, "He who travels can anticipate certain inconveniences." I wouldn't say that this slide shows an example of one of our inconveniences in traveling since we had a private van, and a private driver! We stayed in some marble palaces in Italy and some of the restored chateaus in France and they were great trips. On these trips, I also had an opportunity to witness the more or less Abraham Lincoln-like equanimity of Dr. Rhoads on some of these occasions. As a matter of fact, one time we sat on split rails for our luncheon, and you may be able to see Dr. Rhoads there in the background of this slide. The only difficulty was that we hadn't selected the place for our luncheon very well. It turned out to be right next to an anthill and not far from a swarm of bees, who I think had more of our lunch than we did. One other difficult problem arose in a little family restaurant in Italy. My wife had a good friend on the faculty of UCLA who traveled to that country almost annually, and she insisted that we visit this little family restaurant in Rome and she stated that we should all sample the wonderful pasta dishes that they had. So my wife turned to the rest of us and said each one of us should order a separate pasta dish, and then we could pass them around so that all of us would have an opportunity to sample these dishes. Well, we were astounded a short time later when two waiters came in bearing heavily laden trays and set down six dishes of pasta before each one of us. Somewhere in the translation our intentions had been lost, and I have to admit that I think that Jonathan was the only one who did a fair job on that meal.

One other episode that comes to mind occurred in our travel along the mountain roads of Tuscany, just outside the little village shown in this slide. One of the lugs on the rear wheel came loose, the car started to shimmy, and the doors rattled; it looked as if not only the car but all of the passengers and luggage were going over the side of the road. We very carefully limped into the nearest village and as the car was being repaired, our strong suspicion that Jonathan had a well-concealed sin was exposed when we noticed that every time that we stopped any place, Jonathan would be seen quietly ambling away from the rest of the group, maybe sometimes attracted by a couple of young ladies as shown in this slide, like our friend, Mr. Gary Hart. But more often we would see him disappear into a little delicatessen or a nearby candy store only to come out a short time later with this very satisfied look on his face and his little cache of candies and sweets having been replenished.

Well, I suppose that one of the supreme tests of a man's character and the trust that his friends are willing to place in him comes on a traveling expedition of this kind when the group pools its funds and selects one of the members of the group to handle the finances. I am happy to report that on at least two occasions, Jonathan has been selected for this test. And I am also happy to report to you that he has emerged from this test with his scruples and his morals intact. Through many other crucial tests of character that I've witnessed over the past thirty years, Jonathan continues to stand tall as a friend and, as a colleague with his unique intelligence, his unfailing loyalty, his ready wit and humor, and with a kind, sound judgment that wins the respect of all of us.

William Longmire, M.D.

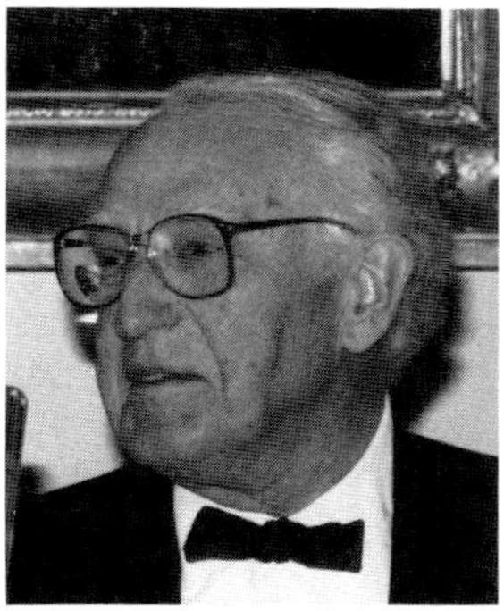

Francis D. Moore, M.D.

JONATHAN AND TERRY, Ladies and Gentlemen. In 1979, Dr. Digby Baltzell, a scholar of our colonial folk ways, published a book entitled *Puritan Boston and Quaker Philadelphia.* Much of the book details the contrasting events in the two rival cities of the British Colonies in the 17th and 18th century. There were bitter rivalries. The book contrasts the ethnic, religious, and cultural mores of the two cities. The author even traces the rise and fall, and later, the expulsion for heterodoxy to a foreign land (as far away as New Jersey!) of certain Quaker families. He tells of the Quakers who came repeatedly to visit and proselytize Puritan New England and were finally hanged because of their religious convictions. This was hardly a hospitable step for the Puritans to take considering their recent loudly stated conviction on religious liberty. The book is a delight for those many of us here tonight who cherish the traditions of these two remarkable communities. It is a very interesting history of the two cities and their rivalry which was so fertile (*i.e.*, a stimulating battle) in both directions in the 16th, 17th, 18th, and 19th centuries. It does open up old sores, and it does point out a couple of embarrassing things. For example, this Philosophical Society was founded in 1742. But in Boston, the American Academy of Arts and Sciences, which was patterned after this great foundation of Benjamin Franklin, wasn't opened until 1782! Pretty sad. Furthermore, the Medical School here was started in 1765 or thereabouts, and Harvard was way behind, coming along in 1782. So in Boston, we have been running along trying to catch up, doing our best while cherishing this interesting rivalry between the two cities.

In the last and final chapter, the author finally gets around to the leading people of the present day, especially those whose ancestry is easily traceable back through these centuries of the growth and flowering of the city of Philadelphia. He writes:

> Dr. Jonathan Rhoads was chosen Provost (of the University of Pennsylvania) by President Harnwell. Dr. Rhoads, the John Rhea Barton Professor of Surgery at Pennsylvania, was on the Board of Haverford College, Bryn Mawr College, A Director of the Provident Mutual Bank, President of the American Philosophical Society, and generally acknowledged to be the City's First Citizen when he received the Philadelphia Award in 1977.

Of such a man do we weave tales of affection and reminiscence tonight. Jonathan was a man not content with the accoutrements or vestments of honors, achievements, and professorships. He took off his suit, donned his scrub clothes, rolled up his sleeves, and delved into the blood and guts, not only of surgical care to alleviate suffering, but of science, to advance knowledge.

I would like to focus on some special aspects: his tenacity in science and his consistent exhibition of two traits, two scientific tastes that are of immense importance for any scientist and that have characterized Jonathan's work over the decades. First, is a taste for simplicity and directness. Possibly this is Quaker in origin. And second, a strong sense of what is important in the advance of human knowledge in the biomedical sciences.

Starting over thirty years ago, working in the Harrison Department of Surgical Research, Jonathan became interested in surgical nutrition. That was also an interest of ours up there at Harvard Medical School in rival Boston. We viewed his work with interest, envy, a sense of rivalry, and sometimes a bit of skepticism. He wrote many articles on hypoproteinemia in rats produced as a result of a low protein diet. We often looked in vain for much about serum protein concentrations, which is what the word means. But never mind the words. These protein-lacking rats of Jonathan's were of major interest. Then, a few years later, he became interested in fostering nutrition by infusing lots and lots of useful soluble nutrient "goodies," but then getting rid of all that extra water with a solute diuresis. At that time, we were trying to do the same thing, providing both calories and a diuresis, with intravenous alcohol.

So, at that time, and I think it was some time in the '50s or early '60s, Jonathan's subjects enjoyed good nutrition, but had to ask the nurse for the urinal quite frequently, or go off down the hall to the bathroom pushing their IV poles before them. Meanwhile, our patients *enjoyed* nutrition and went off blissfully to sleep with smiles on their faces.

And then, finally, his team—many of whom are here tonight, including Dr. Wilmore, Dr. Vars, and Dr. Dudrick—produced that simple experiment in growing puppies that gave the word modern intravenous nutrition; a new term, the "lifeline"; and that masterly contradiction in terms, "total parenteral alimentation."

His were experiments that needed no statistics. There was no complexity. They were simple and direct, right to the point, and very, very significant. They didn't even need large numbers. They just showed that puppies grown on nothing but intravenous nourishment grew normally in every way. There was a sort of a new phenomenology in this, leaving no doubt in anyone's mind.

There are several things that have occurred in science during this century, in which all areas of biology and medicine owe a debt to surgery. There was the pump oxygenator (also a Philadelphia product), allotransplantation of organs (for which Boston might claim some credit), certain aspects of the endocrine treatment of cancer (the Nobelist is with us tonight), microvascular anastomosis (New York is heard from at last?), the use of lasers to repair the retina (surely not the Pentagon here!), and the localization of functional areas in the cerebral cortex (Montreal owns this one). To these epoch-making advances, the kind for which Nobel Prizes are awarded, we must add total intravenous feeding—the product of Jonathan's long and tenacious study.

The world owes this advance to Jonathan Rhoads. It was one of his several peaks. Just as the loftiness of peaks in a mountain range rise as you recede from the range and can see them in perspective, so also this advance of Jonathan's has become clearly more and more preeminent as the years have passed.

As I come down here tonight to the Philosophical Society, from that ancient rival city of Boston, I bring greetings to Jonathan from his many friends and associates in surgery and in all fields of life and from the Dean of the Harvard Medical School, Dan Tosteson, who has worked with Jonathan in several projects.

But I think especially of Dr. Walter Cannon, a Harvard faculty member of an earlier generation. He had no Quaker background. His was an Irish family that came across Canada to central Wisconsin in the late 18th century. But he was tenacious, brilliant, and went for the heart of important concepts by simple experimentations. I bring with me tonight a new biography of Cannon written by our colleague in physiology, Dr. A. Clifford Barger. The book tells of the life work of Dr. Cannon, surely the greatest scientist on the faculty in my medical school days at Harvard, and a close associate of Dr. Otto Folin, the father of Terry Rhoads.

So, both for reasons of its symbolism in science, and of some personal and family comments made in the book, I present to Jonathan and Terry, the biography of Walter Cannon, as a gift from Laurie and me to the Rhoadses. But also, it symbolizes the many friendly gestures between Boston and Philadelphia, despite all those ancient rivalries dealt with in Mr. Balzel's book, and is most fitting for me to present from the Harvard Faculty. As I give it to him, I am moved by the fact that I am giving a biography of Walter Cannon, one of my scientific gods, to the Walter Cannon of American Surgery, Dr. Jonathan Rhoads.

Francis D. Moore, M.D.

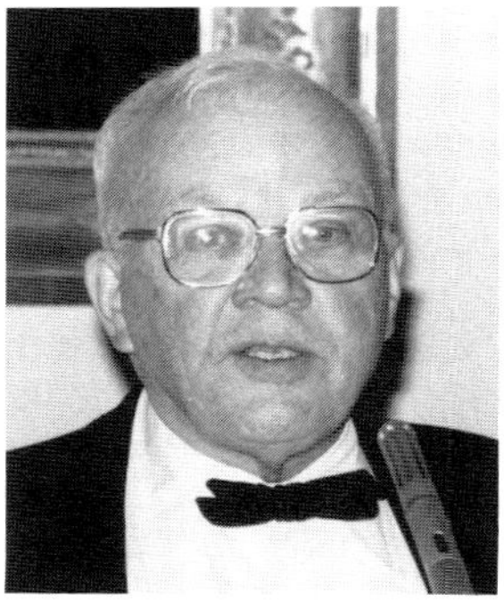

Whitfield J. Bell, Jr., M.D.

AT THE RECEPTION across the street earlier this evening, someone asked "Where are we?" And perhaps you will permit me to answer that we are in the hall of the American Philosophical Society which was erected in 1785, in Franklin's day. This portrait of Franklin on this wall was given to the Society by Charles Willson Peale, when the Society was raising money for this building. Artists like himself, he said, ought to contribute something of their handiwork to the Society rather than pay a subscription for bricks and mortar. So he copied this painting, which was in Franklin's house, and gave it to the Society, where it has been ever since. The portrait of Thomas Jefferson on that wall was made at Monticello when Jefferson was 79-years-old. What a marvelous face that is for a man of 79. I might also have pointed to the portrait of George Washington, ordered by the Society from Gilbert Stuart a few weeks after Washington's death, but it is on exhibition in another building in connection with the bicentennial of the Constitution. So much for where we are.

It is a welcome task for me, but not an easy one, to join in paying a tribute of respect and affection to our friend and to do it in terms that are appropriate, ample, simple, and deserved. Had I been one of Jonathan's patients or were I speaking as their representative, I would say to him and to you, (as I have said often to other people) that if I were seriously ill and Jonathan simply walked through my room, I would feel better. For in addition to abilities and wisdom and personal integrity, he has "reserve force." That word was used more than a century ago of George Bacon Wood, who like Jonathan, was also a professor in the University of Pennsylvania Medical School and president of the College of Physicians of Philadelphia and president of the American Philosophical Society. And if it be objected that Wood was a physician and Jonathan is a surgeon, then let me mention William W. Keen, like Jonathan a distinguished surgeon and teacher of surgeons, and like Jonathan and Wood a president of the College of Physicians of Philadelphia and of the American Philosophical Society. Their portraits hang on these walls, as Jonathan's will when his modesty can be sufficiently overcome to allow us to have it painted. Thus, in this place tonight, Jonathan is surrounded by well-wishers of this and former generations.

He was elected president of this Society in 1977. Now, the president of the Society is ex-officio a member of practically every committee (and that is a great many), and as is to be expected, presidents vary in the extent and intensity of the interest they take in committee business. What kind of president Jonathan would be I learned at the first meeting of the Library Committee after his election. On that day ten years ago, Jonathan was attending a professional meeting in Texas. He certainly could not be expected to attend our little meeting, but he flew up from Texas that morning, attended the meeting of the Library Committee, attended another meeting of the Society, and then flew back to Texas, where he delivered a Presidential Address to a surgical society that evening. Reporting this afterward in amazement and admiration to one who knew him then better than I, I was told that that performance was nothing unusual, as indeed I soon learned it was not. Which brings me to his schedule.

Each week we received a mimeographed sheet or two listing his appointments and engagements. Just to read this document, one member of our staff exclaimed, made her tired; while another, having examined several of these schedules over several weeks, announced that Dr. Rhoads had apparently discovered how to live without food or sleep. As president of the Society, he acquainted himself with every aspect of its work. Give him an agenda, a committee report, a budget, a suggestion, or a proposal and he would screw his face into a squint, frown, and read it carefully item by item, missing nothing and forgetting nothing, least of all the objectives of the exercise. In particular, he understood the peculiar nature of the American Philosophical Society. It was, of course, a matter of satisfaction to him that its finances were no cause for worry or alarm. Members of the finance committee readily admitted that he had the best financial judgment of any of them; it would often happen that after the bankers and the brokers and lawyers had considered what they should buy or sell, the chairman would turn to Jonathan and ask, "Dr. Rhoads, what is your judgment"? and he might reply in his slow, deliberate way, "I wouldn't put my money in it," and that settled it.

He knows about bottom lines, but he knows also that in a scholarly enterprise like a college or a learned society, the bottom line is measured in new knowledge and understanding, in new books and experiments, in young careers and the confidence and imagination to support them. He never expected the final accounting to be rendered on the next December 31. He conducted our meetings in the solid Quaker way: inviting ideas, tolerating even rambling irrelevances, and then in a few words, summing up the consensus, which everyone recognized, of course, as the only sensible action to take. Every few years, for example, some members of the American Philosophical Society become exercised over its very large number of aged members, and suggestions would fly back and forth for bringing in what is called "new blood." Jonathan once brought such a discussion back to basics by observing quietly that, with respect to the nonogenarians, time and nature would soon restore the balance. He is never hurried, always wise, sometimes witty; one of the most surprising and delightful sights is to see that great face break up into laughter at one of his own jokes.

As president of the Philosophical Society, he was sometimes called upon for a service none of his predecessors had performed, unless it be Wood or Keen, that of unofficial medical consultant. If some member of the staff falls ill with something serious or recalcitrant, Jonathan is asked for reassurance, advice, or the name of a specialist. Once, at a meeting of the Executive Committee, our legal counsel remarked that his knee was troubling him. "Roll up your trousers and I'll look at it," Jonathan ordered, and he did.

What was said of George Bacon Wood may be said with equal appropriateness of Jonathan Rhoads: he possesses capacity of a high order and has a methodical and mathematical mind, a striking feature of which is in its strong common sense. With this is united the greatest, perhaps, of all talents, steady and unwearied application.

Whitfield J. Bell, Jr., M.D.

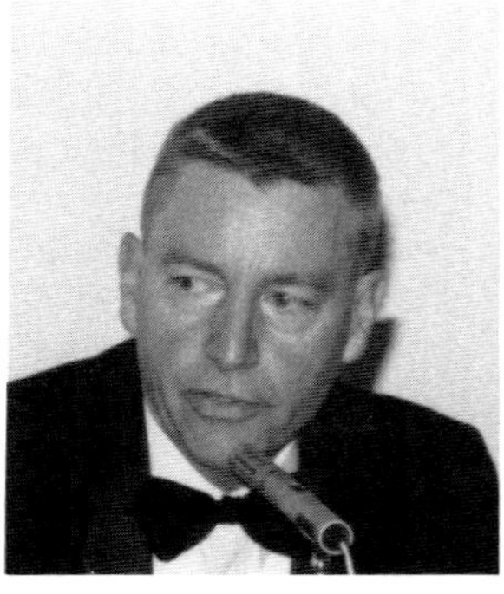

Clyde F. Barker, M.D.

AFTER THE AMERICAN Philosophical Society has been represented by Whitfield Bell, great schools of surgery in Baltimore and Los Angeles by Bill Longmire and the one in Boston by Francis Moore, I am intimidated by the assignment of representing the University of Pennsylvania. First, I want to express the gratitude of the Department, to our loyal graduates and to Dr. Rhoads' many friends for traveling to Philadelphia and for making this such a marvelous day and evening. We hope you will agree to come and do it again in another eighty years.

In this great hall of the American Philosophical Society, it seems mandatory to consider Jonathan Rhoads' career in historical perspective. With regard to the Department of Surgery of the University of Pennsylvania, many of us feel that he *is* the Department and indeed we can relate Dr. Rhoads' career to almost a third of this venerable Department's history. To do this we will have to exclude the earliest years of the School of Medicine, which dates to 1765, and begin in 1805 when Philip Syng Physick, was appointed Professor of Surgery. Philip Syng Physick was, after all, an old-timer. He was John Marshall's doctor and Andrew Jackson's doctor, and he was the Department's first real Professor of Surgery, since prior to his time it had been a Department of Anatomy and Surgery. If we jump only 80 years forward to 1885 when D. Hayes Agnew was Professor of Surgery, we can already make an association with Jonathan Rhoads, since his father served that year as a house officer under Agnew at HUP, which opened the year before. Four years after Dr. Rhoads' father was an intern at the new University Hospital, Thomas Eakins' Agnew Clinic was unveiled at the commencement exercises in which William Osler gave the Valedictorian address *Aequanimitas* just before leaving our faculty for that other school in Baltimore. Forty-seven years later, Jonathan Rhoads was a house officer at HUP. Thus, we find that Dr. Rhoads himself spans about a third, and he and his father collectively more than half of the Department's history.

However, such considerations are far too serious for tonight's happy occasion. We have heard about the accomplishments of Dr. Rhoads and his students during today's scientific program, and this evening, we have heard about his contributions to American surgery, to the Philosophical Society, and to his city. I will now attempt to review some less generally known aspects of his career and to develop the case that as he has approached his 80th birthday, he has actually been getting younger. Figure 1 shows the young Jonathan Rhoads with his father, Agnew's and Osler's intern. In 1921, Jonathan entered Westtown School where Ted Hetzell, one of his classmates, photographed him as shown in Figure 2, already in his Lincolnesque mode.

At Haverford College, he must have had a rather carefree and wonderful time. Mentioned on this page from the Haverford yearbook of 1928 (Figure 3) are his college nicknames, "Colossus" and "Johnny," neither of which I've heard anyone use lately, although I submit that one of them is apt. The rest of the text from the yearbook page reads as follows:

> "Place: The eighth entry of Lloyd, [which I assume is one of the dormitories] Time: anytime day or night. Enter Rhoads preceded by his after dinner war whoop. There follows a business of raising hell accompanied by loud shrieks from the victims and the turmoil concludes with the forcible eviction of Jonathan or the miraculous escape of everyone else. Jonathan's accomplishments are many and varied, he is always the first in the dining room, has never been known to complete a chemistry experiment, knows more math than anyone, never studies until the day before an examination. He has the distinctions of aptly defining philosophy as saying things that everybody knows in words that no one can understand and of lifting his huge bulk 11 ft. in the air with the aid of a bamboo pole. Where he will end up we hesitate to say but he will probably succeed in inventing a radio controlled auto if premature death is not incurred through his indulgence in experimental aeronautics" [which I suggest is what he has been doing in his automobile all of these years]

Dr. Rhoads once told me a wonderful story about his college days. On May 21, 1927, he was competing in a track meet at Union College where things were going quite well for him in his event, the pole vault. At this point, Dr. Rhoads remembers that the announcement of the news of Lindbergh's transatlantic flight so distracted the crowd that they lost interest in the results of the pole vaulting. He did, in fact, clear 11 ft. 9 in., which might not sound like much in these days of the fiberglass pole, but he then missed, a very close miss, at 12 ft. 1 in., which would have been a Middle-Atlantic record.

After college, his career probably provided fewer carefree days. His chief, Dr. Ravdin, had high expectations of everyone and could not have been an easy man for the youthful Jonathan Rhoads to work for, first as a house officer and then as a young faculty member (Figure 4). However, these two developed a warm relationship. They are also shown in Figure 5 a few years later, perhaps at about the time when the young Jonathan Rhoads, only recently finished with his residency, was chosen by Dr. Ravdin to operate upon him when Rav developed acute cholecystitis. His activities, however, were evidently not totally confined to hard work, and Jonathan and Terry soon began their large and wonderful family.

They are shown in Figure 6 in 1938 with their children. I was reminded in the next photograph (Figure 7) [which Terry provided]) of a song in a musical by Steven Sondheim. The lyrics go something like this, "Here I am with my feet on the ground and you in the air." Certainly, Jonathan's feet are on the ground and Terry's are in the air, but it is evident from the expression on their faces that they are happy and very much in love.

Eventually, in 1959, Dr. Rhoads became John Rhea Barton Professor and Chairman. The next 13 years must have been an especially demanding time in his life, but the outcome of his effort was one of America's great departments of surgery. A plaque outside his office listed the names of his faculty: I. S. Ravdin (at that time Emeritus), Julian Johnson, Henry Royster, Bill Fitts, Clete Schwegman, Brooke Roberts, Robert Ravdin, Peter Randall, Jack Mackie, Bugs Lehr, Bill Inouye, Bob Crichlow, Len Miller, Horace MacVaugh, John Waldhausen, Frank Rosato, Ralph Hamilton, Dutch Dyson, and Stan Dudrick and myself.

Even more impressive, perhaps, was his record as Director of the Harrison Department of Surgical Research. Under his stewardship, the genesis of much of the work described earlier today took place and, of course, this included the crucial experiments on hyperalimentation, a story told so well this evening by Dr. Moore (Figure 8).

Perhaps the most impressive tribute to his performance as a chairman is the subsequent record of the chief residents he turned out. Suffice it to say that 62 of his residents now hold academic appointments in 34 different American medical schools: 28 are full professors and 11 have become chairmen (Table 1).

In 1972, Dr. Rhoads stepped down as Chairman. We know that this would not by any means relax him, but one might say that after this, he seemed to attack life with a slightly more casual intensity. While he was Chairman, my fellow residents and I would swap stories, a good many of which we've heard today, concerning his aggressiveness behind the wheel of an automobile and in the operating room. We imitated the timbre and inflections of his measured speech, but did this never in his presence. It never occurred to us that anyone would ever tease him about an idiosyncrasy. However, after he was finished with the chairmanship, he seemed a bit different, more approachable, and the younger residents, while deeply respecting him, did things those of my generation would never have considered. Sometimes, he even became the subject of cartoons drawn by the residents, such as this one shown in Figure 9. He continued to travel more than any other faculty member, still had a large surgical practice, still took notes at scientific meetings, and discussed papers with authority. But, at the same time, he became a more relaxed and skillful after-dinner speaker, a genuine raconteur. Indeed, he seemed to have become younger.

Also during this period, he found himself with time to attend the reunions of Provosts of the University. In Figure 10, we see him with Elliot Stellar, the new President of the American Philosophical Society, and Vartan Gregorian and the other recent provosts who succeeded him. He also attended reunions of the Presidents of the American College of Surgeons, a number of whom are with us tonight (Figure 11). He had time to receive the congratulations of the country's presidents, such as Jimmy Carter and Ronald Reagan (Figure 12). He had time to receive honorary degrees from many universities. A revealing story goes with the degree given to him by Georgetown. In 1981, Dr. Rhoads was on his way to Washington from a meeting in Europe, and during the transatlantic flight, he realized that he had developed thrombophlebitis. However, he was not deterred from appearing at the commencement by this inconvenience nor even by his additional self-diagnosis shortly thereafter of a pulmonary embolus. After accepting the degree (Figure 13), he caught the train to Philadelphia, came directly to the Hospital, and gave himself up for heparin treatment over the next several weeks. His priorities are well-illustrated by this episode. One can't help admiring his stoicism while at the same time wishing that he would show more concern over his health.

We hope that during these recent years he has been able to spend more time with Terry (Figure 14). My impression is that he has generally been having a good time, and this has certainly been well-deserved.

It has been mentioned tonight that Dr. Rhoads received the Philadelphia award a few years ago. In his acceptance speech, he referred to Benjamin Franklin saying, "His breadth of interest, his belief in the role of private citizens in advancing the public interest, his sagacity and his amazing capacity for getting things done by avoiding self aggrandizement are characteristics exemplified by many generations of Philadelphians." I submit that these are characteristics not commonly exemplified by Philadelphians or anyone else, but that they are exemplified by Jonathan Rhoads. For 55 years at the University of Pennsylvania, he has been a man for all seasons. We wish that we could have 55 more like these.

Since my thesis tonight was that the recent years have made Dr. Rhoads seem younger, I'll close by showing a series of photographs in reverse chronological order: Karsh's photograph of him now (Figure 15A), as a member of the Haverford Board (Figure 15B), as a senior faculty member (Figure 15C), as a young faculty member (Figure 15D), as a house officer (Figure 15E), and finally, getting back to a time that must have been an especially good one, his college days, a photograph, which I have spent the last two weeks searching for and about which I'd like to create a little suspense. If I were to give Dr. Rhoads a birthday present, it would have to be in the form of a wish. Since he has achieved virtually everything in life, it is difficult to wish something for him that he hasn't already had. Thus, my wish for him is for one more sunny Saturday afternoon in May of 1928, a fiberglass pole, and another crack at that 12 ft. 1 in. collegiate record in the pole vault (Figure 16).

Addendum: Dr. Rhoads confided to me the day after the symposium that his third attempt at 12 ft. 1 in. was made after his coach, in smoothing out the runway, inadvertently erased the marks Dr. Rhoads had carefully made after the previous jumps. What impact the need to replace these reference points had on his last unsuccessful try he doesn't know but, he remembered with a shrug, "It didn't help."

Clyde F. Barker, M.D.

Illustrations of Dr. Barker's Sketch

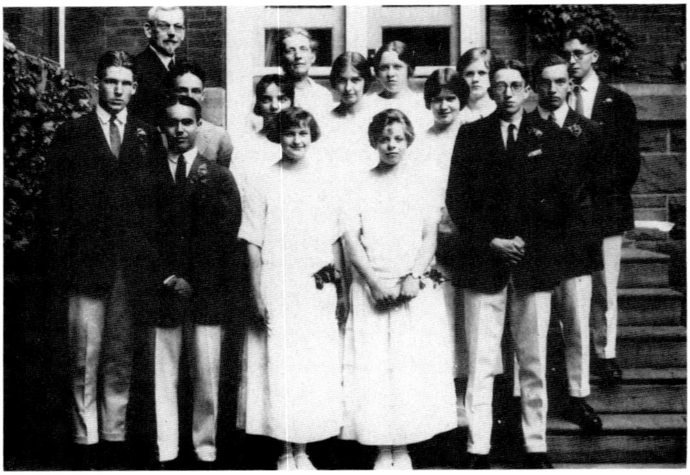

Figure 1. Dr. Edward Rhoads (Dr. Jonathan Rhoads' father who served as a house officer at HUP under Agnew and Osler), Mrs. Rhoads, Jonathan (at far left), *Ted Hetzel next to JER, and other Westtown School classmates on Commencement Day in 1924.*

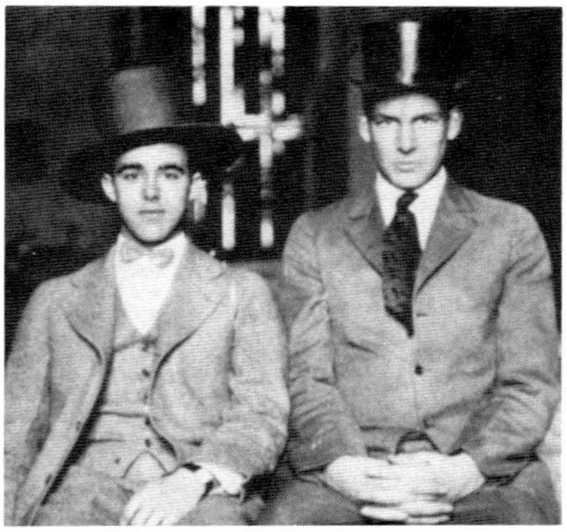

Figure 2. Dr. Rhoads as a high school senior in 1924 with Westtown School classmate Ted Hetzel.

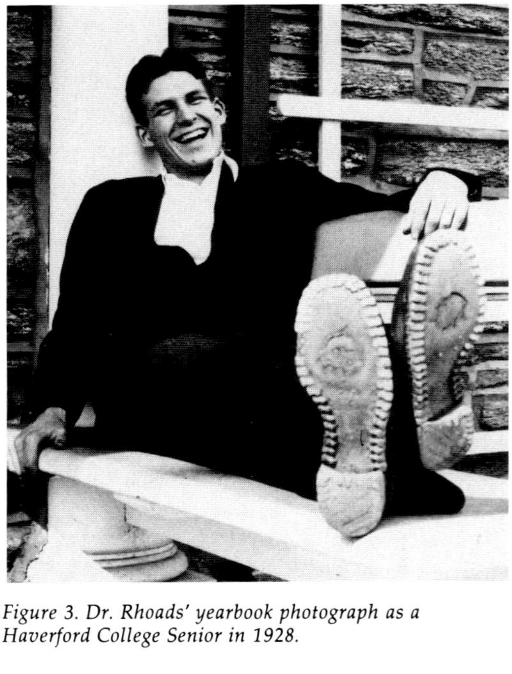

Figure 3. Dr. Rhoads' yearbook photograph as a Haverford College Senior in 1928.

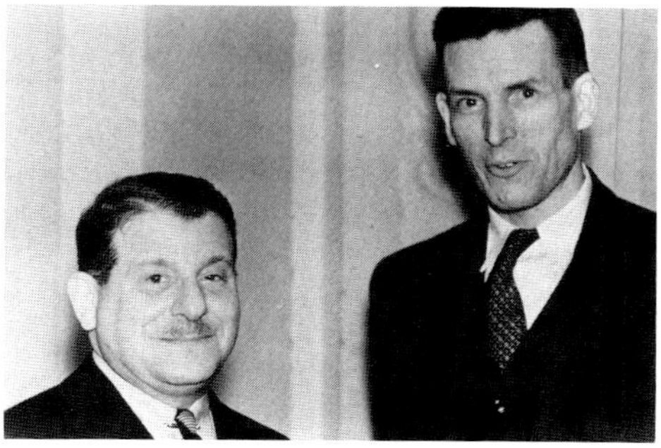

Figure 4. Dr. I. S. Ravdin with the young Dr. Rhoads.

Figures 5. Dr. Rhoads discusses a case with his chief, I. S. Ravdin.

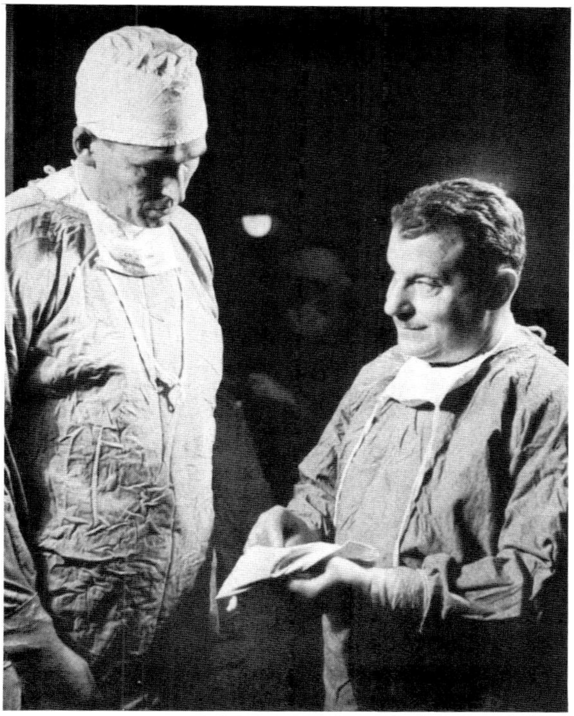

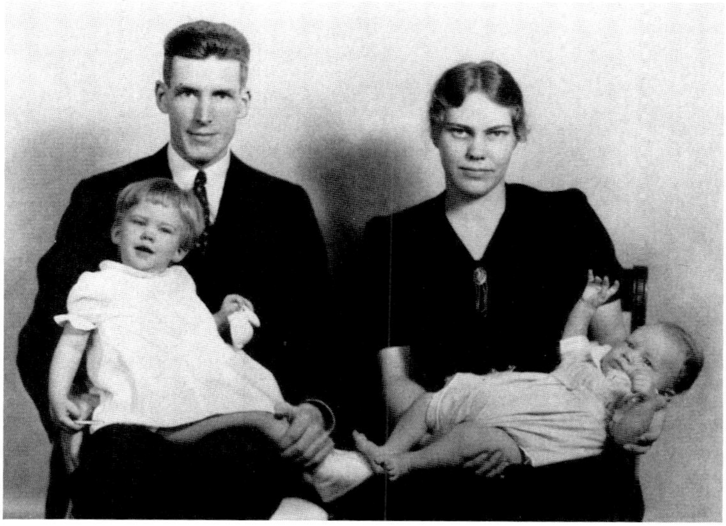

Figures 6. Dr. and Mrs. Rhoads in 1938 with their children, Margaret and Jonathan, Jr.

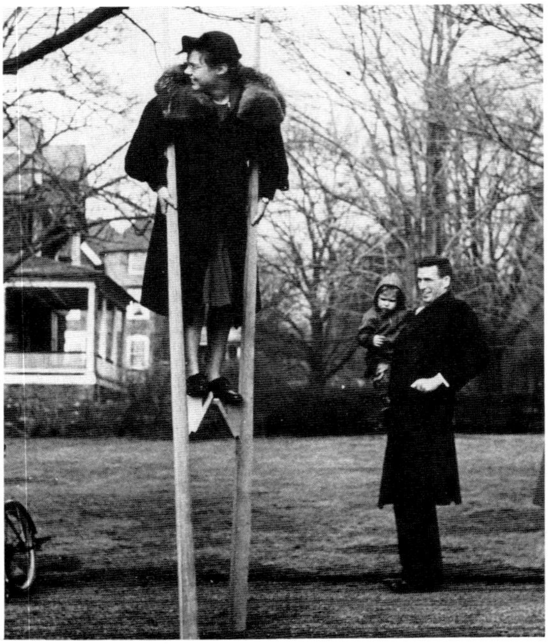

Figures 7. Dr. and Mrs. Rhoads and their son George in an informal moment at their home in 1942.

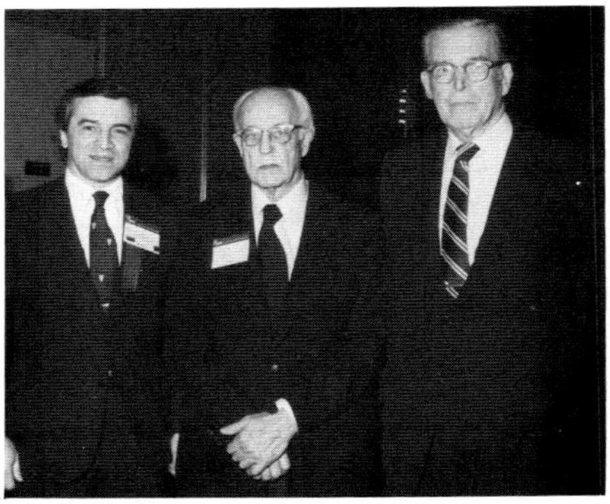

Figures 8. Dr. Rhoads in 1982 with his colleagues in the development of hyperalimentation, Drs. Harry Vars and Stan Dudrick.

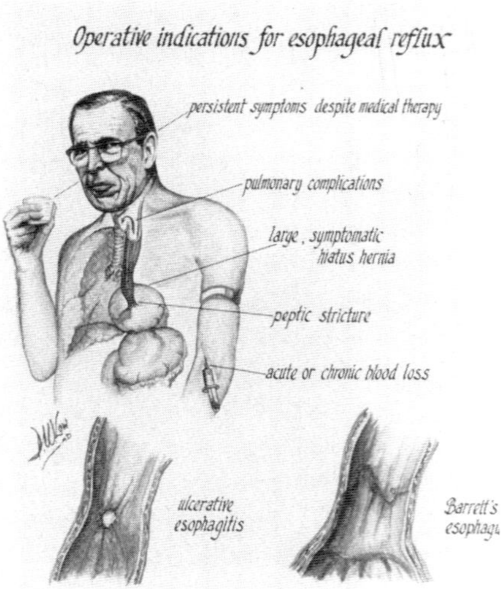

Figures 9. Cartoon of Dr. Rhoads by Dr. David Low, a gifted medical illustrator who was HUP Chief Resident 1985–86.

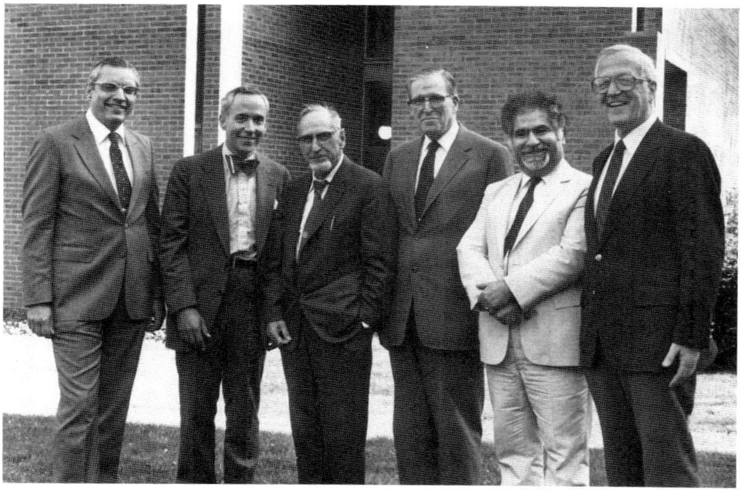

Figure 10. Dr. Rhoads with other recent provosts of the University of Pennsylvania. (Left to right): Curtis Reitz, Thomas Ehrlich, David Goddard, Jonathan E. Rhoads, Vartan Gregorian, and Elliot Stellar.

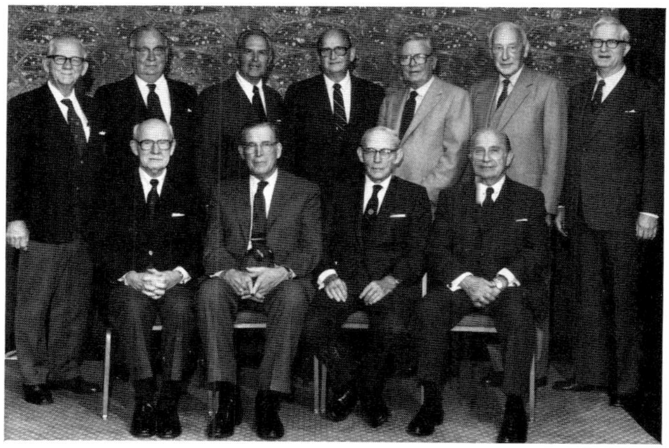

Figure 11. Past Presidents of the American College of Surgeons, five of whom attended the Rhoads Birthday Symposium. (Seated, left to right): Charles W. McLaughlin, Jr., Jonathan E. Rhoads, Warren H. Cole, and Robert M. Zollinger. (Standing, left to right): William A. Altemeier, Frank E. Stinchfield, H. William Scott, Jr., William H. Muller, Jr., Wiliam P. Longmire, Jr., Claude E. Welch, and James D. Hardy.

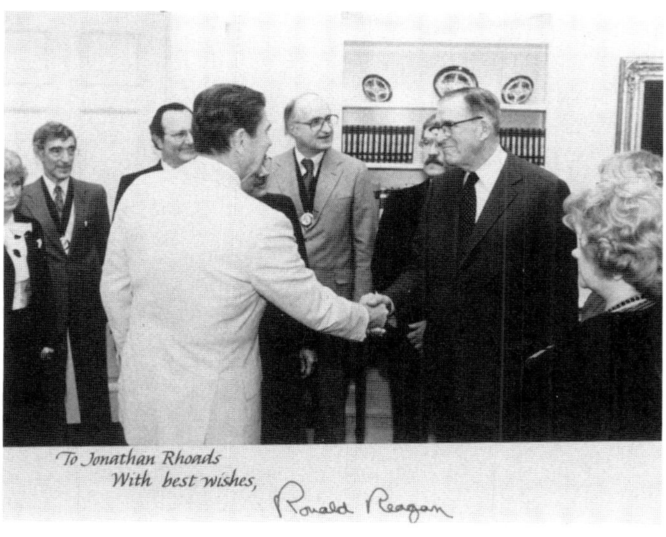

Figure 12. Dr. Rhoads with President Reagan.

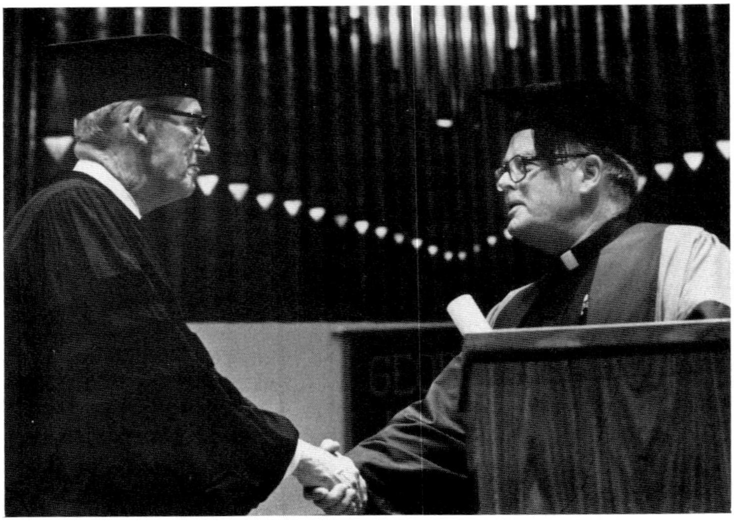

Figure 13. Dr. Rhoads receiving his honorary D.Sc. degree in 1981 from Georgetown President Timothy S. Healey, shortly after having self-diagnosed a pulmonary embolus.

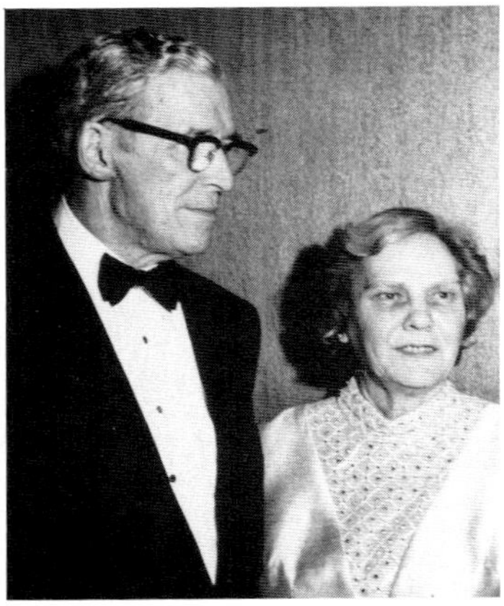

Figure 14. Dr. and Mrs. Rhoads in 1972.

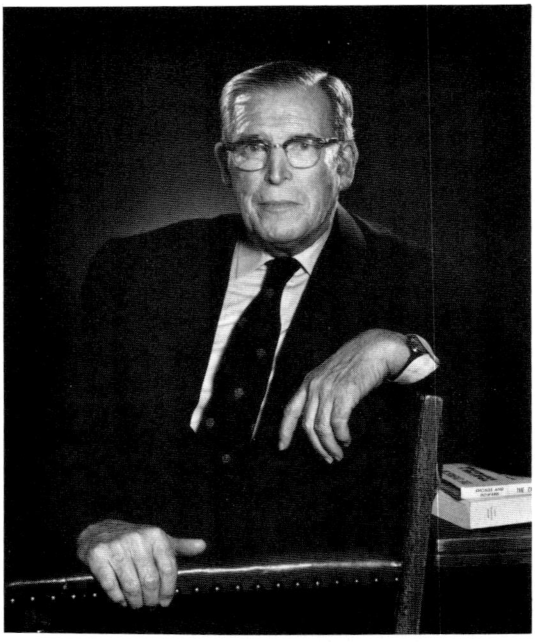

Figure 15A. Dr. Rhoads in 1983 as photographed by Yousuf Karsh.

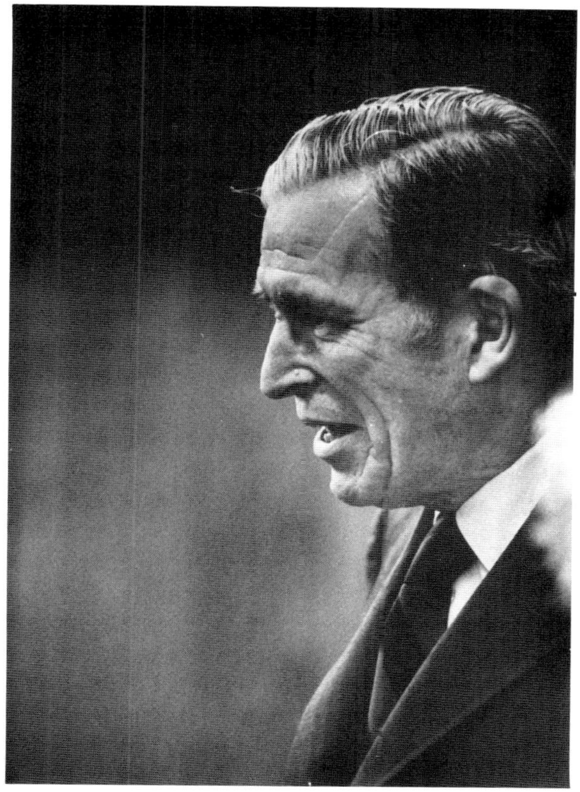

Figure 15B. Dr. Rhoads at a Haverford College Board Meeting.

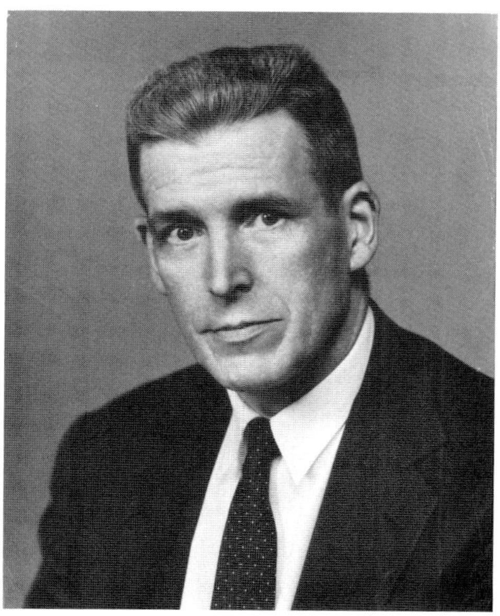

Figure 15C. Dr. Rhoads as a senior faculty member.

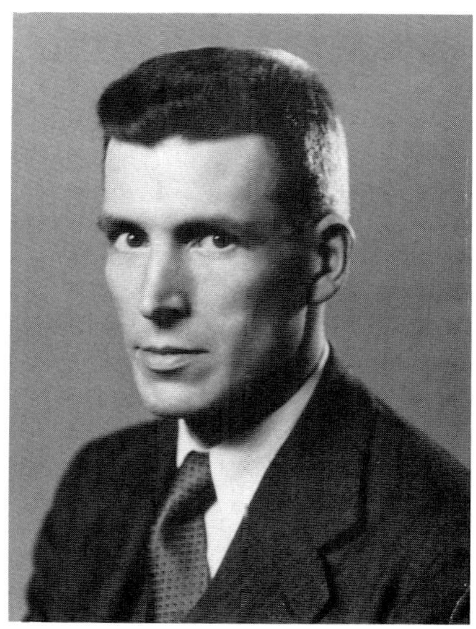

Figure 15D. Dr. Rhoads as a young faculty member.

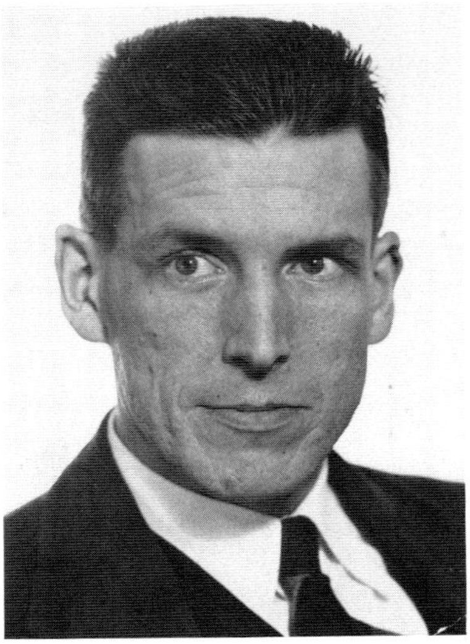

Figure 15E. Dr. Rhoads as a house officer.

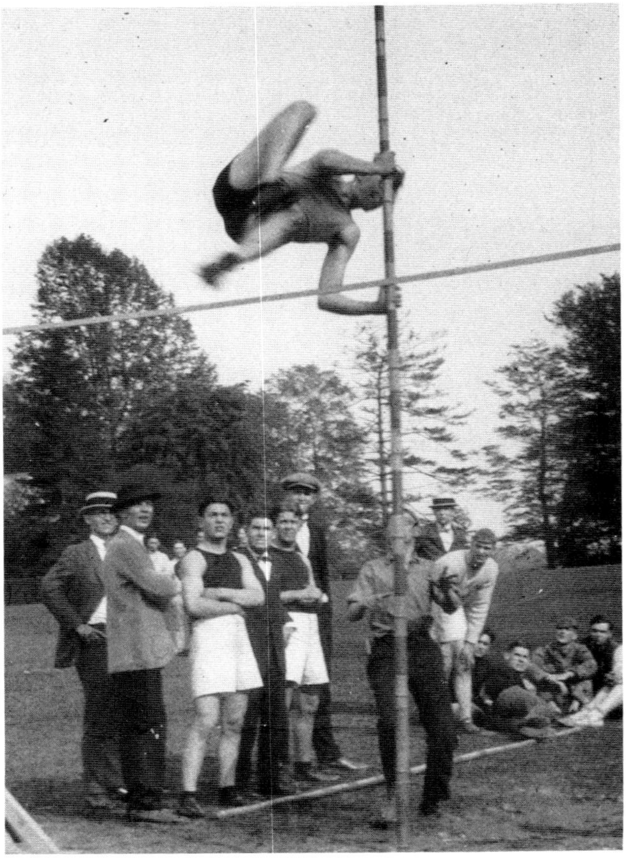

Figure 16. Dr. Rhoads as a pole vaulter for Haverford College in 1928.

TABLE 1

Chief Residents at HUP During Dr. Rhoads' Chairmanship

1959–60

Davis, Arnold V. O.
Dexheimer, Frank R.
Gyorgy, Tilbert R. M.
Muir, William R.
Orr, Jack T.
Wolferth, Charles C., Jr.

1960–61

Akin, John M., Jr.
Hood, Frederick R., Jr.
Inouye, William Y.
Light, Harry G.
Patterson, Lewis T.
Smart, Charles R.

1961–62

Danielson, Gordon K.
Johnson, LeRoy L.
Kessler, Frederick B.
Nightingalte, David S.
Timmis, Hilary H.

1962–63

Barnes, Anne U.
Berggren, Ronald B.
Crichlow, Robert W.
Heisterkamp, Charles A.
Jannetta, Peter J.
Nelson, Harry M., Jr.

1963–64

Barker, Clyde F.
Hardesty, William H.
Mac Vaugh, Horace III
Miller, Leonard D.
Myint, Maung Kyaw

1964–65

Hartzell, George W.
Johnson, Charles J.
Spagna, Paschal M.
Talman, E. Armistead

1965–66

Hamilton, Ralph W.
Nance, F. Carter
Reis, Robert L.
Rosato, Francis E.

1966–67

Dudrick, Stanley J.
Jones, Rayford S.
Kaplan, Edwin L.
Noto, Joseph A.
Weiner, Leonard J.

1967–68

Boruchow, Irwin B.
Curreri, P. William
Neiby, C. Paul
Rosato, Ernest F.
Tyers, G. Frank O.
Vibul, Santi

1968–69

Berkowitz, Henry B
Copeland, Edward M., III
Hanson, Victor A.
Knecht, James W.
Park, C. Dick
Pierce, William S.

1969–70

Diaco, Joseph F.
Lundy, Barbara S.
Noble, Raymond
Reber, Howard A.
Saik, Richard P.

1970–71

Appel, Sidney D.
Attkiss, Michael J.
Finnegan, James O.
Noone, R. Barrett
Perloff, Leonard J.
Seltzer, Murray H.
Staroscik, Rudolf N.
Wilmore, Douglas W.

1971–72

Agnes, Robert F.
Allen, Tery R.
Coller, John A.
Friedman, Jerald N
Long, James M., III
Lynch, Dennis J.
Nicholas, Gary G.
Silberman, Howard

Assistant Residents at HUP During Dr. Rhoads' Chairmanship

Agris, Joseph
Brown, Arthur S.
Butler, Charles J.
Caplan, Howard S.
Cayten, C. Gene
Davis, Robert M.

Edynak, Eugene M.
Ellman, Barry R.
Gittleman, Mark A.
Goodwin, Cleon W., Jr.
Gray, Dennis C.
Jacobs, William E.

Kellet, Cyril F., Jr.
Kyger, E. Ross, III
Levin, John M.
Mac Fayden, Bruce V., Jr.
Mayer, Lawrence J.
McClure, John M., III

Mullen, James L., Jr.
Mullis, William F.
Naji, Ali
Reckard, Craig R.
Ruberg, Robert L.
Samuels, Garth A. S.

Saxena, Naresh C.
Shesol, Barry F.
Shumate, George R.
Steiger, Ezra
Sugerman, Harvey J.
Thomas, James H.

Tomasello, Donald N.
Wallack, Marc K.
White, Raleigh R., IV
Williams, Gary A.
Ziegler, Moritz M.

Response by Jonathan E. Rhoads, M.D.

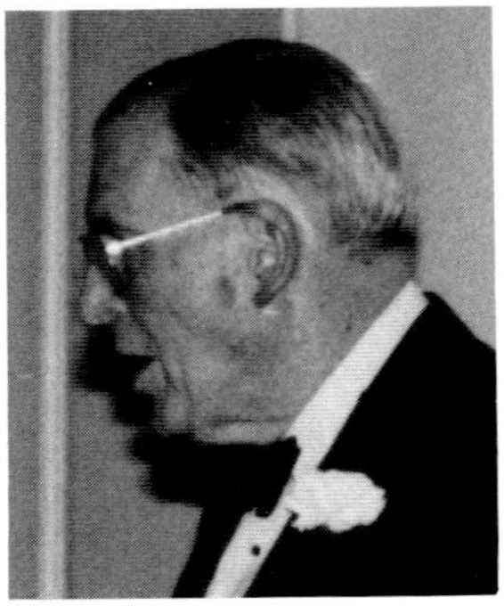

LADIES AND GENTLEMEN, this is an extraordinary experience for me. I have had experiences of a different kind in the course of university life, as all of you can imagine. But anyhow, I won't deny that I've enjoyed it, and I'll try not to take it too seriously. I think perhaps I should start off with a story that I was going to end up with. I think that of all the American surgeons, perhaps the one that had the most delicious sense of humor was Englebert Dunphy. When he described his retirement dinner, he said that he'd been officially appointed Emeritus Professor of Surgery, and there had been a note in the newspaper about it. The Dean reported that several patients had written to him and congratulated the Dean on having gotten him this appointment as Emeritus Professor. They mostly described how well he had taken care of them. But one particular woman whom he had cured wrote to the Dean in praise of him, and at the end of the letter, she said there was just one thing she could not understand and that was why the University had not made him emeritus long ago.

I am most grateful to Clyde and Dode Barker for all they did to arrange this wonderful weekend and wonderful day and wonderful evening. I am deeply appreciative to all of you for the great effort you have gone to to come, and I hope it has been a chance to renew old acquaintances and make some new ones with younger members of the present staff. I thought the scientific program was really superb, but I can only give partial recognition to the important efforts of others who were not speaking today. And, of course, the program does not recognize the nonresearch contributions which all have made and which are so important. We, in turn, are part of a larger fraternity or perhaps several fraternities represented by such bodies as the American College of Surgeons, the Association of Academic Surgeons, the Society of University Surgeons, the American Surgical Association, and several international societies to which a goodly number of you belong. We are fortunate, too, to have lived in a half century when the whole field of medical science has been moving and moving swiftly. We live, too, in an era of broad public appreciation of progress in the health sciences.

At a meeting in London in 1958, I met Charles Huggins, and he told me that a person devoted to research was much like an actor on the stage, he needed an audience. I was rather shocked by this statement at the time, but I have since had to admit, grudgingly, however, that there is an element of truth in it. My former professor of philosophy, Rufus Jones, had a somewhat different approach. He noted that in various eras of history there were a succession of outstanding figures, such as Shakespeare among playwrights in the 16th and 17th centuries, Beethoven among musicians in the 18th century, and Darwin among the interpreters of natural history in the 19th century, and that in each instance, by enquiry, one found that their pinnacles of achievement were carried out against the background of a broad interest by society at large, and whereas many people remembered only one name, there actually were considerable groups of people active in the same field. For instance, Marlowe in the case of Shakespeare, a number of great musicians in the days of Beethoven, and Wallace and others in the time of Darwin. Another example he used to cite was that the great cathedrals were built in an era when numerous cities in different countries were building cathedrals. We are living in an era of great discoveries in the biomedical sciences, and even if we cannot all achieve positions of preeminence, we can be part of the total movement on which great achievements are built.

On a very personal note, I arrived at the age of 80 this morning at about 8:00 a.m., which is the hour I was FOB in Germantown in 1907. I cannot help being impressed by the large role that fortune plays in one's career. Just to mention a few of the favors that fortune has dealt me, there have been a half-dozen auto crashes without so much as a broken bone; perhaps eight anesthesias without a mishap; tuberculosis, but not until the year that streptomycin became available; appendicitis that Dr. Eliason, one of the most skillful of our surgeons, brought me through; a parotid tumor that Henry Royster operated on that turned out to be benign; angina pectoris without any measured myocardial loss; and a pulmonary embolus you've already heard about. There have been seven carcinomas, but all have been confined to the skin.

On a quite different level, I was blessed with loving parents, excellent educational opportunities, and a wonderful relationship with Dr. Ravdin. Dr. Ravdin convinced me that I had abilities that I had been convinced I didn't have. That was one of his extraordinary gifts. We used to say he was a one-man employment agency. People would call him up, and he would suggest somebody to them that sometimes seemed unlikely, but it always seemed to work out. Then I had a fine opportunity with Walter Estell Lee, who introduced me to other hospitals and to many other opportunities in Philadelphia and in American surgery. And I am deeply grateful to Jack Gibbon, my next door neighbor for a number of years, who put me on the *Annals of Surgery* board and sponsored me for the Society of Clinical Surgery; to Gaylord Harnwell, President of the University, who gave me the opportunity of serving as Provost of the University, which led to my becoming a member and later, as you heard, President of this venerable institution in which we sit; to Julian Johnson, whose support was a *sine qua non* for the years I spent as Chairman of the Department of Surgery, and to whom I owe a special debt of gratitude; and to Drs. Mackie, Schwegman, Roberts, Royster, Randall, Kirby, Bob Ravdin, and others who were earlier members of our group. Then there is my wife who has loved me in my better moments, her parents who graciously tolerated me and her willingness to sacrifice a very promising professional career so that we could have a large family, and her support of our six children, particularly during the year that I was laid up with TB. It was during this year, while pregnant, that she developed a dominant breast lump that very fortunately proved to be benign. After that, the fact that I had just discovered the tuberculosis the previous month seemed indeed unimportant. However, when the pregnancy terminated in twins, who are here tonight, we were both more concerned than we had expected to be.

Having commented on the extent to which I am the embodiment of good luck, I cannot help but reflect a bit on the pleasures of old age. In the book of *Ecclesiastics* is the statement, "the years of man are three score and ten and if by reason of strength they be four score years what thank have ye." In contrast with this pessimistic statement, I've found much to be thankful for in my eighth decade. There has been travel: the Far East, Australia, India, some of the Near East, a bit of Africa, much of Europe, six countries south of the border, as well as three or four of the Caribbean Islands. It has allowed time for the addition of various nonessential items to my bibliography, and it gave me two more years on the National Cancer Advisory Board, during which I think we did something to improve the contract program as well as to up the total appropriations for the Institute. It provided an opportunity to help Bill Altemeier found the Surgical Infection Society, which meets here next week, and to strengthen the American Trauma Society and the International Federation of Surgical Colleges of which Bill Longmire is the current President.

More importantly, it has supported an opportunity to see many of our former residents recognized in academic life: some as chairmen, some as professors, and some as holders of significant offices. For instance, I would count rather high on the list the fact that Doris Bender Maxwell, who could not be here, practicing surgery in the small city of Greensburg, PA, was elected President of the Pittsburgh Surgical Society. You should all know that the surgeon for the Miami Dolphins (Dr. Leonard Miller told me this) is Joe Diaco. HUP has produced another Surgeon General in C. Everett Koop, and Chick has done a great deal to reestablish the importance of this position in the public health service. He has further advanced knowledge of the dangers of cigarette smoking, a field in which our former Vice President, Luther Terry, played such a key role. He has now taken the lead in educating the public about AIDS.

Through the kindness of William Fitts, Leonard Miller, Brooke Roberts, and Clyde Barker, and with the vital support of Julius Mackie and Clete Schwegman, I have continued as an active member of the faculty in the Department of Surgery, although I plan to stop operating at the end of this academic year.

A long life certainly provides one a longitudinal view of life in general and of families. I have met six generations in one line of mine. It emphasized the fact that in medicine, one's most productive ideas are apt to come during student and training days and, perhaps, the first several years after one finishes his training. It reinforces the view that these periods of so-called preparation for life are actually life itself and no less important than the years that follow. For a teacher, it provides a time to observe the accomplishments of one's students and gives a progressive perspective on the role which social organizations, such as universities, scientific societies, and branches of government, play in the larger frame of things. One sees the operation of the Peter Principle, according to which some people who do one thing well, may fail in the next larger job. It reinforces one's respect for hard work, as the amperage which multiplied by the voltage of ability produces the watts or the total work which is the output of a human life. It makes one aware of the tremendous debt we owe to the founders of this Country for the extraordinary combination of conservatism and adaptability which they built into the constitution. It makes one conscious of some of the failures of our form of government in not stimulating the less advantaged people in our population, with the result of unemployment and poverty.

History is written largely in terms of political change, and in one sense, the constitution does represent political change, but it is also based on a rather profound philosophy. In general, however, I have been convinced that it is the innovative thinkers in our society, such as Dalton, Newton, Pasteur, Lister, Farraday, Jefferson, Edison, Bell, Marconi, Kelvin, Einstein, and in our own university, Mauchly and Eckert, who have really shaped the course of history rather than the Julius Caesers and the Napoleans. Perhaps the difference is that the great political leaders see their objectives and the results of their efforts, whereas the great thinkers cannot possibly foresee the results of their discoveries. However, when Farraday showed his model of the dynamo to a member of Parliament, he was asked of what use is it. He told the politician that he could not foresee what its use would be, but he was quite sure that politicians would be able to tax it.

You may have noticed that I have avoided commenting on today's scientific papers. To do so would be unfair because my evaluation of them would mainly reflect my own interests. Thus, I did some peritoneal dialysis, as it was called, having had a long-standing interest in renal failure. We even tried one extracorporeal dialysis when Dr. Saltonstall was at the Pennsylvania Hospital in the early '40s, but none of these efforts were great successes. So I suppose my great interest, as Francis Moore suggested, was nutrition, and I'm especially grateful to all who took the nascent ideas of Dr. Ravdin and myself and developed hyperalimentation as we know it. This effort was led by Stanley Dudrick with Harry Vars and advanced with valuable input by Douglas Wilmore, Ezra Steiger, Robert Ruberg, Dennis Laws, and many others. Earlier, Dr. Cecilia Riegel, Dr. Lehr, Dr. Spagna, and my son Jack had given this a push, and still earlier, Martin Rhode working with Harry Vars had done so. Bob Crichlow and Harry Nelson also contributed, as did John Daly when he was a student.

Dave Cooper's group, with the backup of Otto Rosenthal, made more basic contributions in the identification of the P450 enzyme of the liver and some of the roles which it plays. Len Miller's work on 2-3 diphosphoglycerate was spectacular, as was his work with Henry Berkowitz on renin substrate and renal function. Looking back, we have missed many opportunities, but because of all of the resident group and the staff group, other opportunities have been seized, and important additions to both science and practice have been made. The recognition that I have received belongs rather to many of you, and in the broader sense, to all of you collectively, and tonight gives me an opportunity of acknowledging it.

One of the greatest satisfactions of all, however, has been to see the present activity in the Department. This has been achieved in no small part by recruitment, and of the names on our office door, a minority now stem from the time I was Department Chairman and the majority have been added by thoughtful appointments made by my successors. On visits to the Harrison Department today, one finds a hive of activity that occupies most of a floor of the Medical Education Building and parts of the Hospital itself. So, thank you all so very much for being here. There can be no greater satisfaction than to see your tremendous success in contributing to your patients, to your profession, and to the science of surgery. I thank particularly those who have come from a distance. It was very, very gracious of you.

To Doctor Rhoads:

THE RHOADESIAN

'Round Philly are many new faces
And many new places to see,
But one man remains almost constant,
Amazing as that seems to be!

But Quinnie, for one, knew for certain
That young Jonathan would some day go far,
But who would have guessed way back then
That Jonathan would become J.E.R?

For now he's an octagenarian—
A man of great wit and so wise.
He's still just as active as ever,
A fact that his own age belies.

So lift a toast to our chairman,
Who's as fresh these days as artesian.
True surgeon, true scholar, true teacher,
The consummate chief—the Rhoadesian!

With sincere regards and great admiration, we are genuinely sorry we could not be there for the celebration. Many thanks for your leadership, counsel, and support over the years!

Jim, Vicky, Andrew, and Jonathan Long

May 9, 1987

Reminiscences of the Surgical Service of the Hospital of the University of Pennsylvania From 1931 to 1935

CHARLES W. McLAUGHLIN, M.D., F.A.C.S.

THERE ARE VERY FEW remaining who served on one of the surgical services of the Hospital of the University of Pennsylvania between 1931 and 1935. With the exception of Jonathan Rhoads, whom we honor on this occasion, Bill Erb, Claus Jordon, and myself, that is perhaps the lot to the best of my knowledge, since the recent death of Julian Johnson.

It seemed worthwhile for this special event to paint a word picture, as memory permits, of the state of surgical training, surgical practice, and a word about the senior surgeons at the time Jonathon entered his fellowship at Penn.

In the late 1920s and early 1930s, opportunities for advanced training in general surgery and its specialties were much less than those available today. It is true that residency programs were then well established in centers such as Hopkins, Harvard, Washington—St. Louis, Michigan, Rush, Yale, and a considerable number of the older State University Medical Centers, but many of these latter departments were small and operated on very limited budgets. The Mayo Clinic offered a standard three-year fellowship, retaining a few for an extra year or two who might be selected for permanent staff. One- and two-year periods of training were available at the Cleveland and the Lahey Clinics, and were largely sought by those with limited previous surgical training or others dropped from the pyramidal systems.

I left Washington University—St. Louis for an internship at the Montreal General Hospital in 1929 with the idea of obtaining a firm background in internal medicine under Campbell Howard, one of William Osler's outstanding students and then Professor of Medicine at McGill. At that time, the Montreal General Hospital offered a one-year residency in either surgery or internal medicine, but prior to being accepted in either, one was required to have a full year of pathological training following internship. A second year spent in pathology was a rare experience in a teaching hospital of 600 active beds with a superb staff in which postmortem examinations were done on 98% of those who died in hospital.

Having decided upon surgery as the field of my choice, I very naturally looked to Philadelphia because of the long-standing exchange of medical fellows between McGill and Pennsylvania, although there has been no similar exchange in surgery. It was somewhat discouraging to learn that they had never awarded a non-Pennsylvania graduate a Surgical Fellowship, but it was my good fortune to attain an appointment for a three-year training period on the "C" service under Dr. Eldridge Eliason beginning July 1, 1931.

"Coming in from the cold" into the close-knit environment of the University of Pennsylvania at that time was quite an experience. In all fairness, they proved to be wonderful people, and in no time, I found acceptance.

The surgical services then consisted of four units: A, B, C and D. The overall chief and chairman was Dr. Charles Frazer, head of Neurosurgery and surgical service "A". His second in command and associate was Dr. Chubby Grant. Dr. George Mueller directed the "B" service, Dr. Eliason the "C" service, and Dr. Isadore Ravdin had the "D" service together with his duties as head of research for the entire surgical department.

Dr. Frazer had one fellow on Neurosurgery serving for a three-year period and one fellow on the thyroid service with a one-year appointment. Strangely enough, the thyroid services

From the University of Nebraska Medical Center and the Nebraska Methodist Hospital Foundation, Omaha, Nebraska.

was still under Dr. Frazer's complete control. Thyroid surgery was done one day each week, and General Surgical fellows wishing to have experience in this field needed to have this especially arranged by their chief with Dr. Frazer. There were two fellows on the Mueller service, two on the Eliason service, and one on the Ravdin service, each of whom were serving for a three-year period.

Beds in General Surgical were evenly divided between "B" and "C" services, and each had approximately 50 beds. The "D" service under Dr. Ravdin was much smaller with approximately 10 active beds at that time. Dr. Charles Johnston was Ravdin's fellow in the early 1930s, and he later served with distinction as the Professor and Chairman of the New Department of Surgery at Wayne University in Detroit.

Dr. Frazer had his own operating rooms, and in General Surgery, we had little contact with this service except when we were able to be assigned for a period to thyroid service. At that time, Dr. Frazer had operated upon over 1100 individuals with tic douloureux using the procedure he had developed with Dr. Spiller with such striking success.

Dr. Mueller's service operated three days per week, and Dr. Eliason's service did likewise, using the same operating room facilities three mornings per week. Using a single operating room of huge dimensions, one case was operated under the main lights in the front of the theatre and moved to the rear for closure, while the next case, previously anesthetized in an anteroom, was moved under the front lights and the procedure carried out with a second set of assistants. Thus, the normal seven- or eight-case schedule could be completed without difficulty.

The senior fellow on each of the surgical services initially did any case the chief did not choose to operate. During his first year, the new general fellow gradually assumed his operative burden with the beds assigned to him. Dr. Eliason never assisted either of his fellows although he would usually sit in the operating room and was always available for advice during a morning schedule.

Surgery started promptly at 8:00 AM on each operative morning, with the senior fellow always having made rounds on all patients before this hour. He would have noted particularly those patients about whom any questions might be asked and called the chief at his home 30 minutes before 8:00, including Sunday. This was an absolute rule, and it made no difference if you had been up operating until 5:30 or 6:00 that morning. Rounds by fellows and interns were always made on all patients late each evening.

Both Dr. Eliason and Dr. Mueller placed great trust in their fellows and gave them a great deal of responsibility. In return, fellows were held strictly responsible for their performances in the absence of the chief in handling all emergencies and surgical problems.

The surgical fellows lived outside the hospital and were not provided with board or room. Salary during this three-year period was $1200, $1500, and $1800 per year. Beginning in 1931, however, following the depression, everybody took a 10% cut in the above salary. Each of the chiefs, and I speak specifically for my chief Dr. Eliason, spent many hours advising, counseling, and practically treating each of the fellows as a son. It was in many respects a truly ideal system for training a surgeon, but, of course, it is impossible in today's much more complex and large institutions.

What are some of the striking differences in the practice of surgery 50 plus years ago in the University Hospital as contrasted with today? Immediately one remembers that at that time neither sulfa nor any of the many other commonly used antibiotics had come over the horizon. Prontosil was the first of the miracle intravenous drugs available, but this came about only in the late 1930s and was followed by the sulfonamides and the succession of miracle drugs. Penicillin did not become available until the fall of 1943 and was initially limited to the military.

Anesthesia by the early 1930s was primarily provided with gas ether and, on occasion, ethylene. Spinal anesthesia was employed for some procedures, but it was not widely utilized. None of the relaxant drugs were available, and what a difference that often made in obtaining exposure.

Blood banks did not come into general use until World War II. Bob Elman did not introduce Amigen, the first protein supplement for intravenous feeding, until some years later, and reliable intravenous nutrition, which was developed by Stan Duderick and Jonathan Rhoads in this department, did not appear for almost another 40 years.

Duodenal ulcer was a very common surgical problem, and the standard operative procedure was a gastroenterostomy. Gastrectomy was then restricted almost entirely to cancer of the stomach. The general technique in biliary surgery has changed little except that table-cholangiography was not used because of the explosiveness of anesthetics and poor grounding in operative theatres. Hernias were done by the Ferguson and Bassini technique, and McFay had not yet described his modification.

All services did staged drainage of lung abscesses, which were quite common, and empyema thoracis was handled by both closed or open drainage. I do not recall seeing a single case of primary lung carcinoma during the three years I spent at Penn nor did I post one in a series of over 300 autopsies done at McGill.

The "C" service of Dr. Eliason did all the fracture and joint surgery at University Hospital. Orthopedics limited themselves to congenital deformities and nontraumatic problems. We had extensive experience with all types of fractures, but the pinning technique for fractures of the hip had not been well developed at that time. All open reductions were done with meticulous "no touch" Lane technique with the constant hazard of infection.

A year or so after I arrived at Penn, a tall, young Quaker lad, having graduated from Hopkins, came up to Philadelphia for his internship. This was a two-year rotating service at that time. It was here that I first met Jonathan Rhoads, a soft-spoken, very pleasant, almost retiring young man, but on association, one immediately sensed what a fine gentleman was inside this quiet self-effacing person. Perhaps I felt some special kinship because he too was not a Penn Graduate.

As Jon's internship moved toward completion, I felt very strongly that he should apply for a surgical fellowship and confided this to Dr. Eliason who encouraged me to pursue it with Jonathan. On a beautiful spring evening, we walked for an hour or so under the trees on Hamilton Walk, which some may recall used to be behind the University Hospital and in front of the library and the research building. Every argument I could think of was presented to convince Jonathan to apply for a fellowship, and with some hesitation, either because of this or for some other reason, he ultimately accepted this advice. Perhaps I had a hand in making a major contribution to American Surgery. Jonathan did apply, he did become a Surgical Fellow, and I need not tell you what a career he built on that Foundation. We have remained close friends during these intervening 55 years. I salute him on this special occasion for the luster that he has brought to this great University and to its Department of Surgery.

10th Anniversary Presidential Address: Parenteral Feeding (1966–1986)—Growth and Development of an Individual, a Scientific Discipline and an Organization

JOHN M. DALY, M.D.

A PRESIDENTIAL ADDRESS can serve many purposes; it can be generalized or specific, political or socialistic, a review of the past or a prediction of the future! In his erudite presentation yesterday, Dr. Stanley Levenson described the events leading to the implementation of total parenteral nutrition in this country in 1967. In view of this 10th anniversary of the A.S.P.E.N. Clinical Congress and our need to relate past to present and present to future, my address will review some of the scientific achievements related to parenteral feeding which have been described in the literature from 1966 to the 1980s. Recognize that there is inherent selection bias in this review, and that these are my personal reflections on the scientific development of parenteral nutrition. Because of time constraints I cannot acknowledge every major contribution, and many of the reports were chosen because of personal involvement.

The subtitle of my talk "Growth and development of an individual, a scientific discipline and an organization" is taken from a hallmark publication by Wilmore and Dudrick in 1968 entitled "growth and development of an infant receiving all nutrients exclusively by vein."[2] This paper revolutionized the care and management of pediatric patients by convincingly demonstrating body tissue growth in an infant receiving all nutrition exclusively by vein. The work described in this publication dramatically altered my life, for I was at that time a college student, who worked under Drs. Wilmore, Dudrick, Vars, and Rhoads at the Harrison Department of Surgical Research. I watched these men place this child's catheter, mix solutions, add electrolytes, and begin parenteral feeding. I watched this child grow.

From 1967 to 1975, explosive growth in laboratory and clinical research occurred in the field of nutritional support leading to widespread applications of this advancing technology, reports of spectacular success and occasional words of caution. In 1975 the American Society for Parenteral and Enteral Nutrition was conceived and formed by a dedicated group of individuals. During the past 10 yr the Society has grown and prospered.[3] It has become a leading force in organized medicine to promote clinical care, education, and research in a burgeoning medical discipline.

Some description of the evolution and current status of our Society at present is needed since we are an indirect reflection of the current art and science of nutrition. It is hoped by this review that you obtain a sense of where we as nutritionists, nurses, dietitians, pharmacists, students, PhDs and physicians have come from. Armed with this sense of history, we can plan where we should be going.

First Five Years (1966–1970): Widespread Application of a New Technology

In 1966 Lyndon Johnson was president of the United States, the Beach Boys reigned in California, and I was a college student with a summer job installing and removing telephones for the Bell Telephone Company. In Sweden, Hallberg, Schuberth and Wretlind

From the Department of Surgery, University of Pennsylvania School of Medicine, Philadelphia, Pennsylvania.

Delivered at the 10th A.S.P.E.N. Clinical Congress on February 11, 1986 in Dallas, TX.

TABLE 1.

Reference	1966–1971
Wretlind et al	New fat emulsion
Dudrick et al (6, 7)	TPN: Methods + use
Duke & Kinney	Metabolic results
Scribner et al (13)	Home TPN

described experimental and clinical studies with a new fat emulsion for intravenous nutrition.[4] The following summer an infant born with intestinal atresia was chosen for central venous catheter placement and institution of total parenteral nutrition.[2] The new fat emulsion described by Wretlind was unavailable so fatty plasma was intermittently infused to provide trace metals and essential fatty acids. Dudrick et al[6] reported the first effective total parenteral nutrition requirements and their methods and techniques of administration, but others raised a note of caution about prolonged venous catheterization as a cause of sepsis.[7] Duke et al[8] documented the metabolic utilization of intravenous high calorie/nitrogen solutions in patients, and several authors demonstrated the efficacy of this new technique in a wide variety of pathologic states such as trauma, inflammatory bowel disease, intestinal fistulas, and other catastrophic illnesses.[9–12] Scribner[13] even attempted to maintain patients at home using A-V shunts for fluid administration (Table 1).

Despite these successes, reports of bacterial and fungal infections prompted investigations as to causation by or association with the long-term use of catheters and hypertonic dextrose solutions.[14] As these first 5 yr drew to a close, it was clear that science, technology, and a clear clinical need had come together to improve medical care.[15,16] High risk procedures became routine. New industries would develop built on imagination and nurtured in this new technology.

On a personal note, I continued to work at the Harrison Department of Surgical Research part-time during school and full-time during the summer. I had progressed from college student to medical student. Nutrition was not taught as a formal course in my medical school even though it was within a radius of 10 miles from the University of Pennsylvania. Total parenteral nutrition was used only sporadically since clinical protocols required physician interest for their initiation. The multidisciplinary approach to nutritional support to improve efficacy and reduce complications was just being developed.

Second Five Years (1971–1975): Identification of Efficacy and Recognition of Morbidity

This second half-decade was marked by greater than a 4-fold increase in published manuscripts related to parenteral nutrition. The techniques of central venous cannulation were investigated and refined (Table 2).[17–19] Methods of fluid administration, use of pumps and filters and the joining together of nurse, pharmacist, dietician, and physician became standardized in efforts to reduce the complications of hypertonic solution administration. Mechanical, infectious and metabolic complications were reported and alternatives were described to reduce morbidity with this developing technique.[17–20]

Iatrogenic complications were noted with dampened enthusiasm in some and opened new avenues of research for others. In 1971 Ruberg et al[21] described hypophosphatemia with hypophosphaturia while Travis et al[22] demonstrated changes in red blood cell oxygen transport as a result of hypophosphatemia. Brenner et al[23] noted the increasing incidence of hyperosmolar non-Getotic coma in surgical patients receiving TPN and recommended steps to reduce the occurrence of this problem. In fact in a letter to the editor of the *New England Journal of Medicine,* Duma[24] admonished against members of industry and overaggressive users of this technique so as not to "do harm."

In the pediatric population, complications of parenteral nutrition such as hyperchloremic metabolic acidosis and essential fatty acid deficiency were described and recommendations were made to avoid these complications.[25–27] Despite these problems even larger series of pediatric patients were treated using peripheral or central parenteral nutrition.[28]

In adults the effects of prolonged catabolism due to sepsis and trauma were well recog-

TABLE 2.

Reference	1971–1975
Recognition of morbidity	
Ryan et al (19)	Catheter complications
Ruberg et al (21)	Hypophosphatemia
Brenner et al (23)	Hyperosmolar coma
Heird et al (26)	Metabolic acidosis
Caldwell et al (27)	Essential fatty acid deficiency
Clarification of efficacy	
McNamara et al (29)	TPN for combat casualties
Wilmore et al (30)	TPN for burned patients
Long et al (31)	TPN: glucose *vs.* fat
Blackburn et al (32)	Peripheral protein sparing
Wilmore and Dudrick (34)	Essential AA for renal failure
Abel et al (38)	Randomized clinical trial
Fisher et al (37)	Metabolic encephalopathy
Wolfe et al (40)	Fistula output
MacFayden et al (41)	Fistula closure
Solassol et al (44)	Home TPN

nized. Experience with casualties during the Vietnam conflict led to more frequent use of parenteral nutrition in injured patients.[29,30] Long et al[31] demonstrated greater nitrogen-sparing efficacy of infused glucose calories compared with fat emulsion calories. This report set off a controversy which was to last well into the early 1980s. Blackburn et al[32] described a concept of "protein-sparing" by administration of amino acid solutions without glucose or fat calories in traumatized patients. This study set the stage for a multitude of clinical trials to evaluate this hypothesis.

Organ system failure, an all-too-often-consequence of major trauma and sepsis, was recognized as altering parenteral nutrient requirements. Earlier, Giovannetti and Maggiove[33] had reported using a low nitrogen diet with proteins of high biologic value for severe chronic uremia. Wilmore and Dudrick[34] demonstrated that patients with acute renal failure could be administered hypertonic dextrose and a mixture of essential L-amino acids in order to reduce the frequency of dialysis or obviate it altogether. Abel et al[35,36] carried this work further in patients with acute renal failure culminating with a prospective randomized trial which demonstrated a lower mortality in patients given hypertonic dextrose and essential amino acids compared with those given hypertonic dextrose alone. Fisher et al[37] suggested that metabolic encephalopathy was caused by alterations in protein metabolism with synthesis of false neurotransmitters. Specially formulated amino acid infusions were then designed to treat this condition. Similarly, the advantages of parenterally feeding malnourished patients with cardiac dysfunction were described.[38]

In the area of gastrointestinal disease, Wilmore et al[39] demonstrated experimentally the benefits of TPN in allowing maximal adaptation of the small intestine following massive resection. This concept of "bowel rest with adequate host nutrient supplementation" led to numerous reports on the use of parenteral feeding in patients with inflammatory bowel disease and those with intestinal fistula.[40] Prognostic criteria for fistula closure and mean time to closure were determined by trial and error and TPN was used in large numbers of these severely ill patients.[41–43] Experience continued to grow with patients who required long-term *home* parenteral nutrition.[44] Technology continued to improve and so did the need for more precise dietary formulations. Finally, the increase in published scientific literature demanded cumulative reviews, with textbooks just around the corner.[45,46] The single most critical event during this period was the joining together of physician, nurse, pharmacist, and dietitian as never before in order to improve clinical care. It became clear that the team's collective strength was greater than the sum of its individual members. Patient care improved.

This explosive growth in a recent therapeutic innovation, recognition of its attendent morbidity if not used properly and lack of a cohesive body to provide education to health

TABLE 3. *A Team Approach and Clinical Trials*

Reference	1976–1980
Skoutaskis et al (50)	Team approach
Blackett et al (52)	Subclavian catheter trial
Border et al (53)	Muscle fuel deficit
Long et al (54)	TPN—septic patients
Hill et al (55)	TPN and total body nitrogen
Shizgal et al (56)	Exchangeable sodium/potassium
Bistrian et al (66)	Nutrition and immunity
Mullen et al (68)	Prognostic index
Holter et al (69) and Williams et al (70)	Prospective trials in surgical patients
Fleming et al (72)	TPN in inflammatory bowel disease
Heymsfield et al (77)	Internal hyperalimentation
Ladefoged et al (84)	Home TPN + quality of life

professionals led to the founding of the American Society for Parenteral and Enteral Nutrition on June 5, 1975. The Society served to educate its members in this developing treatment modality, to provide an open forum for involvement among all members of the nutrition team collectively and to provide seminars, guest speakers and on-site technical assistance to institutions establishing new nutrition programs. By September 30, 1975 the first treasurer's report revealed $750 collected with another $250 pledged.[3] Dr. Stanley J. Dudrick agreed to serve as the Society's first President and preliminary plans were made for a speaker's bureau and a society-sponsored journal.

On a personal note, I completed medical school during this time period and was well along in my surgical training at the University of Texas Medical School at Houston where I saw firsthand the increasing use of parenteral nutrition in patients with a variety of severe illnesses. Our animal studies on malnutrition and colonic wound healing came to fruition with presentation before the Surgical Forum in 1970, 1972, and 1973.

A New Era Begins (1976–1980): Use of a Team Approach and Prospective, Randomized Clinical Trials

At this midway point in the eighth decade of the 20th century, nutritional support technology was acclaimed as "the fourth coming," but editorials regarding TPN also attempted to separate fact from fancy.[48,49] The team approach to parenteral feeding had been previously described (Table 3), but renewed efforts were made to create multidisciplinary teams for the nutritional support of patients.[50,51] Use of the team approach reduced technical and mechanical complications of TPN so that more emphasis could be placed on research into endogenous and exogenous substrate metabolism.[52] Border et al[53] suggested a peripheral muscle energy deficit in sepsis while Long et al[54] emphasized the importance of calorie to nitrogen ratios in hypermetabolic patients. Hill et al[55] and Shizgal et al[56] described unique, sophisticated methods for determining body composition by direct measurement of total body nitrogen using prompt gamma neutron activation and calculation of total body exchangeable sodium and potassium using isotope dilution methods. These tools would be utilized extensively in a research setting to define malnutrition and the relative efficacy of various means of therapy. Later Jeejeebhoy et al[58] would determine that a proper history and physical examination by a trained individual would correlate extremely well with these advanced methods of measuring body composition. Intravenous fat emulsions became available for general use. Prospective metabolic studies in man noted similar relative protein-sparing abilities of intravenous fat and glucose emphasizing differences between fasting normal volunteers and stressed hospitalized patients. However, Askanazi et al[60] cautioned against large glucose loads in stressed patients with pulmonary compromise and suggested a mixed fuel approach to parenterally feeding the seriously ill patient.[57,59]

Use of the peripheral route for administration of nutrients was defined in the pediatric age group and new synthetic amino acid solutions designed for infants and children were tested.[61,62] In adults, "protein-sparing" using only amino acid solutions was deemphasized as use of glucose and fat emulsions were shown to improve utilization.[63–65]

In surgical patients, the relationship of immunocompetence to nutritional status was reestablished and prognostic implications of malnutrition in patients undergoing major operations were determined.[66-68] These retrospective observations led to a series of randomized, prospective clinical trials to evaluate the effectiveness of perioperative nutritional support to reduce postoperative complications.[69-71] In this way, proper, scientific clinical studies were used to test hypotheses built upon large numbers of retrospective reports.

In GI diseases, long-term TPN was suggested as primary therapy in certain cases of inflammatory bowel disease, but acute acalculous cholecystitis became recognized as an entity associated with long-term parenteral support and "bowel rest".[72-74] Hepatic dysfunction was reported to be caused by and yet ameliorated with parenteral nutrition.[75,76] For this reason and because of lower costs, a resurgence of enteral nutritional support occurred using diets which varied from blendarized food to chemically-defined formulas.[77,78] Nasointestinal tubes became softer (siliconized) and smaller for improved patient comfort, while use of weighted tips promoted passage into the jejunum to reduce pulmonary aspiration. Needle-catheter jejunostomy feedings were popularized as an alternative to postoperative TPN.[79,80] Coordinated care by the nutritional team continued to be required for feeding of hospitalized patients and became even more important as the indications for home nutritional support expanded.[81] Experience had documented the reality of providing long-term nutritional support in the home setting.[82] Metabolic studies of patients receiving home TPN were carried out to identify vitamin, trace element, and mineral deficiencies, but to its credit, the profession also worried about the "quality of life" in patients on permanent home parenteral nutrition.[83,84] Humanism was inexorably bound to the technology of nutritional support.

The extent of the growth and development of nutritional support was recognized by the National Institutes of Health in 1980 when a Consensus Conference was held inviting experts to share their scientific data and their opinions. Out of this workshop future directions for research, patient care, and education grew.

On a personal note, I completed my surgical residency training and began my first faculty appointment as an Assistant Professor of Surgery at the University of Texas Medical School at Houston and the MD Anderson Hospital and Tumor Institute. Our laboratory research into the etiologies of cancer cachexia, the manipulation of tumor growth by changing dietary intake and the improvement in tumor responsiveness and drug pharmacokinetics by nutritional support continued to be productive. We began prospective clinical trials evaluating parenteral nutrition at our institutions to define both metabolic and clinical efficacy. Finally, my own surgical practice in patients with complex oncologic problems allowed frequent interplay of the art and science of nutrition and continual reevaluation of contemporary medical ethics.[85-93]

A.S.P.E.N.

Growth Phase

Yesterday, at the opening session I described the founding and early growth of A.S.P.E.N. which from 1975 to 1981 increased in membership from 100 to 2,700 and increased its budget from $750.00 to $750,000.00. As important, the Society increased its credibility among the medical profession. The Clinical Congress continued to promote the exchange of basic knowledge, but in addition advanced seminars in complex metabolic subjects were developed and the scientific short papers sessions increased in quantity and quality. The need for frequent regional seminars on basic concepts of nutritional support decreased as the "team concept" of providing nutrition within institutions flourished. At least one goal of the founding members had been accomplished.

Development Phase

In 1982, Barney Sellars had been appointed as the Society's Executive Director and the National Office staff underwent revitalization. A series of short and medium range goals were formulated to improve the financial status of the organization, to redesign the Society's administrative structure and function, to expand the benefits for A.S.P.E.N.s members, to reemphasize the multidisciplinary nature of our Society and to improve the opportunities for communication and participation within the organization (Table 4).

Starting in 1982, the A.S.P.E.N. Board of Directors began a process intended to substan-

TABLE 4. *A.S.P.E.N. Activities*

Research
Primary Activities—OASIS + direct member surveys
Secondary Activities
Clinical Congress short papers
Vars, Dudrick, and Rhoads Awards
Research workshop
Liaison with government research agencies
Education
Clinical Congress
Fall postgraduate course
Discipline seminars
JPEN and *Nutrition In Clinical Practice*
Monographs, tapes, and self-assessment tests
Professional development
National Board of Nutrition Support Certification
Home and hospital standards of practice
Chapters
Public policy
Hopkins report on "the impact of DRGs"
Changes in ICD-9 cm and ICD-10 cm codes, JCAH standards
Nutrition societies
National
International

tially overhaul the internal workings of the organization in order to influence the Society's capacity to become an increasingly important contributor to health care in this nation. That process succeeded so well such that in 1985 the Society eliminated a historic debt and a modest reserve was established for unexpected emergencies. More importantly, however, the Society developed an improved capacity to respond to the needs of its membership in a much more efficient and effective manner. Membership dues were maintained at a constant level since 1980 despite both rapidly rising and falling inflation. This reflected the commitment of the Board of Directors to expand benefits and activities while controlling membership charges.

Improvement in communication within the organization has been a major goal. A new chapters' program was organized which now recognizes five chapters around the country. The nominations process were made more democratic, and the number, size, and rotation requirements for committees were formalized. Specific efforts by nursing, dietetics, and pharmacy members have expanded participation in their disciplines.

With regard to communicating with the larger medical and public community, A.S.P.E.N. has become a leader in creating the Confederation of Clinical Nutrition Societies, and the International Council of Parenteral and Enteral Nutrition. Indeed, the Society hosted meetings of both these coalitions during its 10th Clinical Congress.

Finally, the Society has substantially increased its investment to influence the development of government policy which affects nutrition support. Specifically, this enhanced government focus has involved:

(1) White papers on hospital malnutrition, and reimbursement for nutrition support;

(2) Briefings on nutrition support for Congress and agencies of the Federal Executive Branch;

(3) Contracting with Johns Hopkins University for a major study of nutrition support and the DRG reimbursement program; and

(4) Development of proposals to change ILD-9 and 10 coding systems used as the basis for disease classification as well as for procedure identification.

Our rededication to assuring maximum involvement of all segments of our Society can first be seen in the makeup of our membership. A.S.P.E.N. is truly multidisciplinary. That basic characteristic is reflected increasingly at the highest levels of the organization in a way which I think is remarkable. For example, consider the following constituent representation in the leadership of the Society: the 15-member Board of Directors for 1986 includes three chairpersons representing pharmacy, nursing and dietetics; a GI specialist chairing our

Education and Professional Development Committee; a physician chairing our Chapters Committee; and a nurse chairing our Publications Committee. Our Executive Committee, which is composed of five Board members, has a nephrologist as Treasurer and a research dietitian serving as Secretary. Our other committees include a pediatric nutrition specialist chairing our Abstract Review Panel and a GI specialist and general surgeon cochairing the 11th Clinical Congress Committee. JPEN is edited by a surgeon and Nutrition in Clinical Practice is edited by a multidisciplinary editorial group headed by a pharmacist. The National Board for Nutrition Support Certification, also multidisciplinary, is chaired by a dietitian. Finally, our first book, the Nursing Core Curriculum Study Guide, was edited by a nurses' committee headed by a registered nurse.

I think you see my point. And my point is that for an organization to be as complex and as representative as we are and to still have a very high level of effectiveness is a tribute to the dedication of its leaders and membership.

We have improved the frequency and content of education programs and benefits. New events at the Clinical Congress include roundtables, cinema, physician consultations, discipline luncheons with experts, workshops, nutrition practice posters; all of these being clinically oriented activities. Each Clinical Congress presents a substantially new faculty. When scientific papers are presented, there is no program competition. Our exhibit program has expanded substantially. With regard to other meetings, we now have a regular fall postgraduate course and a discipline conference in the spring. Our continuing education programs have received approval for the longest periods allowed for CE provider programs, a mark of highly acceptable continuing education efforts in the Society.

We have taken steps to begin the collection of national data on parenteral and enteral nutrition services through the development of the OASIS data collection system in cooperation with the Oley Foundation.

We have created programs to recognize research in Parenteral and Enteral Nutrition including the VARS award, the Rhoads Lecture, and the new Stanley Dudrick Research Scholar Award (Fig. 1). We have created the Research Workshop as a mechanism for bringing together the best clinical and scientific minds on subjects of controversy.

Finally, during this 4-yr period we have taken important steps to improve patient care through efforts to increase the level of professional practice in the field. These steps have included: publication of standards of practice for patients in hospitals and at home; discipline-specific standards of professional practice; preparation of a proposal to amend the JCAH Hospital accreditation manual; creation of the national board of nutrition support

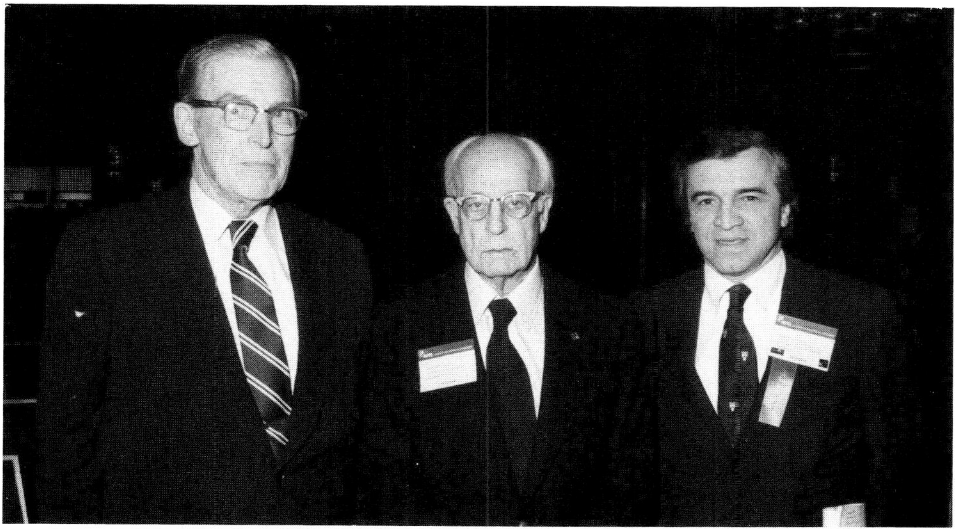

FIG. 1. A.S.P.E.N. Awards and Lectures are named in honor of: Jonathan E. Rhoads, M.D. (*left*), Harry M. Vars, Ph.D. (*center*), and Stanley J. Dudrick, M.D. (*right*).

certification and administration of a certification exam for nurses; and the development and administration of the first self-assessment test.

The development of parenteral nutrition during the past 20 yr has had widespread implications not only for direct patient care, but for us as providers of that care, for the health care industry, for third-party payors and for the government. The ability to completely nourish a human being by vein spread an awareness of malnutrition in our hospitals, created a need for multiple professions to join forces to improve patient care and spawned avenues of research previously impossible. Interestingly, the development of parenteral nutrition prompted a resurgence of enteral nutrition support. It created the need for a new Society and new research forums within older Societies.

As we enter the second-half of this ninth decade, we have a tendency to be overly confident in our ability to provide medical care because of advances in current technology. For example, there are pumps for self-control of analgesia, pumps that are implanted subcutaneously to infuse chemotherapy and pumps that are implanted to replace the human heart. Yet a new disease, acquired immune deficiency (AID) results in a most severe degree of malnutrition and stresses our abilities to restore nutritional status to normal. This illustrates our need to continue to support biomedical research. As individuals in clinical practice we need to support those efforts within our institutions. We must recognize that clinical practice and clinical research are *not* divergent goals. The semiprivate room, the intensive care unit, the operating room, and the outpatient area must remain laboratories of the highest order. While prospective, randomized clinical trials should be the ultimate goal, few of us have the patients, money, and personnel to accomplish this effort. Nevertheless, proper data management of ongoing care can provide meaningful information. In addition, the rigors of this effort provide the fuel for that spark of curiosity which makes us all strive to learn. As an individual within the A.S.P.E.N. organization, I ask that you support our survey efforts to learn more about your practice of nutritional support in hospitalized and home patients. Through these efforts our Society can continue as an effective and representative voice to our government organizations. The legislators clearly need our help, and we must be able to provide them with up-to-date accurate information. Support our Society's two journals: first, by reading them; second, by submitting a manuscript if you can; and third, by letting their editors know where they have succeeded and where they may have fallen short of your expectations. Be cognizant of ways to provide nutrition outside the hospital setting using support personnel, family, and resources to their maximum. Be prepared to deal with "fad" diets and outright nutrition quackery which may be practiced in your region. Know the costs of various products you use, their indications, and relative value in given clinical situations. We must be responsible for holding down health care costs, yet we must always strive to provide the best care for our patients. With conscientious effort this can be done, but we should be the leaders and not the followers in this constant struggle.

As a Society, we must know and respond to the current health care marketplace—government, industry, third-party reimbursers, health care providers, and patients. Standards of care for each of our disciplines must be established. Traditional education methods should be expanded to include video technology. Self-assessment tests and home study programs are popular means of professional development and should be expanded. The Society must become more open to health care professionals who work for profit-making companies. This should be done in a fair, thoughtful fashion. The Society should support efforts by groups such as the Hastings Center to evaluate medical ethics in areas of developing technology. This is a complex area which truly requires a multidisciplinary approach. A.S.P.E.N. must act in a determined manner in areas of public policy and in governmental interactions. We must lead rather than simply respond or react to a changing environment. We are neither a self-interest nor a lobbying group, but a scientific society, yet we must recognize what is going on around us. The Gramm-Rudman Act was passed to force attempts at a balanced budget. Should this mean a loss of social programs with continued military budget escalation to 42% of our total tax dollars? As an individual, I might think I count very little, as 4000 individuals within A.S.P.E.N., we count more, but with the support of many individuals among our many medical societies we will count a lot. We must make our voice heard.

The past 20 yr have been an explosive time for development of nutritional support. Specialized enteral and parenteral formulas are now commonplace, but were only imagined

20 yr ago. Interactions between immune and metabolic responses to injury offer an opportunity to modulate those responses. Vitamins and trace metal requirements need to be redefined, and nutrition individualized by age, disease process, nutritional status, and organ function. This is truly an exciting time in the continuing development of parenteral and enteral nutrition. The future holds great promise to improved care for patients based on sound scientific principles. Let us catch up with the advances in biology as Dr. Douglas Wilmore described so well yesterday to make further advances in clinical care.

REFERENCES

1. Blackburn G. Presential address: Interaction of the science of nutrition and the science of medicine. JPEN 1979;3:131–136.
2. Wilmore D, Dudrick SJ. Growth and development of an infant receiving all nutrients exclusively by vein. JAMA 1968;203:860–864.
3. Seltzer M. A.S.P.E.N.: The genesis. JPEN 1986;10:9–16.
4. Hallberg D, Schuberth O, Wretlind A. Experimental and clinical studies with fat emulsion for intravenous nutrition. Nutr Dieta (Basel) 1966;8:245–281.
5. Durnin JV, Rahaman MM. The assessment of the amount of fat in the human body from measurements of skinfold thickness. Br J Nutr 1967;21:681–689.
6. Dudrick JS, Wilmore DW, Vars HM, Rhoads JE. Long-term total parenteral nutrition with growth, development, and positive nitrogen balance. Surgery 1968;64:134–142.
7. Smits H, Freedman LR. Prolonged venous catheterization as a cause of sepsis. N Engl J Med 1967;276:1229–1233.
8. Duke JH Jr, Kinney JM, Broell JR, Long CL. Metabolic evaluation of high calorie alimentation in surgical patients. Surg Forum 1970;21:74–76.
9. Gimpel A, Schilling JA. Long-term hyperalimentation in ulcerative colitis. J Okla State Med Assoc 1970;63:371–375.
10. Johnson DG. Total intravenous nutrition in newborn surgical patients: A three-year perspective. J Pediatr Surg 1970;5:601–605.
11. Vinnars E, Furst P. The nutritive effect in man of non-essential amino acids infused intravenously (together with the essential ones). 3. Different ratios of essential-non-essential amino acids. Acta Anaesthesiol Scand 1970;14:259–271.
12. Dudrick SJ, Steiger E, Long JM, Rhoads JE. Role of parenteral hyperalimentation in management of multiple catastrophic complications. Surg Clin North Am 1970;50:1031–1038.
13. Scribner B, Cole JJ, Christopher TG. Long-term total parenteral nutrition. JAMA 1970;212:457–463.
14. Ashcraft KW, Leape LL. Candida sepsis complicating parenteral feeding. JAMA 1970;212:454–456.
15. Wilmore D. Total intravenous feeding. N Engl J Med 1970;283:152–153.
16. Morgan A, Filler RM, Moore FD. Surgical nutrition. Med Clin North Am 1970;54:1367–1381.
17. Bernard RW, Stahl WM. Subclavian vein catheterization: A prospective study: I. Noninfectious complications. Ann Surg 1971;173:184–191.
18. Bernard RW, Stahl WM. Subclavian vein catheterization: A prospective study. II. Infectious complications. Ann Surg 1971;173:191–197.
19. Ryan JA, Abel RM, Abbott WM, et al. Catheter complications in total parenteral nutrition: A prospective study of 200 consecutive patients. N Engl J Med 1974;290:757–761.
20. Goldmann DA, Maki DG. Infection control in total parenteral nutrition. JAMA 1973;223:1360.
21. Ruberg RL, Allen TR, Goodman MJ, et al. Hypophosphatemia with hypophosphaturia in hyperalimentation. Surg Forum 1971;22:87–88.
22. Travis SF, Sugarman HF, Ruberg RL, et al. Alterations of red-cell glycolytic intermediates and oxygen transport as a consequence of hypophosphatemia in patients receiving intravenous hyperalimentation. N Engl J Med 1971;285:763–767.
23. Brenner WI, Lanzlay Z, Engelman RM, Stahl WM. Hyperosmolar coma in surgical patients: An iatrogenic disease of increasing incidence. Ann Surg 1973;178:651–656.
24. Duma RJ. First of all do no harm. N Engl J Med 1971;285:1258–1259.
25. Chan JC. The influence of synthetic amino acid and casein hydrolysate on the endogenous production and urinary excretion of acid in total intravenous alimentation. Pediatr Res 1972;6:789–796.
26. Heird WC, Dell RB, Driscoll JM Jr, et al. Metabolic acidosis resulting from intravenous alimentation mixtures containing synthetic amino acids. N Engl J Med 1972;287:943–948.
27. Caldwell MD, Jonsson HT, Othersen HB Jr. Essential fatty acid deficiency in an infant receiving prolonged parenteral alimentation. J Pediatr 1972;81:894–898.
28. Lloyd-Still JD, Schwachman H, Filler RM. Intravenous hyperalimentation in pediatrics. Am J Dig Dis 1972;17:1043–1052.
29. McNamara JJ, Molot MD, Wissman D, et al. Intravenous hyperalimentation. An important adjunct in the treatment of combat casualities. Am J Surg 1971;122:70–73.
30. Wilmore DW, Curreri PW, Spitzer KW, Pruitt BA Jr. Supranormal dietary intake in thermally injured hypermetabolic patients. Surg Synecol Obstet 1971;132:881–886.
31. Long JM, Wilmore DW, Mason AD Jr, Pruitt BA Jr. Fat/carbohydrate interaction: Nitrogen sparing effect of varying caloric sources for total intravenous feeding. Surg Forum 1974;25:61–62.

32. Blackburn GL, Flatt JP, Clowes G, et al. Protein-spring during periods of starvation with sepsos or trauma. Ann Surg 1973;177:588–593.
33. Giovannetti S, Maggiove Q. A low nitrogen diet with proteins of high biologic value for severe chronic uremia. Lancet 1964;1:1000–1003.
34. Wilmore DW, Dudrick SJ. Treatment of acute renal failure with intravenous essential L-amino acids. Arch Surg 1969;99:669–675.
35. Abel RM, Abbott WM, Fischer JE. Acute renal failure. Treatment without dialysis by total parenteral nutrition. Arch Surg 1971;103:513–514.
36. Abel RM, Beck CH Jr, Abbott WM, et al. Improved survival from acute renal failure after treatment with intravenous essential L-amino acids and glucose. N Engl J Med 1973;288:695–699.
37. Fisher JE, Yoshimura N, James H, et al. Plasma amino acids in patients with hepatic encephalopathy. Effect of amino acids infusions. Am J Surg 1974;127:40–45.
38. Abel RM, Fisher JE, Buckley MJ, Austen WG. Hyperalimentation in cardiac surgery: A review of sixty-four patients. J Thorac Cardiovasc Surg 1974;67:294–299.
39. Wilmore DW, Dudrick SJ, Daly JM, Vars HM. The role of nutrition in the adaptation of the small intestine after massive resection. Surg Synecol Obstet 1971;132:673–680.
40. Wolfe BM, Beltner RM, Willman VL. Intestinal fistula output in regular, elemental, and intravenous alimentation. Am J Surg 1972;124:803–806.
41. MacFayden BV, Dudrick SJ, Ruberg RL. Management of gastrointestinal fistulas with parenteral hyperalimentation. Surgery 1973;74:100–105.
42. Fisher JE, Foster GS, Abel RM, et al. Hyperalimentation as primary therapy for inflammatory bowel disease. Am J Surg 1973;125:165–171.
43. Aguirre A, Fisher JE, Welch CE. The role of surgery and hyperalimentation in therapy of gastrointestinal-cutaneous fistulae. Ann Surg 1974;180:383–398.
44. Solassol C, Joyeux H, Etco L, et al. New techniques for long-term intravenous feeding: An artificial gut in 75 patients. Ann Surg 1974;179:519–524.
45. Moore FD, Brennan MF. Intravenous feeding. N Engl J Med 1972;287:862–864.
46. Freeman JB, MacLean LD. Intravenous hyperalimentation: A review. Can J Surg 1971;14:180–194.
47. Daly JM, Steiger E, Vars HM, Dudrick SJ. Postoperative nutrition and colonic wound healing, serum protein metabolism and body weight. Surg Forum 1972;23:38–40.
48. Stevens JC. Surgical nutrition: The fourth coming [letter]. JAMA 1978;239:192.
49. Felig P. Editorial: Intravenous nutrition: Fact and fancy. N Engl J Med 1976;294:1455–1456.
50. Skoutaskis VA, Martinez DR, Miller WA, Dobbie RP. Team approach to total parenteral nutrition. Am J Hosp Pharm 1975;32:693–697.
51. Biebuyck JF. The hyperalimentation unit—the collaboration of clinician, biochemist, pharmacist and nurse. S Afr Med J 1976;50:1724–1725.
52. Blackett RL, Bakran A, Bradley JA, et al. A prospective study of subclavian vein catheters used exclusively for the purpose of intravenous feeding. Br J Surg 1978;65:393–395.
53. Border JR, Chenier R, McManamy RH, et al. Multiple systems organ failure: Muscle fuel deficit with visceral protein malnutrition. Surg Clin North Am 1976;56:1147–1167.
54. Long CL, Crosby F, Geiger JW, Kinney JM. Parenteral nutrition in the septic patient: Nitrogen balance, limiting plasma amino acids, and calorie to nitrogen ratios. Am J Clin Nutr 1976;29:380–391.
55. Hill GL, Bradley JA, Smith RC, et al. Changes in body weight and body protein with intravenous nutrition. JPEN 1979;3:215–218.
56. Shizgal HM, Milne CA, Spanier AH. The effect of nitrogen-sparing, intravenously administered fluids on postoperative body composition. Surgery 1979;85:496–503.
57. Barker JP, Detsky AS, Wersen DE, et al. Nutritional assessment: A comparison of clinical judgement and objective measurements. N Engl J Med 1982;306:969–972.
58. Jeejeebhoy KN, Anderson GH, Nakhooda AF, et al. Metabolic studies in total parenteral nutrition with lipid in man. Comparison with glucose. J Clin Invest 1976;57:125–136.
59. Wolfe BM, Culebras JM, Sim AJ, et al. Substrate interaction in intravenous feeding: Comparative effects of carbohydrate and fat on amino acid utilization in fasting man. Ann Surg 1977;186:518–540.
60. Askanazi J, Rosenbaum SH, Hyman A, et al. Respiratory changes induced by the large glucose loads of total parenteral nutrition. JAMA 1980;243:1444–1447.
61. Filler RM, Coran AG. Total parenteral nutrition in infants and children: Central and peripheral approaches. Surg Clin North Am 1976;56:395–412.
62. O'Neill JA, Meng HC, Caldwell MD, Stahlman MT. Metabolic evaluation of a synthetic amino acid mixture for parenteral nutrition in infants and children. J Pediatr Surg 1976;11:979–985.
63. Greenberg GR, Marliss EB, Anderson GH, et al. Protein-sparing therapy in postoperative patients. Effects of added hypocaloric glucose or lipid. N Engl J Med 1976;294:1411–1416.
64. Hoover HC Jr, Grant JP, Gorschboth C, Ketcham AS. Nitrogen-Sparing intravenous fluids in postoperative patients. N Engl J Med 1975;293:172–175.
65. Freeman JB, Stegink LD, Wittine MF, Thompson RG. The current status of protein sparing. Surg Gynecol Obstet 1977;144:843–849.
66. Bistrian BR, Blackburn GL, Scrimshaw NS, Flatt JP. Cellular immunity in semistarved states in hospitalized adults. Am J Clin Nutr 1975;28:1148–1155.

67. Carpentier YA, Druart ML, Delespesse G. Influence of total parenteral nutrition (TPN) on some immune parameters in malnourished surgical patients. Acta Chir Belg 1981;80:149–155.
68. Mullen JL, Gertner MH, Buzby GP, et al. Implications of malnutrition in the surgical patient. Arch Surg 1979;114:121–125.
69. Holter AR, Rosen HM, Fischer JE. The effects of hyperalimentation on major surgery in patients with malignant disease: a prospective study. Acta Chir Scand [Suppl] 1976;466:86–87.
70. Williams RH, Heatley RV, Lewis MH. Proceedings: A randomized controlled trial of preoperative intravenous nutrition in patients with stomach cancer. Br J Surg 1976;63:667.
71. Abel RM, Fischer JE, Buckley MJ, et al. Malnutrition in cardiac surgical patients. Results of a prospective, randomized evaluation of early postoperative parenteral nutrition. Arch Surg 1976;111:45–50.
72. Fleming CR, McGill DB, Berkner S. Home parenteral nutrition as primary therapy in patients with extensive Crohn's disease of the small bowel and malnutrition. Gastroenterology 1977;73:1077–1081.
73. Petersen SR, Sheldon GF. Acute acalculous cholecystitis: A complication of hyperalimentation. Am J Surg 1979;138:814–817.
74. Mullen JL, Hargrove WC, Dudrick SJ, et al. Ten years experience with intravenous hyperalimentation and inflammatory bowel disease. Ann Surg 1978;187:523–529.
75. Sheldon FG, Peterson SR, Sanders R. Hepatic dysfunction during hyperalimentation. Arch Surg 1978;113:504–508.
76. Ames FC, Copeland EM, Leeb DC, et al. Liver dysfunction following small-bowel bypass for obesity. Nonoperative treatment of fatty metamorphosis with parenteral hyperalimentation. JAMA 1976;235:1249–1252.
77. Heymsfield SB, Bethel RA, Ansley JD, et al. Enteral hyperalimentation: An alternative to central venous hyperalimentation. Ann Intern Med 1979;90:63–71.
78. Lickley HL, Track NS, Vranic M, Bury KD. Metabolic responses to enteral and parenteral nutrition. Am J Surg 1978;135:172–176.
79. Russel RI. Elemental diets. Gut 1975;16:68–79.
80. Page CP, Ryan JA Jr, Haff RC. Continual catheter administration of an elemental diet. Surg Gynecol Obstet 1976;141:184–188.
81. Bloch AS. Dietitians play a role in the home training of patients. JPEN 1977;1:160–162.
82. Riella MC, Scribner BH. Five years' experience with a right atrial catheter for prolonged parenteral nutrition at home. Surg Gynecol Obstet 1976;143:205–208.
83. Strobel CT, Byrne WJ, Fonkalsrud EW, Ament ME. Home parenteral nutrition: Results in 34 pediatric patients. Ann Surg 1978;188:394–403.
84. Ladefoged K. Quality of life in patients on permanent home parenteral nutrition. JPEN 1981;5:132–137.
85. Daly JM, Reynolds HM, Rowlands BJ, et al. Nutritional manipulation of tumor-bearing animals: Effects of body weight, serum protein levels and tumor growth. Surg Forum 1978;29:143–145.
86. Daly JM, Copeland EM, Dudrick SJ. Effects of intravenous nutrition on tumor growth and host immunocompetence in malnourished animals. Surgery 1978;84:655–660.
87. Daly JM, Dudrick SJ, Copeland EM. Effects of protein depletion and repletion on cell-mediated immunity in experimental animals. Ann Surg 1978;188:791–796.
88. Daly JM, Dudrick SJ, Copeland EM. Evaluation of nutritional indices as prognostic indicators in the cancer patient. Cancer 1979;43:925–931.
89. Daly JM, Copeland EM, Dudrick SJ. Chemotherapy in tumor-bearing animals: Effects or oral versus intravenous nutrition. Acta Scand (Suppl) 1979;494:178–181.
90. Daly JM, Dudrick SJ, Copeland EM. Parenteral nutrition in patients with head and neck cancer: Techniques and results. Otolaryngol Head Neck Surg 1980;88:707–713.
91. Daly JM, Copeland EM, Dudrick SJ. Intravenous hyper-alimentation: Effect on immunocompetence in cancer patients. Ann Surg 1980;192:587–592.
92. Daly JM, Copeland JM, Dudrick SJ, Delaney JM. Nutritional repletion of malnourished tumor-bearing and non-bearing rats: Effects on body weight, liver, muscle and tumor. J Surg Res 1980;28:507–518.
93. Daly JM, Reynolds HM, Dudrick SJ, Copeland EM. Effects of enteral and parenteral nutrition on tumor response to chemotherapy in experimental animals. J Surg Onc 1981;16:79–86.

Emulsions of Perfluorochemicals as Blood Substitutes

HENRY A. SLOVITER, M.D., PH.D. AND BISWANATH MUKHERJI, PH.D.

THE NEED FOR BLOOD for transfusion in most parts of the world exceeds the supply.[1] This shortage of blood is primarily a shortage of erythrocytes, since several substitutes for blood plasma are available. The development[2] of a method of preserving erythrocytes for long times in the frozen state has, in some places, contributed to the more efficient use of available blood, but the world-wide need for blood still far exceeds the supply. Since it is likely that the demand will increase faster than the supply, the needs will have to be met by substances other than natural blood or its derivatives.

The recent development of preparations of synthetic compounds which can transport oxygen and carbon dioxide may provide the substitutes for the erythrocyte which, in combination with a simulated blood plasma, constitute an "artificial blood." An artificial blood, which is available in unlimited amounts, which is not antigenic and is free of infectious agents, would be an extremely valuable therapeutic agent. Currently, the most promising substitutes for blood are the emulsions of perfluoro compounds. Perfluoro compounds (PFC) are organic compounds in which all hydrogen atoms have been replaced by fluorine atoms. The very strong bond between carbon and fluorine (11 Kcal/mol) makes these compounds very inert chemically.

Certain liquid perfluorochemicals (PFC) can serve as transporters of oxygen because of their high solubility for gases. The PFC are nonpolar liquids which are insoluble in water, and do not dissolve salts, glucose, or other components of plasma. The PFC cannot provide the functions of the plasma. However, emulsions of PFC in a suitable aqueous medium (simulated plasma) can serve as adequate substitutes for the gas transport functions of blood.

Transport of Oxygen by Perfluoro Compounds

Perfluoro compounds (liquid or emulsified) contain about the same amount of oxygen as an equal volume of erythrocytes when equilibrated with 100% oxygen (O_2). However, the oxygen in PFC is entirely in the physically dissolved state, whereas in the erythrocyte most of the oxygen is bound (ligand) to hemoglobin (Hb). The amount of oxygen contained in the PFC is a linear function of the oxygen tension (PO_2) to which it is exposed, which is not the case for Hb in the erythrocyte. Therefore, although the PFC (FC-80 or FC-47) carries about the same volume of oxygen as erythrocytes when exposed to 100% O_2 (PO_2 = 760 torr), when equilibrated with air or alveolar gas (PO_2 = 100 torr) the PFC contains only 15% to 20% as much oxygen as the same volume of erythrocytes. Therefore, with the presently available PFC emulsions, the recipient animal or human should inspire gas which has a higher oxygen concentration than air in order to adequately substitute for blood. A concentration of 60% O_2 is nontoxic for humans even after prolonged inspiration.

Biological Oxygen Transport

The first preparation and use of a PFC emulsion for biological oxygen transport was for the perfusion of an isolated rat brain.[3] This preparation consisted of the skull and its contents with nearly all extracranial tissues removed.[4] It was prepared from a deeply hypothermic rat without need for anesthetic agents, which are known to affect brain metabolism and functions. The spontaneous electrical activity (EEG) of this preparation is a very sensitive crite-

From the Harrison Department of Surgical Research, School of Medicine, University of Pennsylvania, Philadelphia, Pennsylvania.

rion of its functional condition and of the delivery of oxygen to the tissue. If circulation (perfusion) is stopped for one minute, the EEG rapidly becomes flat.

The ability of emulsified PFC to substitute for erythrocytes was first evaluated by comparing the electrical and metabolic activities of the brain perfused with PFC emulsion with that of the brain perfused with a suspension of washed dog erythrocytes, both in the same simulated blood plasma and oxygenated with 95% O_2-5% carbon dioxide (CO_2). Comparison of the EEG recording showed that perfusion with PFC emulsion maintained the electrical activity of the brain just as well as perfusion with a suspension of erythrocytes. In contrast, the isolated brain perfused with oxygenated plasma alone lost its EEG in about 1 minute. These results demonstrate that emulsified PFC can adequately transport and deliver oxygen to brain tissue, which requires more oxygen than most other tissues.

The concentrations of glucose and lactate in the fluids during perfusion of the brains were almost the same for both types of perfusion fluid and the calculated rates of glucose consumption were not significantly different. The values obtained from measurements of the blood gases and pH were nearly the same for both types of perfusion fluid. These results show that the PFC emulsion transported and delivered gases at a rate which adequately supplied the brain with oxygen and adequately removed the carbon dioxide which the brain produced.

Perfluoro compounds are colorless (no optical absorption in the visible and near ultraviolet regions) and do not fluoresce. The use of PFC as an oxygen transport substance permits some optical measurements which cannot be done when erythrocytes are used because of the optical interference by Hb. In the isolated brain perfused with emulsified PFC, the changes in oxidation-reduction state of NADH were measured by surface fluorometry, using quartz fiber optics.[5] The changes in fluorescence and electrical activity of the perfused brain in response to anoxia were about the same as in the brain of the intact rat.

The first demonstration that PFC could provide the major requirement for oxygen in whole animals was the finding[6] that frogs and mice previously infused with PFC emulsion survived much longer than untreated controls in concentrations of carbon monoxide which almost completely blocked the transport of oxygen by hemoglobin. Subsequently, Geyer[7] showed that rats survived after almost complete replacement of blood by PFC emulsion. Clark *et al.*[8] showed that PFC emulsion provided oxygen in the dog by finding that infusion of PFC emulsion caused an increase in the mixed venous oxygen tension.

The first infusion of PFC emulsion in humans was performed by Makowski *et al.*[9] in individuals who were legally dead as a result of severe brain trauma. They observed some changes in vital function after PFC infusion which returned to preinfusion status after several hours. Subsequent studies in humans,[10-13] have indicated that the PFC emulsions are not acutely toxic, although some potentially unfavorable effects were observed. These studies have been done in all cases, except that done by the group in China,[13] with the PFC emulsion Fluosol-DA, manufactured by The Green Cross Corporation of Osaka, Japan. This preparation contains detergent (Pluronic F-68, BASF Wyandotte) as emulsifying agent. This detergent has been reported to have a variety of actions, including effects on blood platelets, blood coagulation and blood viscosity.[14] Therefore, some effects observed after infusion of Fluosol-DA could be due to Pluronic F-68 instead of, or in addition to, the delivery of oxygen by PFC.

Lipid-Coated Perfluoro Compound Emulsions

The PFC have very unusual physical properties because of their extremely low intermolecular forces, which are due to the presence of the many fluorine atoms. One of the unusual properties is the extremely low surface tension of PFC. Therefore, PFC will affect reactions or phenomena in which surface actions are involved. Although PFC are chemically inert, because of their surface activity, they do affect blood platelets and blood coagulation factors.[15,16] Therefore, the use of PFC emulsions as artificial blood poses the potential hazards which may result from disorders of platelet function and blood coagulation.

In order to prevent the effects of the surface activity of PFC on platelets and blood coagulation, we attempted to cover the surface of PFC particles with a material which would mask this activity. We chose for this purpose a mixture of cholesterol and lecithin, in the proportion in which they constitute the major components of the erythrocyte membrane.

The PFC particles coated with this mixture of lipids did not affect aggregation of human blood platelets *in vitro* and did not cause thrombocytopenia when infused in animals[15]; nonlipid PFC emulsion did affect aggregation of platelets and did cause thrombocytopenia. Subsequently, we found that cholesterol was not necessary and that emulsions prepared with lecithin alone were just as satisfactory.

The emulsified PFC remains in the circulation in rats for about 3 days after infusion. We made the hypothesis that the lecithin-coated particles first lost the lecithin coating and were then removed from the circulation. If this were true, then slowing the removal of lecithin from the particles should prolong their retention in the circulation. We attempted to do this by maintaining a high concentration of lecithin in the blood by daily injection of lecithin. We found[17] that 4 days after infusion of lecithin-coated PFC emulsion in rats, no PFC remained in the circulation. In rats so infused and then given daily injections of lecithin, 67% of the PFC remained in the circulation after 4 days and complete removal of the PFC did not occur until about 14 days after infusion. Thus, it appears that the lipid-coated emulsion is safer because it does not affect blood platelets and blood coagulation, and that it is more efficacious because its retention in the circulation, and hence its function as transporter of oxygen, can be markedly prolonged.

Elimination of Perfluoro Compounds

The principal avenue of exit of PFC from the body is *via* the lungs and to a minor extent *via* the skin. No measurable amounts are excreted in urine or feces. The PFC is removed from the bloodstream by the reticuloendothelial organs and accumulates mainly in liver and spleen. Many of the PFC are retained in liver and spleen for many months. Clark *et al.*[18] reported that perfluorotributylamine persisted in liver and spleen of dogs for years after a single infusion. After testing a large number of PFC, Clark *et al.*[11] found that perfluorodecalin was eliminated from liver and spleen relatively rapidly, in a matter of days. However, perfluorodecalin did not form a stable emulsion when treated in the same way as the perfluoroamines. Naito and Yokoyama[19] reported the preparation of a relatively stable emulsion which contained a mixture of 70% perfluorodecalin and 30% perfluorotripropylamine. This preparation is the Fluosol-DA manufactured by the Green Cross Company of Osaka, Japan. This emulsion remains stable only if it is stored in the frozen state and it must be used within one day after thawing. The perfluorotripropylamine contained in this preparation is not eliminated rapidly from the tissues, being retained in the spleen for many months. Our lipid-coated emulsion of perfluorodecalin is stable at room temperature, can be infused directly from its storage container, and is eliminated from the body in a relatively short time.

REFERENCES

1. Surgenor DM, Mierzwa BD. Artificial blood and the national blood policy. Fed Proc 1975;34:1518–1521.
2. Mollison PL, Sloviter HA. Successful transfusion of previously frozen human red cells. Lancet 1951;2:862–864.
3. Sloviter HA, Kamimoto T. Erythrocyte substitute for perfusion of brain. Nature 1967;216:458–460.
4. Andjus RK, Suhara K, Sloviter HA. An isolated, perfused rat brain preparation: Its spontaneous and stimulated activity. J Appl Physiol 1967;22:1033–1039.
5. Mayevsky A, Mizawa I, Sloviter HA. Surface fluorometry and electrical activity of the isolated rat brain perfused with artificial blood. Neurol Res 1981;3:307–316.
6. Sloviter HA, Petkovic M, Ogoshi S, Yamada H. Dispersed fluorochemicals as substitutes for erythrocytes in intact animals. J Appl Physiol 1969;27:666–668.
7. Geyer RP. Fluorocarbon-polyol artificial blood substitutes. N Engl J Med 1973;289:1977–1982.
8. Clark LC, Becattini F, Kaplan S. The physiological effects of artificial blood made from inert oxygen solvents. Alabama J Med Sci 1972;9:16–29.
9. Makowski H, Tentschev P, Frey R, Necek S, Bergmann H, Blauhut B. Tolerance of an oxygen-carrying colloidal plasma substitute in humans. In: Proceedings of Fourth International Symposium on Perfluorochemical Blood Substitutes, Kyoto, 1978. Amsterdam: Excerpta Medica, 1978;47–53.
10. Mitsuno T, Ohyanagi H, Naito R. Clinical studies of a perfluorochemical whole blood substitute (Fluosol-DA). Ann Surg 1982;195:60–69.
11. Clark LC, Becattini F, Kaplan S, Obrock V, Cohen D, Becker C. Perfluorocarbon having a short dwell time in the liver. Science 1973;181:680–682.
12. Tremper KC, Friedman AE, Levine EM, Lapin R, Camarillo D. The preoperative treatment of

severely anemic patients with a perfluorochemical oxygen-transport fluid: Fluosol-DA. N Engl J Med 1982;307:277–283.

13. Xiong RC, Zhang VA, Chen HF, Huang WY, Lou ZP, Chao WZ. Clinical application of fluorocarbon artificial blood in ten cases. Chuang Hua Wai Ko Tsa Chih 1981;19:213–215.
14. Hymes AC, Rob HJ, Margolis RR. Influence of industrial surfactant (pluronic F-68) on human amniotic fluid embolism. Am J Obstet Gynecol 1970;107:1217–1222.
15. Colman RW, Chang LK, Mukherji B, Sloviter HA. Effects of a perfluoro erythrocyte substitute on platelets *in vitro* and *in vivo*. J Lab Clin Med 1980;95:553–562.
16. Lau P, Shankar VA, Mayer LD, Wurzel HA, Sloviter HA. Coagulation defects in rabbits after infusion of dispersed fluorochemicals. Transfusion 1975;15:432–438.
17. Sloviter HA, Mukherji B. Prolonged retention in the circulation of emulsified lipid-coated perfluorochemicals. In: Bolin R, Geyer R, Nemo G, eds. Advances in Blood Substitute Research. New York: Liss, 1983;181–187.
18. Clark LC, Kaplan S, Becattini F. The physiology of synthetic blood. J Thorac Cardiovasc Surg 1970;60:757–773.
19. Naito R, Yokoyama K. An improved perfluorodecalin emulsion. In: Jamieson GA, Greenwalt TJ, eds. Blood Substitutes and Plasma Expanders. New York: Liss, 1978;81–84.

Total Parenteral Nutrition and Fluid/ Electrolyte Therapy in the Home: Nine Years' Experience

EZRA STEIGER, M.D., F.A.C.S., CATHLEEN MAREIN, R.N., B.S.N., PATRICE MISNY, R.N., B.S.N., FAITH SRP, R.N., MEGAN O'NEILL, B.A., AND JANE PAYSINGER, PHARM. D.

Nine years' experience with total parenteral nutrition and fluid/electrolyte therapy in the home are reviewed. A total of 110 patients could not maintain adequate nutrition, hydration, and/or electrolyte balance due to inadequate bowel length or absorption. Nutrition, clinical examination, and blood studies were corrected, and the patient was instructed in catheter care, fluid compounding and administration, self-monitoring, and management of complications. They were out of the hospital during 90% of their involvement in the program; readmissions were primarily related to underlying disease rather than complications. Home parenteral therapy can reduce or eliminate hospitalization for many patients and may allow return to a near-normal life style.

HOME PARENTERAL THERAPY (HPT), including home parenteral nutrition (HPN) and home fluid/electrolyte therapy (HFE), is a means of providing adequate nutrition and hydration in patients with compromised gastrointestinal (GI) tract function.[1-9] HPT is used for a variety of diseases resulting in insufficient bowel length and/or abnormal intestinal absorption which render the GI tract incompetent.[10-16] The advent of HPT has allowed successful management of patients in the home for those diseases which otherwise would have resulted in repeated or prolonged hospitalization for correction of nutritional, fluid, and electrolyte imbalances. Prolonged venous access for administration of customized nutrient and electrolyte solutions is achieved through the use of a Silastic right atrial catheter.[17-21] Complete instruction of the patient and family in aseptic technique for catheter care and admixture and administration of parenteral solutions is mandatory. Continued success at home depends on regular patient follow-up and monitoring and compliance with the program.[22] The purpose of this nine-year retrospective study was to describe the HPT patient population at The Cleveland Clinic Foundation (CCF) to evaluate their clinical course and to determine the efficacy of the program.

Materials and Methods

A total of 110 patients were discharged on HPN or HFE from January 1976 through December 1984 (Table 1). There were 51 males and 59 females in this group, with a mean age of 45.3 ± 15.8 years (range, 14–73 years). Ninety-four patients (85%) required HPN and 16 patients (15%) required HFE. Patients with Crohn's disease, radiation enteritis, and ischemic bowel disease compromised 67% of the total patient population.

A consult to the hospital Nutrition Support Team (NST) initiated the evaluation for candidacy for HPT. The primary members of the NST included a physician, liaison psychiatrist, nurse, pharmacist, dietitian, and social worker who combined their efforts to thoroughly evaluate, prepare, and follow up the patient. Candidacy for HPT was considered only after dietary modifications, enteral supplements, and anti-diarrheal agents had been found to be unsuccessful in reducing fluid loss. The patient's present nutritional status was

From the Departments of General Surgery (E.S., C.M., P.M., F.S.) and Hospital Pharmacy (J.P.), The Cleveland Clinic Foundation. Submitted for publication Feb 1985; accepted May 1985.

This article has been reproduced with permission from the *Cleveland Clinic Quarterly*, Vol. 52, No. 3, Fall 1985.

assessed and base-line laboratory values obtained to estimate fluid, electrolyte, and calorie requirements. The NST also evaluated the patient's emotional state, cognitive ability, motor skills, and readiness to learn. Team members conferred to determine whether HPT was appropriate and feasible in each case. Placement of a Hickman/Broviac right atrial catheter was done after candidacy for HPT was determined.[23] Instruction in catheter care, solution preparation and administration, and self-monitoring techniques by the NST nurse and pharmacist began once the patient was physically and emotionally prepared to learn.[24,25] The instruction period lasted an average of two to three weeks and was considered complete when the patient demonstrated competency and understanding of the HPT procedures and management of possible complications. Patients were stabilized on 1 to 6 L of fluid per day and gradually tapered off from a 24-hour to an overnight infusion schedule during this training period. The patients were discharged once training was complete, home-going solutions were stabilized, and both patient and family were psychologically prepared. While at home, 82 patients (75%) mixed their own HPT solutions and 28 (25%) received pre-mixed solutions from the home supply vendor. Follow-up examinations, review of home self-monitoring records, and blood studies were done at two-week intervals, progressing to once a month based on patient stability. Routine laboratory studies included blood glucose, electrolytes, blood urea nitrogen (BUN), creatinine, calcium, phosphorus, and magnesium levels. Once a month, a complete blood count, prothrombin time, serum zinc level, and liver function tests were done, with vitamins, trace elements, essential fatty acids, and urinary calcium levels being monitored at six-month intervals.

Results

The average length of HPT for all 110 patients in our program was 26.1 months (range, 1–105), totaling 2,435 months (203 years) for HPN patients and 410 months (34 years) for patients receiving HFE (Table 2). The current active patient population, consisting of 39 HPN and 7 HFE patients, has averaged 36 months on HPT. Patients no longer in the program due to discontinuance of therapy or death (Table 3) had been on HPT for an average of 18.5 months.

Eighty-seven patients were rehospitalized a total of 324 times for an average of 3.76 ± 4.52 admissions per patient, totaling 6,661 days of rehospitalization. Twenty-three patients were never rehospitalized. Only 1,793 of the total of 6,661 rehospitalization days were related to HPT (120 admissions), or approximately 15.3 ± 14.2 days per admission. Non-HPT-related admissions totaled 4,868 days (204 admissions), or approximately 24.4 ± 24.1 days per admission. Thus only 27% of admissions were related to HPT. In addition to rehospitalization, we have noted previously that overall mortality was also related to the underlying disease process rather than to HPT.[26] Of 187 catheters inserted, mean catheter life was 15.34 ± 17.57 months (range, 0.25–99). Seventy-one patients (65%) have never required catheter replacement.

Discussion

In reviewing our nine years of experience with the HPT program, we found the minimal rehospitalization time to be noteworthy. Our 110 patients were out of the hospital for 68,790 days, with rehospitalization accounting for only 10% of their time in the program. The most frequent cause for readmission was the patient's primary disease process and its associated complications. The majority of HPT-related rehospitalizations were for actual or suspected catheter sepsis and other catheter-related complications, with only infrequent readmissions for fluid/electrolyte abnormalities. The fact that our patients were able to spend 90% of their time at home is significant and can be attributed to the concerted efforts of the multidisciplinary team, their extensive knowledge of HPT and its complications, and the thorough instruction and follow-up of each patient. Continued work in the study and understanding of HPT and improvement of products and techniques are necessary in order to enhance the efficacy of HPT and further reduce rehospitalizations.

Catheter Insertion and Care

Prior to the operation, one of the NST nurses shows the patient a catheter, explains the insertion technique, and marks the exit site on the patient's skin with gentian violet. The

TABLE 1. *Home Parenteral Therapy (HPT) Patient Data*

	No. of patients	% of total HPT patients	Age (yr) Mean	Age (yr) Range	Sex Male	Sex Female
Crohn's disease	37	33	37	18–64	16	21
Radiation enteritis	24	22	56	40–73	6	18
Mesenteric vascular infarction	13	11	51	15–64	10	3
Small-bowel obstruction secondary to cancer	9	8	52	28–70	3	6
Ulcerative colitis involving the mucosa of other regions	4	4	37	14–69	3	1
Esophagitis secondary to bone marrow transplant	4	4	23	19–32	3	1
Small-bowel obstruction	4	4	53	40–65	2	2
Pseudo-obstruction	3	3	57	45–71	2	1
Malabsorption syndrome	3	3	53	37–66	2	1
Scleroderma of the GI tract	2	2	55	46–63	0	2
Gardner's syndrome (familial polyposis)	2	<2	38	28–48	1	1
Hirschsprung's disease	1	<1	39	. . .	0	1
Diverticulitis	1	<1	66	. . .	0	1
Congenital malrotation of the intestine	1	<1	22	. . .	1	0
Sclerosing cholangitis	1	<1	35	. . .	1	0
Toxic megacolon	1	<1	17	. . .	1	0
TOTALS	110	100	43	14–73	51	59

TABLE 2. *Length of Home Parenteral Therapy*

	1–12 mo	13–24 mo	25–36 mo	37–48 mo	49–60 mo	61–72 mo	73–84 mo	85–96 mo	97–108 mo	Totals
HPN patients	41	16	11	11	6	2	2	1	4	94
HFE patients	10	1	1	1	0	1	2	1	1	16
TOTALS	51	17	12	12	6	3	0	2	5	110

TABLE 3. *Reasons for Discontinuation of HPT*

Diagnosis	Death			HPT terminated	
	HPT associated (No. of patients)	Underlying disease and/or complicating factors (No. of patients)	Concomitant illness (No. of patients)	Bowel continuity surgically restored (No. of patients)	Bowel continuity medically restored (No. of patients)
Crohn's disease	0	3	5	5	3
Radiation enteritis	0	12*	1	3	0
Ischemic bowel	0	1	3	0	0
Small-bowel obstruction secondary to cancer	0	6	0	1	0
Ulcerative colitis involving the mucosa of other regions	0	0	2	1	1
Esophagitis secondary to bone-marrow transplant	0	0	0	0	4
Pseudo-obstruction	0	0	1	0	0
Small-bowel obstruction	0	2	0	1	1
Malabsorption	0	1	0	1	1
Scleroderma (GI tract)	0	1	0	0	0
Congenital malrotation of bowel	0	0	0	0	1
Sclerosing cholangitis	0	0	0	0	1
Toxic megacolon	0	0	0	1	0
Gardner's syndrome	0	0	0	0	1
TOTALS	0	26 (41%)	12 (19%)	13 (20%)	13 (20%)

* Eight patient deaths were attributable to recurrent cancer.

catheter exits to the right or left of the sternum along the nipple line at a level that can be easily seen by the patient. It should not exit near a draining wound or intestinal drainage bag, so as to minimize the possibility of contamination.

We employ a durable silicone rubber catheter (Hickman or Broviac) which is approximately 90 cm long. The two catheters differ in that the Broviac catheter has a narrower internal lumen than the Hickman catheter (1.0 versus 1.6 mm). Both function and are managed in the same manner, but the Broviac catheter is more likely to become occluded,[27] and blood samples may be more difficult to obtain due to collapse of the internal lumen upon aspiration. On the other hand, the Hickman catheter may theoretically be more thrombogenic because of its larger size.

Bilateral subclavian venograms are obtained prior to catheter placement to determine the availability of vessels in the upper thoracic venous system. Veins usually selected for catheter insertion include the cephalic, internal or external jugular, and the muscular branch of the subclavian. In the event of thrombosis involving the superior vena cava, a saphenous approach to the inferior vena cava may be necessary.[28] Subclinical thrombosis of the subclavian vein, occasionally noted on preoperative venograms, would preclude its use for permanent catheter placement; this is seen most commonly in patients who have had multiple temporary catheters placed for inhospital total parenteral nutrition (TPN) or central venous pressure monitoring. Catheter placement into the azygous system via the intercostal vein is a relatively new approach which has reportedly been successful in children.[29] We have also used direct right atrial catheterization via a thoracotomy incision when all other venous access sites have been depleted.[30]

Catheters must be cared for using aseptic techniques in order to prevent contamination and sepsis. Hickman/Broviac dressings are changed daily by the patient, or more frequently if they become soiled or wet. Localized exit site infections are treated by changing the dressing twice a day and administering intravenous (IV) antibiotics. We have been successful in resolving such infections with this protocol if the organism has not invaded the Dacron cuff within the subcutaneous tunnel. Intravascular catheter sepsis is suspected if positive blood cultures are obtained through the catheter and/or no other source of sepsis can be determined. Antibiotics are usually not necessary if the catheter is removed promptly. A new catheter can be placed in five to seven days if two consecutive sets of peripheral blood cultures prove negative. If the catheter must be removed due to confirmed sepsis, catheter care and mixing procedures are reviewed. Subcutaneously implanted venous access devices such as the Port-a-Cath, Infuse-a-Port, and Mediport have recently been reported to be successful for infusion of HPT fluids,[31,32] but require daily skin puncture and have not yet been widely accepted.

To prevent the catheter from becoming occluded, it is flushed with 2 mL of heparin (100 U/mL) at the completion of the infusion. Should occlusion occur, patency may be restored by infusing a dilute solution of streptokinase or urokinase. Streptokinase, a protein derived from group C beta hemolytic streptococci, acts by forming a complex with plasminogen which then converts plasminogen to plasmin. Urokinase, an enzyme produced by the human kidney, directly converts plasminogen to plasmin. In both instances, the plasmin then degrades the fibrin within the clots. Anaphylaxis and systemic fibrinolysis are potential risks associated with the use of streptokinase, however, the use of a very dilute solution and aspiration of any residual drug in the catheter minimizes these risks. Urokinase is considered nonantigenic, but the increased cost of this product outweighs that benefit and makes streptokinase the thrombolytic agent of choice for preventing catheter occlusions. Using a tuberculum syringe, a mixture of streptokinase and normal saline, producing a concentration of 2,500 U/mL of streptokinase, is gently instilled in a volume equal to the internal volume of the catheter. The solution should remain in contact with the clot for 30 minutes, after which repeated aspirations of the residual clot and drug are made every five minutes until patency is restored. If the catheter is not patent after several attempts, the solution is left in the catheter for 24 hours.[33]

To minimize fibrin formation within the catheter and decrease the incidence of venous thrombosis associated with infusion of hypertonic solutions, 1,000 U of heparin is added to each liter of HPT solution. Venogams should be obtained if thrombosis is suspected. Thrombosis can be confirmed if venous obstruction and collateralization are noted upon injection of contrast material. Distension of veins in the shoulder and anterior chest walls, swelling of the arm, and shoulder pain on the involved side are typical of subclavian vein thrombosis. In addition, neck or throat pain, puffiness of the face, extensive tearing, and rhinorrhea may be noted. While heparin has been found to be ineffective in achieving thrombolysis, success may be attained with local infusion of streptokinase.[34,35] However, in most cases, treatment proves futile and the catheter must be removed.

HPT patients are provided with a temporary repair kit and instructed in its use should catheter breakage occur. The kit contains all supplies needed for temporary repair, including a sterile blunted needle whose gauge corresponds to that of the catheter: a 15 gauge for the Hickman catheter, 18 gauge for the Broviac, and 22 gauge for the pediatric Broviac. The catheter is cut with sterile scissors so that the site of the breakage is removed. The blunted needle is inserted into the lumen of the catheter, forming a new end on the original catheter. Patients are told that this repair is only temporary, and that they should make an appointment with the physician who placed the catheter so that it can be permanently repaired; this involves splicing a new end onto the remaining segment of the original catheter. We have not observed any increase in catheter sepsis rates associated with such repairs.[36]

Patient/family Instruction

The goal of the HPT program is to facilitate a smooth transition of the patient from the hospital to the home. In order to achieve the goal, the patient and/or family must be educated to a level of independence and develop a sense of confidence. Thorough evaluation of the patient prior to instruction is needed to determine any cognitive, psychological, and/or physical impairments in order to plan for learning needs and adapt instruction materials as necessary. The patient is trained as the primary care giver; a family member is involved, if willing, but only as a back-up. This not only prevents family members from feeling burdened with the primary responsibility of the patient's care but also helps to alleviate the patient's loss of autonomy and forced dependency. If absolutely necessary, a family member can be taught to be solely responsible, but never anyone who lives outside the home. Some patients may require total care for HPT; and although resources are available, we have found only a limited number of extended care facilities that would except patients requiring HPN or HFE.

Instruction can be expedited with the use of a Cath-Train vest, a teaching tool which simulates the patient's own catheter. The vest allows the patient to become proficient in working with the catheter and permits unsupervised practice between lessons. Instructions need to be written in simple concise sentences employing very basic terminology. A format of instructions written in step-by-step fashion, separate from definitions, complications, and discussions, is easier for the patient to follow than instructions written in paragraph form or intermingled with diagrams. Memorization of procedures is not necessary as it extends the learning time and increases the patient's anxiety. The patient must be able to simply follow the written instructions. One procedure is demonstrated at a time, practice allowed, and competency nearly mastered prior to advancing to the next procedure Evaluation is conducted continuously, with immediate feedback provided and appropriate changes made. Instruction is complete when the learner can perform all procedures independently and can respond appropriately when posed with actual or hypothetical problems or complications.

Solution/additive Preparation and Administration

HPT solutions can be either mixed by the patient or pre-mixed by the home supply vendor. Since pre-mixed HPT solutions did not become available until 1980–1981, prior to this time, all patients had to be instructed in self-mixing procedures At the CCF, most patients who are expected to be on HPT permanently (or at least more than six months) learn to mix their own dialysis solutions; patients and family members who are unable to learn the mixing techniques, or patients who will only require HPT for six months or less, receive pre-mixed solutions through the home supply vendor. The additional cost of the vendor-prepared solutions is offset by the savings associated with a shorter in-hospital stay for training.

The base solutions and additives used for HPT are basically the same as the TPN and fluid/electrolyte solutions used in the hospital. Fluid composition and nutrient requirements

TABLE 4. *Contents of a Typical HPN Solution*

Nutrient	1 L	2 L
FreAmine III 8.5%*	500 mL	1,000 mL
Dextrose 50%	500 mL	1,000 mL
Calcium gluconate injection (0.46 mEq/mL)	9.2 mEq	18.4 mEq
Magnesium sulfate injection (4.06 mEq/mL)	8.1 mEq	16.2 mEq
Potassium chloride injection (2 mEq/mL)	20.0 mEq	40.0 mEq
Potassium phosphate injection (4.4 mEq K/mL)	10.0 mEq	10.0 mEq
Sodium acetate injection (2 mEq/mL)	20.0 mEq	40.0 mEq
Sodium chloride injection (4 m Eq/mL)	50.0 mEq	100.0 mEq
Heparin sodium (1,000 U/mL)	1,000 U	2,000 U
Multiple vitamins (N = 12)	10.0 mL	10.0 mL
Multiple trace elements concentrate	1.0 mL	1.0 mL
Selenium injection (40 μg/mL)	120 μg	120 μg

* American McGaw Laboratories, Irvine, Calif.

are established, based on each patient's individual nutritional assessment, daily weight, intake and output, BUN, and creatinine. HPT patients may require 1–6 L of nutrient/IV crystalloid solutions to maintain homeostasis, depending on the state of functional impairment of the bowel and losses through a GI tract fistula or stoma. While HFE patients require only IV crystalloids, with appropriate additives to maintain fluid and electrolyte balance and adequate renal function, HPN patients need amino acids, dextrose, electrolytes, vitamins, minerals, and trace elements to maintain nutritional homeostasis. Many HPN patients require additional IV crystalloids to control fluid and electrolyte balance when high-output stomas and/or fistulas are present. Most HPN patients must have a minimum of 2 L of nutrient solutions. A typical 2-L HPN formula containing 4.25% amino acids and 25% dextrose as a base solution, along with additives, is shown in Table 4. Vitamins and trace elements are added to HPT solutions in accord with the American Medical Association (AMA) Nutrition Advisory Group recommendations for parenteral use (Tables 5 and 6).[37,38] Since all fat- and water-soluble vitamins except K are contained in the single multivitamin preparation, the patients are instructed to take 10 mg of vitamin K intramuscularly twice a month.

Deficiencies of trace elements such as zinc, copper, chromium, and selenium in patients receiving TPN have been documented.[41–43] Since 1976, our HPT patients have added not only these trace elements but also manganese to 1 L of their daily infusate to maintain adequate levels. Dosages were originally based on the oral recommendations of the recommended dietary allowances guidelines, but have been re-evaluated yearly as more definitive requirements[39] and clinically manifested deficiency states have appeared. Since 1978–1979, when serum trace mineral analysis using atomic absorption spectrophotometry first became

TABLE 5. *Intravenous Vitamin Additives for TPN*

Vitamin	Multiple vitamins (N = 12) (per 10 mL)	AMA guidelines for adults[37]
A	3,300 IU	3,300 IU
D	200 IU	200 IU
E	10 IU	10 IU
K	. . .	. . .
C (ascorbic acid)	100.0 mg	100.0 mg
B_1 (thiamin)	3.0 mg	3.0 mg
B_2 (riboflavin)	3.6 mg	3.6 mg
Niacin	40.0 mg	40.0 mg
B_6 (pyridoxine)	4.0 mg	4.0 mg
Pantothenic acid	15.0 mg	15.0 mg
Folacin	0.4 mg	0.4 mg
B_{12} (cyanocobalamin)	5.0 μg	5.0 μg
Biotin	60.0 μg	60.0 μg

TABLE 6. *Trace Element Additives for TPN*

	Trace element solution (per mL)	AMA guidelines*[38]		
		Stable adults	Catabolic adults	Adults with intestinal losses
Zinc	5.0 mg	2.5–4.0 mg	Additional 2.0 mg	Additional 12.2 mg per L of small-bowel fluid lost; 17.1 mg per kg of stool or ileostomy output
Copper	1.0 mg	0.5–1.5 mg	...	...
Chromium	10.0 g	10.0–15.0 μg	...	20.0 μg
Manganese	0.5 mg	0.15–0.8 mg	...	...

* Multiple trace element concentrate, LymphoMed, Melrose Park, Ill.

available at the CCF, patient monitoring has progressed to include trace metal analysis every six months as a routine protocol. Dosages of the trace minerals described in Table 6 have maintained serum zinc and copper levels within normal limits. While chromium levels in our patients tended to be in the very low normal range, manganese levels were consistently elevated, indicating that AMA recommendations for manganese in HPT patients may be excessive. Manganese deficiency has not been reported in HPT patients to our knowledge. Selenium levels tended to be low. In a previous monograph describing selenium use in adult and pediatric patients receiving HPT,[40] we indicated that 63% of our patients occasionally had low selenium levels. Reviewing a smaller sample of patients (N = 28) revealed that 39% of them maintained normal levels at the prescribed dosage. When the remaining patients were placed on higher doses, only 35% demonstrated increased selenium levels. However, despite low levels of chromium and selenium and elevated manganese levels for varying periods of time, none of the patients seen during the course of our program has demonstrated clinical trace mineral deficiency[41–43] or toxicity. Exogenous administration of iron-dextran complex (Imferon) may be given as required to maintain normal hematologic values. However, test dosages should be given prior to infusion of the therapeutic dose to test for and guard against the occurrence of an anaphylactic-type reaction. Regular insulin should be added directly to the HPN solution, if necessary, to control serum glucose levels during infusion: they should be ≤200–250 mg% during the infusion, and return to normal within two hours postinfusion. The cyclic, eight-to-12-hour overnight infusion schedule necessitates the use of a volumetric infusion pump with appropriate alarm systems, which assures safe and accurate delivery of solutions while the patient is asleep.[44–47]

Final in-line filtration of particulate matter and bacteria is achieved by the addition of a 0.22-μ air-eliminating filter to the infusion system.[48–50] Solutions may be administered using a Y-tube set for a separated 2 L of fluid, admixture of the entire volume of solution into the appropriate size 2- or 3-L bag, or both. Such set-ups will allow the patient to hang the entire volume of solution at one time, allowing for an uninterrupted night's sleep. During the last hour of infusion, the prescribed infusion rate is reduced by half to taper off the quantity of dextrose infused, thereby preventing reactive hypoglycemia.

In the majority of HPT patients requiring high caloric solutions (HPN group), fat must be provided intravenously in addition to dextrose and protein to prevent essential fatty acid deficiency (EFAD). This condition, characterized by an increase of 5,8,11-eicosatrienoic acid, may develop within two weeks of fat-free parenteral nutrition.[51] Symptoms could include eczematous desquamative dermatitis, hair loss, thrombocytopenia, and possibly impaired wound healing and hepatic dysfunction.[52–55] Providing 2%–3% of the patient's total calories as linoleic acid can prevent these sequelae.[56,57] Infusion of 500 mL of 10% fat emulsion over a period of four hours twice a week is generally sufficient for maintaining essential fatty acid levels; however, they should be monitored periodically to adjust for individual patient needs. A 20% fat emulsion is also available for IV use. However, infusion of a 20% fat emulsion over less than the recommended eight hours was associated with priapism in 2 of our male patients. Although vascular thrombosis is suspected, the exact etiology is unclear.[58]

TABLE 7. *Patients With Metabolic Bone Disease*

Case	Age (yr) and sex	Clinical symptoms	Bone biopsy	Urine calcium balance	Serum calcium	Vitamins		Diagnosis
						25-$(OH)_2$ D2	1,25-$(OH)_2$ D3	
1	61, F	Multiple spontaneous fractures	Active osteopenia	NA	Below normal	Normal	Normal	Radiation enteritis following treatment for cancer
2	67, F	Bone pain and fractured vertebrae	Active osteopenia	Negative	Normal	High normal	Low normal	Short bowel syndrome, diverticulitis
3	28, M	Spontaneous hip fracture	Not done	NA	Normal	NA	NA	Crohn's disease
4	26, F	Rib fracture	Not done	NA	Normal	NA	NA	Crohn's disease
5	51, F	Bone pain	Normal	Negative	Low normal	Elevated	Below normal	Radiation enteritis following treatment for ovarian cancer
6	64, F	Spontaneous hip fracture	Inactive osteoporosis	Positive	Normal	Elevated	Below normal	Radiation enteritis following treatment for ovarian cancer
7	19, M	Bone pain and compression fracture	Active osteopenia/osteomalacia	Positive	Normal	Elevated	Elevated	Crohn's disease

Metabolic Bone Disease

Metabolic bone disease, characterized by bone pain and spontaneous fractures (nonattributable to physical mishap) and diagnosed pathologically by osteoporosis and osteomalacia bone histology, has been documented in patients receiving HPN.[59–62] Previous observations[59,60,63] have indicated that HPN is a primary causative factor in the development of these histological abnormalities despite the underlying disease. Review of the medical histories of the 110 CCF patients treated to date revealed metabolic bone disease in 7 (6.4%) (Table 7), documented clinically by bone pain (1 patient), spontaneous fractures (4 patients), or both (2 patients). Patients included 2 men and 5 women, with the latter group including 4 who were post-menopausal and/or had undergone total abdominal hysterectomy at least 10 years earlier; the mean age was 45.5 ± 20.3 years over a range of 26–67. Three patients had gastrointestinal malabsorption secondary to Crohn's disease, 3 had radiation enteritis following treatment for ovarian cancer, and 1 had diverticulitis; all had undergone multiple operations resulting in short-bowel syndrome one to 10 years prior to HPN. Bone pain developed in 3 patients within six months of initial discharge on HPT. Two patients experienced compression fractures of the vertebrae shortly after onset of bone pain. Four patients without previous pain had spontaneous fractures of the hip or ribs eight to 54 months after initial discharge on HPT.

Four women and 1 man in our series underwent tetracycline labeling and subsequent iliac crest bone biopsy to aid in diagnosis and treatment. Biopsy findings, ranging from normal to severe inactive osteoporosis, were correlated with urinary calcium balance and levels of serum calcium, 25-hydroxy vitamin D and 1,25-dihydroxy vitamin D whenever possible. Based on this analysis, recommendations were made for increased IV calcium to maintain a positive urinary calcium balance[64] and/or increased vitamin D supplementation.[62,65] Only one patient receiving increased calcium has demonstrated long-term relief of symptoms.

Just as the exact etiology of metabolic bone disease in HPT has remained a mystery, treatment has been varied and experimental.[59,62,63,65,66]

Length of Therapy

Depending upon their underlying disease, degree of GI tract dysfunction, and length of bowel remaining, patients may require HPT on a permanent or temporary basis. In our experience, patients with radiation enteritis or ischemic bowel disease due to mesenteric infarction usually remain on HPT permanently, whereas patients with Crohn's disease and/or short-bowel syndrome with subsequent bowel adaptation may only require HPT temporarily. Both groups of patients are able to avoid prolonged hospitalization with HPT and can return home. Patients who have catastrophic enterocutaneous fistulas and require prolonged bowel rest for resolution of inflammation prior to surgery have also been managed with HPT; after three to six months, surgery is performed, if necessary, to resect persistent fistulas and/or re-establish temporarily interrupted GI tract continuity.[14,67]

Conclusion

The 110 patients taking part in the CCF HPT program were able to spend a significant length of time at home with a low incidence of morbidity and mortality. All had significant underlying disease that would otherwise have required either repeated or permanent hospitalization. A satisfactory fluid balance and nutritional status can be maintained with an overnight infusion of customized solutions. Accurate record keeping, routine laboratory monitoring, regular follow-up visits, and continued communication between the patient, patient's family, and NST members are essential to ensure patient safety and well-being as well as the success of the program.

REFERENCES

1. Dudrick SJ, Wilmore DW, Vars HM, Rhoads JE. Long-term parenteral nutrition with growth, development, and positive nitrogen balance. Surgery 1968;64:134–141.
2. Ivey M, Riella M, Mueller W, Scribner B. Long-term parenteral nutrition in the home. Am J Hosp Pharm 1975;32:1032–1036.
3. Bordos DC, Cameron JL. Successful long-term intravenous hyperalimentation in the hospital and at home. Arch Surg 1975;110:439–441.

4. Riella MC, Scribner BH. Five years' experience with a right atrial catheter for prolonged parenteral nutrition at home. Surg Gynecol Obstet 1976;143:205–208.
6. Grundfest S, Steiger E, Sattler L, Washko S, Wateska L. The current status of home total parenteral nutrition. Artif Organs 1979;3:156–160.
7. Steiger E, Grundfest S. A review of home hyperalimentation. Contemp Surg 1979;15:33–40.
8. Grundfest S, Steiger E. Experience with the Broviac catheter for prolonged parenteral alimentation. JPEN 1979;3:45–47.
9. Grundfest S, Steiger E. Home parenteral nutrition. JAMA 1980;244:1701–1703.
10. Byrne WJ, Halpin TC, Asch MJ, Fonkalsrud EW, Ament ME. Home total parenteral nutrition: an alternative approach to the management of children with severe chronic small bowel disease. J Pediatr Surg 1977;12:359–366.
11. Dudrick SJ, MacFadyen BV Jr, Souchen EA, Englert DM, Copeland EM III. Parenteral nutrition techniques in cancer patients. Cancer Res 1977;37:2440–2450.
12. Faulk DL, Anuras S, Freeman JB. Idiopathic chronic intestinal pseudo-obstruction. Use of central venous nutrition. JAMA 1978;240:2075–2076.
13. Fleming CR, McGill DB, Berkner S. Home parenteral nutrition as primary therapy in patients with extensive Crohn's disease of the small bowel and malnutrition. Gastroenterology 1977;73:1077–1081.
14. Oakley JR, Steiger E, Lavery IC, Fazio VW. Catastrophic enterocutaneous fistulae: the role of home hyperalimentation. Cleve Clin Q 1979;46:133–136.
15. Stewart GR. Home parenteral nutrition for chronic short bowel syndrome. Med J Aust 1979;2:317–319.
16. Grischkan D, Steiger E, Fazio V. Maintenance of home hyperalimentation in patients with high-output jejunostomies. Arch Surg 1979;114:838–841.
17. Scribner BH, Cole JJ, Christopher TG, Vizzo JE, Atkins RC, Blagg CR. Long-term total parenteral nutrition. The concept of an artificial gut. JAMA 1970;212:457–463.
18. Byrne WJ, Ament ME, Burke M, Fonkalsrud E. Home parenteral nutrition. Surg Gynecol Obstet 1979;149:593–599.
19. Goldberger JH, Deluca FG, Wesselhoeft CW, Randall HT. A home program of long-term total parenteral nutrition in children. J Pediatr 1979;94:325–328.
20. Solassol C, Joyeux H, Etco L, Pujol H, Romieu C. New techniques for long-term intravenous feeding: an artificial gut in 75 patients. Ann Surg 1974;179:519–522.
21. Broviac JW, Cole JJ, Scribner BH. A silicon rubber right atrial catheter for prolonged parenteral alimentation. Surg Gynecol Obstet 1973;136:602–606.
22. Hughes BA, Fleming CR, Berkner S, Gaffron R. Patient compliance with a home parenteral nutrition program. JPEN 1980;4:12–14.
23. Lees CD, Steiger E, Hooley RA, et al. Home parenteral nutrition. Surg Clin North Am 1981;61:621–633.
24. Gulledge AD, Gipson WT, Steiger E, Hooley R, Srp F. Home parenteral nutrition for the short bowel syndrome. Psychological issues. Gen Hosp Psychiatry 1980;2:271–281.
25. Srp F, Steiger E, Montague N, et al. Patient preparation for cyclic home parenteral nutrition: a team approach. Nutr Support Serv 1981;1:31–34.
26. Steiger E, Srp F. Morbidity and mortality related to home parenteral nutrition in patients with gut failure. Am J Surg 1983;145:102–105.
27. Srp F, Montague N, Steiger E, O'Neill M. A comparison of two types of long-term silicone right atrial catheters (RAC) (abst). JPEN 1980;4:597.
28. Wilson SE, Owens ML. Vascular Access Surgery. Chicago, Year Book, 1980, p 24.
29. Newman BM, Cooney DR, Karp MP, Jewett TC Jr. The intercostal vein: an alternate route for central venous alimentation. J Pediatr Surg 1983;18:732–733.
30. Oram-Smith JC, Mullen JL, Harken AH, Fitts WT Jr. Direct right atrial catheterization for total parenteral nutrition. Surgery 1978;83:274–276.
31. Baptista RJ, Lahey MA, Bistrian BR, et al. Periodic reassessment for improved, cost-effective care in home total parenteral nutrition: a case report. JPEN 1984;8:708–710.
32. Goodman MS, Wickam R. Venous access devices: an overview. Oncol Nurs Forum 1984;11:16–23.
33. Hurtubise MR, Bottino JC, Lawson M, McCredie KB. Restoring patency of occluded central venous catheters. Arch Surg 1980;115:212–213.
34. Rubenstein M, Cregar WP. Successful streptokinase therapy for catheter-induced subclavian vein thrombosis. Arch Intern Med 1980;140:1370–1371.
35. Smith NL, Ravo B, Soroff HS, Khan SA. Successful fibrinolytic therapy for superior vena cava thrombosis secondary to long-term total parenteral nutrition. JPEN 1985;9:55–57.
36. Montague N, Srp F, Steiger E. Emergency catheter repairs in the home parenteral nutrition (HPN) patient (abst). JPEN 1980;4:597.
37. American Medical Association Department of Foods and Nutrition. Multivitamin preparations for parenteral use. A statement by the Nutrition Advisory Group. JPEN 1979;3:258–262.
38. American Medical Association. Guidelines for essential trace element preparations for parenteral use. A statement by the Nutrition Advisory Group. JPEN 1979;3:263–267.
39. AMA Department of Foods and Nutrition. Guidelines for essential trace element preparations for parenteral use. A statement by an expert panel. JAMA 1979;241:2051–2054.

40. Steiger E, Helbley M, Zlotkin SH. Selenium in total parenteral nutrition: clinical experience in two medical centers. Melrose Park, Ill., LymphoMed, 1982.
41. Solomons NW. On the assessment of trace mineral nutriture in patients on total parenteral nutrition. Nutr Support Serv 1981;1:13–16.
42. Johnson RA, Baker SS, Fallon JT, et al. An occidental case of cardiomyopathy and selenium deficiency. N Engl J Med 1981;305:1210–1212.
43. Van Rij AM, Thomson CD, McKenzie JM, Robinson MF. Selenium deficiency in total parenteral nutrition. Am J Clin Nutr 1979;32:2076–2085.
44. Goldfarb IW, Slater H. Techniques of administration. Am J Intra Ther Clin Nutr 1981;8:25–34.
45. Fabry J. Infusion monitoring devices. NITA 1981;4:366–367.
46. Pipp TL. Intravenous infusion pump justification and selection and utilization. Infusion 1978;2:45–58.
47. Turco SJ. Mechanical and electronic equipment for parenteral and enteral use: an update. Am J Intra Ther Clin Nutr 1982;9:9–43.
48. Schneider PJ. Should inline filters be used when administering TPN solution? Infusion 1982;6:66–67.
49. National Coordinating Committee on Large Volume Parenterals. Problems and benefits of in-line filtration. Am J Intra Ther Clin Nutr 1980;7:45–47.
50. Lorenzen BA. Final filtration. NITA 1981;4:322–327.
51. Goodgame JT, Lowry SF, Brennan MF. Essential fatty acid deficiency in total parenteral nutrition: time course of development and suggestions for therapy. Surgery 1978;84:271–277.
52. Collins FO, Sinclair AJ, Royle JP, Coats DA, Maynard AT, Leonard RF. Plasma lipids in human linoleic acid deficiency. Nutr Metab 1971;13:150–167.
53. Richardson TJ, Sgoutas D. Essential fatty acid deficiency in four adult patients during total parenteral nutrition. Am J Clin Nutr 1975;28:258–263.
54. Paulsrud JR, Pensler L, Whitten CF, Stewart S, Holman RT. Essential fatty acid deficiency in infants induced by fat-free intravenous feeding. Am J Clin Nutr 1972;25:897–907.
55. Caldwell MD, Jonsson HT, Othersen HB. Essential fatty acid deficiency in an infant receiving prolonged parenteral alimentation. J Pediatr 1972;81:894–898.
56. Tashiro T, Ogata H, Yokoyama H, Mashima Y, Itoh K. The effect of fat emulsion (Intralipid) on essential fatty acid deficiency in infants receiving intravenous alimentation. J Pediatr Surg 1976;11:505–515.
57. Barr LH, Dunn GD, Brennan MF. Essential fatty acid deficiency during total parenteral nutrition. Ann Surg 1981;193:304–311.
58. Klein EA, Montague DK, Steiger E. Priapism associated with the use of intravenous fat emulsion: case reports and postulated pathogenesis. J Urol 1985;133:857–859.
59. Shike M, Harrison JE, Sturtridge WC, et al. Metabolic bone disease in patients receiving long-term total parenteral nutrition. Ann Intern Med 1980;92:343–350.
60. Klein GL, Targoff CM, Ament ME, et al. Bone disease associated with total parenteral nutrition. Lancet 1980;2:1041–1044.
61. Klein GL, Horst RL, Norman AW, Ament ME, Slatopolsky E, Coburn JW. Reduced serum levels of 1α,25-dihydroxy-vitamin D during long-term total parenteral nutrition. Ann Intern Med 1981;94:638–643.
62. Klein GL, Cannon RA, Diament MD, et al. Infantile vitamin D-resistant rickets associated with total parenteral nutrition. Am J Dis Child 1982;136:74–76.
63. Shike M, Strutridge WC, Tam CS, et al. A possible role of vitamin D in the genesis of parenteral-nutrition-induced metabolic bone disease. Ann Intern Med 1981;95:560–568.
64. Wittine MF, Freeman JB. Calcium requirements during total parenteral nutrition in well-nourished individuals. JPEN 1977;1:152–155.
65. Sloan GM, White DE, Brennan MF. Calcium and phosphorus metabolism during total parenteral nutrition. Ann Surg 1983;197:1–6.
66. Ott SM, Maloney NA, Coburn JW, et al. The prevalence of bone aluminum deposition in renal osteodystrophy and its relation to the response to calcitriol therapy. N Engl J Med 1982;307:709–713.
67. Byrne WJ, Burke M, Fonkalsrud EW, Ament ME. Home parenteral nutrition: an alternative approach to the management of complicated gastrointestinal fistulas not responding to conventional medical or surgical therapy. JPEN 1979;3:355–359.

Total Parenteral Nutrition: A Metabolic Role to Increase Tumor Response to Chemotherapy

MICHAEL H. TOROSIAN, M.D.

THE RELATIONSHIP between cancer, nutrition and the metabolic state of the tumor-bearing host is complex. Nutrient administration generally is associated with an increased rate of tumorigenesis and increased growth of established tumors. Protein–calorie restriction inhibits tumorigenesis and retards tumor growth. The degree of protein–calorie deprivation necessary to impair tumor development, however, may be associated with deleterious effects on host metabolism.

In patients with malignancy, extensive changes in energy, carbohydrate, lipid, and protein metabolism have been documented. Significant host alterations include abnormal energy expenditure, inefficient energy utilization, glucose intolerance, impaired insulin sensitivity, abnormal rates of gluconeogenesis, increased lipid mobilization, changes in total body lipid content, nitrogen balance abnormalities, and host nitrogen depletion. The clinical consequence of these nutritional and metabolic abnormalities in the tumor-bearing host is the syndrome of cancer cachexia.

Cancer cachexia is a symptom complex which consists of anorexia, weight loss, severe tissue wasting, asthenia, and impaired organ function. Although the etiology of cancer cachexia is unknown, a multitute of disease and treatment-related factors contribute to the development of this syndrome in patients with advanced malignancy. As early as 1932, Warren recognized a relationship between host wasting and mortality in cancer patients. Thus, nutrition support is frequently administered to cancer patients in an attempt to prevent or delay the onset of cancer cachexia.

Of clinical concern when administering exogenous nutrients to cancer patients, however, is the potential for stimulating tumor growth. Although stimulation of tumor growth is generally considered detrimental to the host, an alternative approach is to induce tumor cell proliferation for potential therapeutic advantage. In our laboratory, we have demonstrated that it is possible to potentiate tumor sensitivity to cycle-specific chemotherapy by administering total parenteral nutrition.

Measuring response of the AC-33 adenocarcinoma in Lewis/Wistar rats to methotrexate, we have demonstrated significant reduction in final tumor volume in animals receiving parenteral nutrition compared to animals receiving intravenous saline. Maximum tumor response to chemotherapy was observed in animals receiving a short pulse (48 hours) of parenteral nutrition with chemotherapy administered two hours after initiating parenteral infusion. A three-fold reduction in final tumor volume occurred in chemotherapy-treated animals receiving parenteral nutrition with no detectable increase in chemotherapy-related toxicity.

The amino acid moiety in parenteral nutrition is primarily responsible for the improved tumor response to methotrexate in this animal model. Final tumor volume was significantly reduced in methotrexate-treated animals receiving amino acids alone or combined with hypertonic dextrose compared to animals receiving normal saline. No significant difference in tumor response was observed between animals receiving hypertonic dextrose and those receiving normal saline (Table 1).

From the Department of Surgery and Division of Surgical Oncology, University of Pennsylvania School of Medicine, Philadelphia, Pennsylvania.

This article has been reproduced with permission from the *Journal of Parenteral and Enteral Nutrition,* Vol. 7, 1983.

TABLE 1. *Tumor Volume*

Parenteral nutrition	N	Initial TV (cm^3)	Final TV (cm^3)	Final TV/body weight (cm^3/kg)
Normal saline	8	1.08 ± 0.41	0.70 ± 0.22	4.84
Dextrose	10	1.05 ± 0.46	0.62 ± 0.40	4.22
Amino acids	10	1.03 ± 0.40	0.37 ± 0.24*	2.69*
Dextrose + amino acids	11	1.14 ± 0.51	0.25 ± 0.18*	1.60*

TV: tumor volume.
* $P < 0.02$ *versus* normal saline group.
Results expressed as mean ± standard deviation.

TABLE 2. *Tumor Cytokinetics*

Parenteral nutrition	S-phase (% tumor cells)	S-phase ("sensitive cells") / Non-S-phase ("resistant cells")
Normal saline	43.7 ± 7.7	0.80 ± 0.25
TPN, 2 h	55.5 ± 9.1*	1.31 ± 0.43*
TPN, 6 h	51.1 ± 8.7	1.10 ± 0.42
TPN, 12 h	48.9 ± 8.5	0.99 ± 0.35
TPN, 24 h	47.9 ± 11.2	1.02 ± 0.61
TPN, 48 h	43.3 ± 4.2	0.76 ± 0.13

TPN: total parenteral nutrition.
* $P < 0.03$ *versus* normal saline group.
Results expressed as mean ± standard deviation.

Subsequent studies were performed in a similar manner to evaluate the effect of total parenteral nutrition on tumor response to additional chemotherapeutic agents. Adriamycin (doxorubicin), like methotrexate, is a cycle-specific chemotherapeutic agent which is toxic to cells actively synthesizing DNA. Cyclophosphamide is a cycle-nonspecific agent which effects cells at all stages of the cell cycle. Total parenteral nutrition was found to increase tumor response rate to Adriamycin but not to cyclophosphamide.

To determine the mechanism of this phenomenon, growth kinetics of the AC-33 tumor were studied after parenteral nutrient administration. Using flow cytometric study, total parenteral nutrition was found to significantly alter tumor cytokinetics. After only 2 hours of total parenteral nutrition, a significant increase occured in the percentage of tumor cells in S-phase (*i.e.*, period of active DNA synthesis). The ratio of sensitive/resistant tumor cells to chemotherapy directed against cell synthesizing DNA was significantly increased in animals receiving total parenteral nutrition compared to controlled animals (Table 2).

Thus, these studies indicate that total parenteral nutrition can be used effectively to increase tumor response to chemotherapy. This phenomenon occurs independent of changes in host nutritional status and represents a role of total parenteral nutrition in altering tumor metabolism for therapeutic advantage. Although these results cannot be directly extrapolated to the treatment of patients with cancer, these initial studies demonstrate sensitization of tumor tissue to chemotherapy with no exacerbation of host toxicity. The potential for altering the complex tumor–host relationship clearly exists and may be used in the future to increase the efficacy of antineoplastic therapy in human malignancies.

BIBLIOGRAPHY

Buzby GP, Mullen JL, Stein TP *et al.* Host–tumor interaction and nutrient supply. Cancer 1980;45:2940–2948.

Cameron IL, Rogers W. Total intravenous hyperalimentation and hydroxyurea chemotherapy in hepatoma-bearing rats. J Surg Res 1977;23:279–288.

Daly JM, Copeland EM, Dudrick SJ. Effect of intravenous nutrition on tumor growth and host immunocompetence in malnourished anials. Surgery 1978;84:655–658.

Holroyde CP, Gabuzda TG, Putnum RC *et al.* Altered glucose metabolism in metastatic carcinoma. Cancer Res 1975;35:3710–3714.

Mullen JL, Buzby GP, Gertner MH *et al.* Protein synthesis dynamics in human gastrointestinal malignancies. Surgery 1980;87:331–339.

Oram-Smith JC, Stein TP, Wallace HW *et al.* Intravenous nutrition and tumor–host protein metabolism. J Surg Res 1977;22:499–503.

Ota DM, Copeland EM, Strobel HW *et al.* The effect of protein nutrition on host and tumor metabolism. J Surg Res 1977;22:181–188.

Steiger E, Oram-Smith J, Miller E *et al.* Effects of nutrition on tumor growth and tolerance to chemotherapy. J Surg Res 1975;18:455–461.

Stein TP, Oram-Smith JC, Leskiw MJ *et al.* Tumor-caused changes in host protein synthesis under different dietary situations. Cancer Res 1976;36:3936–3940.

Torosian MH, Buzby GP, Presti ME *et al.* Reduction of methotrexate toxicity with improved nutritional status. Surg Forum 1982;33:109–112.

Torosian MH, Mullen JL, Miller EE *et al.* Enhanced tumor response to cycle-specific chemotherapy by parenteral amino acid administration. J Parenter Enteral Nutr 1983;7:337–345.

Torosian MH, Tsou KC, Daly JM *et al.* Alteration of tumor cell kinetics by total parenteral nutrition; potential therapeutic implications. Cancer 1984;53:1409–1415.

The Current Crisis in AIDS

C. EVERETT KOOP, M.D., Sc.D.

The following is an address by C. Everett Koop, M.D., Sc.D., Surgeon General of the U.S. Public Health Service, U.S. Department of Health and Human Services. It was presented on March 24, 1987 to the members of the National Press Club in Washington, D.C.

I AM PLEASED TO HAVE THE CHANCE to speak to an audience of journalists about acquired immune deficiency syndrome (AIDS) and about my report on AIDS. You perform an enormously valuable service for the American people in regard to this disease. The only agent that can halt the spread of this disease right now is the change of behavior on the part of those Americans who are at risk, and they won't change, unless they know the danger they are in. The best and quickest way we have to inform them of that danger is through the media—the press. Those of us in public health, therefore, see the press as a major partner in the fight against AIDS. I know that many of you are not comfortable about being a partner with government in *anything*. I recognize the special nature of your feelings, as journalists, and I have come—grudgingly—to respect them. Nevertheless, if we want to have an informed public doing things that are necessary for their health and their survival, we must have an engaged press following this story. I want you informed. I want you engaged. I want you interested. And so I am here today to share some thoughts with you and, later, to answer your questions.

First, a note of caution. We have a major research effort underway to unlock the secrets of the AIDS virus. The public is naturally interested in any progress made by research, and sometimes the news has been—and will be—very good. But we need to keep in mind that all of the signs so far indicate that the research effort is going to be long and extremely difficult. And money alone can't change that. The development of a vaccine—which, for *any* viral disease, is a long process—has barely begun in the case of AIDS. Some of you may remember that it took 19 years to develop the hepatitis B vaccine—and that was a comparatively easy virus to understand. The AIDS virus, however, is much more difficult. Today, it is our hope that we will have a safe and effective AIDS vaccine generally available sometime toward the end of this century—say, the late 1990s—and that's about as optimistic as we can reasonably be. I hope that you carry this information back to the people who write the headlines over your stories. They are frequently over-stated and at variance with the facts presented in the stories themselves.

We are not doing as well as we would like to in vaccines, but I have to say that we are not doing very well in drugs either. The only drug we have now, azidothymidine (AZT), provides some relief and even a few more months, or maybe years, of life for AIDS patients with *Pneumocystis carinii* pneumonia. But AZT does not cure anyone of AIDS itself. A few other drugs in the investigational pipeline may turn out to do the same thing: that is, treat the symptoms of an AIDS-related disease but probably not AIDS itself. We must remember that our experience with AIDS is barely 6 years old. It all began with only five reported cases in June 1981 and has now reached a cumulative total, as of last week, of nearly 33,000 cases of people with AIDS *and over half of them have already died of the disease.* Most of the rest apparently *will*. Last year more than 13,000 new cases were added to the total, and this year we expect another *23,000* cases. By the middle of 1991, a decade after those first few reports came in, we expect that a quarter of a million Americans will have contracted AIDS—a disease that, so far, has a mortality rate of 100%. Make no mistake about it: AIDS *is* fatal and it *is* spreading.

The other thing we know with some certainty is that the AIDS virus tends to concentrate in body fluids which also carry large concentrations of infected lymphocytes. In most body fluids, such as tears, saliva, or perspiration, for example, the virus particle count is very low or absent altogether. On the other hand, large numbers of virus particles are found in blood and semen. That fact explains why two-thirds of all AIDS victims are homosexuals or bisexual men. Some sex practices among these men not only produce semen but they can also cause bleeding. As blood and semen are exchanged between partners, the virus may be transmitted. The second largest group of AIDS carriers, which is one-fourth of the total, are drug abusers who borrow dirty intravenous needles or other contaminated paraphernalia from other addicts who already have AIDS. The epidemiological evidence indicates that one-third of these drug abusers also happen to be homosexuals—men who have vastly increased their risk of an early death.

Homosexuals, bisexual men, and intravenous drug abusers comprise the vast majority of AIDS victims so far, but this is no longer an exclusive club. Lately, there has been a rise in the number of AIDS cases reported among *heterosexual* men and women who are *not* intravenous drug abusers. In fact, the evidence so far suggests that their *heterosexual* activity *alone* seems to be their single risk factor. As of last week, about 4% of all AIDS reports so far involved heterosexual men and women, which is about 1,200 cases. You might say, "That's not much." However, while the *overall* number of AIDS cases will probably increase ninefold over the next 5 years, the number of AIDS cases involving *heterosexuals* will increase about *20*-fold. As the disease spreads more and more among heterosexuals, we will continue to expand our information and education efforts well beyond the communities of homosexuals and drug addicts.

Another fact that is emerging with more clarity is the incidence of the disease among Blacks and Hispanics. In the population generally, one of every eight Americans is Black, but among Americans with AIDS, one of every four is Black: 24% of the total cases reported so far. One of every 12 Americans is Hispanic, but one of every seven Americans with AIDS is Hispanic. Also, about one-third of all Black and Hispanic AIDS victims are intravenous drug abusers, which is also disproportionate. In addition, more than one-half the number of infants with AIDS are Black and another 24% are Hispanic. Again, these are highly disproportionate figures. And nine out of ten of those Black and Hispanic children with AIDS got the virus from their infected mothers either *in utero* or during delivery. And just to increase our sense of horror at this catastrophe occurring in the Black and Hispanic communities, we suspect that the numbers of cases are vastly under-reported.

What do all these pieces of information suggest? I think they mean that the *geography* of the disease of AIDS is changing. At one time we were concerned primarily—almost exclusively—with the populations at risk in San Francisco, Los Angeles, and New York City, and these cities still have the highest numbers of AIDS cases. But they're no longer alone. Other cities and states are showing a rise in cases, too. Here are some examples of the spread:

Houston had 77 cases in 1983, but it reported 428 last year.
Dallas had only 26 AIDS cases in 1983; it had 284 last year.
Atlanta had 25 in 1983; it had 221 last year.
Boston had 38 in 1983 and 187 last year.

In all, 15 cities have each reported more than 300 cases of AIDS since the counting began in 1981. As of today, at least one or more cases have been reported in all 50 states, Guam, the Trust Territory, the Virgin Islands, and the District of Columbia. Colorado, for example, had 176 new cases during the past 12 months, from March 1986 to March 1987. Ohio had 179 during the same period, Arkansas had 32, and Mississippi had 28, and so on.

We have all been watching the slow but apparently unrelenting spread of this disease over the past 6 years. It is reaching further and further into our society, and we simply aren't yet able to slow it down, much less stop it altogether. It would appear that this might be the time for representatives from all levels of government—federal, state, and local—as well as from all concerned interests in the private sector to sit down together and look at two very serious issues for the future. First of all, the costs of this disease to our society are already high and they are going to get astronomical. The present costs of research and patient care are already running in the hundreds of millions. Before another decade passes, they could be in the tens of billions. How will this money be raised? How will it be spent? What kinds of priorities should we set for ourselves? A related question is the role of insurance. With a disease such as AIDS and with its enormous potential for bankrupting a community's health care system, we need to talk about the role that insurance ought to play *or* ought not to play. In the case of insurance, as throughout this issue of financing the costs of AIDS, we dare not have decisions made by default or by indecision.

Secondly, I think we have to take another look at how we care for terminally ill patients with AIDS. We can't continue indefinitely to set aside beds for them in our acute care and general hospitals. The costs—in both dollars and personnel—will simply overwhelm our hospital system. Yet, we know that the period of debilitation and dying can be prolonged, and that each AIDS patient requires some kind of care every remaining day of his or her life. We need to determine just what levels of care are needed and how we will provide that care in a compassionate, professional, and resource-effective manner. Right now, we are doing a great deal of experimentation in the matter of patient care, and I have nothing but total admiration for the dedicated health personnel who have been involved so far. But we have to make sure that these different approaches are recognized and understood, and when they are seen together in context, that they point us in some helpful and hopeful directions.

I believe that the time may now be upon us to engage in this kind of national dialogue on finances and patient care because—with the help of the press, I might add—the American people are gaining a clearer understanding of the threat posed to them by this disease and are, themselves, trying to work through the issues. It was, by the way, for that very purpose —that is, to increase public understanding—that President Reagan asked me, back in February 1986, to pull together everything we knew about AIDS and put it all down in a plain-English report to the American people. For 8 months (February through September of last year), I met quietly and privately with individuals and groups from across the spectrum of society: groups like the National Education Association and the National Parent-Teacher Association; The Christian Life Commission of the Southern Baptist Convention and the Synagogue Council of America; the National Coalition of Black and Lesbian Gays and the Washington Business Group on Health; and the representatives of local, county, state, and territorial health officials. There were 26 groups in all, and they were all extraordinarily helpful. Each one pledged to do whatever was necessary to distribute my report across the length and breadth of America. And many of them already have. After 8 months of listening and writing, I delivered my report to the White House late last September. The Domestic Policy Council accepted it, and of course, the President accepted it. I want to assure you that at no time in this high-level review process did anyone tinker with it. The final published report I released on October 22nd was the exact same report that I personally wrote between February and September of last year.

The report has accomplished two things: first, it has impressed the country *generally* that AIDS is indeed everybody's problem. Some people did not want to believe that. Now they must. Second, the report makes clear that, in order to end the chain of transmission of this disease once and for all, we need to teach our young people the facts about AIDS and about their own sexuality. The objective is to make them a lot more responsible in their relationships than their elders have been.

What might such an education program say? Who should say it? Who should hear it? And when? Most educators agree that any educational program in this area ought to be part of a comprehensive curriculum in school health education. Such a curriculum usually includes information on nutrition, dental health, physical fitness, accident prevention and so on. The information that is AIDS-related ought to be every bit as factually correct and personally sensitive as the rest of the curriculum is. Science and government can help provide the factually correct information. But in our American tradition, judgments as to the sensitivity and morality of a particular curriculum are left to families and communities to decide.

I do have some observations, however, that are drawn from the collective experience of health and mental health experts who have been working in this area for a long time. With many of them I share the same discomfort with the term "sex education." It has, by now, fairly limited connotations in the public mind. People hear the phrase, "sex education," and they immediately think of class hours devoted to human reproductive biology or what many young people call "organ recitals." Most schools now offer this minimum kind of sex education some time during the junior high or middle school years and that's a good thing, although it might be a little late. I have urged that the material be presented earlier, among 9-, 10-, and 11-year-olds. Of course, developmental age is more important than chronological age, and, again, community standards must be taken into account, and these vary from place to place.

Young children are extremely curious about themselves, as they shape their own identities. They are also kinder and more generous than older children, or even than most adults, for that matter. They are, above all, susceptible to being loved and to offering much love in return. And sex education without the concept of love and responsibility is like a piece of pie that is all crust and no filling. My own preference, therefore, is to have our children introduced to the subject of reproductive biology within a more general discussion of the nature of sensitive and affirmative human relations. That is easier to say than to do, I know. And furthermore, some parents get uneasy about having a school impart certain values to their children. They think that such instruction should be done at home, and actually, I thoroughly agree. In fact, a great deal of instruction does go on in the home, but it is not the kind we want. Not long ago, I received some data on that very subject, and I will share it with you now.

Researchers at Michigan State University took a look at the kind of television shows and movies watched by 9th- and 10th-grade children. They found that a substantial number of teenagers watch mid-day soap operas in which sexual intercourse between unmarried partners is shown or discussed on an average of 1.56 times an hour. These children also watch prime-time shows at night in which acts of unmarried intercourse are shown or discussed on an average of once an hour. The Michigan State team also found that 60 to 70% of these young people saw the year's top 5 "R"-rated films, in which sexual intercourse between unmarried partners occurred on an average of 8 times per film. In most of these cases, no one gets hurt, nobody gets pregnant, and no one takes responsibility. That is really a terrible way for children to learn about sexuality and human relationships. Clearly, this is where parents need to step in. Unfortunately, many parents don't. That is why I believe there is a compelling social need for our schools, churches, synagogues, and other communal institutions to do whatever they can to provide our children with the most helpful kinds of information. Their health—and their very lives—may be at stake.

As I indicated earlier, I think sex education ought to take place within the context of learning about adult relationships that are loving, caring, respectful, and considerate. Such relationships include some fulfilling sexual activity, but they are not defined only by that activity. There is much more to human relationships than just "good sex," and young people ought to be told that. Everyone dreams of such a relationship. The novelist calls it "true love," the sociologist calls it "marital fidelity," and the surgeon general calls it "monogamy." From a public health point of view, the best defense against AIDS, short of total abstinence, is to maintain a faithful, monogamous relationship—the kind of relationship in which you have only one continuing sexual partner *and* that person is as faithful as you are. To paraphrase Mr. Lee Iacocca, I say, "If you have a monogamous relationship, *keep* it. If you don't have one, *get* it." My advocacy of monogamy may sound like a morality lesson, but I didn't come here today to preach to you. Nevertheless, in our battle against AIDS, it just so happens that, in addition to education, you can count science *and* morality as our most powerful allies. For individuals who don't yet have a faithful monogamous relationship for whatever reason, I advise abstinence. And my advice is straightforward enough: If you don't know what you're doing, or with whom you're doing it, then *don't do it.* I believe that's not only good public health doctrine, it's also good science. And there are some who might argue it was good morals as well.

Finally, there are many individuals who *don't* have a monogamous relationship and who *won't* remain abstinent. To them I strongly advise that they take every precaution to protect themselves and their partners from the risk of getting AIDS. If you are one of these individuals, you need to *know with absolute certainty* that neither you nor any of your sexual partners are carrying the AIDS virus. If you are not absolutely certain, then you *must take precautions.* For example, don't have sex with someone who already has AIDS. That ought to be obvious. Don't have sex with someone who indulges in high-risk behavior. That would include homosexuals, intravenous drug users, and prostitutes and others who have many different sex partners. Obviously, the same message goes to any of *those* high-risk individuals as well. And finally, if you *do* decide to have sex with such an individual anyway—a decision carrying profoundly serious health consequences—then, if you're a man, at least use a condom from start to finish. If you're a woman, make sure your male partner uses a condom. A condom won't provide 100% protection—few things in life *do*—but condoms seem to offer the best protection short of monogamy and abstinence. If sexually active people will heed these messages, they will achieve a high degree of protection and most likely won't be infected with the AIDS virus.

I'm sharing these thoughts with you today because I believe that each of us—in our homes or in our schools—has the responsibility to pass that information on to our children. I know that in this room there are dozens of people who will not only do that in their own homes but can do it in their jobs as well. And I hope you *do*, especially if you feel as I do that young lives are at stake. This has been a grim message and I guess I'm a grim courier. I only hope that every American who hears or reads my message will believe it and do his or her part to stop the spread of AIDS; protect and save the lives of people at risk, including unsuspecting young people; and return human sexuality back to its rightful place: part of the total complex of human, caring, interpersonal relations.

Thank you.

Management of Cutaneous Melanomas of the Female Breast

BURT M. GREENBERG, M.D., RALPH HAMILTON, M.D.,
DOUGLAS M. ROTHKOPF, M.D., MICHAEL BALK, B.A.,
WALLACE H. CLARK, JR., AND DONATO LAROSSA, M.D.

Primary melanomas of the skin of the breast are uncommon lesions. Fifty-four patients were surgically treated for this lesion during a 13-year period, accounting for 3.8% of a total of 1431 patients with cutaneous melanoma. Nineteen patients were female and 35 were male. Most recently, in patients with high-risk lesions, such as those exhibiting an aggressive vertical growth phase or a Clark level IV or V, attempts at curative resection have utilized wide and deep excision to the level of the pectoralis fascia with axillary lymph node dissection in selected cases. Reconstruction of the significant breast deficit in five female patients utilized the latissimus dorsi myocutaneous flap. This technique results in an improved aesthetic appearance when compared to primary closure or skin grafting. Donor site morbidity is minimal. Long-term cancer surveillance is not impeded and all five patients expressed satisfaction with the reconstruction. Four of the five female patients currently are alive with no evidence of disease with a mean follow-up of 55 months after definitive therapy.

PRIMARY MELANOMA arising in the skin of the breast is a relatively uncommon occurrence. Ariel and Caron,[1] in reviewing 2824 patients with melanoma, reported an incidence of 0.28%. Lee *et al.*[2] report a 4.8% incidence. Roses *et al.*[3] reported 1140 patients with melanoma, of whom 1.8% were treated for primary melanoma of the breast with wide excision of skin and breast tissue. Closure in these cases was achieved either primarily or with a skin graft.

The reconstructive problems inherent in rebuilding the female breast are not shared by melanomas elsewhere. Adequate treatment of the primary site is one of the most significant factors in determining prognosis.[5] Although past treatment has included mastectomy,[6] current accepted and recommended therapy for high-risk lesions involves wide and deep excision of the primary site including the underlying breast down to and including the pectoralis major fascia.[3] Typically, clinically these high-risk lesions include those exhibiting a vertical growth phase or ulceration.[4] High-risk lesions histologically include those with a Clark level of III or higher.

Treatment of standard low-risk lesions, such as a superficial spreading melanoma of low or intermediate thickness and exhibiting radial growth kinetics, is less controversial. These breast lesions routinely are treated as they would be elsewhere, namely with a 1 cm or 2 cm margin (radius) and either primary closure or skin grafting.

The treatment of the axillary lymph node region is less well defined. Polk and associates,[7] using statistical analysis, showed the probability for benefit from prophylactic removal of the nodes outweighs the morbidity when the chance of metastases to the lymph nodes was 20% or greater. Dellon and Ketcham[8] stress that prophylactic nodal dissection resulted in a 10% to 20% increase in survival. Skeptics believe that the difference in survival rates between those having wide excision alone and wide excision plus lymphadenectomy is not significant.[9] Virtually all authors[10] concur that internal mammary node dissection does not improve survival rate.

From the Division of Plastic Surgery and the Department of Dermatology of the University of Pennsylvania, Philadelphia, Pennsylvania.

This article has been reproduced with permission from *Plastic and Reconstructive Surgery*, Vol. 80, No. 3, September 1987.

Materials and Methods

From February 1972 through May 1985, a total of 1431 patients (737 female, 694 male) with cutaneous malignant melanoma were treated by the Pigmented Lesion Group of the Hospital of the University of Pennsylvania. A retrospective study of the 1431 patients revealed 54 patients with primary melanoma of the skin of the breast (3.8%). For this study the boundaries of the breast are a line 3 cm inferior to the clavicle, the sternum, the anterior axillary line, and the inframammary fold.

All patients were white. The average age was 42.6 years, with the youngest being 16.2 years and the oldest 84.6 years at the time of definitive therapy. Nineteen patients were females with an average age of 38.9 years. Thirty-five were males with an average age of 44.7 years. The average period of follow-up was 58 months after tumor resection (range, 3–128 months). The average period of follow-up for all patients currently living was 65 months. Thirty-eight of the 54 patients were followed for greater than 2 years postoperatively (70.4%), 23 of the 54 patients were followed for greater than 5 years postoperatively (42.6%), and 11 of the 54 patients were followed for greater than 8 years (20.4%). No patient has been lost to follow-up. The Clark and Breslow patient classification are depicted in Table 1. The majority of melanomas (70%) were superficial spreading type.

The site distribution of cutaneous melanoma in our study revealed 25 right-sided (46.3%) lesions and 29 left-sided lesions (53.7%). In 17 of the 19 female patients (89%) the melanoma was located at or superior to a horizontal line transversing the nipple (Fig. 1). The melanomas were more evenly distributed in the 35 male patients (Fig. 2) with 20 occurring at or above this line. One melanoma (in a male) arose from the skin of the nipple.

The resection margins ranged from 10 mm to 99 mm with the average resection margin being a 35.6 mm radius. Twelve of the 52 patients (23.1%) treated with wide and deep excision also had complete axillary lymph node dissections. Six of these 12 dissections were performed in patients with positive clinical nodes and therefore were considered to be therapeutic. Six axillary dissections were prophylactic and the majority of these were performed before 1979. The method of wound closure which was utilized (Table 2) varied. Twenty-seven of the 52 melanomas (51.9%) treated with wide and deep excision underwent primary closure of the remaining breast. Sixteen excisions (30.8%) were closed with split-thickness skin grafting technique. Four wounds (7.7%) were closed with local advancement flaps. Two male patients underwent excisional biopsy only, one of whom presented with metastatic disease. None of the 54 patients received additional therapy at the primary site, but two of the males received adjuvant systemic chemotherapy after metastatic disease became evident.

Five of the female patients underwent latissimus dorsi myocutaneous flap reconstruction. This report reviews the clinical usefulness of the latissimus dorsi flap in reconstruction of the partial mastectomy defect obtained after treatment of a high-risk melanoma of the breast. The site of lesion, level of tumor, and mode of treatment in five reconstructed patients is shown in Table 3. A typical case report is presented.

Case Report

A 28-year-old woman presented after a black nodular lesion appeared on the upper outer quadrant of her left breast and began enlarging. The lesion exhibited a characteristic nodular

TABLE 1. *Tumor Classification by Clark and Breslow Criteria*

Level (Clark)	Patients Total	Patients Males	Patients Females	Thickness (mm) (Breslow)	Patients Total	Patients Males	Patients Females
II	20	10	10	<0.76	20	8	12
III	23	4	19	0.76–1.50	16	5	11
IV	9	4	5	1.50–3.65	15	4	11
V	1	0	1	>3.65	1	0	1
Unclassified	1	1	0	Unclassified	2	2	0
Total	54	19	35	Total	54	19	35

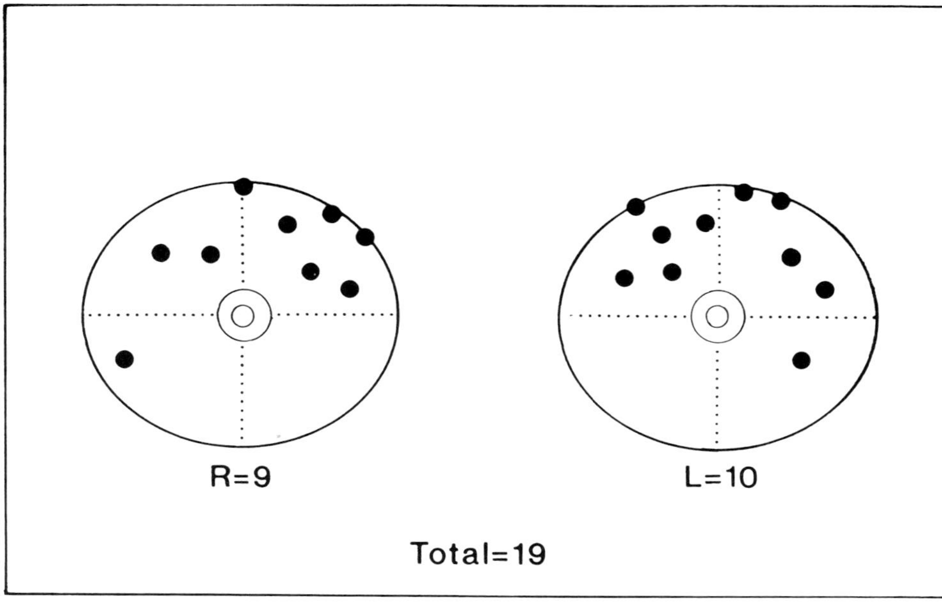

FIG. 1. Site distribution of melanoma: females. Notice that 89% of primary melanomas in females are located at or superior to a horizontal line traversing the nipple.

pattern, but did not ulcerate, nor was there a history of pruritis, discharge, or bleeding. The patient denied the presence of a precursor pigmented lesion or a history of dysplastic nevi. There was no family history of cutaneous melanoma or abnormal nevi, and the patient did not have a previous history of melanoma. The lesion (Fig. 3) measured 3.0 mm × 2.0 mm and exhibited the characteristic findings of melanoma. The remainder of the breast examination was negative. Several palpable nodes were noted in the left axilla and a 2-cm lymph node was present in the left supraclavicular region. The preoperative chest radiograph was

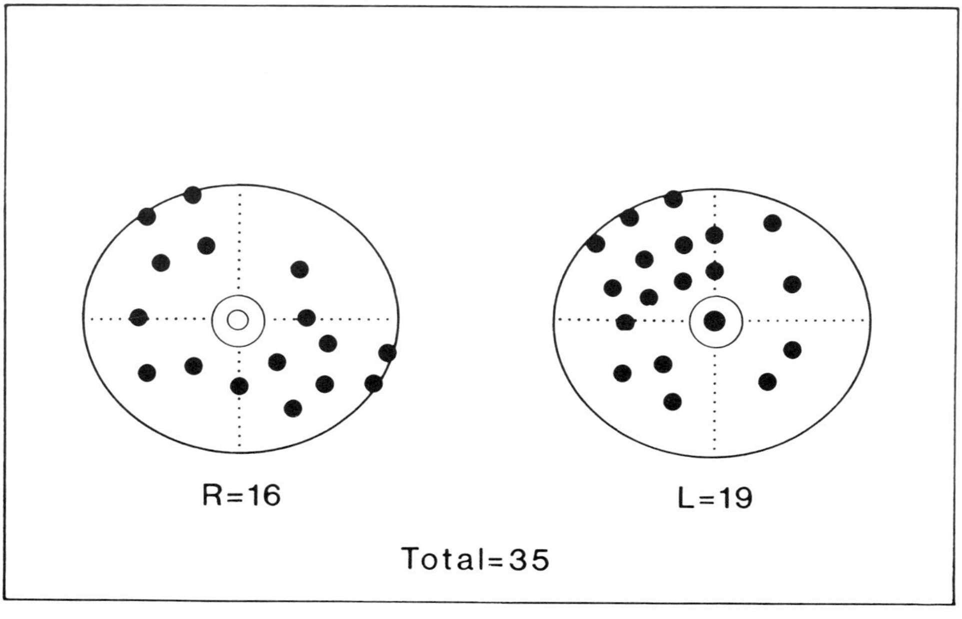

FIG. 2. Site distribution of melanoma: males. Notice the relatively even distribution of breast melanoma in males.

TABLE 2. *Method of Wound Closure*

Primary closure	27
Split thickness skin graft	16
Advancement flap	4
Latissimus flap	5
Excisional biopsy	2
Total	54

unremarkable. Resection of a large segment of the superior aspect of the breast, a limited supraclavicular node dissection, and a therapeutic axillary dissection was performed. Reconstruction was achieved utilizing the latissimus dorsi myocutaneous flap which was tunneled through the pectoralis muscle (Fig. 4) and inset into the defect (Fig. 5). Care was taken to suitably enlarge the tunnel to obviate against vascular compression. The late cosmetic result attained is shown (Fig. 6) and the donor site scar and morbidity are negligible. The pathologic report noted a Clark's level IV nodular melanoma which was 1.19 mm thick; the 18 lymph nodes were histologically free of tumor. The patient is doing well with no evidence of disease at 78 months postoperatively.

Results

Accurate long-term follow-up has been achieved in 100% of our patients. Of the five patients reconstructed with latissimus dorsi flaps, four are alive with no evidence of disease. One patient died of visceral spread of melanoma less than 9 months after partial mastectomy and therapeutic node dissection. Pathologic examination in this instance revealed a Clark level IV lesion (Breslow thickness of 3.65 mm) and one of 14 positive nodes. There was no local recurrence. Reconstruction did not interfere with follow-up examination. The long-term aesthetic results of the latissimus dorsi reconstructed breasts have been excellent. Specifically, contour irregularities and asymmetric size differences as compared to the contralateral breast have been eliminated. There have been minimal donor site morbidity and functional motor problems in utilizing the latissimus dorsi myocutaneous unit. Since the muscle maintains its innervation *via* the thoracodorsal nerve, postoperative atrophy has been uncommon. A slight overcorrection is performed during the initial reconstruction to allow for transient muscle edema which is seen during muscle transposition.

During the early years of this retrospective review six patients underwent prophylactic axillary node dissection. Five patients had no evidence of axillary involvement. One patient with prophylactic dissection had one of 17 sampled nodes positive. Therapeutic axillary dissections were performed in the presence of palpable lymph nodes. Of the six patients who underwent therapeutic axillary dissection, three were disease-free and the remainder contained one of 14 nodes positive, four of 21 nodes positive, and 38 of 42 nodes positive, respectively. Of the four patients with positive nodes histologically, three are dead of disease. Three of the eight patients with negative nodal metastases (37.5%) are dead of disease, four (50%) show no evidence of disease, and one patient is alive with current disease.

Thirty-nine of the 54 patients (72.2%) retrospectively studied with melanoma of the breast are alive with no evidence of disease. Eleven patients are dead of disease secondary to visceral spread of melanoma (20.4%) and two patients died of unrelated causes. Two

TABLE 3. *Five Female Patients With Latissimus Dorsi Myocutaneous Flaps*

Age	Site	Level	Thickness	Margin	Lymph nodes	Status
42	Inf–Lat	II	0.66 mm	3.5 cm	(Not removed)	NED at 78 mo
25	Sup–Lat	III	1.50 mm	3.0 cm	0/12 (prophylactic)	NED at 58 mo
46	Inf–Lat	IV	1.14 mm	3.0 cm	0/17 (therapeutic)	NED at 1 mo
20	Sup–Lat	IV	3.65 mm	4.0 cm	1/14 (therapeutic)	DOD at 9 mo
28	Sup–Lat	IV	1.19 mm	5.0 cm	0/18 (therapeutic)	NED at 76 mo

NED: alive, no evidence of disease (melanoma); DOD: dead, died of disease (melanoma); Inf: inferior, Lat: lateral.

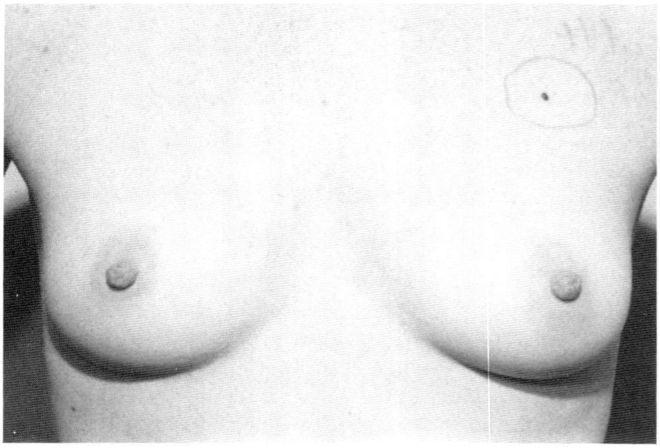

FIG. 3. Nodular melanoma measuring 3.0 by 2.0 cm, level IV 1.19 mm in thickness (case report patient).

patients currently are alive, but with disease; one has visceral spread and the other clinically has regional node involvement. No patient treated with ablation and latissimus dorsi flap was found to have recurrent disease in the margin of resection.

Discussion

The breast represents an uncommon location for cutaneous melanoma, and reconstruction of the partial mastectomy defect presents an unusual challenge. Goals of treatment are

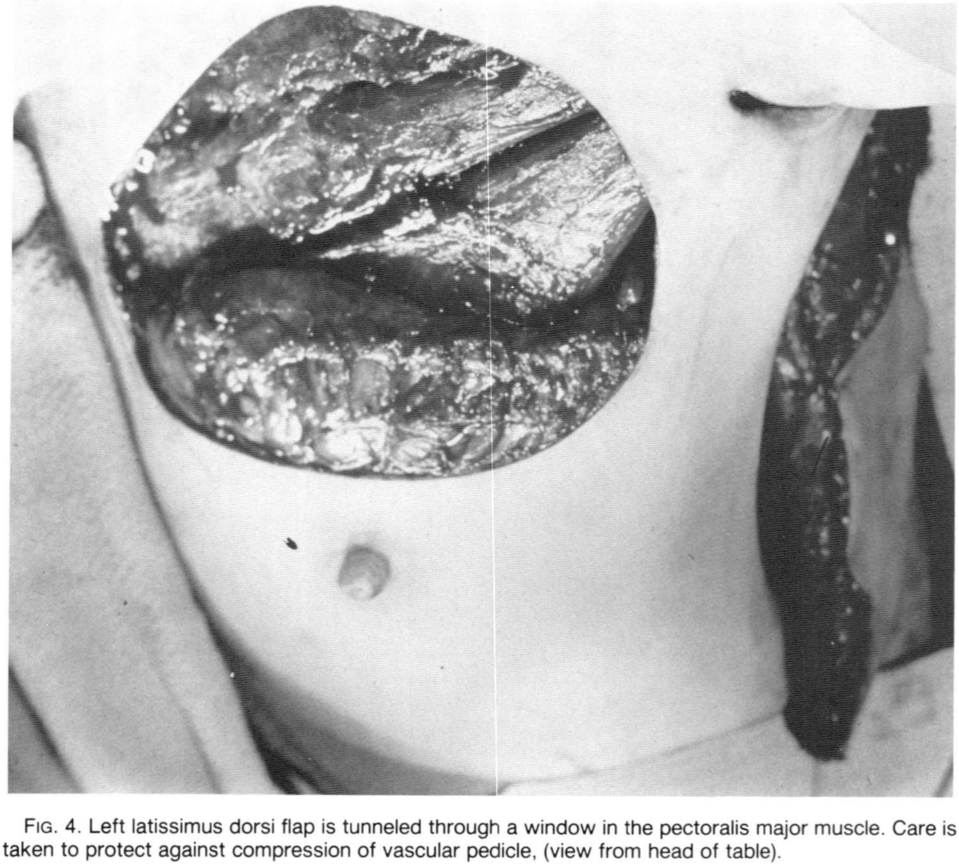

FIG. 4. Left latissimus dorsi flap is tunneled through a window in the pectoralis major muscle. Care is taken to protect against compression of vascular pedicle, (view from head of table).

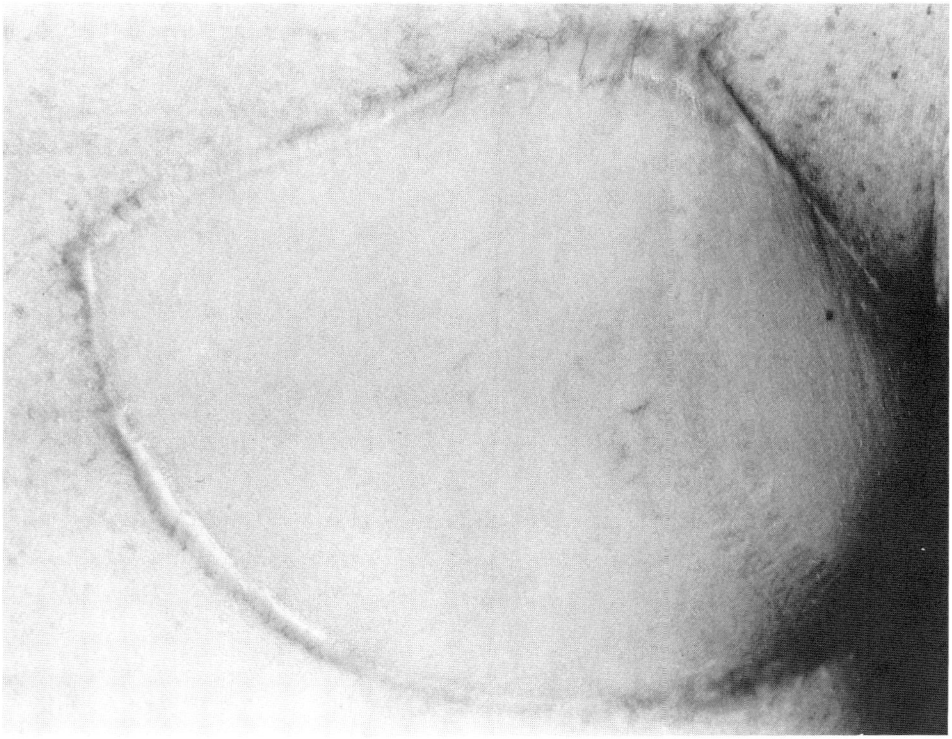

FIG. 5. Inset of latissimus flap into resected chest wall defect.

to restore the natural contour and mobility of the breast, attain symmetry with the contralateral breast, and utilize autogenous tissue. These goals are best met with a myocutaneous flap.

The latissimus has been used for years in the treatment of the breast defect resulting from a modified radical mastectomy. The technique has been well described in the literature.[11,12] The elevation of the muscle skin flap generally is oriented at 90° to the proposed transfer. The thoracodorsal vascular leash is identified posterior–laterally. Further length may be achieved in the reconstruction of the superior breast defect by extending the vascular dissection to the subscapular artery and by detaching the muscle from its humeral insertion. Care is taken in the elevation to preserve the long thoracic nerve to the serratus anterior muscle in order to prevent a winged scapula deformity. The flap contains sufficient bulk to replace the quadrant or hemibreast resected without the need for a prosthesis. It is particularly advantageous to avoid prosthetic implantation and its potential attendant complications such as capsular contracture, implant rupture, and periprosthetic infection.

Our approach at this time is to perform an axillary lymphadenectomy in the presence of palpable axillary nodes, if the tumor lies over the tail of the breast or if a thick lesion (Clark III or IV) is located in the lateral quadrants of the breast. If nodal dissection is elected, it may be performed easily before muscle transfer. The muscle pedicle may be extended superficial to the pectoralis muscle or be placed through the underlying pectoralis to provide bulk superiorly as well as to preserve the anterior axillary fold. Patient satisfaction has been excellent and a natural breast contour was achieved. None of our patients evidenced histologic invasion of the ductal system, although certainly in this specific situation, a simple mastectomy and immediate reconstruction may be considered

Conclusion

Treatment of malignant melanoma of the breast presents a unique challenge. Currently accepted treatment of the high-risk lesion includes partial mastectomy with wide excision of

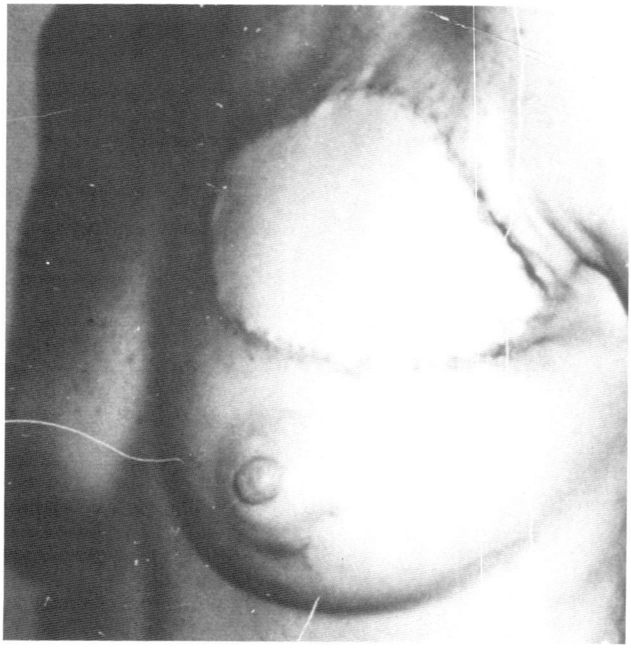

FIG. 6. Results seen three years postoperative. Contour and breast symmetry are achieved (circled lesions are dysplastic nevi that underwent biopsy).

the primary lesion and axillary dissection in selected patients. We recommend latissimus dorsi reconstruction for the defect and believe it provides the optimum aesthetic result with minimal functional defect. It can be performed at the same operation as the ablative surgery with or without axillary dissection and future cancer surveillance is not impaired.

REFERENCES

1. Ariel IM, Caron AS. Diagnosis and treatment of malignant melanoma arising from the skin of the female breast. Am J Surg 1972;124:384.
2. Lee YN, Sparks FC, Morton DL. Primary melanoma of the skin of the breast region. Ann Surg 1977;185:17.
3. Roses DF, Harris MN, Stern JS, Gumport SL. Cutaneous melanoma of the breast. Ann Surg 1979;189:112.
4. Clark WH, Elder DE, Van Horn M. The biologic forms of malignant melanoma human pathology. Hum Pathol 1986;17:153.
5. Davis NC. Cutaneous melanoma: The Queensland experience. Curr Probl Surg 1976;13:1.
6. Attie JN, Khafif RA. Melanotic Tumors. Springfield: Charles C. Thomas, 1964;191.
7. Polk HC, Cohn JD, Clarkson JG. An appraisal of elective regional lymphadenctomy for melanoma. Curr Top Surg Res 1969;1:121.
8. Dellon AL, Ketcham AS. Surgical treatment of Stage I melanoma. Arch Surg 1973;106:738.
9. Conrad FG. Treatment of malignant melanoma: Wide excision alone *versus* lymphadenectomy. Arch Surg 1972;104:587.
10. Lise M, Kinne DW, Fortner JG, Grabstall H. Internal mammary node dissection for melanoma of anterior chest wall. Proc Am Assoc Cancer Res 1974;15:193.
11. Cohen BE, Cronin ED. Breast reconstruction with the latissimus dorsi musculocutaneous flap. Clin Plast Surg 1984;11:287.
12. Bostwick J III, Nahai F, Wallace JG, Vasconez LO. Sixty latissimus dorsi flaps. Plast Reconstr Surg 1979;63:31.

Results in Suprahyoid, Modified Radical, and Standard Radical Neck Dissections for Metastatic Squamous Cell Carcinoma: Recurrence and Survival

WINSTON CHU, M.D., F.A.C.S. AND JOSEPH G. STRAWITZ, M.D., F.A.C.S.

REGIONAL METASTATIC DISEASE is found in approximately 6 to 85 per cent of all patients with squamous cell carcinoma of the head and neck, depending upon the primary site.[1-3] Surgical attempts at control date back to the early twentieth century when Crile[4] described the radical neck dissection.

Operations less radical than this classic neck dissection have been condemned as being inadequate by Martin et al.[3] Consequently, in most institutions this operation is standard for neck metastasis in patients with squamous cell carcinoma of the head and neck. Radical neck dissection is not without significant liabilities. Among other problems, distortion of ipsilateral shoulder function produces significant disability. Furthermore, invoking this handicap in patients with clinically false-positive findings is not rational. A report by Bocca and Pignataro[5] showed the possibility of obtaining optimum control using a less radical operation circumventing the above objections. The present study evaluates the results of our experience with suprahyoid, modified radical, and classic radical neck dissections in controlling cervical metastatic disease.

Material and Methods

A retrospective study was done on all patients treated at the American Oncologic Hospital, Fox Chase Cancer Center between 1943 and 1974 inclusive who presented with clinically enlarged cervical lymph nodes in association with squamous cell carcinomas of the lip, oral cavity, pharynx, and larynx or unknown primary. Three hundred forty-two patients were treated by removal of the clinically enlarged lymph nodes using suprahyoid, modified radical, and standard radical neck dissections. Analysis for age, sex, site of primary tumor, size of primary lesion, apparent cervical lymph node involvement, and pathologic lymph node involvement was done.

Two hundred seventy-one patients had clinical cervical lymph node involvement above, but not including, the juguloomohyoid group of lymph nodes. Seventy-one patients with histologically positive nodes at and below the juguloomohyoid groups were excluded from the study for purposes of standardization. Patients who died postoperatively were eliminated from the statistical analysis. Using the sampled permutation test method, a statistical analysis for recurrence rates within the neck and for survival rates were made for patients treated with each operation. Patients with histologically negative nodes were evaluated separately from those with positive nodes above the juguloomohyoid group. Regular follow-up data were available for at least twenty-four months or until death in all evaluable patients and for sixty months or until death in 95.5 per cent of patients.

From the Department of Surgery, American Oncologic Hospital, Fox Chase Cancer Center, Philadelphia, Pennsylvania. This work was supported in part by funds from Public Health Service Research Grant No. R25 CA 23229-01 from the National Cancer Institute.

Presented at the Joint Meeting of the American Society for Head and Neck Surgery and the Society of Head and Neck Surgeons, Toronto, Ontario, Canada, May 29–31, 1978. (Residents' Award winning essay.)

This article has been reproduced with permission from the *American Journal of Surgery*, Vol. 136, 1978.

Selection of Type of Operation

The choice or extent of operation usually depended upon the judgment of the operating surgeon. However, the following criteria ordinarily served as guidelines. Suprahyoid operations were done for mobile, clinically detectable lymph nodes above the jugulodigastric group, in conjunction with an ipsilateral hemimandibulectomy. When the jugulodigastric lymph nodes were palpable and mobile with or without palpable nodes within the submaxillary group a modified radical neck operation was done in some patients. During this operation, the juguloomohyoid nodes were examined, and if suspicion of tumor was confirmed by frozen section histologic study, the operation was converted to standard radical neck dissection. This latter radical operation was always performed for nodal involvement at or below the juguloomohyoid group. The technics of each of these operations are described elsewhere.[3,5,6] The suprahyoid operation is the simple upper neck dissection. The modified radical neck dissection differs from the classic radical neck dissection only in the preservation of the jugular vein, sternocleidomastoid muscle, and accessory nerve. In all instances of unknown or laryngeal primaries, radical neck dissection was performed.

Results

Two hundred sixty-one patients were evaluable after the ten who died postoperatively were eliminated.

Age and Sex Distribution

Two hundred nineteen men and forty-two women ranging in age from thirty-three to eighty-seven years were included in the study. The age and sex distribution according to the type of operation, primary site, and pathologic nodal status is tabulated in Table 1.

Pathologic Correlation With Clinical Cervical Lymphadenopathy

This study did not include patients undergoing elective neck dissections, and therefore, all pathologically negative nodes were considered clinically false-positive; the figures are 68 per cent, 61.9 per cent, and 30.5 per cent for the suprahyoid, modified radical, and standard radical neck dissections, respectively. No false-negative data are available for the two latter operations, but a false-negative result can be assumed to have occurred whenever the suprahyoid node was histologically negative at dissection and a neck lesion recurred in a lymph node group below the level of dissection. The false-negative incidence was ten of thirty-four patients (29.1 per cent). These patients may represent examples of skipped metastases.

Recurrence Rates Within the Neck

Of the patients with histologically negative nodes, ten of thirty-four (29.1 per cent) had a recurrence after a suprahyoid operation, none (of 13 patients) had a recurrence after a modified radical neck operation, and two of fifty-seven (3.5 per cent) had a recurrence after a classic radical neck dissection. These results show a significantly lower rate of neck recurrence after a modified radical neck operation ($p = 0.05$) and after a classic radical neck dissection ($p = 0.01$) compared with the rate after the suprahyoid operation. No statistical significance was noted when the modified radical neck operation was compared with classic radical neck dissection.

In the group with histologically positive nodes, the recurrence rates were 31.2 per cent, 12.5 per cent, and 30.5 per cent for the suprahyoid, modified radical, and classic radical neck dissections, respectively. (Table 2.) No statistical significance was noted on comparing each operative group with the other.

Survival Rates

Five year survival rates were 63.8 per cent, 60.5 per cent, and 56.3 per cent for the suprahyoid, modified radical, and classic radical neck dissections, respectively, in the group with histologically negative nodes, and 49.2 per cent, 28.9 per cent and 39.1 per cent, respectively, in the group with histologically positive nodes. There was no statistically significant difference in survival.

TABLE 1. *Age and Sex Distribution According to Primary Site, Type of Operation, and Pathologic Nodal Status*

Primary	Type of Operation	Nodal Status	Age Range (yr) (mean)	Sex	
				Male	Female
Anterior lesions*	SH	Negative	46–86 (60)	24	5
		Positive	46–81 (65)	12	1
	MRND	Negative	55–87 (67)	7	3
		Positive	53–80 (70)	5	2
	RND	Negative	39–78 (59)	30	8
		Positive	33–83 (59)	70	12
Posterior lesions†	SH	Negative	52–74 (59)	4	1
		Positive	64–67 (65)	2	1
	MRND	Negative	49–61 (54)	3	0
		Positive	55	1	0
	RND	Negative	47–78 (59)	15	4
		Positive	35–74 (59)	38	4
Larynx	RND	Positive	49–64 (57)	3	1
Unknown	RND	Positive	42–68 (58)	5	0
Total				219	42

Note: SH = suprahyoid neck dissection; RND = standard radical neck dissection; MRND = modified radical neck dissection.
* Oral tongue, floor of the mouth, gingiva, buccal mucosa, and lip.
† Fauces, retromolar trigone, tonsil, and pharynx.

Outcome of Failures After Suprahyoid Dissection

Those ten patients with histologically negative nodes from the suprahyoid group who had a recurrence showed recurrent disease below the level of the previous dissection. Eight patients underwent subsequent standard radical neck dissection, which resulted in three postoperative deaths. In five patients the disease was controlled, with an average survival of 13.6 years after the second operation. Five patients with recurrence after a suprahyoid operation and having histologically positive nodes initially all had unresectable lesions and died from extension of disease.

Status of Primary Tumor in Patients With Neck Recurrences

Suprahyoid operation: Only two of ten patients with initial histologically negative lesions and with neck recurrences had uncontrolled primary tumors, but two of five patients with initial histologically positive lesions and neck recurrences had uncontrolled primary tumors.

Modified radical neck operation: The only patient with neck recurrence in this group also had a recurrence at the primary site.

Radical neck dissection: Of those with histologically negative tumors, both patients with recurrence also had uncontrolled primary tumors, and of those with histologically positive tumors, twenty-three of forty-one with neck recurrences also had uncontrolled primary tumors.

These data further emphasize the importance of control of tumor at the primary site and may be also an indication of the biologic aggressiveness of these recurrent tumors.

Comments

Farr and Arthur[1] brought to our attention the biologic seriousness of the development of cervical metastases in cancer of the head and neck. They also showed that survival rates declined as the level of lymph node involvement descended from the submaxillary group (47 per cent at 5 years with no evidence of disease) to the supraclavicular group of lymph nodes (0 incidence) in sixty patients with pathologically positive nodes. Cancer ablation should be designed in proportion to the tumor burden. For example, total glossectomy is not an appropriate operation for T1 cancer of the tongue. Similarities can be drawn in designing operations for neck metastases.

Our results appear to confirm the practice of performing an operation proportional to the extent and degree of metastatic disease. In patient groups that are roughly comparable, less radical removal of tissue results in statistically similar survival rates at equivalent levels of lymph nodal group involvement (tumor burden). Recurrence rates are also comparable in histologically positive node groups. But the recurrence rates are significantly higher after suprahyoid operations than after either modified radical or formal radical neck dissections in patients with histologically negative nodes. Frequently, these recurrences are within the lymph node group adjacent to or just below the level of dissection encompassed by the suprahyoid operation. This may be the result of faulty staging inherent in this particular operation. Salvage of these patients with recurrence, although still possible, is not encouraging (5 of 10 patients). The two patients with unresectable lesions and the three patients who died after a salvage radical neck dissection (postoperative deaths) had low tumor burdens initially and therefore were potentially curable had they originally undergone either a

TABLE 2. *Local Recurrences According to Type of Operation and Nodal Status*

Type of Operation	Nodal Status	No. of Patients	Patients with Recurrence
SH	Negative	34	10 (29.1%)
	Positive	16	5 (31.2%)
MRND	Negative	13	0
	Positive	8	1 (12.5%)
RND	Negative	57	2 (3.5%)
	Positive	133	41 (30.5%)

Note: SH = suprahyoid neck dissection; MRND = modified radical neck dissection; RND = standard radical neck dissection.

modified radical neck operation or standard radical neck dissection. All patients with recurrence in all three operative groups with histologically positive nodes had very poor salvage either related to an uncontrolled primary or to the biologic aggressiveness of the primary tumor.

The preferred less extensive neck dissection is therefore modified radical neck dissection. This operation is adequate for the removal of tumor-bearing lymph nodes when the disease is confined within the nodes. The wide excisional nature of cancer surgery is preserved without sacrificing functional and cosmetic end results. The recurrence and survival rates also compare favorably with those of radical neck dissection; although the latter is performed on some patients with slightly greater tumor burdens, it is confined to the lymph node groups above the juguloomohyoid group. This modified operation also seems to provide satisfactory information for staging the level of lymph node involvement within the neck, as we routinely rely on frozen section histologic sampling at and below the juguloomohyoid group during the operation for guidance as to whether or not to proceed with radical neck dissection. We have abandoned the suprahyoid operation because of the significantly higher local recurrence rate observed in patients with histologically negative nodes and because, unlike the experience with modified radical neck dissection, inaccurate staging results in the loss of potentially highly curable patients.

The standard radical neck dissection still has a role in the control of neck metastases in our institution. However, the lesser dissections are useful when lower postoperative morbidity and mortality are desired (all postoperative deaths followed radical neck dissections in this series), especially when combined primary and neck dissections are contemplated in the absence of clinically detectable neck involvement. As the incidence of head and neck cancers increases in women because of more liberal consumption of alcohol and tobacco, the modified radical neck operation may be preferred in the treatment of limited disease. Since follow-up examinations have not been a major problem in our relatively homogeneous patient population, this operation can be used more frequently. Hopefully, as the knowledge expands in the field of cell kinetics and as predictability of cancer behavior becomes more accurate, tailoring therapy to disease will become more precise.

Summary

Two hundred sixty-one patients who underwent three types of neck dissection for cervical lymphadenopathy in association with squamous cell cancer of the head and neck are analyzed retrospectively. Patients were grouped into those with histologically negative nodes and those with histologically positive nodes. Statistical analyses for neck recurrence and survival rates were made using the sampled permutation method. The results show that suprahyoid neck dissection is associated with an unusually high recurrence rate in the neck in patients with histologically negative nodes. Modified radical neck dissection and standard radical neck dissection are equivalent with regard to recurrences in the neck and five year survival rates when the disease is above the juguloomohyoid lymph node group. The study suggests that simple upper neck dissection is contraindicated in patients with negative or positive nodes and that modified radical neck dissection can be used in selected patients instead of the formal radical neck operation.

REFERENCES

1. Farr HW, Arthur K. Epidermoid carcinoma of the mouth and pharynx 1960–1964. Elective radical neck dissection. Clin Bull 1971;1:130.
2. Jesse RH, Lindberg RD. Evolution of clinically negative neck. Squamous cell carcinoma of the oral cavity and faucial arch. JAMA 1971;217:32.
3. Martin H, Del Valle B, Ehrlich H, Cahan WG. Neck dissection. Cancer 1951;4:441.
4. Crile G. Excision of cancer of the head and neck. JAMA 1906;47:1780.
5. Bocca E, Pignataro O. A conservation technique in radical neck dissection. Ann Otol 1967;76:975.
6. Blair VP, Moore S, Byars LT. Cancer of the Face and Mouth. St. Louis, C. V. Mosby, 1941, p 579.

Oncologic Surgical Aspects of Immediate Breast Reconstruction

THOMAS G. FRAZIER, M.D. AND R. BARRETT NOONE, M.D.

IN JANUARY OF 1977, with the increased realization that progress in the treatment of carcinoma of the breast had become limited more by systemic therapy than by local therapy, the authors began to develop an interest in the potential for immediate reconstruction of the breast at the time of mastectomy for initial treatment.

In looking at the advantages of immediate reconstruction, our belief was that the patient would have an immediate breast form; it would require only one anesthetic, and there would be an obvious psychological advantage to the patient to have this done on an immediate basis rather than delaying or living with a defect for an extended period of time.

The Team Concept

The dual authorship of this report underscores the essential team approach required for a successful program of immediate reconstruction. Although a medical oncologist is included in the care of many patients, the essential personnel in every case are the oncologic surgeon and the plastic surgeon. For ultimate benefit of the patient, from the standpoint of both tumor care and reconstructive result, it is essential that close cooperation and clear lines of responsibility are established between these surgical specialists. The oncologic surgeon must have complete control over surgical treatment of the tumor. Although modifications in approach can be suggested by the plastic surgeon, the responsibility rests with the oncologic surgeon to provide optimal cancer care for the patient. The oncologic surgeon also is in the unique position to evaluate candidacy of patients for immediate reconstruction, and to introduce this concept to a large number of women who otherwise would not have this opportunity. He has been demonstrated to be the primary stimulating influence for the great majority of women who receive reconstruction immediately.[1]

Unless the plastic surgeon is prepared to manage the diagnosis and treatment of the complete range of breast disease, benign and malignant, and maintain a proficiency in all aspects of breast cancer, he should not perform the extirpative procedure of mastectomy. Likewise, the oncologic surgeon should direct all aspects of the reconstructive procedure to the plastic surgeon.

One concern frequently expressed involves the scheduling difficulties implicit in any team approach. Whereas the temporal relationships of the oncologic surgeon and plastic surgeon may be awkward at the beginning, such matters generally are well-resolved as the program develops. If the combined procedure is performed in the oncologic surgeon's operating room as the last on his schedule, he may then, at the completion of mastectomy, address the family and leave the operating suite or hospital. He finds the subsequent time required in postoperative hospital and office visits slightly less, since wound care is largely assumed by the plastic surgeon. The plastic surgeon, however, may schedule his portion of the procedure between cases or during completion of ongoing work in another room, especially if residents or surgical assistants are available to help with closure and dressings of the immediate reconstruction. The authors have discovered that rather than constrict their operative schedule on a given day, the immediate reconstruction program has actually increased their case load.

From the Departments of Surgery and Plastic Surgery, The Bryn Mawr Hospital, Bryn Mawr, Pennsylvania; Department of Plastic Surgery, Lankenau Hospital, Philadelphia, Pennsylvania; the Thomas Jefferson University Hospital, Philadelphia, Pennsylvania; and the School of Medicine, University of Pennsylvania, Philadelphia, Pennsylvania.

Diagnosis and Evaluation by the Oncologic Surgeon

Early diagnosis and proper treatment remain the most important factors in improving prognosis from breast cancer. The diagnosis can be aided by noninvasive techniques such as breast self-examination, mammography, ultrasonography, and thermography. However, a two-step approach to the ultimate tissue diagnosis and treatment of breast cancer is used by the authors. The first step consists of either a fine-needle aspiration cytology, tru-cut needle biopsy, or open excisional biopsy. Fine-needle cytology is the best single diagnostic test of a palpable lesion, short of open biopsy. At Bryn Mawr Hospital, Bryn Mawr, Pennsylvania, an accuracy of 97.5% in our first 1000 cases was reported.[2] A positive cytologic finding for malignancy is considered conclusive. If there is a question on cytologic results, then the patient undergoes open biopsy, usually as an outpatient under local anesthesia. The importance of hormone receptor analysis for both prognostic and therapeutic guidance cannot be overemphasized. Every specimen is taken to the pathology laboratory, preferably within 30 minutes of removal, and a portion saved for hormone receptors. In situations of less than 5 mm of tumor, immunoperoxidase staining is used with 85% correlation.

When open biopsy is used for diagnosis, the biopsy for most patients is planned with the thought that they may choose to undergo primary radiation therapy rather than total mastectomy. Therefore, the biopsy serves as a segmental resection unless a very strong family history, multicentricity, or other factors by mammography suggest that the only possible treatment would be modified radical mastectomy with or without immediate reconstruction. This decision may be obviated somewhat by a positive cytologic finding on fine-needle aspiration, or the patient's own informed decision to have a total mastectomy with immediate reconstruction. In these latter instances, the biopsy incision is planned with reconstruction in view. For most biopsies, incisions outlined in the National Surgical Adjuvant Breast Project (NSABP) Protocol B-06 are used.[3] These are radial incisions below the transverse line of the nipple, and circumferential areolar incisions for tumors above the nipple. These incisions allow for creative planning of skin flaps to include resection of the biopsy site and nipple–areolar complex in preparation for immediate reconstruction.

Decision for Mastectomy

The publication of the NSABP Protocol B-06 has given patients a choice for primary therapy in the treatment of tumors 4 cm and less with clinically negative nodes. In general, disease-free survival and survival are essentially the same for all patients regardless of the method of local treatment of the breast. Therefore, a number of different factors determine the decision between mastectomy and segmental resection with radiation therapy. These include patient factors, tumor factors, and treatment factors.

If multifocal disease or diffuse disease is present in the breast, then the patient probably is not a good candidate for anything less than a total mastectomy and axillary dissection. In addition, if there is an associated lobular carcinoma *in situ*, or if there are multiple areas of calcification by mammography, the patient is not a good candidate for radiation therapy. Other factors of importance are a previous history of radiation to the breast, or strong genetic factors suggesting that this may in fact be a diffuse disease and not necessarily a disease isolated to a specific area of the breast.

The patient factors play an equally important role. Some patients will not agree to a total mastectomy, regardless of the possibility of a good result with reconstructive surgery. These patients will almost always opt for one of the breast conservation procedures, regardless of a logical approach in terms of other factors even if immediate reconstruction is offered. The treatment factors themselves may be limited by whether or not the patient is able to receive radiation therapy of sufficient quality, or by the availability of good surgical treatment. For the most part, however, tumor factors are the single most important factors in influencing primary treatment.

Preoperative Evaluation by the Oncologic Surgeon

Patients are divided into three major categories, which will affect their preoperative evaluation and assessment. These are based on the size of the tumor, whether or not lymph nodes are clinically palpable and suspicious, or whether there are no clinically palpable nodes.

The authors' experience has been that with smaller tumors under 2.5 cm with no clinically palpable nodes, the decision on preoperative scanning can be made simply on the basic laboratory evaluations. If the lactate dehydrogonase (LDH) and alkaline phosphatase are normal, the patient has no elevation of her serum calcium, and is asymptomatic, then no scans are indicated. If the patient has a larger tumor, greater than 2.5 cm with symptoms or with positive laboratory values, then preoperative evaluation includes both bone and liver scans. The patient's age and smoking status is somewhat important in deciding candidacy for immediate reconstruction. Age is not a deterrent to immediate reconstruction if health factors allow the procedure. Because of potential skin flap ischemia and necrosis in women who are heavy smokers, these patients are cautioned to discontinue smoking for approximately 2 weeks before surgery and to continue this abstinence for 2 weeks after surgery.

The psychological evaluation of the patient with breast cancer is an important part of the holistic health concept and the various factors regarding patient acceptance of mastectomy is important in the preoperative evaluation of those people who would be good candidates for simultaneous mastectomy and reconstruction.

Cooperative Preoperative Marking and Planning

It is recommended that the plastic surgeon be involved in the marking of the pattern of the skin for extirpation. Proper surgical treatment of invasive breast carcinoma demands both a wide and local excision of the biopsy site and its contaminated tract as well as excision of the pigmented nipple–areolar complex. The oncologic surgeon determines the extent of the wide local excision, determining the amount of skin which will be removed with the underlying tumor. This extent will vary with the attitude and training of the surgeon. The authors favor at least a 1-cm margin around the biopsy site if an excisional biopsy was done, and inclusion of the nipple–areolar complex with the resection. The remainder of the incision is more of an aesthetic import than oncologic. Any excision of traditional "dogears" tissue should be postponed at the time of extirpation and left to the plastic surgeon during the final skin closure. In this fashion, medial extension of the mastectomy scar into the exposed V-neck area can be avoided largely by directing "dogear" excisions inferiorly in all but the occasional upper inner quadrant lesion. If no other benefit accrues than the avoidance of unsightly hypertrophic scarring in this region, then the collaboration of the plastic and general surgeon is adequately justified.

Again, access to the axilla can be kept low and transverse with virtually no encumbrance to axillary dissection. In performing the marking, the areolar border is lightly outlined. A circular excision is then indicated about the biopsy site of a diameter appropriate to the size of the primary lesion. In the case of early T1 lesions, this diameter usually is less than 6 cm. The patterns for nipple–areola and tumor are then blended together by parallel connecting tangents. An extension is indicated in the lateral direction to the subaxillary tissues. The inframammary fold is marked to act as a guide during surgery.

It is appropriate that the oncologic surgeon avoid the excision of the pectoralis minor muscle or division of the pectoral nerves, the thoracodorsal nerve and neurovascular bundle and, preferably, the branches of the intercostobrachial nerve. There is no advantage to removal of the pectoralis minor since in our experience the number of axillary nodes dissected has been no higher in the Patey or Handley modified radical mastectomies than in total mastectomy with axillary dissection alone. The goals of immediate reconstruction cannot be met if subsequent muscular wasting and infraclavicular depression is inflicted on an encouraging early appearance.

Oncologic Considerations of Immediate Reconstruction

Acceptance of immediate reconstruction after prophylactic mastectomy was almost universal. One of the delays in accepting reconstruction immediately after modified radical mastectomy for cancer were the concerns expressed by general surgeons, oncologists, and plastic surgeons about a number of potential or theoretically possible limitations on cancer cure, adjuvant treatment, detection of recurrence, or treatment of recurrent tumor. It remained for these concerns to be answered directly before widespread acceptance of immediate reconstruction could be expected. Specifically the following areas needed attention.

Compromise of the Completeness of Mastectomy

The two-team approach to mastectomy and reconstruction still gives the surgeon the opportunity to perform the complete mastectomy which would be done in the absence of reconstruction. Although the skin incisions are planned as a team preoperatively, the general surgeon has the ultimate decision regarding the margin to be used surrounding the biopsy site of the primary tumor and the extent of skin to be resected. The nipple–areolar complex is considered part of breast tissue and always is removed with the breast. The immediate reconstruction allows ample exposure of the axilla for complete axillary dissection, the extent of which is determined by the oncologic oncologic. The pectoralis fascia is removed. Deep tumors which invade the pectoralis fascia may require muscle resection. In such instances, reconstruction by the use of the local muscle flap techniques or by distant myocutaneous flaps would be indicated.

Inference With Host–Tumor Immunologic Response

Concerns have been expressed that the placement of a silicone prosthesis could have a detrimental effect on the immune response in the host and adversely effect the ability of the body to inhibit recurrent or metastatic disease. There is no clinical evidence to date which would indicate an impairment of the immunologic response because of the presence of silicone protheses. Experimental data on mammary implants done in the rat laboratory model indicate no adverse immunologic effects.[4,5]

Delay in Adjuvant Treatment

Our own experience with immediate reconstruction in clinical Stage I patients revealed involvement of axillary lymph nodes in approximately one third of the patients.[6] This group of patients, as well as some patients who were node-negative with negative estrogen receptors or with large primary tumors were offered systemic adjuvant chemotherapy after wound healing. No alteration in either the initiation or duration of treatment occurred because of the immediate reconstruction, and no complications of the reconstruction were attributable to the adjuvant therapy. Oncologists generally agree that it is most important to begin administration of adjuvant drugs early in the postoperative period. It is our opinion that there should be no justification for delay in beginning treatment, even if the prosthesis would seem to be at risk. In fact, if these women had elected to undergo delayed reconstruction it would be done after completion of chemotherapy, and hence delayed even further.

Inhibition of Detection of Recurrences

Concern that the placement of the silicone prosthesis in the submuscular space would either introduce tumor cells into a new plane of dissection, or would inhibit detection of recurrences in the local chest wall tissue also has been expressed. When they occur, local chest wall recurrences are found in the skin or subcutaneous tissue superficial to the pectoralis muscle plane.[7] Detection of such recurrences, therefore, should not be obscured by the placement of the prosthesis behind the pectoralis muscle. The development of such local recurrences is not increased by the immediate reconstructive effort.

We recently reviewed a combined series of 185 consecutive patients undergoing immediate mastectomy reconstruction, based on experience in two institutions.[8] This group of 185 patients has now been followed for a minimum of 2 years, and a maximum of 9 years after mastectomy. The mean follow-up period was 51 months, when reviewed for publication. During this time, 11 local recurrences, six regional metastases, and 13 systemic metastases were noted as the initial demonstration of recurrent disease. This represents an overall recurrence rate of 16%. Those presenting as local recurrences totaled 6%. In all patients except one, the local recurrence in the patient was treated by resection, chemotherapy and/or radiation therapy without adverse effects on the reconstruction. One patient desired removal of her prosthesis during the period of treatment of the local recurrence. This would not have been necessary for treatment, however, but was done because of the patient's own desire and later was reinserted. Twelve patients have died from their breast disease. The major studies of Rosen *et al.* can be cited to place these figures in perspective,[9,10] and show no increase in recurrence.

Conclusion

It is our opinion that immediate reconstruction is a safe and effective alternative for the patient treated by mastectomy. Using a two-team approach, it can be done safely with as complete a mastectomy as in those patients who do not have reconstruction. Cure has not been compromised and local recurrences have not been increased. We continue to embrace this positive approach to treating the patient with breast cancer, and strongly recommend this as an option in primary therapy.

REFERENCES

1. Noone RB, Frazier TG, Hayward CZ, Skiles MS. Patient acceptance of immediate reconstruction following mastectomy. Plast Reconstr Surg 1982;69:632.
2. Frazier TG, Rowland CW, Woolery CT, Ryan SM. Cooperative value of aspiration cytology and the diagnostic evaluation of breast masses. J Surg Oncol 1979;8:353.
3. NSABP Protocol B-06: A protocol to compare segmental mastectomy and axillary dissection with and without radiation of the breast and total mastectomy and axillary dissection. May 22, 1980.
4. Harris HI. Surgery of breast implants from the point of view of carcinogenesis. Plast Reconstr Surg 1961;28:81.
5. Schuler FA, Rosato FE, Horton CE. Silicone prosthesis and anti-tumor immunity. Plast Reconstr Surg 1978;61:762.
6. Noone RB, Murphy JB, Spear SL, Little JM III. A 6-year experience with immediate reconstruction after mastectomy for cancer. Plast Reconstr Surg 1985;76:258.
7. Gilliland MD, Larson DL, Copeland EM. Appropriate timing for breast reconstruction. Plast Reconstr Surg 1983;72:335.
8. Rosen PP, Saigo PE, Braun DW *et al.* Predictors of recurrence in Stage I (T1N0M0) breast carcinoma. Ann Surg 1981;193:15.
9. Rosen PP, Saigo PE, Braun DW *et al.* Prognosis in Stage II breast cancer. Ann Surg 1981;194:576.

Immediate Reconstruction After Mastectomy for Cancer: Reconstructive and Psychological Considerations

R. BARRETT NOONE, M.D. AND THOMAS G. FRAZIER, M.D.

THE SIGNIFICANT emotional distress accompanying the loss of a woman's breast to mastectomy has stimulated a search for alternatives to this procedure. This distress becomes more apparent as the incidence of breast cancer increases, with one in 11 American women expecting to contract the disease in her lifetime.[1] Faced with the thought of a mutilating procedure, many women express an option for breast-conserving procedures such as lumpectomy and irradiation or for immediate reconstruction. As techniques to restore feminine form by breast reconstruction on a delayed basis after mastectomy have improved in the last 15 years, acceptance of the use of these techniques at the time of mastectomy is growing.

Immediate reconstruction was introduced by Hueston and McKenzie[2] in Australia at about the same time that delayed reconstruction was begun in the United States.[3] Immediate reconstruction was slow to gain acceptance in this country for a number of reasons. General surgeons were concerned that the addition of reconstruction at the time of mastectomy would compromise their ability to provide the most complete surgical procedure possible and would increase the surgical complication rate after mastectomy. Oncologists expressed the opinion that immediate reconstruction would limit their ability to provide adjuvant therapy after treatment of the breast cancer and would perhaps delay or inhibit the detection of local or regional recurrences of the tumor in the follow-up period. Psychiatrists were concerned that psychological sequelae would occur associated with a mastectomy before entering the reconstructive phase. Plastic surgeons, in addition to the above, had concerns that the aesthetic quality of the reconstruction would not be as good and that the patient would not appreciate the reconstruction as well as she would have if she were forced to "live with" the deformity for a period of time before undergoing reconstruction.

These concerns delayed introduction and acceptance of immediate breast reconstruction in this country during the 1970s at a time when the technical advantages in breast reconstruction were being advanced. The widespread acceptance of the silicone prosthesis as a breast substitute and the development of safe and effective techniques in its placement, mainly the submuscular breast reconstruction technique during prophylactic mastectomy,[4–8] paved the way for wider acceptance of mastectomy reconstruction in general, and allowed the introduction of basic techniques to the patient as an alternative at the time of mastectomy. As facility with the reconstructive techniques using the silicone implant increased, the introduction of the major myocutaneous flaps in breast reconstruction for augmenting or replacing deficient tissues led to the application of these techniques in the patient in the immediate mode.[9–13]

The authors began to address the above concerns in 1977 at the Bryn Mawr Hospital, Bryn Mawr, Pennsylvania.[14] The content of this report is based on personal experience with over 250 immediate reconstructive procedures.

As other centers also contributed to the immediate reconstruction experience in the last 5 to 10 years, a growing acceptance of this procedure in the plastic surgery community has

From the Department of Surgery, University of Pennsylvania School of Medicine, Philadelphia, Pennsylvania; the Departments of Plastic Surgery and Surgery, Bryn Mawr Hospital, Bryn Mawr, Pennsylvania, and the Department of Plastic Surgery, Lankenau Hospital; Philadelphia, Pennsylvania; and the Thomas Jefferson University School of Medicine, Philadelphia, Pennsylvania.

been seen.[15–22] In 1984 it was estimated that approximately one third of the 98,000 mastectomy reconstructions performed in the United States were done on an immediate basis.[23]

Advantages of Immediate Timing

Advantages of immediate timing for breast reconstruction are many. They can be grouped into four categories: (1) enhanced aesthetic results; (2) various forms of economy; (3) psychological advantages; and (4) availability.

Aesthetic Results

Aesthetic results actually are enhanced for a given patient facing surgical treatment of breast cancer because the extent of deformity can be controlled and minimized by the general surgicalplastic surgical collaboration. Lesser procedures for reconstruction can be planned for immediate timing. In addition, there is a considerable advantage to immediate reconstruction in working with unscarred tissue such that muscles can expand more freely at the time of dissection without the partial denervation and internal and external scarring that inevitably accompany the postoperative phase of healing after mastectomy.

Economic Time Considerations

The economies of immediate timing are as obvious for breast reconstruction as any other category of reconstruction. They include an economy of finances in limiting the extirpative and reconstructive procedures to a single general anesthetic with a single hospital admission. This hospital stay when immediate submuscular reconstruction is used is no longer than that for mastectomy without reconstruction. The authors have noted a mean hospital stay of 6.9 days when immediate reconstruction is added to mastectomy.[14]

In 1980 the average length of stay for patients younger than 70 years who underwent mastectomy for cancer without reconstruction was 8.9 days. This is a reported statistic of the Federal Register governing rules and regulations for implementation of fiscal reimbursement to hospitals under the diagnosis-related groups (DRG) program.[24] Although two or more subsequent operations might be required to complete the reconstructive project, including the nipple/areolar reconstruction and secondary revision, these usually are performed on an outpatient basis with minimal hospitalization cost.

An economy of time is equally important. As more and more women find themselves pursuing careers in the work place and as family economies are dependent on such contributions, the clear impact of two major hospitalizations and recoveries compared to one is obvious. Time away from families and small children can essentially be halved with the immediate approach to timing. A major concern of many educated patients facing such surgery is the general aesthetic with its attendant risks. Limiting the need for general anesthesia to a single procedure is seen by many women as a major advantage. The postoperative morbidity of both procedures, particularly the expected discomfort, can be combined in a single recovery period rather than be faced on two occasions.

Psychological Impact

Initial assumptions about a negative psychological impact of immediate reconstruction have been shown to be largely false. Psychological studies support a facilitation to recovery and rehabilitation to women having the immediate procedure, as is discussed later. It might not be far afield to suggest that a psychological boost at the time of facing the major life crisis that breast cancer represents might have a positive overall effect not only on surgical treatment, but perhaps on tumor–host relationship. If psychological influences affect the course of any malignancies, it can be proposed that they are likely to do so in the case of chronic malignancy of breast cancer.

Increased Availability

A final advantage must be seen as that of increased availability to women as a whole. Within the entire population of women facing mastectomy there is a subgroup that are by nature unassertive and unselfish. For them, an elective decision to reenter the hospital to initiate a course of breast reconstruction with additional major surgery and recovery is an unlikely event. Immediate timing essentially makes the benefits of breast reconstruction available to these women who otherwise would be effectively denied them if forced to elect a delayed operation.

Plastic Surgery Consultation

If the option for treatment of the breast cancer is removal of the breast with immediate reconstruction, preadmission consultation with the plastic surgeon in his office is scheduled. This usually is done within a week of the positive biopsy diagnosis. In an effort to render as realistic a result as possible, photographs of unreconstructed and reconstructed patients are shown. This gives the patient who has never seen a mastectomy deformity an opportunity to appreciate the deformity and to obtain an impression of the limitations of reconstruction, as well as the benefits.

Choice of Technique

The goal of the surgical team is eradication of the tumor and reconstruction of the breast using the procedure or series of procedures which will give the best aesthetic result accompanied by the least morbidity.

Basic techniques used in immediate reconstruction include the following: (1) submuscular silicone prosthetic reconstruction; (2) tissue expander placement at the time of mastectomy followed by delayed replacement with a prosthesis; (3) primary reconstruction with the transverse rectus abdominis musculocutaneous (TRAM) flap; and (4) latissimus dorsi musculocutaneous flap. The latter procedure has been limited to those who need skin coverage because of large tumor resections, salvage mastectomies, or other reasons for skin deficiency when the TRAM flap is unable to be used or is not desirable.

The choice of technique is determined by a number of factors including age; breast size; body habitus; tumor location, size, and pathologic type; size, configuration, and future surgical plans for the opposite breast; ancillary health indications such as a history of heavy cigarette smoking; and socioeconomic and lifestyle considerations.

In the great majority of patients, submuscular reconstruction with the conventional prosthesis alone is utilized. The reasons for this preference are many. When the general surgeon and plastic surgeon plan the extirpation and reconstruction together, consistently good results are achieved with a lower rate of complications.

As with any foreign body reconstruction, a number of patients will develop undesirable effects such as symptomatic scar capsule contracture, leading to a second procedure for correction. The submuscular reconstructive technique is performed expeditiously at the completion of the extirpative session, rarely extending operative time more than 1 hour with practiced teams. Masking of early local recurrence is virtually eliminated by this approach, and this assurance may be offered to surgical and medical oncologist alike. One assesses the suitability of the simple procedure during the physical examination. Here the overall volume and shape of the involved breast is evaluated, taking into account the size of the primary tumor that underwent biopsy. In general, the patient with the quite small breast and larger tumor will require more complicated approaches. Occasionally a moderate-size breast with a large tumor which will require a major resection of skin might indicate the same. In general, such situations will require the addition of tissue brought in from a distance.

Both the latissimus dorsi musculocutaneous flap with the continued use of the mammary prosthesis as well as the transverse lower rectus musculocutaneous flap, as described below, alone remain the available options. A final alternative remains the use of tissue expanders in these individuals. In obese patients with large breasts or those whose skin flaps might be compromised by cigarette smoking, a two-staged expander-prosthesis route may be chosen. The routine use of expanders in large numbers of patients appears to the authors unnecessary and counterproductive, committing the patient to further surgery which might need to be delayed until after chemotherapy is completed, and perhaps defeating the psychological benefits of a one-stage procedure.

Complications of Submuscular Reconstruction and Their Management

The well-described complications of skin necrosis, hematoma, seroma, and infection might occur after any mastectomy without the addition of immediate reconstruction. With a prosthesis in place, these problems can lead to loss of the prosthesis and the accompanied surgical and psychological trauma of an operation for its removal. Therefore, preoperative and intraoperative goals are directed toward prevention of the occasion for complication. Preoperative instruction against ingesting blood-coagulation inhibitors such as aspirin is given, and a standardized list of these medications is included with preoperative instructions. During surgery, total muscle cover of the prosthesis is the single most important factor in prevention of prosthesis loss.

Marginal Skin Necrosis

Marginal skin necrosis is the most frequent problem seen, with a small rim of skin loss in the central portion of the skin closure seen in approximately 15% of patients.[14] However, as noted below, prosthesis salvage is possible in all but a few.

Hematoma

Hematoma can be avoided by meticulous attention to hemostasis and the placement of suction catheters at the time of surgery. Major hematomas have been a rare occurrence in the authors' experience, seen in 2% of immediate reconstructions.[14]

Seroma

Seroma, or fluid collections secondary to lymphorrhea, are seen as frequently as 12% postoperative, despite routine use of suction catheter drains. These are usually in the axillary area of the breast, in the lateral gutter or inframammary fold, and might require frequent aspiration with the use of some form of intracatheter needle. Tolerance of small fluid collections can lead to fibrosis of the overlying skin, usually in the lower pole of the breast where drawn by gravity. This fibrosis, although softening over time, can detract significantly from the final result.

Cellulitis

Cellulitis of the skin is an occasional problem, usually responding to appropriate antibiotic coverage. It has not lead to prosthesis loss in the absence of skin necrosis or hematoma.

Prosthesis Loss

Loss of prosthesis is the most serious complication after immediate reconstruction. Fortunately, with attention to meticulous details, this should be a rare event, with an incidence of 3% in experience with over 250 procedures by the authors. It might follow infection, skin necrosis, or hematoma. The loss of an immediate prosthesis is a significant emotional event, since the patient might experience this as "mourning" for the loss of the breast. The grief exhibited by these patients seems greater than any other mastectomy patient.

Capsule Formation

Capsule formation is discussed preoperatively with the patient as an expected sequel and not as a complication. It is stressed with all patients that capsule formation is normal for formation of the breast mound, but only a certain percentage of patients have significant capsule formation requiring secondary surgery. A symptomatic capsule contracture rate of 10% to 15% remains consistent with the experience of the authors in delayed reconstruction with submuscular prostheses and is not dissimilar from that reported after subcutaneous or prophylactic mastectomy.[4,5]

Other Complications

There are other complications of extirpative surgery which frequently are pointed out by the patient and might require full wound maturity to resolve. These may include painful neuromas within the axilla, as well as arm and shoulder weakness sometimes associated with neuropraxic injury to the nerves within the axilla. Shoulder stiffness and lateral thoracic neuromuscular pain is seen. Massage is encouraged with vitamin E. A significant amount of the pain and discomfort which is experienced initially by the patient tends to resolve with time. These rarely become a major problem requiring surgical intervention.

Aesthetic Results

As experience with breast reconstruction grows, physicians and patients have become more critical of the aesthetic results from all forms of reconstruction. Therefore, when done in the immediate setting, the aesthetic goals should be essentially the same as those planned for the delayed reconstruction. Accordingly, the preoperative selection of the patient and technique depends on aesthetic considerations regarding chest size, overall weight and body build of the patient, and the size and configuration of the contralateral breast. Early objections to immediate reconstruction stated that the aesthetic results would not be as good as those with delayed reconstruction. This view is not shared by the authors who believe that given the ability to coordinate planning and proper incisions with the general surgeon, and given the opportunity to work with unscarred, fresh muscle and skin, the immediate results of prosthetic reconstruction should essentially be the same, if not better, than delayed reconstruction. There appears to be no difference in aesthetic results between patients who have a temporary tissue expender at the time of the immediate procedure or a flap reconstruction if it is needed, when these procedures are compared with delayed reconstruction.

Although there is some feeling that the patient in the immediate situation might "expect less" from her result and be pleased with the procedure, nevertheless, there is no reason that the reconstructive surgeon should expect a less than desirable result if done at the time of mastectomy.

Psychological Aspects of Immediate Reconstruction

It is well known that a mastectomy for breast cancer is a profound psychological stress for the patient, as well as being a major surgical procedure.[25] The impact of mastectomy, added to the fear of recurrence of the cancer, produces alterations of mood, body image, sexuality, feminity, and social and occupational functioning.

Psychological theories related to loss and bereavement had provided a major area of resistance to immediate breast reconstruction.[26] These theories suggested that a woman must mourn the loss of her breast by experiencing the absence of the breast before being able to adapt to the other aspects of her life.[27] The mourning process includes a sequence of denial, anger, depression, despair, and hopefully eventual acceptance. Those treating breast cancer believed that women who sought reconstruction were having difficulty in completing the mourning process by not adapting to the loss of the breast and eventually accepting this loss.[28]

The theories of reaction to loss and the necessity for bereavement have been challenged in recent years. The psychiatric literature began to support the view that reconstruction is the only solution to the real disfigurement caused by a mastectomy.[29] Plastic surgeons suggested that even planning the reconstruction with the patient before her mastectomy, to allow her to expect the reconstruction after she had healed after surgery, reduced the negative psychological consequences of the mastectomy.

Clifford evaluated signs of depression and distress in postmastectomy patients and found that the expected signs were not present in those who had undergone immediate reconstruction.[30]

Stevens and co-workers[31] compared patient groups with respect to the timing of reconstruction and found that patients undergoing immediate reconstruction expressed less change and feelings of attractiveness in femininity as well as a noticeable absence of the sense of mutilation which was expressed by patients who had delayed reconstruction. They suggested that immediate reconstruction does not alter the mourning process since mourning for the breast loss begins in both groups even before the mastectomy with the anticipation of the breast loss. They also noted that patients seem to be satisfied with the cosmetic result regardless of the time of mastectomy. However, the reconstructed breast seemed to be better integrated into the body image when immediate reconstruction was performed, being experienced as a "restoration" for the removed breast rather than a "replacement."

Dean and co-workers also emphasized the psychological salutary effects of immediate reconstruction, showing the less psychiatric morbidity was present in patients undergoing immediate intraoperative repair than those who delayed their reconstruction.[32]

Goin and Goin evaluated the psychological impact of immediate reconstruction in patients who had previous mastectomies and delayed reconstructions on the opposite side and concluded that no psychological benefit was present in a delayed environment.[33] They found that many expressed a wish that reconstruction could have been done at the time of mastectomy.

Noone and co-workers directed attention at patient acceptance of the procedure after immediate reconstruction, showing that it was not necessary for patients to experience the deformity of a mastectomy in order to be satisfied with the results following reconstruction.[34]

Noone and Little also have evaluated the psychosocial correlates of immediate versus delayed reconstruction in a combined patient series.[35,36] Psychological evaluation of nine major areas of functioning included somatization, obsessive–compulsive reactions, interpersonal sensitivity, depression, anxiety, hostility, phobic anxiety, paranoid ideation, and psychoticism were determined in groups of immediate and delayed reconstruction patients. The results of this study questioned a number of previous assumptions about breast reconstruction. Contrary to an earlier prejudice that women who search breast reconstruction are maladapted and "unable to accept their defect,"[28] both groups of patients studied were normal on psychological testing and were very similar in most respects to a normative group of adult females of comparable age. With respect to timing and sociodemographic features, it was demonstrated that it was not only the younger, single, or more highly educated woman who sought immediate reconstruction. To the contrary, requests for immediate procedures came from a group entirely comparable to that opting for conventional, delayed timing. Such requests for immediate reconstruction, then, depend on the knowledge of availability as presented to the patient by the general surgeon or physician initially concerned with the cancer care.

Another assumption challenged by these findings is that the patient benefits from "living with her deformity" and that her satisfaction is "enhanced by such exposure."[37] There was no significant difference between the immediate and delayed group, with 96% of the former and 89% of the latter reporting satisfaction with the breast reconstructive procedure.[35,36] There is, in fact, clinical evidence that a woman who undergoes immediate reconstruction is more likely to incorporate her new breast into the body image and thereby achieve a higher level of comfort and satisfaction from the onset.[31] Reduction in the psychological distress of the mastectomy appears to be a major benefit of immediate reconstruction.

In the experience of the authors, patients undergoing reconstruction, either immediate or delayed, experience a cancer diagnosis and, as a result, a major body alteration. It appeared that women who had immediate reconstruction did not experience the magnitude or duration of psychological symptoms and seemed to experience an earlier return to former psychological equilibrium than women who lived for a time with a deformity of mastectomy. When asked to recall the emotional distress toward the cancer surgery experience, the women in the immediate group reported significantly less distress than those who had delayed reconstruction. It appears that the maintenance of a breast contour throughout the mastectomy might lessen the trauma of the ablative experience and might influence subsequent adjustment in a positive manner. Perhaps the end point of breast reconstruction might be the same for both the immediate and delayed group, with a facilitated return to normal psychological function. However, the presence of a breast contour created at the time of mastectomy might ease the type of magnitude of the burdens carried by the patient in the journey toward the end point.

Summary

Experience with immediate reconstruction of the breast after mastectomy for cancer has led to acceptance of the psychological benefits of this approach and to refinement in techniques sufficient to produce aesthetic results comparable to delayed reconstruction. This experience has diminished concerns about the safety and efficacy of immediate reconstruction. In the rapidly changing area of breast cancer treatment, the woman desiring preservation of feminine form has the clear additional alternative of immediate reconstruction if mastectomy is selected for her treatment.

REFERENCES

1. Cancer Facts and Figures, 1985. American Cancer Society, 1985; 5–7.
2. Hueston JT, McKenzie G. Breast reconstruction after radical mastectomy. Aust NZ J Surg 1970;39:367.

3. Snyderman RK, Guthrie RH. Reconstruction of the female breast following radical mastectomy. Plast Reconstr Surg 1971;47:565.
4. Jarrett JR, Cutler RG, Teal DF. Subcutaneous mastectomy in small, large, or ptotic breasts with immediate submuscular placement of implants. Plast Reconstr Surg 1978;62:702.
5. Woods JE, Irons GB, Arnold PG. The case for submuscular implantation of prostheses in reconstructive surgery. Ann Plast Surg 1980;5:115.
6. Gruber RP, Kahn RA, Lash H, Maser MR, Apfelberg DB, Laub DR. Breast reconstruction following mastectomy: A comparison of submuscular and subcutaneous techniques. Plast Reconstr Surg 1981;67:312.
7. Dinner MI, Labandter HP. Total mammary adenectomy with histologic evaluation and immediate reconstruction. Plast Reconstr Surg 1981;68:505.
8. Jarrett JR, Cutler RG, Teal DF. Aesthetic refinements in prophylactic subcutaneous mastectomy with submuscular reconstruction. Plast Reconstr Surg 1982;69:624.
9. McCraw JB, Dibbell DG, Carraway JH. Clinical definition of independent myocutaneous vascular territories. Plast Reconstr Surg 1977;60:341.
10. Schneider WJ, Hill HL, Brown RG. Latissimus dorsi myocutaneous flap for breast reconstruction. Br J Plast Surg 1977;30:277.
11. Muhlbauer W, Olbrisch R. The latissimus dorsi myocutaneous flap for breast reconstruction. Chirurg Plast (Berlin) 1977;4:27.
12. Dinner MI, Labandter HP, Dowden RV. The role of the rectus abdominis myocutaneous flap in breast reconstruction. Plast Reconstr Surg 1982;69:209.
13. Hartrampf CR, Scheflan M, Black PW. Breast reconstruction with a transverse abdominal island flap. Plast Reconstr Surg 1982;69:216.
14. Noone RB, Murphy JB, Spear SL, Little JW III. A 6-year experience with immediate reconstruction after mastectomy for cancer. Plast Reconstr Surg 1985;76:258.
15. Rosato FE, Fink PJ, Horton CE, Payne RL. Immediate postmastectomy reconstruction. J Surg Oncol 1976;8:277.
16. Georgiade GS, Georgiade NG, McCarty KS Jr, Ferguson BJ, Seigler HF. Modified radical mastectomy with immediate reconstruction for carcinoma of the breast. Ann Surg 1981;193:565.
17. Watts GT, Caruso F, Waterhouse JA. Mastectomy with primary reconstruction (Letter to Editor). Lancet 1980;2:967.
18. Georgiade GS, Georgiade N, McCarty KS, Seigler HF. Rationale for immediate reconstruction of the breast following modified radical mastectomy. Ann Plast Surg 1982;8:20.
19. Georgiade GS *et al.* Long-term clinical outcome of immediate reconstruction after mastectomy. Plast Reconstr Surg 1985;76:415.
20. Wilkinson LH, Peloso OA, Dail WG Jr. Modified radical mastectomy with immediate breast reconstruction. Arch Surg 1982;117:579.
21. Watts GT. Reconstruction of the breast as a primary and secondary procedure following mastectomy for carcinoma. Br J Surg 1976;63:823.
22. Webster DJT, Mansel RE, Hughes LE. Immediate reconstruction of the breast after mastectomy: Is it safe? Cancer 1984;53:1416.
23. American Society of Plastic and Reconstructive Surgeons, Inc. 1984 Media Survey.
24. Rules and Regulations, Department of Health and Human Services, Health Care Financing Administration. Federal Register 1983;39881.
25. Renneker R, Cutler M. Psychological problems of adjustment to cancer of the breast. JAMA 1952;148:833.
26. Parkes MC. Bereavement Studies of Grief in Adult Life. London: Pelecan Books, 1972.
27. Klein R. A crisis to grow on. Cancer 1971;28:1660.
28. Goldsmith HS, Alday ES. Role of the surgeon and the rehabilitation of the breast cancer patient. Cancer 1971;28:1672.
29. Asken MJ. Psychoemotional aspects of mastectomy: A review of recent literature. Am J Psychiatry 1975;132:56.
30. Clifford E. The reconstruction experience: The search for restitution. In: Georgiade NG, ed. Breast Reconstruction Following Mastectomy. St. Louis: Mosby, 1979.
31. Stevens LA, McGrath MH, Drus RG, Kister SJ, Gump FE, Forde KA. The psychological impact of immediate breast reconstruction for women with early breast cancer Plast Reconstr Surg 1984;73:619.
32. Dean C, Chetty U, Forrest AP. Effects of immediate breast reconstruction on psychosocial morbidity after mastectomy. Lancet 1983;26:459.
33. Goin MK, Goin JM Psychological reactions to prophylactic mastectomy synchronous with contralateral breast reconstruction. Plast Reconstr Surg 1982;70:355.
34. Noone RB, Frazier TG, Hayward CZ, Skiles MS. Patient acceptance of immediate reconstruction following mastectomy. Plast Reconstr Surg 1982;69:632.
35. Wellisch DK, Schain WS, Noone RB, Little JW III. Psychosocial correlates of immediate *versus* delayed reconstruction of the breast. Plast Reconstr Surg 1985;76:713.
36. Schain WS, Wellisch DK, Pasnau RO, Landsverk J. The sooner the better: A study of psychological factors in women undergoing immediate *versus* delayed breast reconstruction. Am J Psychiatry 1985;142:40.
37. Luce EA. Breast reconstruction after mastectomy. South Med J 1983;76:190.

Immunizing and Tumor-Promoting Properties of Two Structurally Similar Alkylating Agents

ELIZABETH E. MILLER, PH.D. AND KWAN C. TSOU, PH.D.

This work was carried out in collaboration with Dr. Kwan C. Tsou, who designed and synthesized the alkylating agent, N,N′-diallyl β-aziridinoproprionamide (DAAP), based on an enzyme rationale. N,N′-dimethyl β-aziridinoproprionamide (DMAP) was prepared in order to determine the alkylating activity of the β-aziridino group, and these compounds differed only in the diallyl and dimethyl moieties. The DAAP was found to have a very low toxicity for dogs and to be a very effective anticancer agent against Dunning Leukemia in rats. The DAAP then was used in a rat lymphoma system, resulting in complete tumor regression and subsequent immunity when a challenge inoculation of live tumor cells was given. The current report describes a comparison of the effects the two alkylating agents, DAAP and DMAP, in this rat lymphoma system. For these experiments female Lewis inbred rats were implanted with Lymphoma 8 using tissue fragments. Untreated tumor-bearing controls died consistently from the tumor in 9 to 12 days. Because of the low toxicity, DAAP and DMAP were injected daily for 2 weeks. The DMAP, like DAAP, caused complete regression of the lymphoma, and immunity was demonstrated when a challenge injection of live tumor cells was given. The rats treated with DMAP and DAAP appeared to be normal and healthy over an extended observation period, but at about 9 months rats treated with DMAP, including normal drug treated controls, developed multiple tumors of types other than lymphoma, principally mammary tumors. No tumors appeared in any DAAP-treated rats or in any normal or sodium chloride-treated controls at this time. Because of the structural differences in the two compounds, it appeared that tumor regression with subsequent immunity was associated with the β-aziridinoproprinonamide portion of the molecule. The results of these studies clearly indicate that anticancer drugs can be designed that will be effective in causing tumor rejection and at the same time allow the host to mount an effective immune response. In addition, it is shown that very small structural differences are responsible for tumor induction.

STILL TODAY there exists the need for less toxic and more effective chemotherapeutic agents for the treatment of lymphoproliferative diseases.[1] Taking advantage of enzyme differences between normal and neoplastic cells, N,N′-diallyl β-aziridinoproprionamide (DAAP) was synthesized by Tsou *et al.*[2] with the expectation that it would have a low toxicity, and it was found to be effective against Dunning Leukemia in both the solid and ascites forms. A preliminary Stage I trial with this alkylating agent was carried out on 13 terminal cancer patients, and relatively low toxicity was found.[3] Studies using another rat tumor, Lewis Lymphoma 8,[4] showed that this compound caused complete tumor regression with subsequent immunity to reimplantation of the tumor.[5] A compound with a structure similar to that of DAAP, dimethyl β-aziridinoproprionamide (DMAP) also was prepared in order to compare the alkylating effect of the β-aziridino group.[2] This report describes the results of studies over a long period of time with these two alkylating agents in the rat lymphoma system.

From the University of Pennsylvania, Philadelphia, Pennsylvania.

Proceedings of the First Beijing International Symposium on Cancer Treatment, September 1986, Beijing, China.

Since Dr. Tsou is deceased (1985) his name appears on this paper with the permission of his wife, and he shares equally in any credit. However, the first author assumes full responsibility for the results.

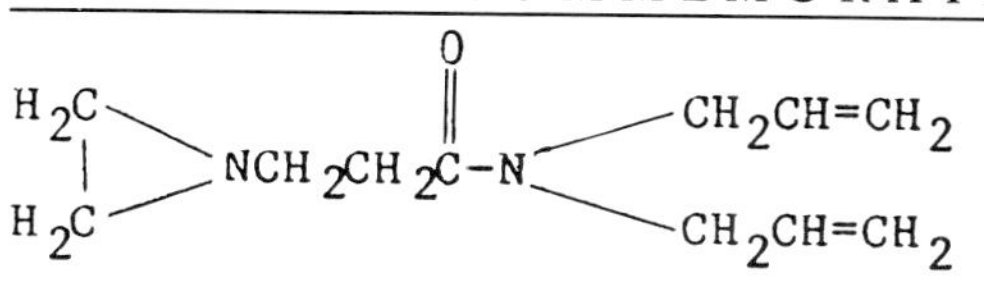

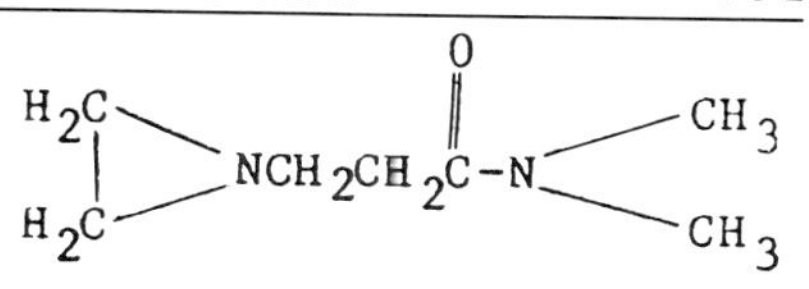

FIGS. 1A AND 1B. The molecular structure for (A, left) DAAP and (B, right) are shown.

Experimental Methods

The synthesis, physical properties and rationale for the design of DAAP and DMAP (Figs. 1A and 1B) were described previously.[2] The two compounds were identical except for the diallyl and dimethyl moeities.

Lymphoma 8[4] was a lymphosarcoma, histologically similar to the human type, which arose spontaneously in the Lewis inbred rat strain. These experiments were designed to observe animals in which drug treatment was effective over a long period of time. Therefore, control groups of nontumor-bearing animals were included, which served later at 9 to 10 months to test the viability of the challenge lymphoma transplant. Rats were distributed into experimental groups on the basis of litters, so that each group was homogeneous genetically. Females weighing 180 to 235 g were implanted subcutaneously with six tumor fragments approximately 2 mm in size. Later, when the lymphoma challenge transplants were given, the dose was increased four times because of the age of the rats.

The compounds were injected intraperitoneally in 0.9% sodium chloride (NaCl) daily for 2 weeks starting on the second day after tumor implantation. The DAAP was given at a concentration of 20 mg/kg of body weight, and injected in a volume of 1 ml for each 100 g of body weight. The concentration used for DMAP was 14 mg/kg, which was calculated to be the molecular equivalent of DAAP. For comparative purposes, a few rats were injected with Cytoxan (cyclophosphamide) 10 mg/kg, since this was a widely used alkylating agent. Observations were made over a period of 2 years for the recurrence of lymphoma and signs of drug toxicity. Animal weights were measured and tail blood collected. Tumor size was measured with calipers and calculated according to the formula $\sqrt[3]{d_1 \times d_2 \times d_3}$.

Results and Discussion

As was found with DAAP, the lymphoma regressed in all rats treated with DMAP, whereas all NaCl-treated or untreated rats died of lymphoma. These lymphoma-bearing control rats, as well as the normal rats which later served as controls for the lymphoma challenge transplant, all died 9 to 12 days. None of the rats died of drug toxicity.

Figure 2 shows the regression of the initial lymphoma transplant in rats treated with DMAP. Lymphoma did not recur during an observation period of 9 months. At this time the surviving rats were given a second lymphoma transplant, and it was found that rats treated with DMAP, like those treated with DAAP, were immune to the lymphoma challenge, whereas NaCl or untreated nontumor-bearing controls died.

Coincidentally, it was noted that tumors other than lymphoma started to appear around the face, neck, or mammary tissue in rats that had been treated with DMAP, both those that had lymphoma which had regressed and normal rats that had been treated with DMAP. Histologically these tumors were mammary adenocarcinoma or papilloma, a thyroid adenoma, squamous cell papilloma, and a fibrosarcoma. Immunity to the lymphoma did not affect the progressive growth of these tumors and did not prevent the growth of a transplantable tumor of another type (Sarcoma MCI) indicating that the immunity was specific. As can be seen from the previous figure, the lymphoma in drug-treated rats grew to a larger size than that in the controls before it started to regress, and it is possible that this experience with the tumor aided the host in establishing immunity. Other factors responsible for the ability of the host to evoke a protective immune response may be the low toxicity of these two alkylating agents, as evidenced by the mild effects they had on body weight and blood components. Figure 3 shows that, although DAAP caused a slight drop in weight during the injection, the normal rate of weight gain was reestablished as soon as the injections were

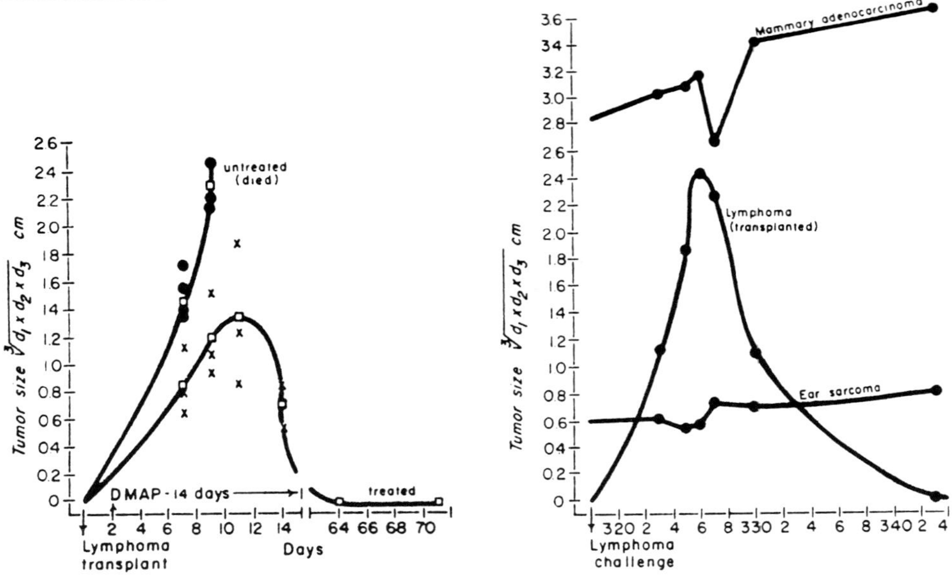

FIG. 2. Growth curves (plotted on average values) of rats treated with DMAP (left). Growth curves of two spontaneous tumors and the lymphoma challenge transplant in a rat previously treated with DMAP (right).

stopped. This was not true for Cytoxan-treated tumor-bearing rats, even though the tumors regressed much faster than those in the DAAP-treated rats. Although there was a slight leucopenia during treatment of rats with DAAP, it was not as severe as in those treated with Cytoxan and returned to normal when the drug treatment was finished.

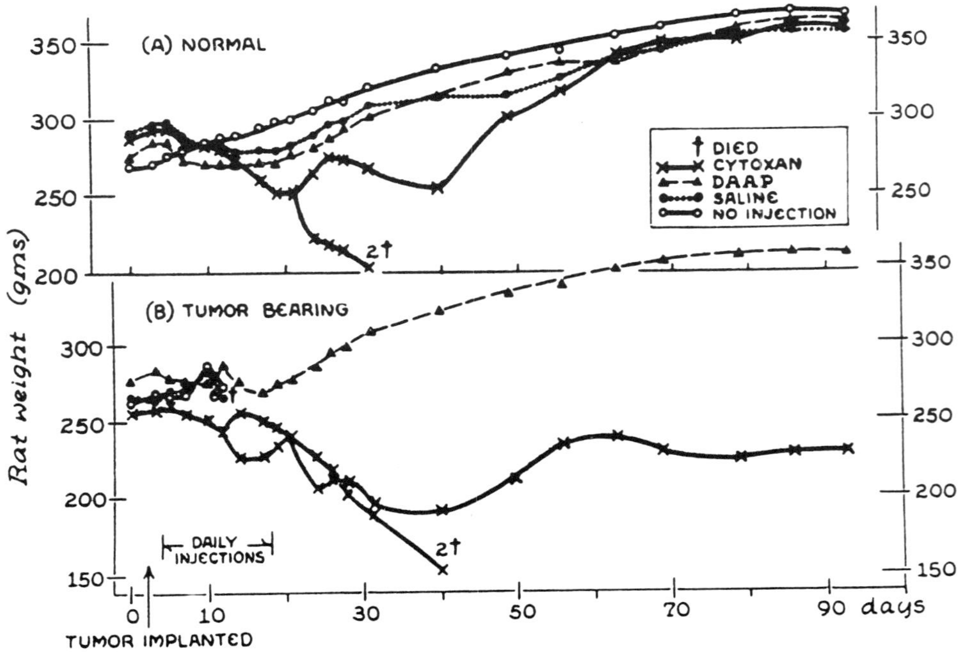

FIGS. 3A AND 3B. Weight curves (plotted on the average of three values) of normal rat (A) and lymphoma-bearing rats (B) treated with drugs, 0.9% NaCl (saline) or untreated. Littermates were distributed equally into the different groups.

In conclusion, our results show that (1) DMAP, as well as DAAP, caused complete regression of Lewis Lymphoma 8 in inbred rats and subsequent specific immunity to lymphoma reimplantation; (2) DMAP female rats developed tumors of types other than lymphoma at about 9 months, whereas DAAP treated rats survived for almost 2 years; and (3) both compounds were found to have very low toxicity with respect to causing permanent weight loss or severe leucopenia.

REFERENCES

1. Pattengale PK, Lukes RJ, Taylor CR. In: Lymphoproliferative Diseases: Pathogenesis, Diagnosis, Therapy. Dordrecht, Holland: M. Nighoff, 1985.
2. Tsou KC, Damle SB, Crichlow RW, Ravdin, RG, Blunt HW. Synthesis of possible cancer chemotherapeutic agents based on enzyme rationale. J Pharm Sci 1967;56:484–488.
3. Benson GS, Weinstein JD, Groff RA, Tsou KC, Ravdin RG. Unpublished data. Harrison Department of Surgical Research, Annual Report, 1970;30–32.
4. Lewis MR. A transplantable lymphoma in rats. Science 1953;118:355–357.
5. Miller EE, Tsou KC. Immunity to lymphoma induced by diallyl B-azridinoproprionamide in inbred rats. Cancer Res 1967;27:1496–1497.

Improvement in Disease-Free Survival of Melanoma Patients in Conjunction With Serologic Response in a Phase Ia/Ib SEG Trial of Vaccinia Melanoma Oncolysate

MARC K. WALLACK, M.D., JERRY A. BASH, PH.D., EVELYN S. DARNELL, A.A.S., AND A. BARTOLUCCI, PH.D.

THE CONCEPT of adjuvant immunotherapy of melanoma has generated much interest as well as criticism over the past 20 years.[1-3] The specific active immunotherapeutic approach has theoretical advantages over nonspecific stimulation since the possibility exists to amplify and focus the hosts responses against tumor specific tumor cells and to establish in the host the capacity to generate an anamnestic response against recurrence.

Specific active immunotherapy is based on the assumption that tumor-associated antigens exist and are sufficiently immunogenic to elicit a response in patients against their own tumors. Although a wide variety of melanoma-associated antigens have been described using murine monoclonal antibodies[4,5] and several antimelanoma responses have been documented in patients,[6-8] the high incidence of metastatic recurrence suggests that the host's natural responses are inadequate.

A variety of means, therefore, have been sought to enhance the immunogenicity of melanoma cells.[9] One method of achieving this is by infection with oncolytic virus.[10] We have been particularly interested in vaccinia virus because of its proven efficacy in animal models[11-13] and its documented safety in mass smallpox immunizations. Therefore we have produced vaccinia melanoma oncolysates (VMO) and performed a series of clinical trials[14-16] with VMO. An early observation from these studies was that melanoma patients treated with VMO produced melanoma-restricted antibody. In the current study preliminary evidence was obtained to relate the efficacy of VMO treatment with antimelanoma antibody production.

Patients and Methods

Patient Selection

Patient eligibility was based upon criteria of histologically confirmed nonrecurrent malignant melanoma, read as Clark's Level IV or V and Breslow Level greater than 1.5 mm depth of invasion (DOI), which was histologically node-positive after regional node dissection. Patients with high-risk Stage I disease, *i.e.*, Breslow Level of 3.0 DOI or greater, were eligible without node dissection. The primary tumor must have been surgically excised with a wide margin and patients had to be disease-free at the time of being placed on study. Exclusion criteria included previous malignancy and previous therapy. The study included one high-risk Stage I and 38 Stage II patients with a male/female ratio of 23/16 and a median age of 44 years.

Vaccinia Melanoma Oncolysate Preparation

The VMO used in this study was prepared at Institut Merieux, Lyon, France, by a method which has been described in detail elsewhere.[14] Briefly, four allogeneic melanoma cell lines

From the Mount Sinai Medical Center, Miami Beach, Florida, and the University of Alabama, Birmingham, Alabama.

Presented at the 5th International Conference on Adjuvant Therapy of Cancer, Tucson, Arizona.

This article has been reproduced with permission from *Adjuvant Therapy of Cancer V*, Grune & Stratton, Orlando, Florida.

were infected with vaccinia virus for 20 hours at 37°C. The pooled cell suspensions were centrifuged at low speed and the resulting pellet (1) was sonicated and recentrifuged. The pellet was discarded and the supernatant (2) retained. The original supernatant (1) was centrifuged at high speed for 2 hours. The supernatant was discarded and the pellet (2) was combined with supernatant (2) to make the oncolysate. The preparation was sonicated and homogenized to eliminate intact cells and the final product was adjusted to 2 mg/ml total protein concentration. Viral content was monitored and the presence of intact melanoma-associated antigens was confirmed by radioimmunoassay.[17]

Vaccinia Melanoma Oncolysate Immunotherapy

Each patient received a smallpox booster 1 week before initiation of VMO therapy. The VMO then was administered intradermally near sites of regional lymphyatics, excluding the site of regional node dissection. Injections of 2.0 mg VMO in 1 ml were given once weekly for 13 weeks followed by injections every other week for 1 year or until recurrence. A dose escalation schedule based on negative melanoma-reactive serological response in the Staphylococcus protein A (SpA) assay was included and consisted of incremental 2.0 mg increases after each 3-month evaluation.

Staphylococcus Protein A Assay

Serum obtained from patients before treatment and every 3 months after treatment was tested in a SpA assay modified from the method of Pfreundschuh *et al.*[18] as described in detail elsewhere.[14] Briefly, melanoma line (MEL 4) target cells were seeded into multiple wells of Terasaki plates (Falcon, Oxnard, CA) , at a density which resulted in 50% to 75% confluence after 24 hour incubation at 37°C. Serum diluted 1:10 were added to washed monolayers for 1 hour at 37°C. The plates were washed and incubated for another hour with SpA-conjugated human O-positive erythocytes. The monolayers were washed and then scored positive or negative for rosettes. Positive wells contained greater than 50% rosettes which were defined as target cells with 50% or more of their surface bound by erythrocytes.

Enzyme-linked Immunosorbant Assay

An enzyme-linked immunosorbant assay (ELISA) was performed directly in flat-bottomed microtiter plates (Dynatech, Alexandria, VA) which had been used to culture target cells. Target cells were plated 24 to 48 hours before the experiment at a density which would result in 95% to 100% confluent monolayers at the time of the assay Monolayers were washed repeatedly to remove serum-containing medium and then fixed with 0.0037% glutaraldehyde (Sigma, St. Louis, MO) for 15 minutes. After thorough washing of monolayers with phosphate-buffered saline (PBS), serial dilutions of patient sera was incubated with target cell monolayers for 1 hour at room temperature. After thorough washing, a second 1-hour incubation was performed with horseradish peroxidase-conjugated goat anti-human IgG or IgM F(ab')2 (Tago, Burlingame, CA). After washing away unbound conjugate, o-paradiethylamide substrate was added for 15 to 30 minutes and absorbance at 490 nm was measured with an automated ELISA reader (Dynatech MR600).

Human Leukocyte Antigen (HLA) Microcytotoxicity Screening

Standard microcytotoxicity techniques were performed by South Florida Blood Services, Miami, to screen patients' sera for anti-HLA antibodies. Pretreatment and treatment sera of 25 patients were tested against a panel of 50 HLA-typed lymphocyte donors. A,B,C screening was performed against unseparated peripheral blood lymphocytes and DR, DQ. Screening was performed against B-cell enriched targets. After incubation with rabbit complement, eosin-stained cells were scored and reactions were interpreted.

Statistical Methods

Significance of extended disease-free survival of the 39 VMO-treated patients was obtained through comparison with controls which were randomly selected from patients who received either BCG or *Corynebacterium parvum* adjuvant therapy. Controls consisted of 39 melanoma patients with the same stage of disease matched according to the priority of

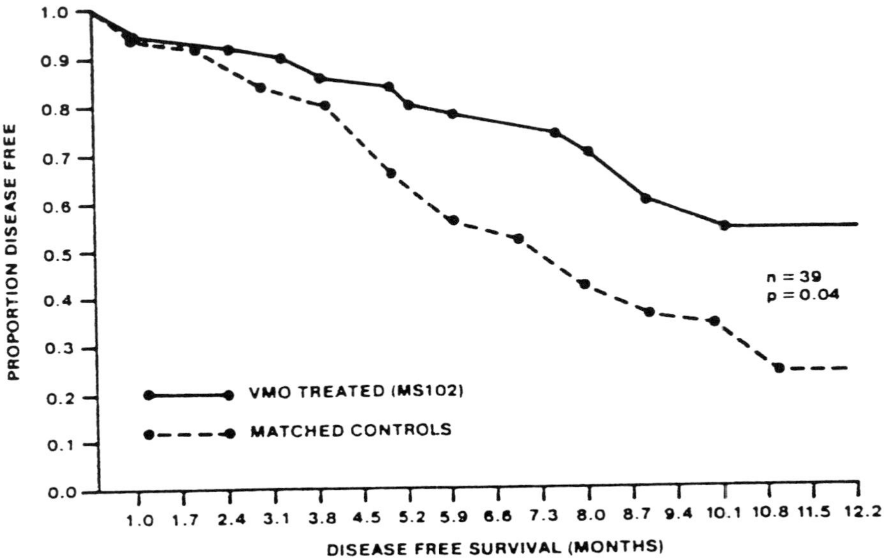

FIG. 1. Disease-free survival of VMO-treated patients compared to matched controls.

number of nodes positive, number of nodes excised, age, and sex. The matched controls were randomly selected from patients who received either Bacillus Calmette-Guerin (BCG) or *C. parvum* adjuvant therapy.

Results

Disease-Free Survival

As of the latest update (December 1986) 21 of 39 patients show no evidence of disease, with a median disease-free survival of 18.5 months. As seen in Figure 1, comparison of the disease-free survival of all patients in this trial with that of matched controls from previous BCG or *C. parvum* trials demonstrates a significant advantage ($P = 0.04$) for the VMO-treated group.

SpA Results

As seen in Table 1 none of the patients' pretreatment sera was positive in the SpA assay for melanoma-binding antibody. At 3 months of treatment, however, 17/33 (51%) had become positive and this percentage increased at each 3-month interval of testing.

Enzyme-Linked Immunosorbant Assay Results

To further document the serologic responses of the patients in this study an ELISA procedure was used to detect IgG and IgM antibodies reactive with melanoma lines. This assay proved to be more sensitive than the SpA assay. Moreover, when the ELISA reactivity of patient sera was tested against the melanoma lines used in VMO preparation (Fig. 2) sera from patients who recurred had lower activity than sera from patients who remain free from disease.

Human Leukocyte Antigen (HLA) Screening Results

In order to monitor development of anti-HLA antibodies in the serum of patients undergoing VMO treatment, pretreatment and treatment serum from 25 patients were screened for anti-HLA antibodies. Both HLA-A,B,C and DR/DQ reactivity was tested. Although many samples showed broad nonspecific cytolytic activity against target cells both before and during treatment, none of the treatment sera demonstrated specific DR/DQ antibodies and only one showed selective anti-HLA A/B reactivity against one of the cells in the panel.

TABLE 1. *Staphylococcus Protein A Results*

Patient	Time serum samples obtained				
	Pre	3 mo	6 mo	9 mo	12 mo
1.	–	+	R		
2.	–	+	R		
3.	–	+	+	R	
4.	–	+	–	–	–
5.	–	+	R		
6.	–	–	+	+	+
7.	–	+	+	+	+
8.	–	+	–	R	
9.	–	–	+	+	+
10.	–	+	+	+	+
11.	–	+	+	+	+
12.	–	–	–	–	–
13.	–	+	+	–	–
14.	–	–	–	NA	–
15.	–	–	+	+	+
16.	–	–	–	+	+
17.	–	+	+	+	+
18.	–	+	+	+	+
19.	–	–	+	+	+
20.	–	+	+	R	
21.	–	–	–	–	–
22.	–	–	–	–	–
23.	–	+	+	R	
24.	–	–	–	–	NA
25.	–	–	–	–	R
20.	–	+	+	+	+
27.	–	+	+	NA	+
28.	–	–	–	–	+
29.	–	+	+	–	+
30.	–	–	R		
31.	–	–	R		
32.	–	+	–	+	–
33.	–	–	–	–	–
+/Tested	0/33	17/33 (51%)	16/28 (57%)	14/23 (61%)	14/22 (64%)

R: recurrence; NA: sample not available; Pre: before.

Discussion

This study represents the latest in a series of trials in which viral oncolysates have been used to treat melanoma.[14–16,19,20] Cassel *et al.*[19] used Newcastle Disease Virus oncolysates to treat melanoma and reported dramatic success in halting progression of the disease as compared to historical controls. More recently, Hersey *et al.*[20] performed a large study with a vaccinia oncolysate similar to ours. The results of that study also demonstrated increased survival of oncolysate-treated patients by comparison with historical controls and suggested a relationship between serologic responses and clinical benefit.

The results obtained in the current study suggest an association between IgG antibody detected in ELISA and favorable clinical outcome. Jones *et al.*[7] found that IgM antibody produced during the natural course of melanoma had prognostic significance. In the current study IgM antibodies were not detected before treatment and showed no clear correlation with clinical status during treatment (data not shown). The difference in class of the antibodies relevant to disease-free survival may have resulted from hyperimmunization. Although a direct role for antibody in prevention of recurrence is difficult to establish, Hersey *et al.*[8] have demonstrated that leukocyte-dependent antibody activity has prognostic significance. We also have shown that antibody produced by long-term disease-free survivors can bind to autologous melanoma and mediate antibody-dependent cell-mediated cytotoxicity *in vitro* (unpublished observations).

The majority of patients undergoing VMO treatment developed antimelanoma reactivity

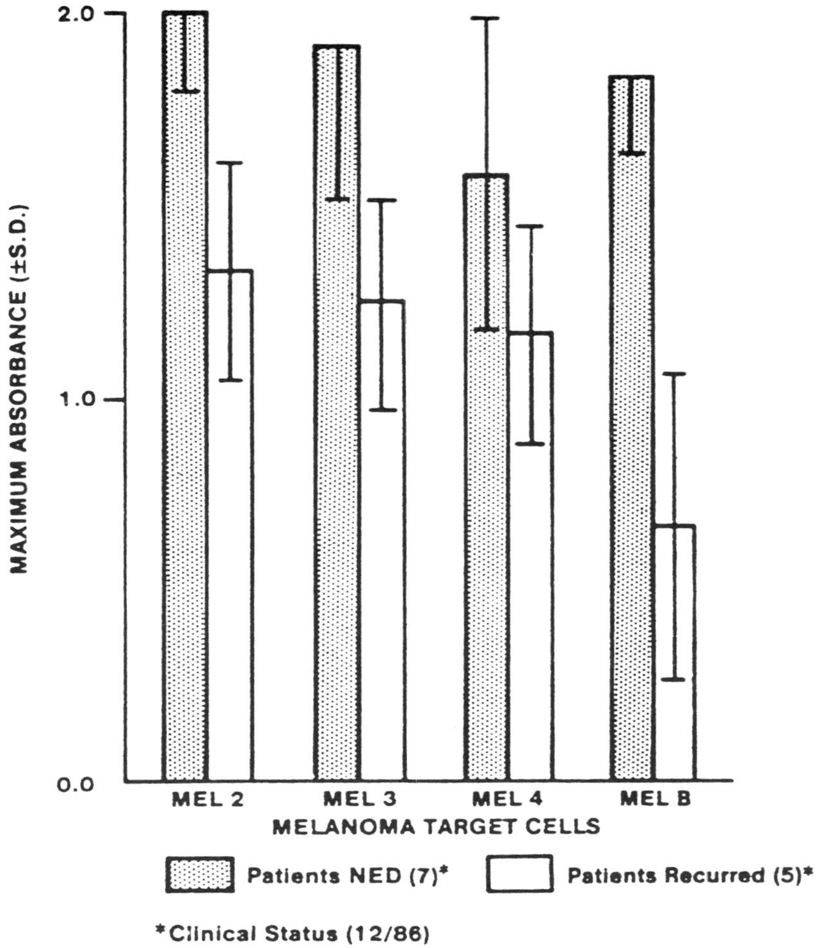

FIG. 2. ELISA measurement of antibody (IgG) reactive with melanoma cell lines.

in the SpA assay, yet there was no correlation of SpA results with clinical course (Table 1). One explanation for this may lie in the selective binding of IgG subsets by SpA in contrast to the binding of all subsets by the goat anti-human IgG conjugate used in the ELISA. In addition, the sensitivity of the ELISA allowed better quantitation of antibody than in the SpA which was scored positive or negative at 1:10 dilution only. It also should be noted that the SpA was performed against the MEL 4 line which was the least discriminatory in the ELISA assay.

Since the oncolysate used in this study was prepared from allogeneic cell lines, screening of patients' sera for anti-HLA antibodies against a panel of HLA-typed lymphocytes was performed and the results support the conclusion that there is no relationship of anti-HLA responses to the antimelanoma-associated antibody response of the majority of VMO-treated patients. We also have confirmed this directly in other experiments (data not shown) in which we have absorbed out anti-HLA activity with pooled platelets and B-cell lines without removing antimelanoma reactivity. Although Livingstone *et al.*[21] failed to demonstrate melanoma-restricted responses to allogeneic vesicular stomatitis virus (VSV)-melanoma oncolysates, Savage *et al.*[22] demonstrated production of antitumor membrane-restricted antibodies to allogeneic Newcastle disease and vaccinia melanoma oncolysates. A goal of our future studies is to identify and characterize the antigen(s) which are relevant to induction of prolonged disease-free survival.

The results of this study provide preliminary evidence that VMO treatment may extend disease-free survival of high-risk melanoma patients in the adjuvant setting. Further evidence for clinical efficacy and the significance of antimelanoma antibody production will be determined in an upcoming randomized double-blind prospective study.

ACKNOWLEDGEMENTS

This study was sponsored by the Southeastern Cancer Study Group and included the participation of Drs. Charles Balch and Marshal Urist at the University of Alabama, Birmingham, AL, Dr. Hilliard Seigler at Duke University, Durham, NC, Dr. Kirby Bland at the University of Florida, Gainesville, FL and Dr. Harold Wanebo at the University of Virginia, Charlottesville, VA.

REFERENCES

1. Mavligit G, Gutterman JU, McBride C *et al.* Tumor directed immune reactivity and immunotherapy in malignant melanoma: Current Status. In: Immunology of Cancer: Progress in Experimental Tumor Research vol. 19. Karger: Basel, 1974;222–252.
2. Terry WD. Immunotherapy of malignant melanoma. N Engl J Med 1980;30:1174–1175.
3. Hersey P, Balch CM. Current status and future prospects for adjuvant therapy of melanoma. Aust NZ J Surg 1984;54:303–315.
4. Koprowski H, Steplewski Z, Herlyn D *et al.* Studies of antibodies against human melanoma produced by somatic cell hybrids. Proc Natl Acad Sci USA 1978;75:3405–3409.
5. Real FX, Houghton AN, Albino AP *et al.* Surface antigens of melanomas and melanocytes defined by mouse monoclonal antibodies: Specificity analysis and comparison of antigen expression in cultured cells and tissues. Cancer Res 1985;46:4401–4411.
6. Morton DL, Malmgren RA, Holmes E *et al.* Demonstration of antibodies against human malignant melanoma by immunofluoresence. Surgery 1968;64:223–240.
7. Jones PC, Sze LL, Liu PY *et al.* Prolonged survival for melanoma patients with elevated IgM antibody to oncofetal antigen. J Natl Cancer Inst 1981;66:249–254.
8. Hersey P, Edwards A, Murray E *et al.* Prognostic significance of leukocyte-dependent antibody activity in melanoma patients. J Natl Cancer Inst 1983;71:45–53.
9. Kobayashi H. Modification of tumor antigenicity in therapeutics: Increase in immunologic foreignness of tumor cells in experimental model systems. In: Mihich E, ed. Immunological Approaches to Cancer Therapeutics. John Wiley & Sons, 1982;405–440.
10. Austin FC, Boone WB. Virus augmentation of the antigenicity of tumor cell extracts. Adv Cancer Res 1979;30:301–345.
11. Wallack MK, Steplewski Z, Koprowski H *et al.* A new approach in specific active immunotherapy. Cancer 1977;39:560–564.
12. Wu KS, Ueda S, Skaue Y *et al.* Prevention of syngeneic tumor growth in vaccinia virus-modulated tumor cells. Biken J 1981;24:153–158.
13. Shimizu Y, Fujiwara H, Ueda S *et al.* The augmentation of tumor-specific immunity by virus help: II. Enhanced induction of cytotoxic T-lymphocyte and antibody to tumor antigens by vaccinia virus-reactive helper T cells. Eur J Immunol 1984;14:839–843.
14. Wallack MK, Meyer M, Burgoin A *et al.* A preliminary trial of vaccinia oncolysates in the treatment of recurrent melanoma with serologic responses to the treatment. J Biol Resp Modifiers 1983;2:586–596.
15. Wallack MK and Michaelides MC. Serologic responses to human melanoma line from patients with melanoma undergoing treatment with vaccinia melanoma oncolysates. Surgery 1984;96:791–799.
16. Wallack MK, McNally KR, Leftheriotis E *et al.* A Southeastern Cancer Study Group Phase I/II trial with vaccinia melanoma oncolysates. Cancer 1986;57:649–655.
17. Herlyn M, Clark WH, Mastrangelo MJ *et al.* Specific immunoreactivity of hybridoma secreted monoclonal antimelanoma antibodies to cultured cells. Cancer Res 1980;40:3602–3609.
18. Pfreundschuh MG, Ueda R, Rauterberg EW *et al.* Comparison of multiple rosetting assays for detecting antibody reactivity of different immunoglobulin classes against surface antigens of benign and malignant tissue culture cells. J Immunol Methods 1980;37:71–81.
19. Cassel WA, Murray DR, Phillips HS. A phase II study on the postsurgical management of Stage II malignant melanoma with a Newcastle disease virus oncolysate. Cancer 1983;52:856–860.
20. Hersey P, Edwards A, D'Alessandro G *et al.* Phase II study of vaccinia melanoma cell lysates (VMCL) as adjuvant to surgical treatment of Stage II melanoma: II. Effects on cell mediated cytotoxicity and leukocyte dependent antibody activity. Immunological effects of VMCL in melanoma patients. Cancer Immunol Immunother 1986;22:221–231.
21. Livingstone PO, Albino AP, Chung TJC *et al.* Serological responses of melanoma patients to vaccines prepared from VSV lysates of autologous and allogeneic cultured melanoma cells. Cancer 1985;55:713–820.
22. Savage HE, Rossen RD, Hersh EM *et al.* Antibody development to viral and allogeneic tumor cell-associated antigens in patients with malignant melanoma and ovarian carcinoma treated with lysates of virus-infected tumor cells. Cancer Res 1986;46:2127–2133.

Mammography and Palpable Cancer of the Breast

STANLEY EDEIKEN, M.D.

This statistical analysis determines the accuracy of mammography in diagnosing a palpable cancer of the breast. All of the women were treated by the author, had mammography after discovery of the cancer which was subsequently proven by biopsy, and had cancer which did not involve the skin. All mammograms that demonstrated any abnormality in the area of the cancer were deemed to be positive. This study demonstrates that 22% of the women who have a palpable cancer of the breast will have a false-negative mammogram; 44% in women 50 years of age and younger, and 13% in women older than 50 years. Mammography is detrimental if used to avoid biopsy when there is a persistent mass, especially in the younger woman. Biopsy should be performed on every undiagnosed persistent dominant mass without consideration of the mammogram.

MAMMOGRAPHY in asymptomatic women, as a screening test to find unsuspected cancer, has been demonstrated to be the best practical test and the majority of those cancers found by mammography only are minimal cancers with a high 5-year and 10-year survival rate. Unfortunately, this test is underutilized because many physicians do not recommend mammography for screening and many patients fear the theoretical unproven consequences of radiation in low dosage. To find one cancer in an asymptomatic woman, 200 studies must be done.[1]

This study is a statistical analysis to determine the diagnostic accuracy of mammography in women with a palpable cancer of the breast.

Methods

All of the women treated by the author from 1976 to 1985 who had mammography in the presence of a palpable cancer of the breast were included in this study. Cancer was proven by biopsy subsequent to mammography. The mammograms that were interpreted as showing malignancy, suspicion of malignancy, or an abnormality in the area of the carcinoma have been classified as positive. Most of the mammograms were performed on one of six different dedicated machines and read by one of ten radiologists. All of the mammograms were reviewed by the author. Excluded from this study were patients who did not have mammography subsequent to discovery of the mass and tumors producing edema, retraction, or ulceration of the skin.

Results

From 1976 to 1985 there were 499 patients who had a palpable carcinoma and mammography, 78% had a positive mammogram and 22% were negative. One hundred thirty-nine patients were younger than 51 years and only 56% had a positive mammogram. Three hundred sixty were older than 50 years and 87% had a positive mammogram. There was no difference in the accuracy of mammography between the early and later years of this study (Table 1). The size of the tumor did not effect the sensitivity of mammography (Table 2).

Discussion

Sensitivity is positivity in disease.

$$\text{Sensitivity} = \frac{\text{Total positive}}{\text{Total positive} + \text{false negative}} \times 100$$

From the Jersey Shore Medical Center, Neptune, New Jersey.

TABLE 1. *Sensitivity of Mammography*

	No. of palpable cancers	No. + MAM (%)	No. − MAM (%)	Sensitivity
1976–1985	499	391 (78%)	108 (22%)	78%
Women < 51 yr	139	78 (56%)	61 (44%)	56%
Women > 50 yr	360	313 (87%)	47 (13%)	87%
1976–1981	293	233 (80%)	60 (20%)	80%
Women < 51 yr	73	39 (53%)	34 (47%)	53%
Women > 50 yr	220	194 (88%)	26 (12%)	88%
1982–1985	206	157 (76%)	49 (24%)	76%
Women < 51 yr	66	39 (59%)	27 (41%)	59%
Women > 50 yr	140	119 (85%)	21 (15%)	85%

MAM: mammograms.

Table 3 contains studies[2–6] which show the sensitivity of mammography when a palpable cancer is present. All cancers found on mammography only have been excluded to determine the true-positive and false-negative rates for mammography when there is a palpable carcinoma. This demonstrates that the false-negative rate is much higher than usually is reported in the literature and that mammography is far less sensitive than advertised. The Breast Cancer Detection Demonstration Project (BCDDP)[1] had 87% of the cancers demonstrated by mammography but there is no computation of sensitivity; occult cancers were included and 12 of the 29 centers had 100% sensitivity of palpable cancers on the first screen (Table 3).

If all of the patients with palpable cancers, multicentric cancers, and cancers detected by mirror-image biopsy were used to calculate the sensitivity of mammography, the figure would be much less than 50%. Physical examination would also have a low sensitivity.

Unfortunately, delay in biopsy of a persistent mass at medical centers and in the communities, continues to occur because of a false-negative mammogram. A persistent mass is a

TABLE 2. *Sensitivity of Mammography in Cancers 1 cm or Less*

	No. of palpable cancers	No. + MAM (%)	No. − MAM (%)	Sensitivity
1976–1985	64	45 (70%)	19 (30%)	70%
Women < 51 yr	21	11 (52%)	10 (48%)	52%
Women > 50 yr	43	34 (79%)	9 (21%)	79%

TABLE 3. *Sensitivity of Mammography*

Reference	No. of palpable cancers	No. + MAM (%)	No. − MAM (%)	Sensitivity
Strax[2]	80	58 (73%)	22 (27%)	73%
Feig *et al.*[3]	98	60 (61%)	38 (39%)	61%
McClow and Williams[4]	156	135 (87%)	21 (13%)	87%
Lesnick[5]				
Women <45 yr	50	21 (42%)	29 (58%)	42%
Egeli and Urban[6]	520	412 (79%)	108 (21%)	79%
Women <51 yr	154	108 (70%)	46 (30%)	70%
Women >50 yr	366	304 (83%)	62 (17%)	83%
Edeiken 1976–1985 (current report)	499	391 (78%)	108 (22%)	78%
Women <51 yr	139	78 (56%)	61 (44%)	56%
Women >50 yr	360	313 (87%)	47 (13%)	87%

MAM: mammograms.

lump which does not decrease in size or disappear in 1 to 2 months. Mann *et al.*[7] analyzed women who had cancer of the breast which was not demonstrated on the mammogram and found that there was a delay, attributable to the false-negative mammogram, of 3 to 24 months in 50% of the patients. Although the study of Mann *et al.* was reported in 1983, delay still exists in a high percentage of patients and additional education of physicians is mandated until the delay is eliminated. Martin *et al.*,[8] after reviewing interval cancers from four Breast Cancer Centers, stated that the major reasons for the false-negative mammograms are poor technique, obvious oversight by the radiologist, lack of recognition of subtle radiographic signs, and absence of radiographic criteria of cancer. I believe that the latter two are the common reasons. A negative mammogram should never obviate surgery when a persistent dominant mass is palpable or other signs of cancer are present. This is especially true in the younger woman.

Mammography can play an important role in avoiding delay in biopsy of a dominant mass thought to be due to fibrocystic disease when the physician elects to reexamine the patient after one or two menstrual cycles before advising biopsy; under these circumstances, if the mammogram is suspicious for carcinoma, surgery should be performed without delay. This is the only valid change in diagnostic thinking that should occur as a result of the mammogram when a mass is present. Therefore under no other circumstance should the mammogram influence the decision to perform biopsy of the dominant lump. Without doubt, biopsy should not be obviated by a negative mammogram.

Then why is mammography important to the surgeon when a mass is present? The answer is three-fold: (1) to find an unsuspected cancer in either breast which should be biopsied at the time of surgery; the palpable mass could be benign and accompanied by a nonpalpable cancer in either breast; (2) to find an unsuspected second cancer in the ipsilateral breast when breast conservation surgery is contemplated; and (3) to obtain another estimate of the size of the tumor when breast conservation therapy is contemplated.

Although mammography is of very limited value when a mass is present, it has unsurpassed value as a screening test to find unsuspected cancers at an early stage of the disease.

Mammography and physical examination have high false-negative rates but they are the only practical ways of detecting cancer of the breast. Used together as complementary examinations, with realization of their limitations, provides the patient with her best chance of cure of cancer of the breast.

Conclusion

Mammography can confirm the presence of a suspected cancer but its sensitivity rate is too low to rule out cancer, especially in the young woman. Failure to biopsy the persistent dominant mass because of a negative mammogram can be a lethal mistake. The important rule is as follows: Biopsy should be performed on every persistent dominant mass without consideration of the mammogram.

REFERENCES

1. Beahrs OH, Shapiro S, Smart C *et al.* Report of the Working Group to Review the National Cancer Institute–American Cancer Society Breast Cancer Detection Demonstration Projects. J Natl Cancer Inst 1979;62:640–709.
2. Strax P. Control of breast cancer through mass screening. JAMA 1976;235:1600–1602.
3. Feig SA, Schwartz GF, Nerlinger R, Edeiken J. Prognostic factors of breast neoplasms detected on screening by mammography and physical examination. Radiology 1979;133:577–582.
4. McClow MV, Williams AC. Mammographic examinations. Ann Surg 1973;177:616–619.
5. Lesnick GJ. Detection of breast cancer in young women. JAMA 1977;237:967–969.
6. Egeli RA, Urban JA. Mammography in symptomatic women 50 years of age and under, and those over 50. Cancer 1979;43:878–882.
7. Mann BD, Guiliano AE, Bassett LW, Barber MS, Hallauer W, Morton DL. Delayed diagnosis of breast cancer as a result of normal mammograms. Arch Surg 1983;118:23–24.
8. Martin JE, Moskowitz M, Milbrath JR. Breast cancer missed by mammography. Am J Radiol 1979;132:737–739.

Dietary Control of Glutathione Levels to Enhance Radiosensitivity of Malignant Tumors

JAMES M. ROSEMAN, M.D., F.A.C.S.

THIS STUDY EXPLORES the importance of cellular protection and repair of radiation-induced cytotoxicity in a rodent tumor model. It is thought that tumors, like normal cells, require reducing substances, such as glutathione and nonessential protein sulfhydryl (SH) to act as a sink or scavenger of hydroxyl ions and other toxic species produced intracellularly when ionizing radiation interacts with a cell.[1] Accordingly, despite the inherent side effects of SH depletion, drugs which alter nonprotein SH have been employed to enhance normoxic and hypoxic radiosensitivity.[2]

Many radiosensitizers currently under investigation act by interferring with glutathione function. However, they have additional toxic side effects.[3]

Having considerable interest in the treatment of tumors with radiation, we hypothesize that dietary-induced reduction in cellular SH might side-step many of the adverse effects of radiosensitizers currently employed in the treatment of cancer.

Materials and Methods

Female Wistar-Furthe 250 to 300 g rats were used. They received, subcutaneously, an MTW9 transplantable tumor.

This is a malignant mammary tumor that results from intraperitoneal injection of 3′ methylcholanthrene. The rat then is implanted with mammotropin to stimulate growth.

Three tumor subtypes develop in varying numbers. These include type A and type B, which contain estrogen and progesterone receptor proteins, and type D, which contains no detectable receptor protein. Only the type A tumor is hormonally dependent.

After the tumors were implanted subcutaneously into the flank, variable times were needed to detect tumor growth. Once growth was established, 50% of each group served as controls. The remainder received radiation to the tumor in a dose of 300 rad using a cobalt 60 machine.

Tumor measurements then were continued in all animals for an additional seven days. Change in tumor size was expressed as a fractional change with respect to the controls.

In addition, the tumors were analyzed for glutathione content by the technique of Mokrasch and Teschke.[4] Proteins were analyzed by the method of Lowry.[5]

Oxygen consumption was determined on fresh tumor using a standard Warburg apparatus.

In a separate, parallel experiment, C3H mice implanted subcutaneously with C3HB mammary tumors were used.

Once there was definite evidence of tumor growth at the subcutaneous site, the animals were stratified into two groups. The groups, each composed of six animals, varied based on diet. The control population was maintained on a regular diet whereas the test group was fed a low-sulfur diet (Table 1).

The animals were kept on the respective diets for 10 days. They were monitored for the following: (1) weights; (2) tumor size (three-dimensional using Vernier calipers); (3) food

From the Department of Surgery, Eastern Virginia Medical School, Norfolk, Virginia.

Presented in part at the Second International Congress of Neoadjuvant Chemotherapy, Paris, France, February 1988.

TABLE 1. *Sulfur Amounts Per Diet (Mol Sulfur/kg)*

	Regular	Low SO_4
Casein	0.341	0.0341
$CaSO_4$	0.105	0
Cysteine	0.253	0
Methionine	0.383	0
Total sulfur	0.1082	0.0341

$CaSO_4$: calcium sulfate; SO_4: sulfate.

and water consumption; and (4) other observation as may relate to the study, *e.g.*, activity, irritability, or tumor necrosis.

On the tenth day, the animals were killed. Tumors were minced, as were livers and brains. Glutathione and protein measurements were completed on the tumors using the previously indicated methods.

The data was analyzed as a multifactorial analysis of variance[6] for continuous outcome measurements (*e.g.*, weights). The chi-square test for the comparison of M-independent proportions served to analyze all dichotomous outcome variables.[7]

Results

Results are represented in Tables 2 and 3.

Discussion

Sulfur-containing compounds are ubiquitous in nature and are required for growth and development by microorganisms, plants, and animals.[8] Among the significant cellular sulfur-containing compounds, glutathione has an important role in the defence mechanisms against toxic effects of reactive metabolites of oxygen and various zenobiotics.[9]

Dietary sulfur consists of two sources for utilization by animals: organic and inorganic sulfur. The need for organic sulfur is met primarily by the sulfur-containing amino acids, methionine and cysteine (cystine).[10]

Although inorganic sulfate has been shown to be an important dietary constituent for a rat,[11] a need for dietary inorganic sulfate by man has yet to be demonstrated.[12] Although an early study demonstrated cysteine to be an indispensible dietary constituent for the rat,[13] Jackson and Black[14] later established methionine as an essential amino acid. Finkelstein and Mudd[15] investigated the methionine-sparing effect of cysteine and concluding that in rats fed a diet low in methionine and supplemented with cysteine enables methionine to remain in the remethylation pathway or be utilized for protein synthesis.

In view of the sparing effect of cysteine upon methionine, the replacement of cysteine for methionine has been estimated. Animal species will vary; however, cysteine can supply from 17% to 68% of the total sulfur-containing amino acid requirement in rats.[16,17] In humans, cysteine sulfur can replace approximately 80% of the methionine requirement.[18]

Smith[11] demonstrated that dietary inorganic sulfate was an important nutrient for the rat and resulted in the formulation of an optimal level of dietary inorganic sulfate.[19] Based on

TABLE 2. *Results: Correlation of Tumor Glutathione, Oxygen Consumption, and Sensitivity to Ionizing Radiation (Mean Values)*

Tumor	Oxygen consumption (ml/min/mg Prot)	Glutathione (nmol/mg Prot)	GSH per unit oxygen consumption	% Tumor reduction
A	4.41	11.61	2.63	56
B	2.39	7.21	3.02	40
D	1.47	6.60	4.49	25

Prot: protein; GSH: glutathione.

TABLE 3. *Results: Effect of Diet on Tumor Glutathione Levels*

	Regular diet	Low SH diet	Low SH diet
	Control	Preimplant	Post implant
Glutathione (nmol/mg Prot)	189	1[illegible]4	144

SH: sulfhydryl; Prot: protein.

the data reported by Smith,[19] the optimal level of inorganic sulfate for the rat was determined to be 0.02%. Dietary inorganic sulfate is used in the biosynthesis of taurine and chondroitin[20] and is incorporated into cysteine but not methionine. With the observation of the incorporation of sulfate into cysteine, approximately 7% to 9% of the dietary sulfur amino acid requirement of chicks can be met by inorganic sulfate.[21]

Glutathione biosynthesis (synthesis of glutamyl-cysteine) can occur in liver, kidney, biotin, muscle, lens, intestine, and erythrocyte.[22] It is predominantly an intracellular compound that exists in relatively high concentrations (0.5–10 mM). The intracellular concentration of glutathione is much higher than the concentrations of cysteine, cystine, or glutamylcysteine. It has been suggested that glutathione serves as a reservoir of cysteine.[23]

The biosynthesis of glutathione involves the incorporation of glutamate, cysteine, and glycine, forming the tripeptide. The controlling enzyme is glutamylcysteine synthetase, which is controlled by feedback inhibition. The rate of glutathione synthesis may be influenced significantly by the intracellular concentrations of L-cysteine.[22]

In the absence of dietary cysteine or cystine, methionine provides the primary source of cysteine. Finkelstein *et al.*[24] have evaluated the concentration of methionine metabolites in rat tissue. They conclude that hepatic methionine concentration appears insensitive to changes in dietary protein intake; however, cysteine hepatic levels increase with augmented dietary protein. Smith *et al.*[25] have shown body pool sizes of cysteine are approximately four times that of methionine when animals are fed diets containing an optimal level of inorganic sulfate (0.02%) and supplemented with equal molar amounts of cysteine or methionine. These results are consistent when other reports[26,27] indicating that an increased supply of cysteine in the diet should increase glutathione synthesis.

When inorganic sulfate is omitted from the diet, an animal must satisfy its sulfate requirements by the oxidation of amino acid sulfur to sulfate. The oxidation of cysteine sulfur to sulfate has been demonstrated to be a wasteful process. Whittle and Smith[28] reported that rats fed diets low in inorganic sulfate excrete twice as much cysteine sulfur as taurine sulfur when compared to animals fed diets containing 0.1% of inorganic sulfur. Furthermore, the methionine requirement appears to be increased in rats fed diets low in inorganic sulfate.[29] Smith and Acuff[30] concluded that the liver sulfate pool is limited by a combination of the oxidation rate of the sulfur-containing amino acids and the extraction of sulfate from the portal system.

Therefore, animals consuming diets both low in cysteine and inorganic sulfate should have decreased glutathione levels. Furthermore, the inequivalency of methionine and cysteine as dietary supplements[31] would indicate that unless a methyl demand is created, methionine would not leave the remethylation pathway at a sufficient rate to supply the endogenous cysteine required for normal body function.[11,32–34] Smith[11] has presented data to indicate that animals receiving diets containing equal molar amounts of methionine in place of cysteine had decreased levels of both reduced and total glutathione levels in kidney and liver tissues. The supplementation of methionine not only produces less kidney glutathione but also increases the urinary excretion of amino acids. This increase in urinary amino acids may be an impairment of the glutamyl cycle.[35]

Our data supports the following hypothesis: (1) Glutathione levels, when expressed in relation to oxygen consumption, correlate stoichiometrically with sensitivity to ionizing radiation. (2) By altering dietary intake of sulfur-containing amminc acids and inorganic sulfate, one can significantly change tumor levels of glutathione-stimulating hormone (GSH) in a rat/tumor model. (3) The extent of the alteration can be achieved over a relatively short time course and with no overt side effects to the animals. (4) The level of the GSH alteration is adequate to cause significant enhancement to destruction by ionizing radiation.

This was accepted for presentation, in part, at the XIV International Cancer Congress.[36]

Conclusion

At least in a rat and mouse tumor model, there seems to be a direct correlation between tumor levels of glutathione, the degree of oxygen consumption, and the sensitivity to ionizing radiation.

Simple dietary modification altering the tumor glutathione level and ongoing work will establish if that is adequate to enhance radiation-based tumor destruction.

REFERENCES

1. Arrick B, Nathan C. Glutathione metabolism as a determinant of therapeutic efficacy: A review. Cancer Res 1984;44:4224–4232.
2. Stratford I. Mechanisms of hypoxic cell radiosensitization and the development of new sensitizers. Int J Radiat Oncol Biol Phys 1982;8:391–398.
3. Kim JH, Chu F. Chemical radiation sensitizers and protectors: Recent developments. Clin Bull 1981;11:5–11.
4. Mokrasch L, Teschke E. Glutathione content of cultivated cells on rodent brain regions: A specific flurometric assay. Analyt Biochem 1984;140:506–509.
5. Lowry.
6. Winer BJ. Statistical Principles in Experimental Design, ed. 2. New York: McGraw Hill, 1971.
7. Fleiss JL. Statistical Methods for Rates and Proportions, ed. 2. New York: John Wiley & Sons, 1981.
8. Schiff JA. Pathways of assimilatory sulfate reduction in plants and micro-organisms. In: Sulphur in Biology, Ciba Foundation Symposium 12. New York: Excerpta Medica, 1980;49–69.
9. Chasseaud L. The role of glutathione and glutathione-S-transferases in the metabolism of chemical carcinogens and other electrophilic agents. Adv Cancer Res 1979;29:175–274.
10. Young LG, Maw GA. The Metabolism of Sulphur Compounds. New York: John Wiley & Sons, 1958.
11. Smith JT. Inorganic sulfate: An Important Dietary Constituent for the Monogastric Animal, Bulletin 571. Knoxville, TN: University of Tennessee Agricultural Experiment Station, 1977.
12. Swendseid ME, Wang M. Sulfur requirements of the human. In: Muth OH, ed. Symposium: Sulfur in Nutrition. Wesport: Avi Publishing, 1970;209–221.
13. Finks AJ, Jones DB, Jones CO. The role of cystine in the dietary properties of the proteins of the cow-pea, *vigna sinensis*, and of the field pea, *pisum sativum*. J Biol Chem 1922;52:403–410.
14. Jackson RW, Black RJ. The metabolism of cystine and methionine. J Biol Chem 1931;98:465–477.
15. Finkelstein JD, Mudd SH. Trans-sulfuration in mammals. J Biol Chem 1967;216:763–773.
16. Baker DH. Sulfur in Nonruminant Nutrition. West Des Moines, Iowa: National Feed Ingredients Association, 1977.
17. Womack M, Rose WC. The partial replacement of dietary methionine by cystine for purposes of growth. J Biol Chem 1941;141:375–379.
18. Rose WC, Wixom RL. The amino acid requirements of man. J Biol Chem 1955;216:763–773.
19. Smith JT. An optimal level of inorganic sulfate for the diet of a rat. J Nutr 1973;103:1008–1011.
20. Almquist HJ. Sulfur nutrition of nonruminant species. In: Muth OH, ed. Symposium: Sulfur in Nutrition, Westport: Avi Publishing, 1970;196–208.
21. Sasse CE, Baker DH. Sulfur utilization by the chick with emphasis on the effect of inorganic sulfate on the cysteine–methionine interrelationships. J Nutr 1974;104:244–251.
22. Meister H, Tate SS. Glutathione and related-glutamyl compounds: Biosynthesis and utilization. Anal Rev Biochem 1976;45:559–604.
23. Tateishi N, Taneaki H, Naruse A, Nakashima K, Shiozaki H, Sakamoto Y. Rat liver glutathione: Possible role as a reservoir of cysteine. J Nutr 1977;107:51–60.
24. Finkelstein JD, Kyle WE, Harris BJ, Martin JJ. Methionine metabolism in mammals: Concentration of metabolites in rat tissues. J Nutr 1982;112:1011–1018.
25. Smith JT, Acuff RV, Bittle JB, Gilbert ML. A metabolic comparison of cysteine and methionine supplements in the diet of a rat. J Nutr 1983;113:222–227.
26. Tateishi N, Higashi T. Turnover of glutathione in rat liver. In: Sies H, Wendel A, eds. Functions of Glutathione in Liver and Kidney. New York: Springer-Verlag, 1978;3–7.
27. Tateishi N, Higaski T, Shinya S, Naruse A, Sakamoto Y. Studies on the regulation of glutathione levels in rat liver. J Biochem 1974;75:93–103.
28. Whittle B, Smith JT. The effect of dietary sulfur on taurine excretion in the rat. J Nutr 1974;104:666–670.
29. Michels FG, Smith JT. A comparison of the utilization of organic and inorganic sulfur by the rat. J Nutr 1965;87:217–220.
30. Smith JT, Acuff RV. The effect of dietary sulfur on liver inorganic sulfate in the rat. Ann Nutr Metab 1983;27:345–348.
31. Finkelstein JD, Mudd SH. Transsulfuration in mammals: The methionine-sparing effect of cysteine. J Biol Chem 1967;242:873–880.

32. Lombardi B, Pani P, Schlunk FF, Shi-Hua C. Labeling of liver and plasma lecithins after injection of 1-2 C-2 dimethyl aminocthanol and C-methionine-methyl to choline deficient rats. Lipids 1969;4:67.

33. Barnes RH, Fiala G, Kwong E. Prevention of coprophagy in the rat and the growth-stimulating effects of methionine, cysteine and penicillin when added to diets containing unheated soybeans. J Nutr 1965;85:127–131.

34. Stegirek LD, Deri Besten L. Synthesis of cysteine from methionine in normal adult subjects: Effects of route of alimentation. Science 1976;178:514.

35. Meister A. On the enzymology of amino acid transport. Science 1973;180:33–39.

36. Roseman J, Acuff R. Preliminary Correlation of Tumor Response to Radiotherapy with Levels of Glutathione Per Unit Oxygen Consumption. XIV International Cancer Congress, Budapest, Hungary, August 22, 1986.

The Hour Glass of Learning

N. HENRY MOSS, M.D., F.A.C.S.

AS A TRIBUTE to a superb generalist, Dr. Jonathan E. Rhoads, on the occasion of his eightieth birthday, it is a privilege to propose a concept in his honor, the "Hour Glass of Learning." This idea relates to our role as physicians in pursuing our professional careers and our daily lives. It is one that postulates a narrowing down of our personal body of knowledge into a more focused area of specialization and in many instances of superspecialization. Yet, at some useful point in our careers, there is a broadening out into other realms of expertise like an hour glass narrows and then broadens in shape.

The "Hour Glass of Learning" suggests that all of us should be encouraged to reach continuously for elements of general medical knowledge, while we simultaneously are developing expertise in selected areas of medicine. Such persistent efforts will be very helpful in making us better physicians, more eloquent communicators of our professional advice to our own patients and to the public at large, and certainly to the media when the occasion permits.

The fantastic growth of specialization in science, medicine, and technology during our lifetime has provided numerous research breakthroughs in multiple disciplines, increased survival for the general population, and overall better quality of life against man's greatest afflictions. Specialization in medicine began to evolve in the 1920s and 1930s, blossomed in the late 1940s and 1950s, reached a golden age in the 1960s and 1970s, and by now in the 1980s is further fully fragmented into multiple superspecialties within each previous area of specialization. We recognize such developments as advances in medicine, and the appropriate bodies of knowledge now are categorized and superdepartmentalized. Frequently, at a major institution, the patient encounters three to ten physicians, each pursuing his own narrow area of activity and responsibility without flaw. Yet, the patient becomes bewildered, confused, and frustrated when the coordination, communication, and care fail to keep pace with the technological activity.

A balanced interplay of generalism is needed in our delivery system. It is not easy to achieve. Our training programs from medical school through residency training at our major teaching hospitals do not lend themselves to such a process. The halo of the superspecialist is supreme, for the rewards and awards are given to those who achieve a precise and specific advance within a field of endeavor. The greater understanding of one's own field, however, limited, has a fulfilling aspect for every scientist and physician. It is rewarding for one to be up to date completely with the current state of the art and be familiar with all the recent articles within one's specialty. The explosion of the bodies of knowledge within all fields of medicine challenge us to keeping up to date with the literature in one's own field, let alone beyond this. In recent years, there has been a growing recognition of the need for such a balanced generalism in our orientation. The Admissions and Curriculum Committees at the University of Pennsylvania Medical School have altered the premedical requirements for admission and encouraged less early specialization in the curriculum. The American Board of Surgery has resisted further fragmentation toward additional Specialty Boards.

Thus, it is with great respect and admiration that the rare and talented individual like Dr. Rhoads exemplifies the epitome of the superb generalist while maintaining his competence and leadership in his own specialty. He is not only a superb specialist, but also a superb generalist in our time. As a devoted practitioner of the science, technique, and the art of surgery, as an excellent teacher and professor, as a respected Chairman of a well-known Department of Surgery, as a distinguished editor and author, as a national leader in the

From the Department of Surgery, Temple University Health Sciences Center and Albert Einstein Medical Center, Philadelphia, and the Academy of Sciences at Philadelphia, Pennsylvania.

American College of Surgeons, the American Cancer Society, the American Surgical Association, numerous other professional organizations and societies, as the Chairman of the President's Cancer Advisory Committee, and as one of the only physicians ever to be elected President of the oldest scientific organization in the United States, the American Philosophical Society, Dr. Rhoads has no peer. He has done it all, and in doing so has achieved the mark of the superb specialist and superb generalist. He has lived and demonstrated the "Hour Glass of Learning" in his lifetime. It is up to us as his students to aim in this direction and strive for such a cherished goal.

REFERENCES

1. Moss NH. The pursuit of knowledge: Synthesis or fragmentation? Trans NY Acad Sci 1968;30:393–396.
2. Moss NH. Superspecialization: The trend and its impact in American medicine. Ann NY Acad Sci 1971;184.
3. Moss NH. Superspecialization: A surgeons view. Health Affairs: Bulletin of the University of Pennsylvania. Philadelphia: University of Pennsylvania, 1975;6.

Mechanical Support of the Circulation Prior to Cardiac Transplantation

WILLIAM S. PIERCE, M.D., GERSON ROSENBERG, PH.D.,
WALTER E. PAE, M.D., AND JOHN A. WALDHAUSEN, M.D.

During the last 3 years, five patients who were considered to be cardiac transplant candidates had profound circulatory failure before a donor heart was identified. A period of circulatory support ranging from 3 to 31 days was provided with a ventricular assist pump (four patients) and an artificial heart (one patient) designed and constructed at The Pennsylvania State University, Hershey, Pennsylvania. Excellent circulatory support was provided and, at the time of transplantation, each patient was in reasonable condition. Three patients who had circulatory support with the left ventricular assist pump did well after transplantation and are now home and doing well. One patient in whom left ventricular assist assistance was provided developed a coagulopathy and low peripheral vascular resistance at the time of cardiac transplantation and subsequently developed an infectious complication and died. The patient with the artificial heart also had a coagulopathy at the time of cardiac transplantation which was difficult to bring under control. This patient developed organ failure and sepsis and died after transplantation. The authors conclude that mechanical circulatory support or the artificial heart play an important role in sustaining a patient with severe cardiac failure before the availability of a donor heart. When using such a device the surgeon must pay extraordinary attention to the fine line between bleeding and thromboembolic complications. Moreover, such patients are at increased risk for developing sepsis, particularly in association with immunosuppression therapy.

DURING THE LAST TWO DECADES, cardiac transplantation has moved from a laboratory curiosity to a therapeutic and effective form of treatment for patients with end-stage heart disease. Unfortunately, approximately 20% of all patients who are potentially candidates for cardiac transplantation die before a donor organ is obtained. Standard forms of support of the failing circulation before cardiac transplantation include the use of inotropic drugs and the intraaortic balloon. However in some patients, these forms of therapy do not provide adequate circulatory support. Without extraordinary means of treatment, these patients die.

At the University Hospital, The Pennsylvania State University, Hershey, Pennsylvania we have performed 39 heart transplants since 1983. In five instances investigational forms of mechanical circulatory support have been employed to support the circulation of patients with profound circulatory failure who could not be stabilized by the conventionally forms of therapy for end-stage congestive heart failure.[1–3] This report describes the ventricular assist pump and artificial heart that have been developed at The Pennsylvania State University and the clinical experience with the use of these devices before cardiac transplantation.

Materials

Pneumatic Ventricular Assist Device

The ventricular assist device developed at The Pennsylvania State University consists of a flexible segmented polyurethane blood sac positioned within a rigid plastic housing (Fig. 1).[4] An external pneumatic power unit generates pulses of compressed gas and creates a flexing motion within the blood sac. Unidirectional flow is achieved by Björk-Shiley tilting disc valves within the inflow and outflow port of the pump. The stroke volume of the device is 70 ml. When the assist pump is employed in the bridge for transplantation mode, the inflow

From the Division of Artificial Organs, Department of Surgery, College of Medicine, The Pennsylvania State University, Hershey, Pennsylvania.

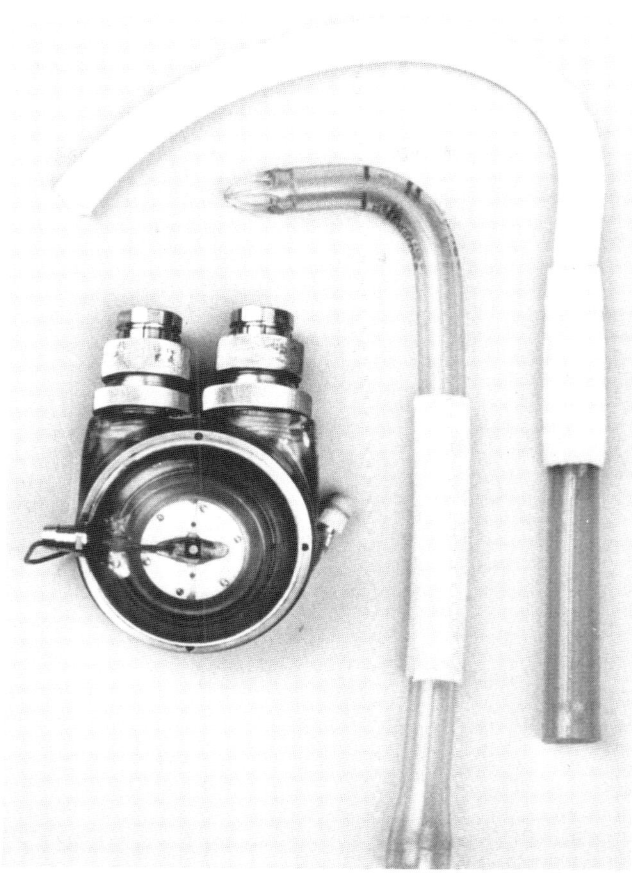

FIG. 1. The pneumatic assist pump has a smooth, segmented polyurethane blood sac and valved inlet and outlet ports. The atrial inflow cannula is a curved Sarns 51F polyurethane coated tube whereas the outlet cannula is a composite segmented polyurethane-woven Dacron tube.

cannula is inserted into the left ventricular apex (Fig. 2). Blood is pumped from the device to the ascending aorta through a segmented polyurethane-woven Dacron prosthetic graft. The ventricular assist device is positioned on the anterior abdominal wall and the cannulas exit the chest below the costal margin.

The pump can operate in either an automatic or manual mode. In the automatic mode, pump systole is initiated when a sensor indicates the blood sac is full. This sensor, a Hall effect proximity switch, is positioned external to the blood sac. In the manual mode, the pump rate is set at any desired value.

Pneumatic Artificial Heart

The artificial heart developed at The Pennsylvania State University is a pneumatically powered device and consists of two pneumatically powered prosthetic ventricles (Fig. 3).[5,6] Each ventricle contains a flexible segmented polyurethane sac positioned within a rigid plastic housing. The internal structure of each prosthetic ventricle is similar to that of the pneumatic ventricular assist device.

The total artificial heart has a built-in automatic control system. For the left pump, the beat rate is set to maintain an aortic pressure within a desired range. If the mean aortic pressure falls below this range, the left pump rate and thus output will increase; conversely if aortic pressure rises, the left pump rate and thus output will decrease. The right pump rate is controlled by the left atrial pressure. As left atrial pressure increases, the right pump rate will decrease, thus lowering left atrial pressure. Accordingly, this control system indirectly senses the patients peripheral vascular resistance and appropriately adjusts cardiac output.

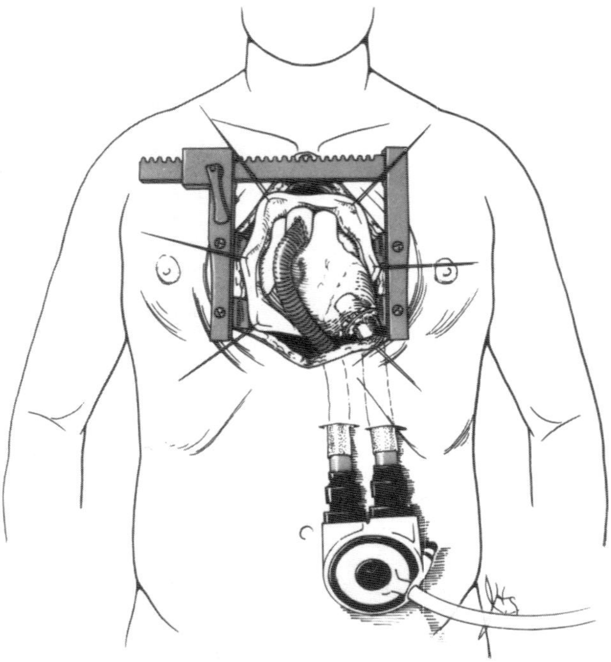

FIG. 2. The assist pump as it is employed in the bridge to transplant application. Blood is taken from the left ventricular apex and pumped into the ascending aorta. The pump is placed on the anterior abdominal wall.

Furthermore the system prevents significant elevation in left atrial pressure, thus avoiding the risk of pulmonary congestion.

The Penn State heart is implanted by excising the native heart at the atrioventricular groove; as much atrial tissue is conserved as possible to facilitate subsequent transplantation.[7] Atrial cuffs, fabricated of polymer-coated stretch fabric, are anastomosed to the native atria. Dacron vascular grafts are anastomosed to the aorta and the pulmonary artery. Both

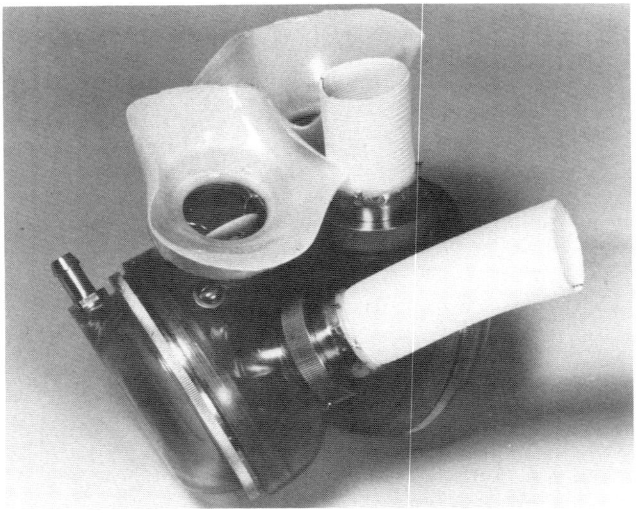

FIG. 3. The Penn State Heart consists of two air actuated ventricles. Björk-Shiley convexo-concave valves with Delrin discs are used to provide unidirectional flow. Hearts of this design have functioned in experimental animals for almost 1 year.

the atrial cuffs and vascular grafts have attached union nut connectors which allow rapid attachment to the prosthetic ventricles. The placement of the artificial heart in the chest is shown in Figure 4.

The pneumatic power assist power unit and control system are contained in a console that is placed alongside of the patient. Two drive lines, 3 m in length pass through the chest wall and link the power unit to each prosthetic ventricle. These tubes are tunneled subcutaneously; in their subcutaneous position, the drive lines are covered with Dacron velour to encourage tissue ingrowth and provide protection against bacterial invasion.

Results

Patient 1

A 24-year-old woman with idiopathic cardiomyopathy was transferred to our institution for evaluation for a heart transplant. Progressive ventricular failure developed despite inotropic support and the insertion of an intraaortic balloon (IAB). Cardiac arrest resulting from ventricular fibrillation occurred 4 days after admission. After resuscitation, the cardiac index was 1.7 l/minute/m^2, despite an infusion of dobutamine (50 μg/kg/minute) and counterpulsation with an IAB. Because of inadequate cardiac output and worsening of the ventricular dysrhythmias, she was taken to the operating room for placement of a left ventricular assist pump (LVAD). Hemodynamic parameters before operation are listed in Table 1. Once the LVAD was in place, right ventricular function was adequate. She did require an infusion of dobutamine (5–10 μg/kg/minute) to be weaned from cardiopulmonary bypass; this was required for 36 hours. Hemodynamic parameters during assist pumping were excellent (Table 1).

Because of hypoxia, she required ventilatory support for 13 days, but thereafter had excellent pulmonary function. Renal function was normal. Liver function was abnormal during the first week (total bilirubin level 11.6 mg/dl, alkaline phosphatase activity 495 U/l, serum glutamic oxaloacetic transaminase [SGOT] 298 U/l) but returned to normal over the next 2 weeks. Plasma hemoglobin level remained at <10 mg/dl throughout her course. A

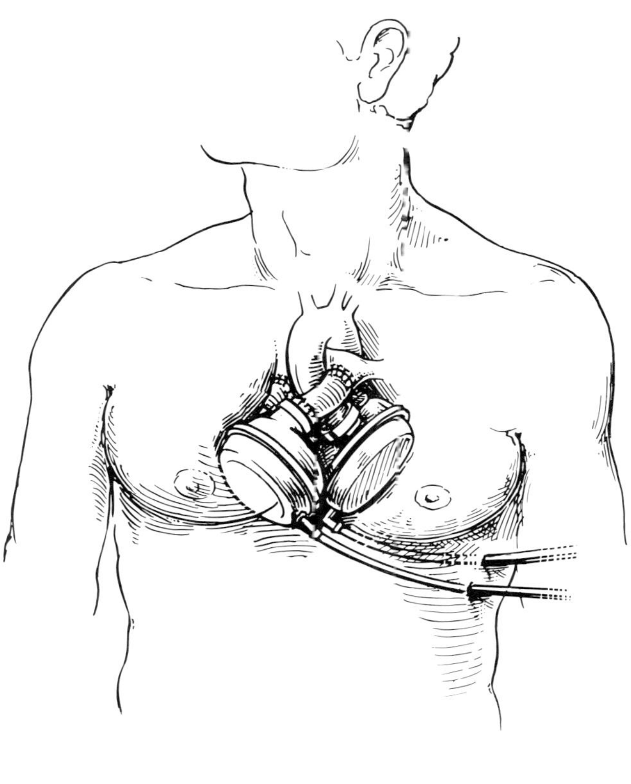

FIG. 4. Pneumatic energy to power the heart required the use of two percutaneous tables. These tables are covered with Dacron velour to encourage tissue ingrowth and firm fixation.

TABLE 1. *Hemodynamic Parameters Before and After Left Ventricular Assist Pump Implanatation*

	BP (mmHg)	CI (l/min/m^2)	CVP (mmHg)	LA (mmHg)
Patient 1				
Before	90/60	1.7	21	32
After	125/65	3.2	11	11
Patient 2				
Before	95/65	1.8	23	33
After	130/70	2.8	16	10
Patient 3				
Before	95/45	2.0	7	30
After	135/85	2.7	6	4
Patient 4				
Before	90/50	N/A	18	30
After	128/70	3.0	13	15

BP: blood pressure; CI: cardiac index; CVP: central venous pressure; PA: pulmonary artery pressure; PCW: pulmonary capillary wedge pressure; LA: left atrial pressure; PVR: pulmonary vascular resistance; N/A: not available; LVAD: left ventricular assist pump; IAB: intraaortic balloon.

Notice that hemodynamic parameters "before" were obtained with the patient on the IAB and inotropic drugs.

superficial infection with *Staphylococcus epidermidis* developed at the percutaneous cannula site after 12 days, which because of the presence of the prosthetic device was treated with both intravenously administered vancomycin and local wound care. Low molecular weight dextran (LMD) was infused at 20 ml/hour to inhibit platelet activation. No anticoagulants were employed.

Orthotopic heart transplantation was done 21 days after implantation of the LVAD. Her postoperative course was uncomplicated. Because of the drive line infection, intravenously administered vancomycin was continued for 2 weeks after surgery. No septic complications developed, and the patient was discharged from the hospital approximately 1 month after receiving the transplant. She has continued to do well 2 years after transplantation.

Patient 2

A 20-year-old man with viral cardiomyopathy was transferred to our intensive care unit because of rapidly deteriorating cardiac function. While he was receiving dobutamine (12 μg/kg/minute), dopamine (2 μg/kg/minute), and counterpulsation with an IAB, the cardiac index was 1.8 l/minute/m^2 (Table 1). Because of abnormal results of liver function tests (prothrombin time 28 seconds, SGOT 2240 U/l, alkaline phosphatase activity 106 U/l, and total bilirubin level 3.2 mg/dl), he was not a candidate for immediate transplantation.

After correction of the prolonged prothrombin time, a LVAD was implanted: the patient weighed only 62 kg and the chest size was too small for an artificial heart. An infusion of isoproterenol (2–4 μg/minute) for support of right ventricular function was necessary for 2 days, but thereafter hemodynamic parameters were excellent without any inotropic drugs (Table 1).

The endotracheal tube was removed 24 hours after operation. Renal function was normal, and liver dysfunction rapidly improved. Low molecular weight dextran was infused at 20 ml/hour, but no anticoagulants were used. The patient had a fever the first day after implantation of the device. A pulmonary artery catheter grew *Pseudomonas aeruginosa,* but blood cultures were negative. He received intravenous gentamicin and ticarcillin therapy and remained without fever, with a normal leukocyte count.

After 11 days with the LVAD, orthotopic heart transplantation was done. Immediately after transplantation, he had hypotension resulting from diffuse bleeding and a low peripheral vascular resistance; later, left ventricular dysfunction developed, which required inotropic support and insertion of an IAB. Cardiac function returned to normal after 5 days, but a *P. aeruginosa* infection developed. Despite drainage of the empyema and antibiotic therapy, renal failure and pancreatitis developed, and he died of septic shock 27 days after transplantation.

Patient 3

A 26-year-old white man, was transferred to our University Hospital with end-stage idiopathic cardiomyopathy for evaluation as a potential cardiac transplant recipient. Despite the intraaortic balloon and inotropic support, cardiac function was inadequate and a left ventricular assist device (LVAD) was implanted. Hemodynamic indices before, and after insertion of the LVAD are shown in Table 1.

A low-grade fever and leukocytosis (leukocyte cell count 15,000–20,000/mm^3) persisted for 2 weeks after LVAD implantation. Cultures obtained at the time of bronchoscopy, performed on the third postoperative day for right upper lobe atelectasis, grew *Streptococcus viridans* and he received a 7-day course of penicillin and clindamycin. His chest roentgenogram rapidly improved after bronchoscopy and all subsequent blood, urine, and sputum cultures were sterile.

Antiplatelet therapy with LMD and dipyridamole was begun on the first day after LVAD implantation. Low molecular weight dextran was discontinued on the tenth postimplant day because of mild hyperamylasemia. Extreme thrombocytosis occurred 2 weeks after LVAD implantation and he was begun on a continuous heparin infusion. He remained on the heparin infusion until the time of transplantation.

Eighteen days after LVAD implantation, he developed visual changes, vertigo, and an occipital headache. Although the clinical diagnosis was bilateral occipital lobe infarcts, a computed tomography scan demonstrated a small frontal lobe infarct. His symptoms resolved completely over 2 days and he was left with no permanent neurologic deficits.

After 31 days of LVAD support a donor organ became available and he underwent orthotopic cardiac transplantation. Multiple thrombi were present in the LVAD system at the time of transplantation. After excising the native ventricles a small vegetation was seen at the junction of the superior vena cava and right atrium. Cultures of the vegetation grew *Candida albicans* and he was treated with amphotericin B and 5-fluorocytosine. Mediastinitis with *C. albicans* and *S. epidermidis* occurred 4 days after transplantation and was treated with mediastinal irrigation. Massive mediastinal hemorrhage secondary to rupture of mycotic aneurysms of the great vessels occurred at both 2 and 4 weeks after transplantation. These were successfully repaired with a bovine pericardial patch. He was discharged from the hospital 67 days after transplantation and is well 5 months later (Figs. 5A and 5B).

Patient 4

A 25-year-old white man, was transferred to the University Hospital with end-stage idiopathic cardiomyopathy for evaluation as a potential cardiac transplant recipient. Progressive hemodynamic deterioration occurred, despite intraaortic balloon counter pulsation and inotropic support, and a LVAD was implanted. Hemodynamic indices before and after insertion of the LVAD are shown in Table 1.

His postimplant course was uneventful. Low molecular weight dextran and dipyridamole were given for the first 2 postimplant days. On the third day, a continuous heparin infusion was begun because of a large left ventricular mural thrombus present at the time of LVAD insertion. A donor organ became available 3 days after LVAD insertion and he underwent orthotopic cardiac transplantation. His hospital course was remarkably uneventful and he was discharged from the hospital 1 month after cardiac transplantation. Currently he is well, 4 months after transplantation.

Patient 5

A 44-year-old man with ischemic cardiomyopathy was admitted to the intensive care unit with severe congestive heart failure. Over the next several days, his cardiac output deteriorated and ventricular ectopy increased. While he was receiving dobutamine (10 μg/kg/minute), dopamine (5 μg/kg/minute), lidocaine (2 mg/minute), and counterpulsation with an IAB, the cardiac index was only 1.8 l/minute/m^2. Because of the low cardiac output and increasing ventricular dysrhythmias, a total artificial heart (TAH) was implanted. The patient weighed 78 kg but had a large chest because of chronic congestive heart failure. Accordingly, the fit of the artificial heart within the thorax was excellent.

After surgery, the cardiac index was easily maintained between 2 5 and 3 l/minute/m^2. Serum creatinine concentration ranged between 1.2 and 1.9 mg/dl, but the patient required

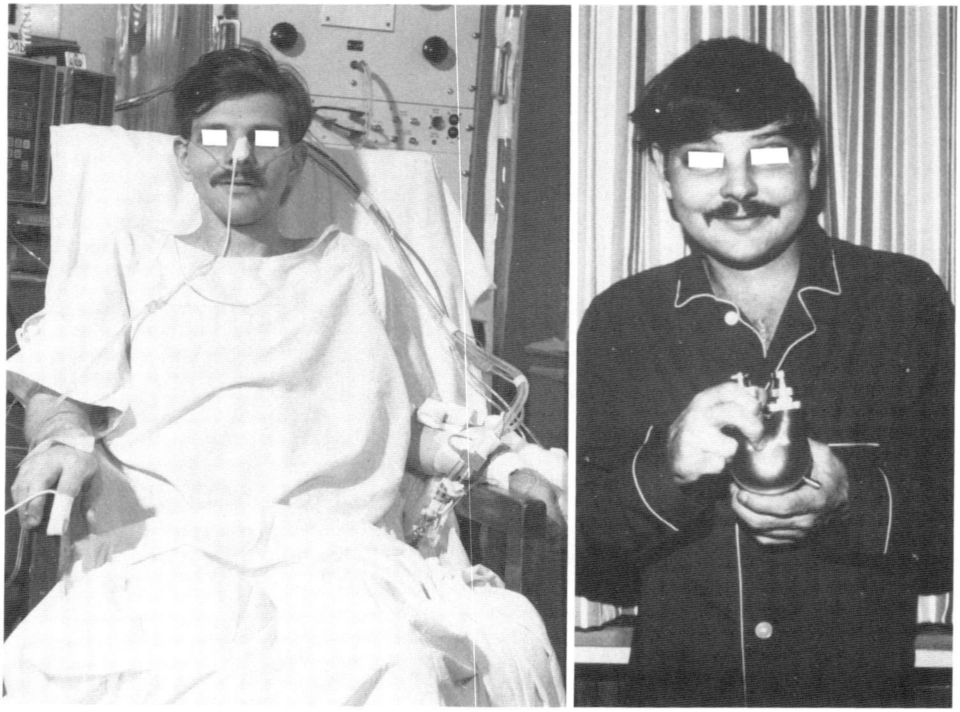

FIGS. 5A AND 5B. Patient 3: (A, left) A left ventricular assist pump was employed to support the circulation before the availability of a suitable donor heart. The patient was extubated, eating, and was out of bed on a daily basis during the "bridge" period. (B, right) The same patient after heart transplantation before hospital discharge. Notice the cushingoid appearance, due to steroid therapy. The patient is now home and continues to do well 4 months after transplantation.

intravenously administered furosemide to maintain adequate urine output. Plasma hemoglobin level was <10 mg/dl. Five days after operation, he developed right upper quadrant abdominal pain associated with elevation of the serum amylase level (226 U/l). The pancreas, liver, and gallbladder were normal by ultrasound study, but, nonetheless, oral nutrition was stopped, and hyperalimentation was started. The abdominal pain resolved, but the serum amylase activity remained elevated (200–350 U/l).

After operation he was alert and lucid, but on the third day after surgery had intermittent fluctuation in mental status. There were no focal neurologic signs, and metabolic studies. Electroencephalogram (EEG), and computed tomographic scan failed to reveal any acute changes. The patient had had a gunshot wound to the right temporoparietal region of the brain at 19 years of age. It was thought that the fluctuation in mental status reflected the effects of sleep deprivation, sedation, and intensive care unit stress in a patient with limited cerebral cortical reserve. Low molecular weight dextran (20 ml/hour) and aspirin (325 mg/day) were given to inhibit platelet activation. Cefamandole was started at the time of TAH implantation and maintained throughout the postoperative period. On the fifth day after surgery, a low-grade fever developed (38.2°C). All cultures were negative, and no temperature elevations occurred thereafter.

Orthotopic heart transplantation was done 11 days after implantation of the TAH. Examination of the artificial heart showed that the connectors, valves, and blood sacs were free of thrombus. Diffuse bleeding occurred at the time of cardiac transplantation which was difficult to control.

After operation, renal failure and pancreatitis developed within 24 hours. Cultures of mediastinal tissue taken at the time of the transplantation operation grew a fungal organism (*Trichosporon beigelii*), and despite therapy with amphotericin B, the patient died of disseminated fungal sepsis 17 days after heart transplantation.

Discussion

Considerable clinical judgment is required to decide on the optimal time for intervention in a patient who is a cardiac transplant candidate who has profound circulatory failure. Such a patient should be on an optimal medical program. Hospital admission and significant curtailment of activity form the first line of defense. Continuous intravenous dopamine administration at levels up 10 mg/kg/minute may provide significant improvement in cardiac output and in renal function. If this is inadequate, percutaneous insertion of the IAB is indicated. The use of the IAB may result in a decrease in inotropic drug requirement. Mechanical circulatory assistance or the artificial heart should be considered for use in a patient who has an inadequate circulation in spite of reasonable use of inotropic agents and the IAB. A cardiac output index less than 1.8 l/minute/m^2, a pulmonary capillary wedge or left atrial pressure >25 mmHg, urine output of <20 ml per minute, a rising blood urea nitrogen (BUN), mental obtundation, or dangerous arrhythmias are indications of an inadequate circulation and help to identify patients who are not likely to survive until a donor organ is identified.

After implantation of the mechanical circulatory support device, significant improvement in cardiac output, reduction in left atrial pressure and improved organ function generally will be dramatic. However, patients in whom a single LVAD has been implanted generally will experience only a modest increase in cardiac output. Small amounts of dopamine or isoproterenol frequently are required to improve right ventricular performance and thus increase overall cardiac output. One patient in our series (Patient 2) experienced an improvement in hepatic function thus considerably improving the chances that a successful cardiac transplant could be performed.

Risk of thromboembolism serves as a major concern in patients with implanted prosthetic devices. Clearly, the major elements associated with safe prosthetic pump use center around device design and high blood flow rates through the device. Whereas these factors alone may be adequate to prevent thromboembolic complications, we believe that some agent should be employed to decrease platelet adhesiveness after adequate hemostasis has been obtained and after coagulation studies have returned to normal levels. Currently, oral dipyridamole (75 mg orally three times daily) is administered beginning after the risk of bleeding has passed. As soon as a potential donor organ is identified, the dipyridamole is discontinued. Platelet transfusions and the use of fresh frozen plasma may be required at the time of cardiac transplantation. Low-dose heparin (5000 U intravenous [IV] every 6 hours) also may be employed. Larger doses of heparin are of concern because of the risk of bleeding. Similarly, we no longer employ LMD in transplant candidates because of the risk of bleeding at the time of cardiac transplantation.

Another area of risk in the patient with a prosthetic device is that of a septic complication, which greatly increase the risks associated with cardiac transplantation and associated immunosuppression. Accordingly special care must be taken with intravenous lines, Swan-Ganz catheters, percutaneous vascular cannula, and drive lines. All percutaneous access sites should be cleaned daily with alcohol, be coated with an iodine-containing cream applied and be dressed sterilely. Persons not familiar with care of such lines should not be permitted access to them. The studies to date suggest that serious infectious complications may occur but with appropriate care, device use can be followed by transplantation and required immunosuppression with an excellent result.

The optimal technique for supporting a patient before cardiac transplantation is not yet known. Clearly, there have been spectacular successes with isolated left ventricular support, biventricular support (using paracorporeal assist pumps) and with the artificial heart. Currently, we favor the simplest system that will do the job. There have been successful outcomes in patients with acute myocardial infarction and with cardiomyopathy using a single left ventricular assist pump. Accordingly, if the patient has isolated left ventricular failure, we favor the implantation of a single assist pump. The cardiopulmonary bypass time required for insertion is brief, the technique of insertion is well described and mediastinal structures are minimally disturbed. Furthermore, at the time of cardiac transplantation, all vascular suture lines associated with the assist pump use can be excised.

If the patient has biventricular failure, both sides of the circulation must be supported. If the chest size is adequate, implantation of a pneumatic artificial heart appears to be a perfectly reasonable course. However, in the patient with a small chest cavity, artificial heart implantation can be disastrous. In those patients two paracorporeal left and right ventricles will provide an excellent result. Only with further experience will it become apparent as to whether there is an advantage in the artificial heart over two paracorporeal assist pumps.

ACKNOWLEDGMENT

The research that ultimately lead to the ventricular assist pump and artificial heart described in the preceding report began in the Harrison Department of Surgical Research Department of Surgery, University of Pennsylvania in 1960. At that time, Dr. Rhoads was Chairman of the Department of Surgery. Because of the excellence of the staff and house officers, and because of the encouragement that I received while a medical student, I subsequently applied for and was accepted as a first year resident in Dr. Rhoads' program. His encouragement continued and the productivity of the artificial heart laboratory at the University of Pennsylvania increased. At times we "out ran" our budget and I was forced to go, hat in hand, to Dr. Rhoads and explain the situation. He never failed to be supportive and to provide the funds required to meet our obligations. My training subsequently included a 2-year tour at Clinic of Surgery, National Heart Institute, National Institutes of Health, and then back to the University of Pennsylvania for the coveted senior residency in the general and thoracic surgical training program. Although my subsequent career has been in Hershey at The Pennsylvania State University rather than in Philadelphia at the University of Pennsylvania, Dr. Rhoads has continued to play an important role in my career decisions. You can only imagine my pride when I called him in 1985 and said "Dr. Rhoads, we just implanted our first artificial heart in a patient."

My best wishes to Jonathan E. Rhoads, M.D., master surgeon, educator and humanitarian on the occasion of his eightieth birthday. May he have many more.

REFERENCES

1. Pennock JL, Wisman CB, Pierce WS. Mechanical support of the circulation prior to cardiac transplantation. Heart Transplant 1982;1:299–305.
2. Pennock JL, Pierce WS, Campbell DB *et al.* Mechanical support of the circulation followed by cardiac transplantation. J Thorac Cardiovasc Surg 1986;92:994–1004.
3. Richenbacher WE, Pae WE, Rosenberg G, Pennock JL, Pierce WS. Experimental and clinical experience with the PSU pneumatic VAD and TAH. Presented at the Cardiostim Conference '86, Monaco, Monte Carlo, France, June 19, 1986.
4. Pierce WS, Parr GVS, Myers JL, Pae WE Jr, Bull AP, Waldhausen JA. Ventricular assist pumping in patients with cardiogenic shock after cardiac operations. N Engl J Med 1981;305:1606–1610.
5. Pierce WS, Myers JL, Donachy JH *et al.* Approaches to the artificial heart. Surgery 1981;90:137–148.
6. Pierce WS. The artificial heart 1986: Partial fulfillment of a promise. Trans Am Soc Artif Intern Organs 1986;32:5–10.
7. Richenbacher WE, Pennock JL, Pae WE Jr, Pierce WS. Artificial heart implantation for end-stage cardiac disease. J Cardiac Surg 1986;1:3–12.

Bi-Caval Obstruction With Budd-Chiari Syndrome Following Transvenous Pacemaker Implantation: Surgical Management

HILARY H. TIMMIS, M.D., F.A.C.S., LYLE F. JACOBSON, M.D., F.A.C.S., AND DAVID PINTAR, S.A.

Thrombotic occlusion of the superior vena cava (SVC) is a well-documented sequela of transvenous pacemaker implantation. A case is reported in which this complication was followed 10 years later by obstruction of the suprahepatic inferior vena cava (IVC). A Budd-Chiari syndrome developed leading to multisystem failure. Reconstruction of the suprahepatic IVC was performed with a pericardial patch. Five-year follow-up confirms a satisfactory clinical status.

DURING THE LAST 25 YEARS, cardiac pacing has been an invaluable adjunct in the management of heart block and other dysrrhythmias.[1] The application of this measure has been enormously broadened by the transvenous technique of permanent pacemaker implantation, which is technically simple and in many instances is performed by a diagnostic cardiologist. However, no invasive procedure is completely innocuous and here, too, a spectrum of complications is well documented.[2–10] The four primary areas of potential morbidity in cardiac pacing have proved to be the physiologic tolerance and cardiac responsiveness of the recipient and the mechanical and functional integrity of the pacing system.[3] Physiologic intolerance to implanted pacemakers is manifested by hematoma, extrusion, infection, myocardial perforation, and thromboembolism. The experience cited here deals with thrombosis, complicating the use of silastic-sheathed catheters within the venous vascular tree.

Occlusion of the superior vena cava (SVC) has been reported with prohibitive frequency after superior caval shunts for hydrocephalus,[3,4] but, much less commonly, when this vessel provides passage for permanent implantation of endocardial electrodes.[6,7] To our knowledge, occlusion of the inferior vena cava (IVC) after implantation of a pacing electrode has not been reported, probably because this vessel rarely is used.

In the following report, first the superior vena cava and then almost 10 years later the inferior vena cava were the sites of initial thrombosis followed by gradual but progressive fibrous occlusion around an unused endocardial transvenous electrode which had been introduced years before. The physiological impact was profound with the development of a Budd-Chiari syndrome and subsequent multisystem collapse.

Case Report

A 65-year-old white man had a transvenous pacing system implanted *via* the right external jugular vein in 1969 for the management of complete heart block. Pulse generator malfunction necessitated replacement of the unit that same year. In 1970, after continuing malfunction of both the new pulse generator and endocardial lead, an epicardial system was implanted. At this time an attempt was made to remove the endocardial system. During the maneuver, the electrode slipped out of the right ventricle and recoiled down through the orifice of the IVC (Figs. 1A and 1B). Further withdrawal apparently was impossible. The electrode then was divided at the level of the cephalic vein and allowed to retract. During routine follow-up in 1973, the patient was noted to have thrombosis of the right cephalic

From the William Beaumont Hospital, Royal Oak, Michigan.

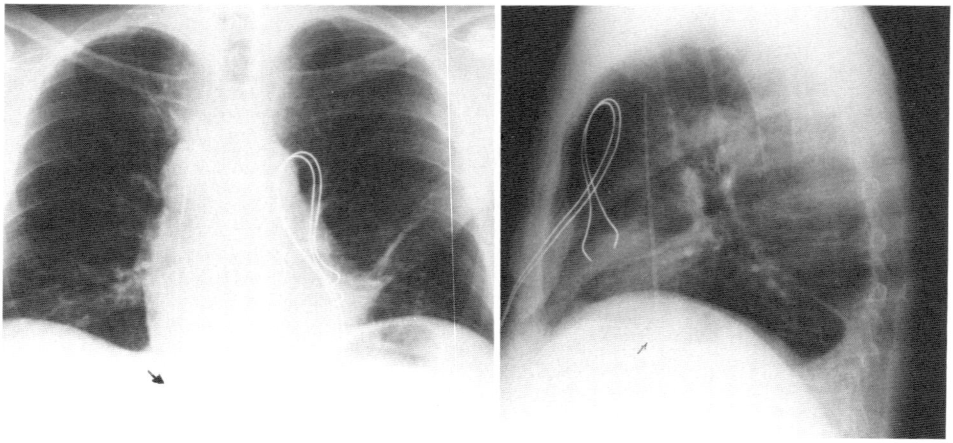

FIGS. 1A AND 1B. (A, left) The remnant of the endocardial lead can be seen in this preoperative chest film along the right heart border. Epicardial electrodes are implanted in the left ventricle. (B, right) Side view of the endocardial lead can be seen extending well below the diaphragm (into the inferior vena cava).

and axillary veins; SVC obstruction was subsequently demonstrated. In 1975, 1976, and 1978 the pulse generator of his epicardial system was replaced.

He was asymptomatic until the autumn of 1980 when he noted increasing abdominal girth and swelling of both lower extremities. These subsided with salt restriction and diuretic therapy. In July of 1982, ascites and edema of the lower extremities recurred and gradually worsened despite anticoagulation with warfarin sodium and vigorous daily therapy with furosemide.

He was referred to the Cardiovascular Service of William Beaumont Hospital, Royal Oak, Michigan, in December of 1982 with dyspnea, severe ascites, and lower extremity edema. A 10-k weight gain was recorded despite a general appearance of inanition and muscle wasting. Roentgenographic examination of his chest revealed a left pleural effusion. A remnant of an endocardial pacing electrode was noted which extended from the SVC into the proximal IVC (Figs. 1A and 1B). Abdominal computed tomography (CT) scan and ultrasound confirmed the presence of fluid but were otherwise uninformative. Cardiac catheterization demonstrated normal pulmonary artery and right atrial pressures and a 22-mm gradient across the suprahepatic IVC. A high-grade stenosis in this region of the IVC was defined by angiography. Pericentesis was performed to remove approximately 4000 ml of straw-colored fluid and after additional supportive measures, the patient was discharged 1 week after admission.

He was readmitted 5 days later with severe recurrent ascites, dyspnea, and back pain. He was afebrile and vital signs were stable. A venogram showed complete obstruction of the IVC, thought to be due to thrombosis. Streptokinase was given intravenously starting with a 100,000-U bolus, followed by 100,000 U per hour for 3 hours and then 18,000 U per hour for 24 hours. Venography was repeated the following day, revealing persistent occlusion of the previously stenotic IVC (Fig. 2). Angioplasty with a balloon catheter was attempted but was unsuccessful, in part due to inadequate balloons. Streptokinase and supportive measures were continued and evaluation was begun for a surgical solution to his desperate problem. However, a precipitous and intractable worsening of hepatic and renal function necessitated immediate operation.

Operative Procedure

The heart was exposed through a median sternotomy and cannulations for cardiopulmonary bypass carried out *via* the femoral and azygos veins and the femoral artery. The body temperature was lowered to 19°C. Dense adhesions between the pericardium and the heart were divided, after which the right atrium was opened and the caval orifices inspected. The

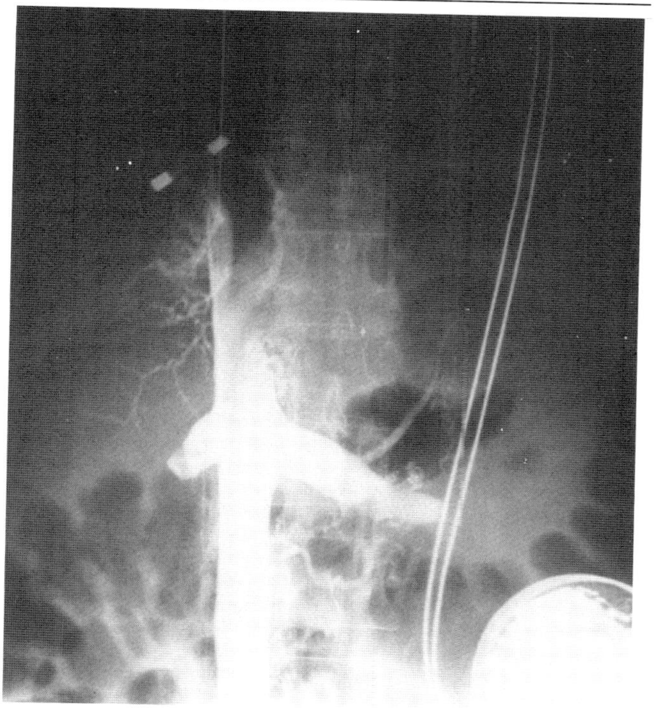

FIG. 2. Preoperative visualization of the inferior vena cava demonstrates complete obstruction at the level of the diaphragm. The distal end of the endocardial electrode extends into the right hepatic vein.

SVC was completely obstructed just above the azygos vein and the inferior vena cava totally occluded at the level of the diaphragm. The sites of caval obstruction were easily visualized and were found to be smooth concavities with no evidence of a recent channel.

The right atrial incision was extended to the level of the diaphragm after which the electrode remnant which was completely imbedded in fibrous tissue, was exposed by sharp dissection from its posterior location and removed. The residual channel was used as a guide for dissection into the suprahepatic IVC. A series of metal dilators were passed as the caval lumen was gradually enlarged by excision of dense fibrous tissue. Eventually the operator's index finger could be inserted into the suprahepatic IVC where the enlarged orifice of the right hepatic vein could be palpated. A small amount of clot was extracted with a large balloon catheter. Dilators up to a 40-French diameter were passed easily after which the IVC was widened with a 2 × 4 cm patch of pericardium from the diaphragm below to the atriocaval junction. After rewarming, cardiopulmonary bypass was discontinued without difficulty. An atrial-ventricular (A-V) sequential pacemaker with epicardial leads was implanted and the patient moved to the intensive care unit.

Postoperative Course

Hepatic and renal function improved dramatically in the early postoperative period and the ascites and peripheral edema lessened almost immediately. Coumadin (warfarin sodium crystalline) and Persantine (dipyridamde) were administered, however on the twenty-fourth hospital day, thrombosis of the caval repair was suspected because of sudden recurrent edema of both lower extremeties. He again received intravenous streptokinase therapy followed by a course of anticoagulation with intravenous heparin sodium. A venogram performed 2 days later confirmed patency of the IVC (Fig. 3). Some residual stenosis was evidenced by the presence of an 8-mmHg gradient across the site of caval reconstruction. Maintenance of adequate nutrition was a major postoperative challenge and was responsible largely for his long hospital course. At follow-up examination 3 months after discharge the patient was free of ascites. Most of his peripheral edema had resolved and he appeared to

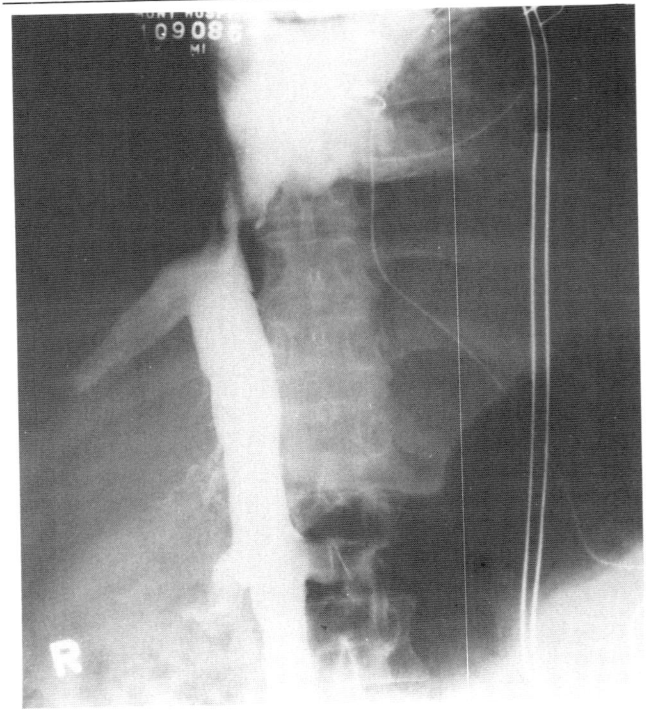

FIG. 3. A postoperative venogram demonstrates flow from the inferior vena cava into the right atrium. Some channeling of contrast is present.

have recovered much of his muscle mass. He was last examined in April 1987, almost 5 years after surgical reconstruction of the IVC. There was no evidence of recurrent caval obstruction.

Discussion

The presence of a nonobstructing intravascular foreign body can produce thromboembolic complications even when covered with a nonwettable, relatively impervious, electrically neutral silicone rubber surface. Venous thromboembolism has dogged the use of silastic ventriculoatrial and ventriculovenous shunts used for the treatment of hydrocephalus.[4,5,13] A similar but remarkably less frequent incidence of caval occlusion has been reported with silastic-sheathed transvenous electrodes for permanent cardiac pacing.[6–12] Fatal pacemaker electrode-induced thrombosis of the SVC was first reported by Kaulbach and Krukonis in 1970.[8] Since then there have been multiple case reports of SVC syndrome of similar etiology managed successfully by surgical intervention in some instances[14–16] and with diuretics, fibrinolysis and anticoagulation in others.[9,11] To our knowledge obstruction of both cavae due to the presence of a pacemaker electrode is unprecedented and had profound physiologic significance because of the intense, congestion of the abdominal viscera leading to a Budd-Chiari-like syndrome and eventually to fulminating hepatorenal failure.

Isolated superior vena caval obstruction was actually well tolerated here over a period of years, producing few signs and no incapacitating symptoms. The advent of inferior caval stenosis precluded the development of effective, compensatory drainage into the brachiocephalic system. Within 6 months he was emcumbered with intractable ascites and very severe truncal and lower extremity edema. After the IVC became completely occluded, serum bilirubin and blood ammonia rose precipitously, renal failure ensued and he became deeply obtunded as metabolic encephalopathy rapidly worsened.

The only reasonable strategy to reverse a certain, lethal clinical course was to decompress his liver and reestablish inferior caval flow. Several techniques to relieve Budd-Chiari-type syndromes secondary to suprahepatic caval obstruction have been defined in the recent surgical literature.[16–20] Portocaval or mesocaval shunts were insufficient here because of the extent of obstruction of his systemic drainage. Bypass with a rigid synthetic fabric graft from the distal IVC to the right atrium was feasible but we feared the likelihood of thrombosis in a prosthetic graft of this length. Consequently we elected to deal with the site of obstruction within the IVC directly. There were several secondary gains: (1) the pathology was visualized; (2) the offending pacemaker electrode was removed; (3) the orifices of the hepatic veins were assessed and found to be patent; (4) residual clot was evacuated which conceivably could have propagated into the hepatic veins; and (5) the opportunity for an anatomic repair was provided. The site of repair has been protected by coumarin anticoagulation and by the use of platelet inhibitors, both of which will be continued indefinitely. So far his therapy appears to be effective as he is successfully completing his fifth postoperative year.

REFERENCES

1. Parsonnet V. Permanent pacing of the heart: 1952–1976. Am J Cardiol 1977;39:250–256.
2. Grogler F, Frank G, Greven G *et al.* Complications of permanent transvenous cardiac pacing. J Thoracic Cardiovasc Surg 1975;69:895–904.
3. Koskowsky B, Barr I. Complications and malfunctions of electrical cardiac pacemakers. Prog Cardiovasc Dis 1972;14:501–514.
4. Friedman S, Berger N, Cerruti M, Kosmoski J. Venous thrombosis and permanent cardiac pacing. Am Heart J 1973;85:531–533.
5. Overton M, Derrick J, Snodgrass S. Surgical management of superior vena cava obstruction complicating ventriculo-atrial shunts. J Neurosurg 1967;25:164–171.
6. Stoney W, Addlestone R, Alford W *et al.* The incidence of venous thrombosis following long term transvenous pacing. Ann Thorac Surg 1976;22:166–170.
7. Matthews D, Forfar J. Superior vena caval stenosis: A complication of transvenous endocardial pacing. Thorax 1979;34:412–414.
8. Kaulbach M, Krukonis E. Pacemaker electrode induced thrombosis in the superior vena cava with pulmonary embolism. Am J Cardiol 1970;26:205–207.
9. Wertheimer M, Hughes R, Castle H. Superior vena cava syndrome: Complication of permanent transvenous endocardial pacing. JAMA 1973;224:1172–1173.
10. Chamorro H, Rao G, Wholey M. Superior vena cava syndrome: A complication of transvenous pacemaker implantation. Radiology 1978;126:377–378.
11. Williams D, Demos N. Thrombosis of superior vena cava caused by pacemaker wire and managed by streptokinase. J Thoracic Cardiovasc Surg 1974;68:134–137.
12. Branson J. Radiology of cardiac pacemakers and their complications with three cases of superior vena cava obstruction. Australas Radiol 1978;22:125–131.
13. Noonan J, Ehmke D. Complications of ventriculovenous shunts for control of hydrocephalus. N Engl J Med 1963;269:70–74.
14. Crook B, Gishen P, Robsinon C, Orams O. Occlusion of the subclavian vein associated with cephalic vein pacemaker electrodes. Br J Surg 1977;64:329–331.
15. Yakiervich V, Alagem D, Papo J, Vidne B. Fibrotic stenosis of the superior vena cava with widespread thrombotic occlusion of its major tributaries: An unusual complication of transvenous cardiac pacing. J Thoracic Cardiovasc Surg 1983;85:632–638.
16. Blair T, Seibel J, Goodreau J *et al.* Surgical relief of thrombotic superior vena cava obstruction caused by endocardial pacing catheter. Ann Thorac Surg 1982;33:511–515.
17. Imaoka S, Okamoto N, Kobayaski T, Fujimote K, Iwanaga T. Treatment of inferior vena cava obstruction producing Budd-Chiari syndrome. Arch Surg 1984;119:965–968.
18. Huguet C, Deliere T, Ollvier J, Levy V. Budd-Chiari syndrome with thrombosis of the inferior vena cava: Long-term patency of meso-caval and cavoatrial bypass. Surgery 1984;95:108–111.
19. Segadal L, Aruesjo B, Halevoses J, Gothlin J, Myking A, Solberg C. Budd-Chiari syndrome with obstruction of the inferior caval vein: Successful treatment by cavosplenoatrial shunt. Surgery 1985;98:63–67.
20. Victor S, Jayanthi V, Kandasamy I, Ratnasabapathy A, Madanagopalan N. Retrohepatic cavoatrial bypass for coarctation of inferior vena cava with a polytetrafluoroethylene graft. J Thorac Cardiovasc Surg 1986;91:99–105.

Long-Term Results of Transluminal Angioplasty of the Iliac and Femoral Arteries

RICHARD K. SPENCE, M.D., DAVID B. FREIMAN, M.D., ROBERT GATENBY, M.D., CHARLES L. HOBBS, M.D., CLYDE F. BARKER, M.D., HENRY D. BERKOWITZ, M.D., BROOKE ROBERTS, M.D., GORDON McCLEAN, M.D., JUAN OLEAGA, M.D., AND ERNEST J. RING, M.D.

One hundred forty-eight iliac artery and 103 femoral artery stenoses were successfully treated using percutaneous transluminal angioplasty (PTA) in 239 patients between January 1978 and January 1981. Patency rates for iliac PTA were 93.4% after one year, 87.2% after two years, and 79.4% after three years. Patency rates for femoral PTA were 79.6% after one year and 74.9% after two years. The PTA procedure can be performed successfully for both claudication and salvage, and its results compare favorably with those of bypass surgery for the treatment of peripheral vascular lesions.

SINCE THE DEVELOPMENT by Andreas Gruntzig of the polyvinyl balloon catheter,[1] the use of percutaneous transluminal angioplasty (PTA) as a means of treating occlusive vascular disease of the lower extremity has become widespread. Within the last three years, reports of experiences in centers across the United States and in Europe have been published in both the radiologic and surgical literatures.[2–8] Many of these, however, suffer in that they have been, by necessity, short-term studies of small numbers of patients. Others fail to examine those aspects that the vascular surgeon uses to evaluate and compare various treatments.

We examined PTA as vascular surgeons, by examining those factors that are known to affect the outcome of surgical treatment of lower-extremity occlusive arterial disease.

Materials and Methods

A total of 282 iliac and femoral artery lesions were dilated in 239 patients between January 1978 and January 1981. Age and sex distribution, as well as associated risk factors, are given in Table 1. The patients were predominately men who smoked, with those undergoing femoral PTA being a decade older. Indications for PTA are as follows: of the iliac dilations, 22 (18.7%) were for salvage and 138 (86.3%) for claudication; whereas of the femoral dilations, 34 (28.6%) were for salvage and 85 (71.4%) were for claudication. Symptoms of claudication were experienced after walking two blocks or less by most patients, and had been present for longer than six months.

All patients treated for limb salvage had rest pain. Eight in the iliac artery group and 15 in the femoral artery group had ischemic ulcers. Four in the iliac artery group and 11 in the femoral artery group had gangrene.

The condition of each patient was initially assessed by history and by results of physical examination, pulse volume recordings, and arteriography. Lesions seen on the last were

Accepted for publication July 10, 1981.

From the Departments of Surgery (Drs. Spence, Hobbs, Barker, Berkowitz, and Roberts) and Radiology (Drs. Freiman, Gatenby, McClean, Oleaga, and Ring), Hospital of the University of Pennsylvania, Philadelphia, Pennsylvania.

TABLE 1. *Patient Population*

	Iliac	Femoral
Age, yr	39–81 (58)*	42–89 (67)
Sex, No.		
M	93	70
F	38	38
Smokers, %	87	70
Diabetes, %	24	27
Hypertension, %	43.5	31.5
ASCVD,† %	32	17.6

* Mean.
† ASCVD indicates arteriosclerotic cardiovascular disease.

categorized by location, extent of calcification, and both the degree and length of stenosis or occlusion. Intravascular pressures above and below stenotic iliac lesions were obtained to demonstrate a pressure gradient whenever a question existed as to hemodynamic significance. Whenever practical, dilation was performed at the time of the initial arteriogram.

Dilations were attempted in a wide variety of patients during the first year of the study. Because of our early experience of relatively poor results and high complication rate with dilation of total occlusions of the iliac and stenoses longer than 10 cm in either the iliac or femoral arteries, these lesions are now dilated only in extremely poor-risk patients with threatened loss of limb Arteriographic and dilation techniques have been previously described by our group.[9]

All patients were given 5,000 units of heparin through the arterial catheter after traversing the stenotic lesion. Long-term anticoagulation was not routinely used postdilation. Patients were placed on a regimen of aspirin, 600 mg orally twice a day, and dipyridamole (Persantine), 50 mg orally three times a day.

Initial success or failure was assessed by angiographic appearance of the dilated vessel, elimination of pressure gradients, and restoration or improvement of distal pulses. Pulse-volume recordings were repeated within several days after dilation. Patients were followed up at three- to six-month intervals by assessment of degree and duration of symptomatic relief and the status of peripheral pulses. Follow-up pulse-volume recordings were obtained when a major change in pulse or pressure indices was observed. On occasion, angiographic examination of the dilated vessel was performed in conjunction with evaluation of disease in other areas.

Distal runoff was assessed and graded for both the iliac and femoral artery dilations, using the following criteria.

Of the iliac arteries, 0 indicates superficial femoral artery (SFA) occluded, profunda occluded; 1, SFA occluded, profunda patent; 2, SFA and profunda patent, but diseased to level of popliteal; and 3, SFA and profunda patent and not diseased to level of popliteal. Of the femoral arteries, 0 indicates popliteal and outflow vessels occluded; 1, isolated popliteal segment or single outflow vessel patent; 2, popliteal patent, two outflow vessels patent; and 3, popliteal patent, three outflow vessels patent.

Analysis of patency rates was performed using the life-table method of Cutler and Ederer.[10]

Results

Definitions

For the purpose of our study, initial failure means inability to dilate a stenotic or occlusive lesion. Successful dilation is defined as improved angiographic appearance, diminution of symptoms, improved pulses, or an increase in pulse-volume-recording indices of greater than 0.15.[11] Late failure is defined as return of symptoms, diminution or loss of pulses, decrease in pulse-volume-recording indices, and angiographic evidence of restenosis after

24 hours that could not be successfully treated by further dilations. Successful redilations of areas of restenosis are not considered failures.

Iliacs

One hundred sixty dilations were attempted in 131 patients. Initial success rate was 92.5%. Twelve dilations were initially unsuccessful. Of these, six were stenoses 5 to 10 cm or more long and four were total occlusions. In one patient, the initial angiographic catheter punctured the wall of the iliac artery, necessitating prompt surgical repair that was performed using a bifurcation graft. Two patients underwent aortic bifurcation grafts after a partial occlusion was converted to a total occlusion. A 1-cm segment of the aorta was dissected locally by the catheter in another patient who subsequently underwent successful grafting. A 1-cm subintimal flap was raised in the iliac artery of another patient. The procedure was terminated, the patient was observed, and, at a later date, the lesion was successfully dilated. No patients in the iliac group underwent amputation.

Patency rates of successfully dilated iliac vessels, as determined by life-table analysis, are given in Table 2 and Fig. 1. Accumulated patency rates were 93.4% at one year, 82.2% at two years, and 79.4% at three years. One third of the failures occurred within the first six months after dilation. All but one occurred within 18 months.

Twenty-nine patients (22%) had multiple procedures, ie, dilations of stenotic areas in other vessels in addition to their iliacs. Twenty had both iliac vessels dilated; 15 had both an iliac and a femoral vessel dilated. Seven patients underwent a total of nine redilations of lesions in the same vessel from two to 18 months after the initial procedure. Of these, five (55.6%) were new areas of stenosis. All but one of the nine stenoses were successfully redilated. There were nine deaths in the group; all were from cardiac or neurovascular causes, except for one patient who died of a stroke after becoming hypotensive during the PTA procedure.

Seventeen patients had iliac artery PTA performed as a preliminary procedure prior to saphenous-vein femoropopliteal bypass grafting. Of these, one patient displayed recurrent symptoms of claudication at five months and another underwent successful redilation of his iliac vessel after nine months. Sixteen of the 17 have now been followed for up to two years and are asymptomatic, with patent vein grafts.

Patency rates for iliac dilations performed for salvage vs claudication are shown in Fig. 2. Patency for salvage was 80.9% at one year and 50.6% at two years. Patency rates according to runoff category are shown in Fig. 3. Groups 0 and 1 are compared with groups 2 and 3, with 53 patients at risk in the former and 90 at risk in the latter. Patency is better for those with good runoff after both one year (97.5%, compared with 85.7%) and two years (85.4%, compared with 73.4%). Of the 22 vessels dilated for limb salvage, nine (41%) had poor runoff. Forty-five of 126 limbs (35.7%) in the claudication group had poor runoff.

Femorals

Percutaneous transluminal angioplasty was attempted on 122 femoral arteries. Of these, 19 were unsuccessful, for an initial success rate of 84.4%. Fourteen of these 19 were lesions of longer than 10 cm. Four long, stenotic lesions were converted to occlusions. Because of extremely calcified vessels, three other stenoses could not be dilated. Sixteen of the 19 PTA failures had poor distal runoff, with no more than one patent vessel below the popliteal. Nine of the patients whose vessels could not be successfully dilated had threatened loss of limbs and seven had gangrene. Five of these seven then underwent prompt amputation, not being candidates for reconstruction. Seven of the remaining ten patients who had claudication underwent femoralpopliteal or femorotibial bypass procedures after the failed dilation attempt.

Thirty-seven patients (34.3%) underwent dilations of other diseased vessels; approximately half of the lesions were proximal to the femoral and half were distal. Seven patients, after successful PTA displayed a recurrence of symptoms and returned for redilation. One patient returned twice for new lesions and twice for restenosis. Overall, ten redilations were done, six for new lesions and four for restenosis. All were successful, and only two eventually failed, both of which were recurrences in lesions longer than 10 cm.

Nine of the initial 122 patients (7.4%) eventually underwent amputation. Five amputa-

TABLE 2. *Iliac Artery Patency Life Table*

Interval, mo	No. at Risk	No. Failed	No. Dead	Not Followed Entire Interval	Interval Failure Rate, %	Interval Patency Rate, %	Accumulated Patency Rate, %
0–6	148	6	3	1	4.1	95.9	95.9
6–12	138	3	4	45	2.6	97.4	93.4
12–18	86	9	3	19	12.0	88.0	82.2
18–24	55	0	0	21	0	100	82.2
24–30	34	1	0	10	3.4	96.6	79.4
30–36	23	0	0	8	0	100	79.4

TABLE 3. *Femoral Artery Patency Life Table*

Interval, mo	No. at Risk	No. Failed	No. Dead	Not Followed Entire Interval	Interval Failure Rate, %	Interval Patency Rate, %	Accumulated Patency Rate, %
0–6	96	9	4	2	9.7	90.3	90.3
6–12	81	8	1	26	11.9	88.1	79.6
12–18	46	1	0	8	2.4	97.6	77.7
18–24	37	1	0	18	3.6	96.4	74.9
24–30	18	1	0	8	7.1	92.9	69.6
30–36	9	0	0	7	0	100	69.6

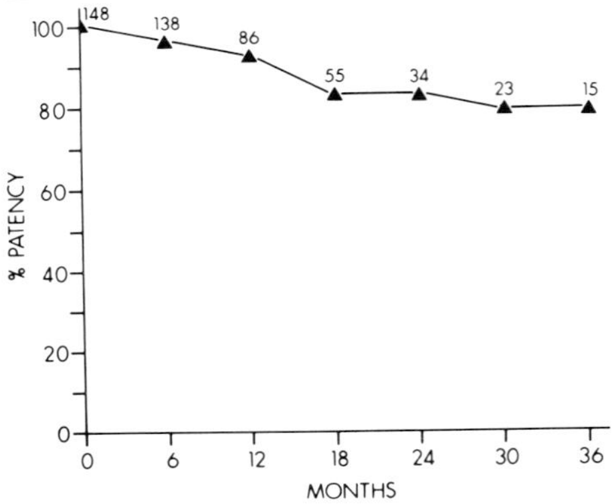

FIG. 1. Iliac artery patency after percutaneous transluminal angioplasty.

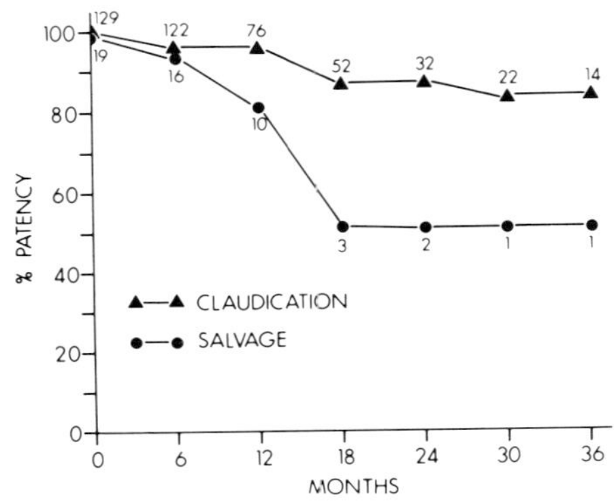

FIG. 2. Iliac artery patency: salvage vs claudication.

tions were performed in patients whose attempted dilation was unsuccessful, leaving only four patients (3.9%) who had limbs amputated after an initially successful femoral PTA. Two of these had poor runoff and gangrene. One other patient underwent femoral dilation to improve chances of healing a planned below-knee amputation. Only one patient who eventually underwent amputation had claudication alone at the time of dilation. She had good relief of symptoms for 12 months, after which time her femoral vessels became thrombotic and she lost her leg.

There were seven deaths in the group, none directly attributable to the dilation procedure. Of four patients who died within six months of undergoing dilation, three had had patent vessels. Of the remaining three who died six to 12 months after PTA, two had already had occluded femoral arteries before death. All deaths were from arteriosclerotic causes, ie, myocardial infarction or cerebrovascular accident (CVA).

Patency rates for femoral PTA are given in Table 3 and Fig. 4. Analysis is given for the combined group of 11 common femoral and 85 SFA dilations and for the SFA group alone. Redilations as separate procedures are not included in the analysis, in keeping with our definition of failure. Patency after one year is 79.6% for the combined group and 78.6% for SFA alone; after two years it is 74.9% for the combined group and 73.4% for SFA alone. There is no significant difference. As Fig. 5 shows, patency rates for claudication and salvage after one year were 79.5% and 76.1%, respectively; whereas after two years they were 72.9% and 76.1%, respectively.

Patency rates for femoral dilations according to runoff are shown in Fig. 6. Respective

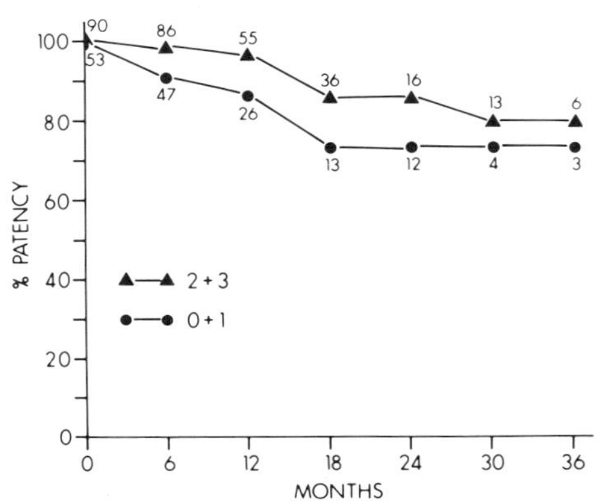

FIG. 3. Iliac artery patency: runoff.

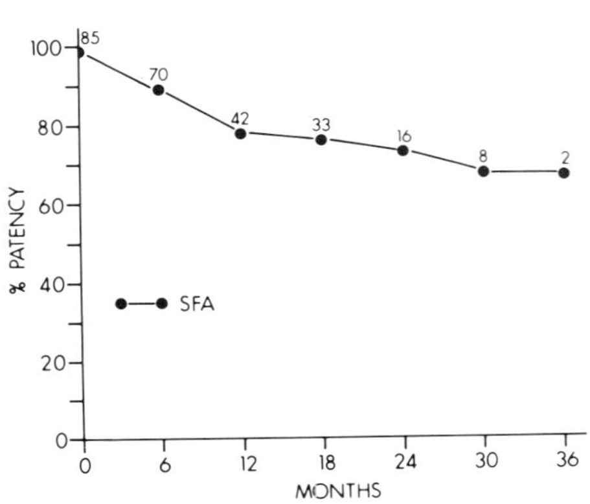

FIG. 4. Femoral artery patency after percutaneous transluminal angioplasty.

one- and two-year patency rates for categories 0 and 1, and 2 and 3, are 76.4% and 80.5%, respectively, after one year, and 69.4% and 76.4%, respectively, after two years.

Figure 7 shows patency rates for diabetic vs nondiabetic patients. Patency rates after one year were as follows: for iliac vessels, 91.7% in diabetics and 93.2% in nondiabetics; whereas for femoral vessels, 53.5% in diabetics and 85.4% in nondiabetics. After two years the patency rates were as follows: in iliac vessels, 91.7% in diabetics and 78% in nondiabetics; whereas in femoral vessels, 53.5% in diabetics and 85.4% in nondiabetics.

Patency rates analyzed according to the length of the lesion dilated are shown in Fig. 8 and 9. Iliac lesions longer than 5 cm were not analyzed because there were only 12 and most of these could not be dilated. Nine lesions longer than 10 cm were encountered in the femoral artery. Five of these could not be dilated and only two of the remaining four were patent up to 24 months. Only ten femoral lesions 5 to 10 cm long were available for analysis, but follow-up for most was 12 months or less. There was one death and no early failures in this group.

Comment

The introduction of the polyvinyl balloon dilation catheter by Gruntzig in 1974 marked the beginning of increased interest and use of PTA.[1] The flexible catheter allows the angiographer to approach and successfully dilate a wide variety of lesions throughout the arterial system. Initial reports of experience with PTA dealt primarily with technical aspects and were limited both in numbers of patients and length of follow-up.[2–8] Interpretations of these results are clouded, since aspects known to affect the treatment of arterial occlusive disease were not reported and different vessels and lesions were often analyzed together.

Since the beginning of our experience with PTA in 1978, we have attempted to record and follow up not only the results of dilations, but a wide variety of aspects that might influence the outcome. By so doing, we hoped to gain answers to the following questions.

Who Should Undergo PTA?

Our patient population, drawn from a large university vascular surgery practice, is similar to those described previously in reports of surgical treatment of aortoiliac and femoropopliteal occlusive disease.[12–18] The incidence of associated diseases and the age and sex distribution are within the standards given by most authors. The average age for the iliac group (58 years) is lower than might be expected.

Dilation has been accomplished with initial success in both those with claudication alone and those in danger of limb loss. The presence of rest pain, ischemic ulcers, or gangrene should not be considered a contraindication per se to PTA. When the severity of the disease is such that operative risk is increased, the decision should be weighted in favor of PTA, even when the vascular lesion is not necessarily a favorable one, ie, a long SFA occlusion with poor distal runoff.

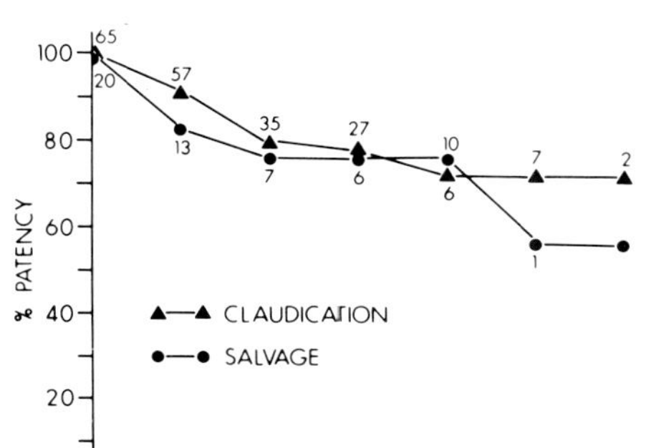

FIG. 5. Femoral artery patency: salvage vs claudication.

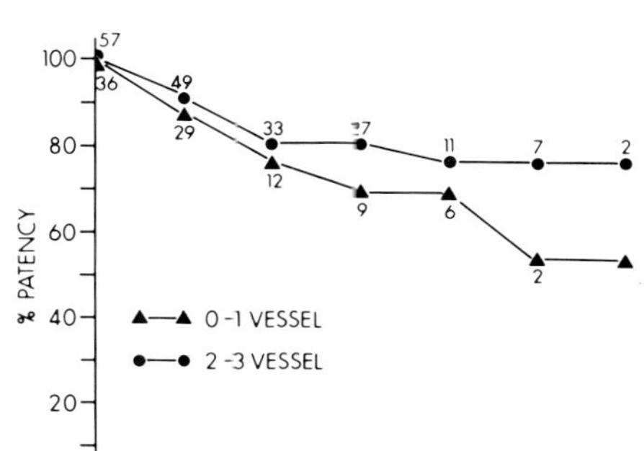

FIG. 6. Femoral artery patency: runoff.

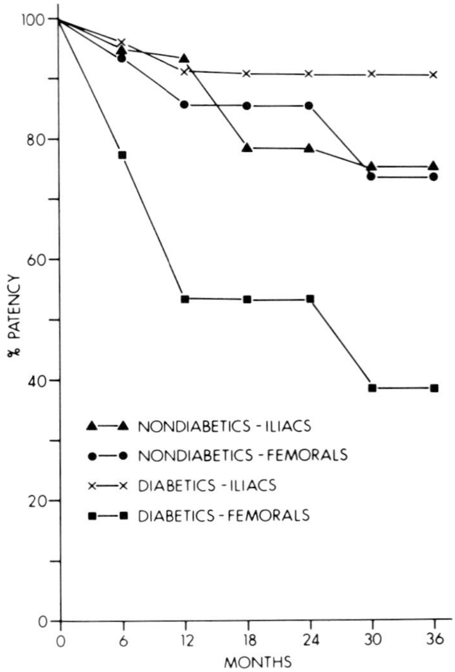

FIG. 7. Iliac and femoral artery patency: diabetes.

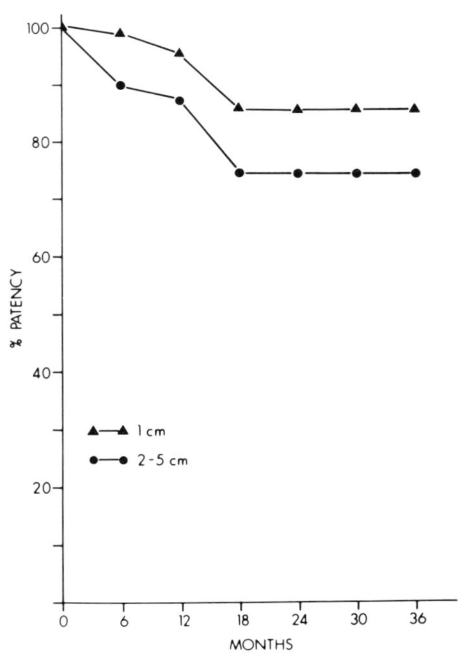

FIG. 8. Iliac artery patency: length of lesion.

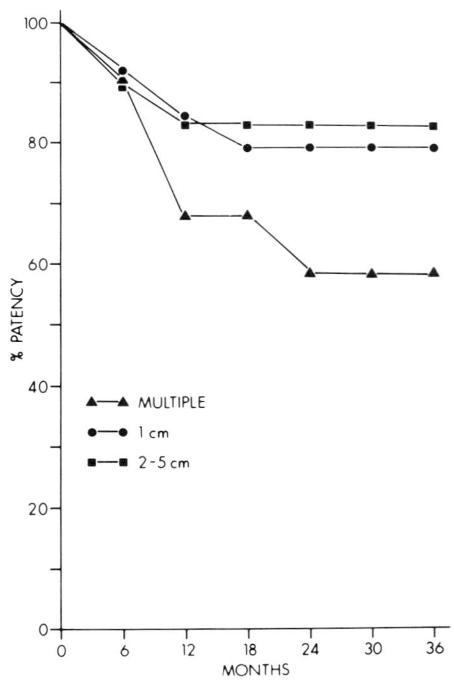

FIG. 9. Femoral artery patency: length of lesion.

Clinical criteria alone should not be the deciding factor in determining who should undergo PTA. Arteriography must be performed to obtain the information needed to decide for or against PTA. It seems, then, that all patients with aortoiliac and femoral occlusive disease should be considered potential candidates for PTA, at least until they have undergone arteriography.

Do Type and Extent of Lesion Influence Outcome of PTA?

Our poor results with dilation of stenoses longer than 10 cm, in both the iliac and femoral arteries, have made us hesitant to attempt PTA of such lesions. However, in the patient with such a lesion and with threatened loss of limb who is too sick to withstand an operation, PTA should be considered despite the high likelihood of failure. Because of a high rate of complications associated with dilation of totally occluded iliac vessels, we have in general abandoned this procedure. Lengthier, more extensive stenoses of both the iliac artery and SFA should be expected to respond less often than discrete, 1-cm lesions. Our results, as shown in Fig. 8 and 9, bear this out. There is no significant difference in results, however, between 1-cm and 2- to 5-cm stenoses in the femoral system. The difference in results between 1-cm and 2- to 5-cm stenoses in the iliac artery is approximately 10% after two and three years. Dilation of multiple lesions have surprisingly comparable early results, but these become significantly worse after one year.

The discrete, 1-cm common iliac stenosis responds very well to PTA and seems to stay open. Patency at one year and two years is the same 85.8%. Long-term patency appears to be inversely proportional to the length of stenosis. Two- to five-centimeter iliac lesions have a 74.6% patency rate two years after PTA. Stenoses longer than 5 cm have much poorer results, as do multiple stenoses. The same seems to hold true for the femoral system.

There is little difference between the long-term patency rates for 1-cm and 2- to 5-cm SFA stenoses, both being around 80%. Multiple lesions in the superficial femoral artery, however, do less well, with a 58.1% two-year patency rate.

Heavily calcified and tortuous, eccentric stenoses are difficult to dilate. Repeated inflations of the balloon may be needed to successfully dilate the former. Passage of the dilation catheter between the eccentric stenosis requires a skillful angiographer. It is, however, possible to treat both types of lesions by PTA.

We were somewhat surprised to find that the runoff status of distal vessels had little bearing on the outcome of the dilation procedure in both the femoral and iliac arteries. There is a slight, but not significant difference in results between good and poor runoff status, especially after two years, with decreased patency in the poor-runoff group.

Does Patient's Associated Disease State Influence Outcome of PTA?

The patient profile for our group is similar to that seen in patients who have undergone bypass surgery.[12–18] Direct comparison with patients who underwent femoropopliteal bypass grafting at our institution, as reported by Naji et al,[15,16] shows similar incidences of associated diseases, with the exception of a lower incidence of cardiac disease in our group.

Only the presence of diabetes seems to have a major influence on patency post-PTA. Our results with femoral PTA in the diabetic patient are significantly worse than those in the nondiabetic. This may be in part artifactual, since the numbers are small (28 diabetics and 46 nondiabetics) and, therefore, may be distorted by life-table analysis. Twelve of the diabetics had either ulcers or gangrene, and 15 had poor runoff vessels. Seventeen had either long (5 to 10 cm) or multiple lesions in the femoral artery—all factors that may have contributed to the poor long-term results. Markedly reduced rates of vein-graft patency in diabetics have been reported by some observers,[17,18] although such has not been our experience. Our results with PTA, however, suggest that diabetics do poorly after femoral artery dilation.

Do Indications for PTA Affect Outcome?

Most of our patients had symptoms of claudication: 86.3% in the iliac group and 71.4% in the femoral group. Patency rates after iliac PTA are much greater, especially after one year, if the procedure is performed for claudication rather than salvage. Once again, the number of patients dilated for salvage is small and not especially suitable for life-table analysis. The indication for dilation (claudication vs salvage) in the femoral artery seems to have little effect on long-term patency.

What Are the Complications of PTA?

We have seen 13 definite complications in all the patients who underwent PTA of the femoral and iliac vessels (roughly 4.6%), as follows: death from hypotension and CVA, one patient; stenosis converted to occlusion, six patients; transient renal failure due to dye overload, three patients; and distal embolization, vessel perforation, and bacterial endarteritis, one patient each. The most common problem was conversion of a stenotic lesion to an occlusion. When this occurred and clot formed in the vessel, the patency of the vessels distal to the lesion was not affected and, consequently, the level of distal anastomosis of subsequent grafts was not changed. Conversion of a stenosis to an occlusion did not jeopardize the patient's limb in any of these cases. The same surgical procedure, ie, aortic bifurcation or femoropopliteal bypass grafting, that would have been performed had the patient not undergone PTA, was performed in each case. Transient renal failure after what proved to be an excessive dye load was seen in three patients, none of whom required dialysis. By staging angiographic procedures and using limited amounts of contrast medium in patients known to have renal disease, this problem can be avoided.

The only patient who died had become hypotensive during an iliac PTA procedure, most likely secondary to a vagal response. The hypotension presumably was worsened by the hematoma that formed in his thigh at the arterial puncture site. He suffered a severe CVA that evening, during another hypotensive episode, and subsequently died. This is the only death we have seen that can be related to a complication of PTA. The mortality attributable to the procedure on the basis of this patient is 0.4%.

We chose early in our experience not to administer anticoagulants routinely to our patients after PTA. By so doing, we believe we have not jeopardized the long-term patency of the dilated vessel. Moreover, by so doing, we have minimized the number of complications seen with systemic anticoagulation, both in the immediate post-PTA period and long term.

When comparing PTA with surgery, one must look at not only patency rates, but also morbidity and mortality. The mortality directly attributable to PTA in our series was 0.4%, a figure that is very much less than the 4% average mortality reported for femoropopliteal surgery.[18] In addition, morbidity for dilation is low: 4.6%. There is no question that the length of hospital stay, recuperative period, and, ultimately, the cost to the patient are very much less with PTA. Our patency rates at one and two years for limbs treated with PTA are comparable with those given by Mehta for femoropopliteal grafts.[18] The fact that they are better than those reported in some series may reflect the small number of patients in the PTA group subjected to life-table analysis. However, with greater numbers and further time for study, we may find that the results change.

How Does PTA Compare to Surgery?

The initial success rate for iliac dilation is 95.9%. Patency rates for one and two years are 93.4% and 82.2%, respectively. Fifteen patients have been followed up for a minimum of three years, and have a patency rate of 79.4%. Brewster and Darling reported a five-year patency rate of 91% for their series of aortoiliac reconstructions.[13] Malone et al reported an immediate patency rate of 99.2% for aortofemoral grafts, with a 4% thrombosis rate each subsequent year.[12] Patency rates for iliac PTA after one year (93.4%) are comparable to those of Malone et al (94%) and only slightly less than those of Brewster and Darling (98%). With time, the failure rate of PTA seems to be higher than that seen with surgery. However, if one looks only at the 1-cm iliac stenotic lesions treated by PTA, the patency rate of 85.8% after three years is comparable with that achieved by Malone et al with surgery.[12]

We have two published series of operations from this institution of patients who underwent femoropopliteal bypass surgery for treatment of claudication[15] and limb salvage.[16] These earlier patients came from the same population as those who underwent PTA. A comparison of results at one, two, and three years, broken down by claudication and salvage, is given in Table 4. Also included in the comparison are figures obtained by Mehta in his review of saphenous vein bypass grafts performed for claudication in 894 limbs and for salvage in 1,420 limbs.[18] Results with PTA for treatment of claudication are not as good

TABLE 4. *Femoral Percutaneous Transluminal Angioplasty (PTA) vs Femoropopliteal Bypass: % Patency*

Years After Procedure	PTA	Bypass	
		Naji et al[15]	Mehta[18]
	Claudication		
1	79.5	86.3	86
2	72.9	81.9	81
3	72.9	79.5	77
	Salvage		
1	76.1	66.6	75
2	76.1	57.5	70
3	. . .	54.1	68

as those attained by femoropopliteal grafting. Taking these factors into consideration, PTA is an acceptable procedure for treatment of lower-extremity vascular disease.

We have two reasons for not considering restenosis of a dilated vessel as a failure. The majority of restenoses were in fact new areas of stenosis in the vessel previously treated. Some were adjacent to the dilated area, others were distinctly separate and, thus, truly new lesions. Since a femoropopliteal bypass graft that becomes stenotic and is successfully repaired is not generally considered a failed graft, by analogy a recurrent or new stenosis in a previously dilated vessel that is successfully treated by PTA is not considered a failure. The PTA procedure can be repeated, if necessary, without additional risk to the patient. If the initial dilation fails and stenosis recurs, successful redilation is the rule rather than the exception. Bypass surgery can be performed without increased risk to the patient if the dilated vessel ultimately occludes.

Having considered these questions, we have come to the following conclusions.

1. The PTA procedure is an effective means of treating certain types of occlusive vascular disease of the iliac and femoral arteries. It compares favorably with bypass surgery when all aspects are considered in this group of patients.
2. The PTA procedure can be used successfully to help patients with either claudication or threatened limb loss.
3. The PTA procedure is very useful in treating iliac lesions proximal to a planned femoropopliteal graft, thereby avoiding a second surgical procedure.
4. Isolated, discrete, short areas of stenosis in the iliac or femoral artery respond very well to treatment with PTA. We believe PTA is the treatment of choice for these lesions.
5. Totally occluded iliac vessels and stenoses of longer than 10 cm in the iliac and femoral vessels currently should not be dilated, except for limb salvage in a patient who is a major surgical risk.
6. Runoff status seems to have less influence on the success or failure of PTA than anticipated.
7. Most recurrent stenoses can be successfully redilated.
8. Diabetics who undergo dilation of femoral artery stenoses respond poorly, when compared with their nondiabetic peers.
9. Complications of PTA are minimal and generally below the range considered acceptable for surgery.
10. Long-term anticoagulation after PTA does not seem to be necessary to prevent progression of disease and vessel occlusion.

On the basis of our experience, we believe PTA is a definite advance in the therapy of many patients with obstructive peripheral vascular disease, and should be in the armamentarium of surgeons who treat such patients. To offer these patients the best possible care, it is imperative that the angiographer and the vascular surgeon cooperate completely. More than any other factor, this report reflects that cooperation, which we have been fortunate enough to foster and maintain.

REFERENCES

1. Gruntzig A, Hopff H. Perkutane rekanalixation chronischer Arterieller: Verschlusse mit einem nellen dilatation-skatheter Modification der Dottertechnik. Dtsch Med Wochenschr 1974;9:2502.
2. Katzen BT, Chang J, Knox WG. Percutaneous transluminal angioplasty with the Gruntzig balloon catheter. Arch Surg 1979;114:1389–1399.
3. Kalman PG, Colapinto RF, Harries-Jones EP. Preliminary results of transluminal dilatation in the treatment of peripheral arterial occlusive disease. Surg Gynecol Obstet 1980;150:865–868.
4. Van Andel G. Transluminal iliac angioplasty: Long-term results. Radiology 1980;135:607–611.
5. Bachman DM, Casarella WJ, Sos T. Percutaneous transluminal angioplasty via the contralateral femoral artery. Radiology 1979;130:617–621.
6. Motarjeme A, Keifer JW, Zuska AJ. Percutaneous transluminar angioplasty of the iliac arteries: 66 experiences. AJR 1980;135:937–944.
7. Waltman AC. Percutaneous transluminal angioplasty: Iliac and deep femoral arteries. AJR 1980;135:921–925.
8. Johnson KW, Colapinto RF, Harries-Jones EP. Transluminal dilatation in the treatment of peripheral arterial occlusive disease. Can J Surg 1980;23:547–548.
9. Alpert JR, Ring EJ, Freiman DB. Treatment of stenosis of the iliac artery by balloon catheter dilatation. Surg Gynecol Obstet 1980;150:481–485.
10. Cutler SJ, Ederer F. Maximum utilization of the life table method in analyzing survival. J Chronic Dis 1958;8:699–712.
11. O'Mara CS, Neiman HL, Flinn WR, et al. Hemodynamic assessment of transluminal angioplasty for lower extremity ischemia. Surgery 1981;89:106–117.
12. Malone JW, Moore WS, Goldstein J. The natural history of bilateral aortofemoral bypass grafts for ischemia of the lower extremities. Arch Surg 1975;110:1300–1306.
13. Brewster DC, Darling AC. Optimal methods of aortoiliac reconstruction. Surgery 1972;84:739–748.
14. Mulcare RT, Royster TS, Lynn RA. Long-term results of operative therapy for aortoiliac disease. Arch Surg 1978;113:601–604.
15. Naji A, Chu J, McCombs PR, et al. Results of 100 consecutive femoropopliteal vein grafts for limb salvage. Ann Surg 1978;188:162–165.
16. Naji A, Barker CF, Berkowitz HD, et al. Femoropopliteal vein grafts for claudication. Analysis of 100 consecutive cases. Ann Surg 1978;188:79–82.
17. Martin C, Foster JH. Femoropopliteal bypass grafts for salvage and claudication: A comparison of long-term results. South Med J 1976;69:420–423.
18. Mehta S. A Statistical Summary of the Results of Femoropopliteal Bypass Surgery. Newark, Del, WL Gore & Assoc Inc, 1980, pp 1–32.

DISCUSSION

W. GRAHAM KNOX, MD, New York: I certainly am encouraged by these conclusions gleaned from a now-significant number of procedures and, more importantly, with a much-needed, longer follow-up.

I and my colleagues first presented our experience at St Vincent's Hospital, New York, with 70 cases of balloon angioplasty at the national meeting of the Society two years ago. At that time, we had had an immediate good result in 35 of 37 iliac stenoses, 17 of 19 femoropopliteal stenoses, and 17 of 18 renal-artery stenoses. We hesitated then to wax too enthusiastic, because we only had a one-year follow-up in 30 of those 70 patients, and at that time PTA was a relatively unknown alternative to the more accepted methods of arterial reconstruction.

We have now performed 370 procedures, and the initial rate of success is 96% in the group of patients with iliac stenoses. Our angiographers, Dr Katzen and Dr Chang, have been loathe to perform procedures on complete iliac occlusions because they have encountered two instances of injury to the arterial wall that needed prompt surgical intervention. Of the femoropopliteal procedures, the initial success rate was approximately 90%; one third of these cases were of occlusion and two thirds of stenosis. Treatment of the renal arteries, in which there were five occlusions and five stenoses, had an immediate success rate of about 90%.

The long-term follow-up period now averages three years, with our longest follow-up being 4½ years. The cases, though few, have been personally evaluated with angiographic studies, as well as with clinical evaluation and Doppler flow recordings.

The drop in the number of patent vessels from the first year to the second in the iliac artery procedures has been from 97% to 91%. In the femoral artery procedures, the decrease in patency was greater, from 87% to 70%. The patency rate for renal angioplasties has stayed about the same, from 88% after one year to 85% after three years.

Our conclusions certainly mirror those of the Philadelphia group, and although we were hesitant in 1979, we are now much more enthusiastic for this technique.

I wish to emphasize the following: (1) This technique requires an expert angiographer. It is not to be performed casually by any radiologist. (2) Like the Philadelphia group, we also have complete and close cooperation between the vascular surgical team and the angiographers. Up to now there has been a constant complication rate of about 4% to 5%. Most complications do not require surgery and, to the best of my knowledge, not one balloon angioplastic procedure has been performed at St Vincent's Hospital without a member of the vascular surgical team being available in case something went wrong.

We are very encouraged with the results of this longer, three- to four-year follow-up. I believe PTA is here to stay.

MAKIS J. TSAPOGAS, MD, Stony Brook, NY: The authors are to be commended for the low incidence of complications related with this procedure and the highly satisfactory results they reported after their follow-up for two years or less.

I was interested to note that the main indication for treatment in the vast majority of their patients was relief of claudication. At the present time, our own criteria for applying this technique are rather stringent.

I wish to emphasize the point that Dr Knox has made: potential candidates for this procedure must be carefully evaluated by a cohesive and well-integrated team. This team should include our radiology colleagues who are fully trained in this area, and vascular surgeons. This joint effort should continue during and after the procedure, as well as the follow-up period. The role of each member should be clearly delineated beforehand. I believe that, at least at this stage of the development of the technique, the team approach is essential to obtaining optimum results.

I was interested to hear that the authors recommend this modality as an initial therapy in patients with peripheral vascular disease. I believe that it is rather early to reach such a conclusion, as this technique is relatively new. We have other well-established procedures that, if applied when the appropriate indications exist, produce reasonably satisfactory long-term results.

Since this procedure was first described, I have not been convinced that the term "angioplasty" is accurate. I suggest that this technique be called "percutaneous transluminal dilation" instead of "angioplasty." After all, this is what the procedure entails. The correct title may have significance beyond the bounds of terminology.

CHRISTOPHER K. ZARINS, MD, Chicago: Over the past three years, I and my colleagues have had experience with more than 120 transluminal angioplasty procedures at the University of Chicago. We used strict criteria of limiting claudication, rest pain, and gangrene, and have not treated cases of mild claudication. Thus, our patient population has more extensive disease than do the patients described by Dr Spence.

In a group of 75 patients, 31% had claudication and 69% had rest pain or gangrene. We considered an ankle pressure index increase of 0.15 or greater to be objective evidence of improved perfusion. Such an increase was seen in approximately 50% of our patients and did not depend on the clinical symptoms, length of segment dilated, or runoff vessel status.

We followed up with 40 patients who had a good clinical result and also had objective evidence of increased perfusion at monthly intervals, with repeated measurement of ankle and sequential pressure indices. All 40 had an increase in ankle pressure index of at least 0.15 and lessening of clinical symptoms after one week. After three months, 71% of the patients continued to have an increase in ankle pressure index of 0.1; after six months, this had decreased to 38% of patients, suggesting that restenosis develops rapidly in most patients. At five to six months, six patients underwent redilation procedures, five of which resulted in an increase in the ankle pressure index. If patients undergoing redilation are counted as displaying continued patency, then the conditions of 63% of the patients were improved after six months, using objective criteria. It is interesting to note that the clinical assessment of results was always better than the objective assessment using the ankle pressure index. This suggests that subjective clinical signs are inadequate measures of vessel patency and that the long-term results of PTA must be documented using objective measures.

This disparity between the clinical and objective assessment of results, can best be illustrated by an example. An active 51-year-old woman was greatly bothered by limiting right calf claudication due to a segmental occlusion of her SFA. Transluminal angioplasty restored vessel patency; her ankle pressure index increased from 0.15 to 1.0, and she was totally relieved of her symptoms. Her ankle index remained unchanged at 1.0 for the next five months, but decreased to 0.55 after six months, with disappearance of her popliteal pulse. She remained totally asymptomatic in that leg and continued to be pleased with the results of PTA on that side; however, she was walking shorter distances because of claudication in the left leg, had adjusted her life-style so that this was not an inconvenience to her, and was not interested in further therapy. I wish to ask Dr Spence how he would classify vessel patency in this patient in his results at six months. Is this a success or a failure? Is there patency or occlusion at six months?

We have also been interested in the mechanism of balloon dilation, and have studied dilation in cadaver SFAs under controlled conditions. In one test, involving a very large atherosclerotic plaque, balloon dilation was performed by fracture of the plaque at its thinnest point, dissection between the intima and the media, and separation of the plaque from the media, very much like an endarterectomy. Increase in lumen area resulted from stretching of media and adventitia, or possibly rupture of the media and containment of the bloodstream by the adentitia. There was no fragmentation of the plaque, which was probably why there is very little distal embolization, and there was no compression of the plaque. Recanalization of totally occluded segment was then performed by catheter dissection between the intimal plaque and the media, rupture of the media, and containment by the adventitia. Such a configuration may not be consistent with good long-term vessel patency.

We believe that PTA is an important therapeutic measure in patients with severe symptoms who are poor operative candidates. However, it should not be used in patients with mild symptoms, and long-term vessel patency will probably not be achieved in most patients.

KENNETH W. JOHNSTON, MD, Toronto: I and my colleagues at the Toronto General Hospital too have used objective criteria to determine the results of 249 dilations. We consider a dilation successful only if all of the following criteria improved: (1) the clinical status; (2) the arteriogram; (3) the pressure gradient measured across the stenosis; and (4) the results of vascular laboratory studies, predominantly Doppler.

Some of our results are less satisfactory than those reported by the authors, and our conclusions are somewhat different, especially when one examines the dilation by site. For 90 common iliac stenoses or occlusions, the accumulated percent success after one year was 86%, and after two years was 80%. Because of the low morbidity of transluminal dilation, we agree that it is a good alternative to surgery if the common iliac lesion is localized, and especially if it is unilateral.

Forty-five external iliac arteries were dilated. The long-term results are not satisfactory and, in general for this site, we do not regard dilation as a good alternative to operation unless the patient's general status is poor. We agree with the authors that the results of dilation of long common and external iliac lesions are not acceptable and probably should only be performed under unusual circumstances.

A total of 70 femoropopliteal procedures were carried out. Forty-four femoropopliteal stenoses were dilated; and at one year the cumulative success rate was 59% and at two years 40%. The results for 26 femoropopliteal occlusions were less satisfactory.

We compared the results of all 70 femoropopliteal dilations with the experience we reported at last year's meeting with 218 femoropopliteal grafts. The cumulative percent of patency for the saphenous vein grafts was 90% and 87% at one and two years, respectively, and in our hands, when a saphenous vein graft is available, we believe that operation clearly gives better long-term results than dilation. Our results for polytetrafluorethylene and umbilical vein grafts were approximately the same as that achieved by dilation.

However, our prosthetic grafts were carried out in patients with severe disease: 67% had rest pain and more than half had no runoff or only one-vessel runoff. Hence, even when a saphenous vein is not available, it is likely that operation gives better long-term results than dilation.

In summary, transluminal dilation is best regarded not as an alternative to operation, but as a form of therapy whose role lies between those of conservative therapy and operation. In our hands, except for isolated common iliac lesions, operation gives better long-term results than dilation.

JOHN L. GLOVER, MD, Indianapolis: When a procedure is as easy to perform as dilation and has such enthusiastic support, especially among angiographers, we must accumulate large amounts of data of the sort just presented to determine if the rate of success justifies the small but appreciable risk.

In our experience with 103 dilations in 70 patients, 15% were initial technical failures and about 30% had other complications: 15% technical (ie, subintimal dissection) and 5% each of hematoma, embolism, and unplanned, urgent operation. One of the problems with analyzing results such as these is that the definition of success varies and that it takes time to determine its durability. Of the 22 patients we observed for longer than six months, only five had sustained hemodynamic improvement, which was quite slight in one. One patient, however, has nearly normal findings two years later. I wish to ask Dr Spence if he is developing criteria to help us select the small group of patients who may obtain lasting improvement with impressively little morbidity.

JOHN J. BERGAN, MD, Chicago: Balloon dilation is with us and we must determine what the natural history of dilation is in each of the vascular beds that is treated. The discussion has brought out the fact that there are different natural histories of each of the vascular beds treated, and has been very valuable on this point.

At Northwestern University Medical Center, Chicago, 44% of femoropopliteal occlusive lesions that were successfully dilated showed restenosis or occlusion, even though the follow-up periods had a mean of 8.5 months. The conditions of many of these patients, as Dr Zarins has shown in his series, were clinically improved, although there was no hemodynamic change in the treated limb.

Dr Fogarty's instrument may allow intraoperative dilation. I stress that all of the observations made on the results of angioplasty, whether they are performed in the angiographic suite or the operating room, must be corroborated by hemodynamic measurements. It is not sufficient today, when we have sophisticated measuring techniques and have made marked advances in vascular surgery, merely to say that the patient is "better." We must have the data. Dr Zarins and Dr Johnston have shown that results based on the data are quite different from the impressions of the treating physicians.

It seems that Dr Spence did not consider need for redilation to be a failure of the procedure. Many of us believe that any need for reoperation is an acknowledged failure of the treatment. Therefore, we should be allowed to know a few things. How many patients who needed redilation were considered to have been treated successfully? Furthermore, as Dr Johnston and Dr Zarins have shown, what were the hemodynamic results of the treatments that were given?

DR SPENCE: Dr Knox, I and my colleagues agree with you that lesions that are completely occluded in both the iliac and the femoral arteries should not be dilated unless there is a threatened loss of limb in a high-risk patient. The numbers you saw with our initial success rate of 92.5% in the iliac artery reflect primarily the early patients who underwent dilation for just this reason, with occlusions of 10 cm or greater. The complication rate is just too high to do this routinely. I commend you on being able to obtain follow-up angiographic studies on all of your patients. We have not done this. We have not thought it necessary, unless, for the reasons I stated, we saw some diminution or change in either pulse or pulse-volume recording status.

Also, I agree that expert angiography and expert angiographers are needed for this procedure, and the cooperation between the vascular surgeons and the angiographers is the keynote for success in the use of percutaneous transluminal angioplasty.

Dr Tsapogas, you mentioned the team approach also, and I and my colleagues agree with you on this entirely. As to the question of "angioplasty" vs "percutaneous transluminal dilation," I believe Dr Szilagyi holds the copyright to the term "angioplasty" and has commented on that in the past. Until the final word on mechanism and what actually happens in the vessel is in, I will reserve the right, if you will, to use "angioplasty," because it is the term which is now in the literature and lessens the confusion.

Around the house we usually call it "the Gruntzig," but we should try to stay away from using eponyms.

Whether it is too early to go ahead and use this procedure routinely is as good a question and a difficult one to answer. Several points should be emphasized. We never said that this procedure is better than surgery. In fact, our results show that it is not. In the long run it may be as good in some areas, but we do not say that now. The major points, however, are two. One, this is a procedure with a very low morbidity and very low mortality. We have had only one death that we think is even indirectly related to the procedure. The length of the hospitalization, the cost to the patient, the discomfort, the recuperative period (one or two days) are all exceptionally low, compared to a femoropopliteal or aortic bifurcation graft. That is one major area where PTA is far better than surgery.

The second major point is that nothing is lost if percutaneous dilation is performed. If you dilate a lesion in the femoral artery and it fails, you can perform an operation that afternoon or the next day. We have had only four patients in the femoral group who have had stenoses converted to occlusions, and none of these have resulted in a more distal anastomosis on a femoropopliteal procedure that was performed afterwards. The same is true with iliac procedures. If you are careful in your dilation technique, you will not create emergent operative situations.

Dr Zarins, your results in the past with the treatment of patients with rest pain and severe claudication are outstanding and prove that this procedure can be used successfully in these patients. We have done this in both patients with claudication and salvage patients. As you saw, about 29% of our femoral procedures were performed for salvage.

Patency should be measured and determined strictly, as both you and Dr Bergan have stated, by objective criteria. We have not considered any patient who is clinically improved as displaying a successful dilation without objective measurement. The measurements we have used are the time-honored laying on of hands and feeling of the pulse that is now stronger, or is present when it was not there before. We followed this with pulse-volume recordings, and, following the work of Dr Bergan's group, we have adhered to an increase either in ankle index or, where this was not measurable in a patient with a gangrenous limb, thigh index pressures of greater than 0.15. By and large, we have seen changes of about 0.3 to 0.4 in the pressure indices.

Dr Johnston, I again emphasize this point, that we have used entirely objective criteria for measuring and following up our patients. The long stenotic lesion, as you say, should not be dilated except under extreme circumstances in a high-risk patient.

Dr Glover, our definition of success is as I have just mentioned. Initial failure was inability to dilate a lesion. Late failure occurring after 24 hours, generally, was diminution of pulse, decrease in pulse volume recordings, or change in angiographic appearance.

We have had patients, as I am sure all of you have had who have performed this procedure, who have been clinically improved, who have been converted from a rest-pain or threatened limb-loss status to a claudication status; this clinically is an improvement in our minds, although we will not say that this definitely constitutes patency of a vessel or success for the procedure.

Dr Bergan, our reasons for not considering a redilation a failure are several. One is that most of the redilations were in fact performed for new stenoses in areas other than the area previously dilated. Whether this has to do with some change in the vessel near the area that is dilated or not, I do not know. About two thirds of the redilations were for this specifically. Of the redilations, two thirds were successful. Some of them were in patients who were dilated three, four, or five times; this requires bringing a patient in, performing an angiogram, dilating the lesion, and sending him out in two days.

I cannot emphasize this point more strongly, that this is a very low-morbidity procedure. You lose nothing if you do it. You can go on to surgery if you wish. You cannot say it is as good as surgery. We do not say that. But what we do emphasize is that it can be performed, again, with no risk, and does not stop you from performing a surgical procedure afterwards.

Surgical Treatment of Abdominal Aortic Aneurysms With the Rigid Intraluminal Prosthesis

PASCHAL M. SPAGNA, M.D.

THE TECHNIQUE utilizing the rigid intraluminal prosthesis has been in use for the last 10 years. This article reports a series using the rigid intraluminal prosthesis for infradiaphragmatic aneurysms. The series includes 29 patients with abdominal aneurysms (including three ruptures). Survey time began in 1982 and is ongoing for 51 months. The mean long-term follow-up is 23 months. The patient age range was 55 to 83 years with a mean age of 67 years. The intraoperative mortality rate was zero; there were two in-hospital, early deaths from myocardial infarction at 3 and 14 days, respectively. There was one late death at 8 months from cancer. There were two thromboembolic complications immediately postoperatively, treated with no residuals. There have been no cases of pseudoaneurysm, spool dislodgement, or hemorrhage.

Since 1984 all patients have been followed with postoperative digital subtraction angiography (DSA) studies.

The author concludes that the rigid intraluminal prosthesis is a safe alternative treatment for abdominal aortic aneurysms with low morbidity and mortality.

From the Medical College of Pennsylvania, Philadelphia, Pennsylvania.

Plasma Sialidase Activity in Acute Myocardial Infarction

VICTOR A. HANSON, M.D., UDIPI R. SHETTIGAR, M.D., RAMESH R. LOUNGANI, M.D., AND MARY D. NADIJCKA, PH.D.

Increased plasma sialidase activity was demonstrated in 25 patients with acute myocardial infarction. Mean plasma sialic acid level after incubation with substrate neuramin lactose was 0.060 ± 0.003 (SEM) μmol/sample compared to 0.017 ± 0.003 in 24 patients without infarction ($P < 0.001$). The erythrocyte endothelial cell adhesion index was highest when both cell types were sialidase treated (0.35 *versus* control 0.00, $P < 0.05$). When sialidase (50 U/ml) was added to whole blood in plastic tubes the mean clotting time was 7.17 ± 1.0 (SD) minutes (n = 8) compared with a mean control of 15.45 ± 3.9 minutes ($P < 0.01$). Sialidase had no effect on prothrombin or partial thromboplastin times. The above studies suggest that increased plasma sialidase activity in patients with acute myocardial infarction may be associated with clumps of desialylated erythrocytes that may alter flow in the microcirculation.

THE PRESENCE OF SIALIC ACID on erythrocyte membranes invites speculation regarding its significance especially since this moiety is responsible for the erythrocyte's net negative surface charge.[1] In a study of the canine pulmonary microcirculation Hanson and associates established the importance of the erythrocyte surface charge in capillary blood flow by demonstrating that a reduction of surface charge was in fact accompanied by erythrocyte clumping and stasis.[2] A reduction of erythrocyte sialic acid and surface charge reported in patients with acute myocardial infarction, stroke, and deep vein thrombosis can be explained by the presence of inflammatory reactants with sialidase activity.[3–6] It is hypothesized that by removing sialic acid residues (responsible for the net negative surface charge) and thus eliminating forces of mutual repulsion of similarly charged membranes, plasma sialidase activity agglomerates the erythrocyte mass.[6] As observed in an animal model, this effect is most pronounced in the microcirculation where erythrocyte clumping is associated with diminished capillary perfusion.[2,3] This study (1) demonstrates increased plasma sialidase activity in acute myocardial infarction, (2) evaluates the role of sialidase erythrocyte–endothelial cell interaction, and (3) studies the effect of sialidase on whole blood clotting times *in vitro*.

Methods

Patients

After obtaining written informed consent from patients suspected of having an acute myocardial infarction within 72 hours of the onset of symptoms, blood was collected by venipuncture in heparinized tubes daily for the first week and then twice weekly until discharge.

The diagnosis of myocardial infarction was established by serial electrocardiograms (ECG) and enzyme determinations.[7] The patients in whom myocardial infarction was ruled out served as controls.

Test for Sialidase Activity

To 100 μl of test plasma (1 ml plasma diluted 1:10 with saline) was added 0.6 ml 15% $K_4Fe(CN)_6 \cdot 3H_2O$ and shaken for 30 seconds; 0.6 ml 30% $Zn(C_2H_3O_2)_2$ was added, shaken

From the Wilmington Veterans Administration Medical Center, Wilmington, Delaware, and Thomas Jefferson University, Philadelphia, Pennsylvania.

This article has been reproduced with permission from the *American Heart Journal*, Vol. 114, No. 1, 1987.

for 30 seconds, and centrifuged at 2400 rpm for 5 minutes; 0.2 ml of supernatant was removed and the thiobarbituric acid determination of Warren[8] was performed. The sialic acid level was compared with 100 μl of test plasma as defined and incubated with 1.0 mg of N-acetylneuramin-lactose and treated as above. The statistical significance of the results of plasma sialidase activity will be compared by the paired Student's t test.

Endothelial Cell Harvest and Culture

Patients who were undergoing abdominal exploration for a variety of reasons were requested to donate a segment of omentum (approximately 2 g). It has been shown that at least 5×10^6 endothelial cells can be obtained from 1 g of omentum.[9] The fat was minced and placed in 10 ml Hanks balanced salt solution (HBSS) without calcium (Ca^{++}) and magnesium (Mg^{++}) with collagenase (4 mg/ml) and bovine serum albumin (BSA) (4 mg/ml). The tissue was incubated with gentle agitation at 37°C for 30 minutes.

The resulting pellet was washed twice in HBSS containing 0.1% BSA and recentrifuged as described above. The final pellet was resuspended in 45% Percoll solution in Dulbecco's cation free buffer (pH 7.4) and centrifuged at $13{,}000 \times g$ for 20 minutes at 4°C. A similar tube of Percoll-containing density marker beads (1.048) were centrifuged simultaneously. The endothelial cell layer was verified by comparison with the density bead layer and harvested.[10] The cells were washed twice in HBSS-BSA solution, centrifuged for 3 minutes at $200 \times g$, resuspended in medium, and plated onto fibronectin coated tissue culture plates. Dulbecco's Modified Eagle Medium/Ham's F12 Nutrient Mixture (1:1) containing 20% FCS, 150 μg/ml endothelial cell growth factor (ECGF) and 100 μg/ml heparin was used as a growth medium for the primary culture. When confluent, the cells were passaged using 0.25% trypsin with 0.04% ethylenediamine tetraacetic acid (EDTA). Once primary cultures were passaged, the ECGF was reduced to 20 μg/ml.

Before being used in an experiment, the cells were verified as endothelial cells by labelling with Dil-Ac-LDL cell marker (Biomedical Technologies, Inc.). At the fourth passage the cells were plated into 35-mm culture dishes at a density of 1.5×10^5 per dish. Forty-eight hours later the confluent cultures were washed twice with HBSS. Fifty percent of the cultures were treated with sialidase (Vibrio cholerae neuraminidase, GIBCO Laboratories, Grand Island, NY) at a concentration of 50 U/ml HBSS. All cultures were incubated for 30 minutes at 37°C in 95% air, 5% carbon dioxide (CO_2) in a humidified incubator.

Human blood was drawn into a heparinized tube and centrifuged at 3800 rpm for 18 to 20 minutes and the erythrocytes were removed and washed twice with HBSS and 50% of their volume incubated with sialidase at a concentration of 50 U/ml for 30 minutes at 37°C. We have used this concentration to demonstrate erythrocyte agglomeration in animal models.[3] At the end of the incubation period both enzyme-treated cultures and untreated erythrocytes were washed twice with HBSS. Erythrocytes were diluted so that a 1-ml suspension was placed into each dish. Quadruplicates of the following experimental combinations were set up: sialidase-treated erythrocytes with untreated endothelium; untreated erythrocytes with sialidase treated endothelium; sialidase-treated erythrocytes with treated endothelium; and untreated erythrocytes with untreated endothelium. All sets were incubated for 30 minutes at 37°C. Each tissue culture plate was washed gently with HBSS five times to remove unattached erythrocytes. Erythrocytes collected from each plate were counted by a Coulter Counter (Coulter Electronics, Hialeah, FL). Before counting, sialidase-treated erythrocytes were washed in 10% dextran 40 (w/v in normal saline) in order to separate the agglomerated cells[3] thereby eliminating counting errors. Counts of the initial number of erythrocytes (both treated and untreated) added to the plates were used to normalize the raw data. Photomicrographs were taken of each plate.

Adhesion Index of Sialidase-Treated Erythrocytes and Endothelial Cells

An adhesion index was assigned by using the following formula:

$$AI = 1 - x_n/k$$

where x_n = the average number of erythrocytes in any one category and k = the average

TABLE 1. *Plasma Sialic Acid (μmol/Sample)*

Method	Group A (n = 25)	Group B (n = 24)
Plasma incubation	Acute myocardial infarction	No myocardial infarction
With substrate	0.060 ± 0.003	0.017 ± 0.003*
Without substrate	0.033 ± 0.006	0.010 ± 0.005

* Compared with Group A with substrate $P < 0.001$.

number of erythrocytes washed from the control plate (untreated endothelium and untreated erythrocytes). The results of this formula represents the relative number of erythrocytes that adhered to the monolayer.

Effect of Sialidase (Vibrio Cholerae Neuraminidase) on Whole Blood Clotting Times

A series of sialidase concentrations, (10–100 U, Gibco Laboratories) was added to 1 ml of whole blood in plastic tubes and incubated for 10 minutes at 37°C. The clotting time was determined using the method of White as follows[11]: (1) Blood was obtained by venipuncture using the "two-syringe technique," *i.e.*, after inserting the needle into a vein and withdrawing a few milliliters of blood, the first syringe disconnected and second clean, dry plastic syringe employed to draw the test sample. (2) Just before venipuncture, three clean Wasserman tubes (3-ml test tubes) were rinsed with saline. Immediately after drawing 5 ml of blood into the second syringe, 1 ml was placed in each tube and a timer started. The tubes were left undisturbed for the next 10 minutes. Then for the next 10 minutes, each tube was tipped to the horizontal at 30-second intervals. The formation of clot was evident when blood failed to flow down the side of the tube. Once the first tube had clotted, the second and third tubes were successfully tipped to obtain average time. One milliliter of blood without sialidase was incubated for 10 minutes at 37°C as a control. The difference between the mean experimental and control clotting times was compared using the paired Student's t test. Fifty units of sialidase were added to each of 10 tubes of citrated control plasma before prothrombin and partial thromboplastin time determinations.

Results

In 25 male patients with acute myocardial infarction (mean age, 60 years) the mean plasma sialic acid level after incubation with neuramin lactose was 0.060 ± 0.003 (SEM) μmol/sample. Before incubation with the substrate the mean plasma sialic acid level in those patients was 0.033 ± 0.006 μmol/sample. In 24 male patients in whom myocardial infarction was ruled out (mean age, 58 years) the mean plasma sialic acid level after incubation

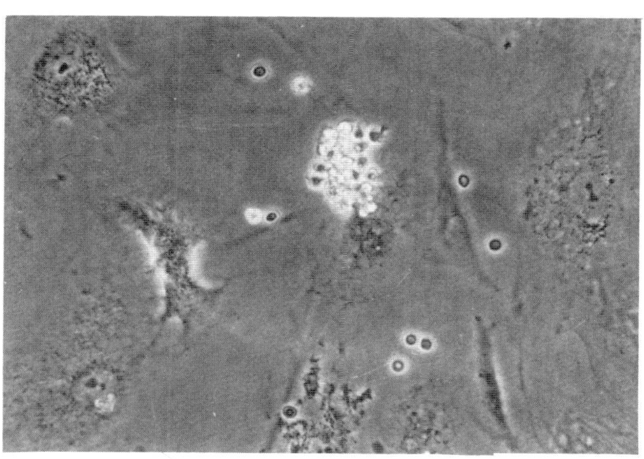

FIG. 1. Treated endothelial cell monolayer with sialidase-treated agglomerated erythrocytes (original magnification ×990).

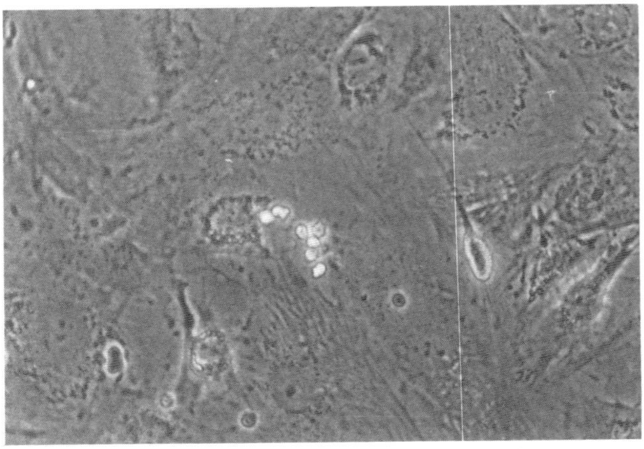

FIG. 2. Untreated endothelial cell monolayer with sialidase-treated agglomerated erythrocytes (original magnification ×990).

with neuramin lactose was 0.017 ± 0.003 μmol/sample. The difference between 0.060 ± 0.003 and 0.017 ± 0.003 is significant with a P value < 0.001. Before incubation with the substrate the mean plasma sialic acid level in this group was 0.010 ± 0.005 μmol/sample (Table 1).

Cellular Interaction in Tissue Culture

Erythrocyte clumping was present only in those experimental groups in which erythrocytes were sialidase treated (Figs. 1 and 2). Treatment of endothelial cells had no effect upon erythrocyte configuration.

Adhesion Index

Table 1 demonstrates the adhesion index, a ratio which expresses the number of erythrocytes which adhere to endothelial monolayer relative to the untreated control. It appears that sialidase treatment of erythrocytes enhances the adherence of erythrocytes to endothelium. However, a significant difference is made only when both erythrocytes and endothelium are enzyme treated. The paired Student's t test was used to compare the normalized values of erythrocytes washed from each plate of the experimental groups with the untreated control group. Only the doubly treated group differed significantly from the control group ($P < 0.05$) (Table 2).

TABLE 2. *Adhesion Index*

Untreated (−)/treated (+)		Adhesion index
Control		
EC	−	0
Erythrocytes	−	
Experimental groups		
EC	+	0.04
Erythrocytes	−	
EC	−	0.14
Erythrocytes	+	
EC	+	0.35*
Erythrocytes	+	

EC: endothelial cells.
* Compared to control data, $P < 0.05$.

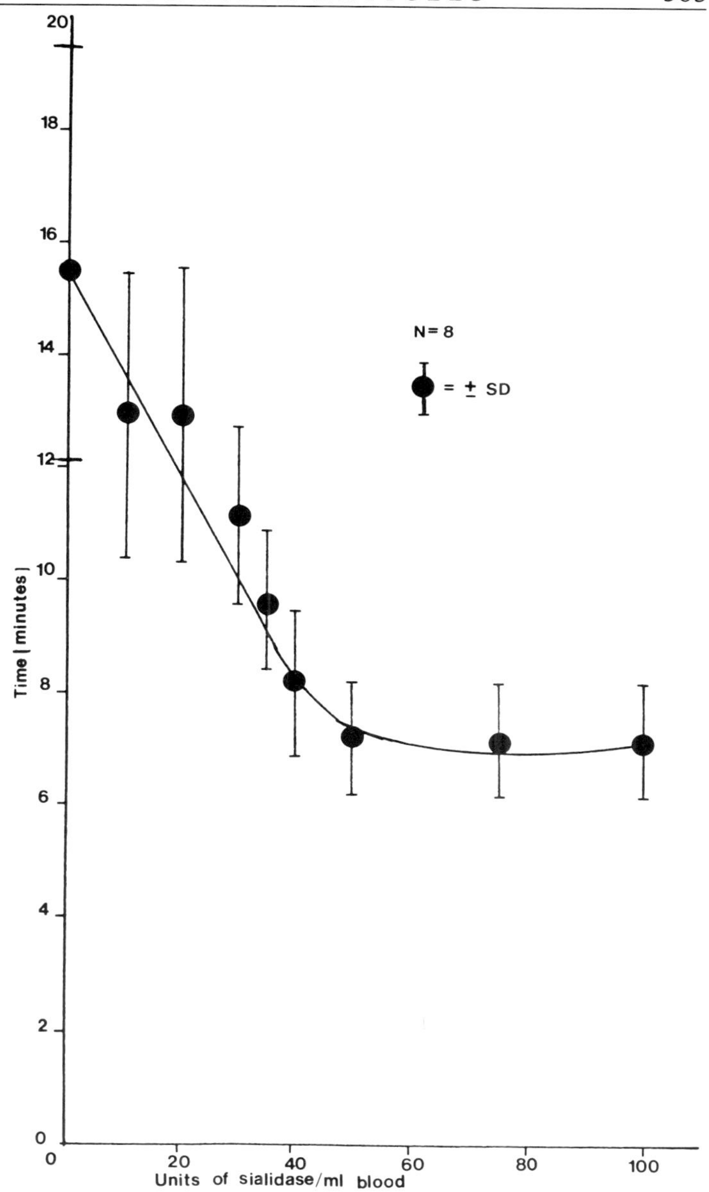

FIG. 3. Effect of sialidase on whole blood clotting time.

Effect of Sialidase on Whole Blood Clotting Time

Sialidase decreased whole blood clotting times in a dose dependent manner with a maximum effect at 50 U/ml (Fig. 3). When sialidase was added to whole blood at a concentration of 50 U/ml the mean clotting time decreased from 15.45 ± 3.9 (SD) minutes to 7.17 ± 1.0 minutes (n = 8) ($P < 0.01$) (Fig. 3).

Discussion

Although depletion of erythrocyte membrane sialic acid during acute myocardial infarction may be viewed as an epiphenomenon, the demonstration of obstructed flow in the microcirculation of the dog lung by clumps of desialylated erythrocytes seriously challenges this view.[3] In this experimental model erythrocyte aggregation occurred after intravenous administration of sialidase (neuraminidase). Similarly, the addition of sialidase to human blood in plastic tubes decreased clotting times in a dose dependent manner without affecting prothrombin or partial thromboplastin times, suggesting that any direct effect upon coagulation factors was indeed remote (Fig. 3). A sialidase concentration of 50 U/ml of whole blood probably results in maximum erythrocyte agglomeration as the flattened curve indicates.

In tissue culture the sialidase-treated erythrocytes clumped in the presence of nontreated endothelial cells (Fig. 2). Since this change in cell–cell interaction occurred in the absence of plasma proteins, one can more readily attribute this to a reduction of electrostatic forces rather than a protein-mediated mechanism. However, the purpose of this study is not to challenge the established role of plasma proteins in erythrocyte aggregation, but rather to demonstrate an additional mechanism of erythrocyte agglomeration. When both erythrocyte and endothelial cells were treated with neuraminidase, the clumped erythrocytes adhered to the endothelial cells. In view of the exceedingly complex nature of the endothelial glycocalyx, interpretation of sialic acid-depleted erythrocytes interacting with desialylated endothelial cells precludes an explanation limited only to a consideration of surface charge alone. The absence of erythrocyte aggregation when only the endothelial cells were treated with sialidase was observed and suggests that a desialylated endothelial glycocalyx has essentially no influence on erythrocyte interaction when the erythrocyte glycocalyx is in tact. However, disruption of both erythrocyte and endothelial cell glycocalyx is associated with maximum, "stickiness" as demonstrated by the adhesion index.

Increased plasma sialidase activity probably contributes to the hypercoagulable state by agglomerating the erythrocyte mass. If in fact desialylated erythrocytes in the human behave like our animal models, perfusion defects resulting from erythrocyte clumping and stasis in the microcirculation may be anticipated.

REFERENCES

1. Eylar E, Madoff M, Brody O, Oncley J. The contribution of sialic acid to surface charge of the erythrocyte. J Biol Chem 1962;237:1992.
2. Hanson V, Wax S, Webb W. Role of the erythrocyte surface charge in the microcirculation. In: Grayson J, and Zingg W, eds. Microcirculation, vol. 1. New York: Plenum Publishing, 1976.
3. Hanson V, Landaw S, Flashner M, Wax S, Webb W. Sialic acid-depleted red cells following acute myocardial infarction. Am Heart J 1980;99:483.
4. Chien S, Cooper G, Jan K *et al.* N-acetylneuraminic acid deficiency in erythrocyte membranes: biophysical and biochemical correlates. Blood 1974;43:444.
5. Resnitsky P, Yaari A, Danon D. Biophysical characteristics of erythrocytes during acute myocardial infarction and venous thrombosis. Thromb Diathes Haemorrh 1972;28:425.
6. Gottschalk A. Glycoproteins. Essex: Elsevier Science Publishers, 1972:381.
7. Report of the Joint International Society and Federation of Cardiology WHO Task Force: Nomenclature and criteria for diagnosis of Ischemic heart disease. Circulation 1979;59:607.
8. Warren L. The thiobarbituric acid assay of sialic acid. J Biol Chem 1971;234:1959.
9. Personal communication, 1987.
10. Marks R, Czerniecki M, Penny R. Human dermal microvascular endothelial cells: An improved method for tissue culture and a description of some singular properties in culture. In Vitro Cell Dev Biol 1985;21:627.
11. Wolf PL. Practical clinical hematology interpretations and techniques. New York: John Wiley and Sons, 1973:55.

Preliminary Characterization of the Procoagulant Material in Human Ascites

V. PAUL ADDONIZIO, JR., M.D.,* AND WILLIAM Y. INOUYE, M.D.†

PERITONEAL–VENOUS (LEVEEN) SHUNTS are used in the treatment of ascites refractory to medical therapy.[1] Although these shunts are considered to be relatively safe, it is recognized that laboratory evidence consistent with disseminated intravascular coagulation (DIC) invariably occurs after shunt placement. In the current study, we isolate the procoagulant material in human ascites, demonstrate its presence in the cellular and fluid fractions, and, on the basis of its substrate requirements, that it is indeed tissue thromboplastin.

Materials and Methods

Approximately 500 ml of ascitic fluid were removed percutaneously from 11 patients with intractable ascites of varied etiology.

Leukocytes were isolated from ascitic fluid by isopycnic centrifugation through Hypaque-Ficoll (Litton Bionetics, Kensington, MD) as described by Rivers *et al.*[2] The ascites fractions were assayed for procoagulant activity (PCA) in a one-stage clotting time assay. The contribution of the protein component of a high-speed precipitate was evaluated by boiling the material to 100°C for 2 minutes before performing the coagulation assays, and the importance of the lipid component was evaluated by incubating the high-speed precipitate for 15 minutes with phospholipase C, 40 μg/ml (Type III from *Bacillus cereus*, Sigma Chemical Co., St. Louis, MO).

Aliquots of high-speed centrifugation pellets were extracted with 20 volumes of chloroform/methanol (2:1 vol/vol). The organic phase was dried under nitrogen and the residue taken for analysis of phospholipid phosphorus and cholesterol, and for thin-layer chromatographic qualitative analysis of phospholipids. Phospholipid phosphorus was determined by the method of Bartlett[3] and cholesterol by the method of Rudel and Morris.[4] Phospholipids were separated on Whatman K5 plates (Whatman International, Ltd., Maidstone, England) as described by Touchstone *et al.*[5] Protein was quantified by the method of Bradford.[6]

Data were analyzed for significant differences using Dunnett's test for comparing multiple treatment groups to a single control group. A P level at <0.01 was considered to be significant.

Results

Native, unfractionated ascites and all fractions prepared from ascites shortened significantly the clotting time of pooled plasma ($P < 0.01$) relative to controls incubated with saline. Ascitic cells and the high-speed precipitate were most effective, shortening the mean clotting time from 260 seconds to 81 and 124 seconds, respectively. The low-speed supernatant reduced the mean clotting time to 160 seconds. The PCA of the high-speed supernatant was similar (mean clotting time, 166 seconds) to that of the low-speed supernatant.

Native unfractionated ascites and all fractions of the ascitic fluid dramatically ($P < 0.01$) reduced the clotting time of Factor VIII-deficient plasma. Again, the ascitic cells and high-

From the University of Pennsylvania School of Medicine, Department of Surgery, Philadelphia, Pennsylvania.

† Dr. Inouye, role model and source of inspiration for surgical house staff from 1961 to 1985, passed away on July 20, 1985. This work is a small tribute to a career of sustained and unparalleled productivity.

* Dr. Addonizio is the recipient of a National Institutes of Health Young Investigators Award HL22346 and a Hartford Foundation Scholarship.

Excerpted from: Addonizio *et al.* Preliminary characterization of the procoagulant material in human ascites. Surgery 1987;101:753–762.

speed pellet were most effective. As observed with pooled normal plasma, ultracentrifugation of the low-speed supernatant resulted in reduced activity of the supernatant solution.

Native unfractionated, as well as all ascitic fractions, failed to shorten the clotting time of Factor VII-deficient plasma. Interestingly, both the low-speed and high-speed supernatant solutions of ascitic fluid lengthened the clotting time of Factor VII-deficient plasma from 100 seconds to 139 and 156 seconds ($P < 0.01$), respectively.

When ascitic cells from two patients were resuspended in buffer, their ability to shorten the clotting time of pooled normal plasma was found to vary directly with the concentration of cells. Beyond 10^7 cells/ml, however, increasing the concentration of cells failed to further alter the clotting time.

Sterol, phospholipid, and phospholipid/sterol ratios were determined. For two patients these were 393 and 488; and 29 and 44 with a phospholipid/sterol ratio of 1.1:1.00 and 1.0:0.89, respectively. Thus, the high-speed pellet of ascitic fluid contained protein, sterol and phospholipid with the predominant polar lipids being lecithin and sphingomyelin, with a lesser quantity of phosphatidylethanolamine. The mean molar ratio of phospholipid to sterol was 1:0.95, which is characteristic of plasma membranes.[7]

The PCA of both the high-speed pellet and our thromboplastin standard was inhibited by heating to 100°C for 2 minutes. Incubating either the high-speed pellet or the tissue factor (TF) standard with phospholipase C for 15 minutes also abrogated the PCA of either preparation. Phospholipase C alone had no effect on observed clotting times (273 seconds with saline *versus* 271 seconds with phospholipase C).

Discussion

The coagulation abnormalities which accompany peritoneal–venous shunting have been well-characterized and include decreased levels of platelets, Factors II, V, VII and X, and fibrinogen with a concomitant rise in plasma levels of fibrin split products.[8] These changes often are reflected in prolonged prothrombin and partial thromboplastin times. Although the exact incidence of overt disseminated intravascular coagulation in this group of patients is difficult to assess because of the presence of underlying liver disease, it is estimated that approximately one third of patients will manifest clinically significant coagulopathy after shunt placement. Virtually all patients will have changes in laboratory tests of clotting. The precise pathophysiology of the coagulopathy is unknown, but various mechanisms have been proposed including bacterial sepsis, absorption of bacterial endotoxin without bacterial sepsis, transfer of nonspecific cellular procoagulant factors, and/or transfer of thrombin, fibrin split products and plasmin.[9] Evidence for the first hypothesis, however, actually is scant in that the presence of bacteria in ascitic fluid has not correlated with induction of hemostatic changes.

The studies reported here indicate that ascitic fluid procoagulant material is present in both the cellular and fluid components of ascitic fluid. Peritoneal macrophages are known to possess the potent procoagulant tissue factor but generally do not express PCA unless stimulated *in vitro* or *in vivo*.[10] Furthermore, although induction of this procoagulant in human monocytes *in vitro* may occur as quickly as 2 hours after stimulation with endotoxin,[11] spontaneous PCA generation (*e.g.*, present *de novo* after isolation of the cells) occurs rarely. However, the ascitic cellular fraction from each patient tested demonstrated procoagulant properties immediately, accelerating the coagulation time of pooled normal plasma to a degree not present (unpublished observations) or expected in circulating leukocytes. Since the procoagulant properties of ascitic cells was present initially, it is unlikely that endotoxin contamination on laboratory plasticware was responsible for the results observed.[11] The factor or factors responsible for the production of this procoagulant activity in ascitic cells are unknown, but it is conceivable that a small amount of endotoxin present in ascitic fluid could serve as the activating agent.

Clearly, a portion of the procoagulant material in the initial fluid phase of the ascites exists in suspension and can be sedimented only by high-speed centrifugation. Peritoneal macrophages activated by endotoxin are known to release into the suspending medium fragments of membrane capable of accelerating coagulation principally through extrinsic pathways of coagulation.[11] Recent studies of tumor cells[12] and human monocytes (Rickles *et al.*, unpublished observations) in tissue culture have revealed the presence of similar membrane vesicles with the properties of tissue factor. Indeed, membrane-bound vesicles were observed in our high-speed pellets. In addition, the procoagulant material precipitated from ascitic fluid is composed of phospholipid, cholesterol, and protein in proportions which suggest a plasma membrane origin.[10] Furthermore, this ascitic material has the characteristics of tissue factor. Like tissue factor, the active component is destroyed by boiling and/or phospholipase C treatment indicating that both the protein and phospholipid components are essential for activity.[13] Like tissue factor, the ascitic material also is dependent upon Factor VII for expression of PCA.[13] It is of interest that the procoagulant properties of the purified apoprotein of tissue factor can be reconstituted with phosphatidylethanolamine,[13] a phospholipid present in excess in our high-speed pellet.

It is tempting to suggest that these findings should have a significant clinical impact. One obvious recommendation is that ascites present at the time of exploration be discarded. It would then be interesting to determine the rate of appearance of procoagulant material in newly formed ascites. A second alternative would be to add a filter to peritoneal–venous shunts. The procoagulant material is sedimentable and therefore should be filterable. Of course, the most important clinical impact of this work is the insights it provides for analogous clinical situations; for example, the thrombotic proclivity which can accompany disseminated malignancies.

REFERENCES

1. Epstein M. Peritoneal venous shunt in the management of ascites and the hepatorenal syndrome. Gastroenterology 1982;82:790–799.
2. Rivers RPA, Hathaway WE, Weston L. The endotoxin-induced coagulant activity of human monocytes. Br J Haematol 1975;30:311–316.
3. Bartlett GR. Phosphorus assay column chromatography. J Biol Chem 1959;234:466–468.
4. Rudel LL, Morris MD. Determination of cholesterol using opthalaldehyde. J Lipid Res 1973;14:364–366.
5. Touchstone JC, Chen JC, Beaver KM. Improved separation of phospholipids in thin layer chromatography. Lipids 1980;15:61–62.
6. Bradford MM. A rapid and sensitive method for the quantification of microgram quantities of protein utilizing the principle of protein-dye binding. Anal Biochem 1976;72:248–254.
7. Rouser G, Nelson GJ, Fleischer S, Simon G. Biological membranes: Physical, fact, function. In: Chapman D, ed. Lipid Composition of Animal Cell Membranes, Organelles and Organs. London: Academic Press, 1968;5.
8. Tawes RL, Rydorak GR, Kennedy PA *et al.* Coagulopathy associated with peritoneovenous shunting. Am J Surg 1981;142:51–55.
9. Phillips LL, Rodgers TB. Procoagulant activity of ascitic fluid in hepatic cirrhosis *in vivo* and *in vitro.* Surgery 1979;86:714–717.
10. Wapnick S, Merskey C, Doebbler TK, Johnson AJ, Owen T, Gliedman ML. Fibrinogen, crossbinded fibrin and their proteolysis products in ascitic fluid. Surg Forum 1982;33:181–82.
11. Niemetz T. Coagulant activity of leukocytes. J Clin Invest 1972;51:307–313.
12. Dvorak HF, Quay SC, Orenstein NS *et al.* Tumor shedding and coagulation. Science 1981;212:923–924.
13. Testy T, Maynard JR, Radcliffe RD, Silverberg JA, Pitlick FA, Nemerson Y. Initiation and control of the extrinsic pathway of blood coagulation in proteases and biological control. Reich E, Rifkin DB, Sheno E, eds. Cold Spring Harbor, NY: Cold Spring Harbor Laboratory, 1975;171.

Review of a Community Hospital Experience With Carotid Endarterectomy

LYDIA G. SLAVISH, B.S., GARY G. NICHOLAS, M.D., F.A.C.S., AND WILLIAM GEE, M.D., F.A.C.S.

Carotid endarterectomy was performed 743 times during 56 months in a community hospital by 24 surgeons. The mortality rate was 2.7% and permanent stroke occurred in 1.8%. Temporary postoperative neurologic deficit occurred in 3.5%. The frequency with which the surgeon performed the procedure did not appear significant in the incidence of postoperative morbidity and mortality.

REPAIR OF CAROTID ARTERY BIFURCATION atherosclerosis was first described in 1954 and two major reviews, in 1968 and 1970, provided the impetus for broad acceptance and application of this procedure.[1-3] Recent reports in the medical literature have presented conflicting information regarding the results of carotid endarterectomy in community hospitals. Carmichael reported a series of 467 carotid endarterectomies performed in a community hospital and found a combined permanent stroke/mortality rate of 2.2%.[4] The combined experience of 11 surgeons in two community hospitals reported by Easton noted a permanent stroke/mortality rate of 21.1%.[5] Coincident to the latter report, a prospective evaluation of all carotid endarterectomies performed at the Lehigh Valley Hospital Center was instituted. The purpose of this study was to test the hypothesis: Carotid endarterectomy can be performed safely in a community hospital. The study began on September 1, 1977, and terminated on May 1, 1982 (56 months).

Methods

Carotid endarterectomy was performed on 743 occasions in the 56-month interval. Twenty-four surgeons performed these procedures. The operations were conducted under general anesthesia and inlying shunts were used. Carotid stump pressures were measured sporadically and electroencephalogram monitoring was not done. All patients were evaluated preoperatively by the surgeon as well as a neurologist or general internist. The patients were also evaluated using noninvasive vascular laboratory techniques.

Each patient underwent ocular pneumoplethysmography (OPG-Gee) on three occasions. At the time of the preoperative test, vascular laboratory personnel reviewed the patient record and pertinent neurologic history and physical findings were noted on the vascular laboratory report. An immediate postoperative OPG was performed in the recovery room. The neurologic status of the patient at that time was recorded on the recovery room OPG report. A physician was available for immediate interpretation of all recovery room OPG tests. The results of any test which suggested thrombosis or serious lumen compromise of the endarterectomy site were communicated immediately by the physician interpreting the test directly to the surgeon. The OPG was again repeated prior to the hospital discharge of the patient, usually the fourth postoperative day. All arteriograms were reviewed jointly by the physician director of the vascular laboratory and the radiologist.

Results

The patients undergoing carotid endarterectomy ranged in age from 40–81 years. The mean age was 65 years. There were 468 males (63%) and 275 females (37%). In 684 cases

From the Department of Surgery, The Milton S. Hershey Center, The Pennsylvania State University, and the Department of Surgery, Lehigh Valley Hospital Center, Allentown, Pennsylvania.

Received May 9, 1983; revision #2 accepted February 10, 1984.

This article has been reproduced by permission of The American Heart Association, Inc, from *Stroke*, Vol. 15, No. 6, November–December 1984.

the endarterectomy was performed as the primary procedure and in 59 cases the carotid surgery was done concomitantly with coronary artery bypass grafting.

The operative procedures were performed by 24 surgeons. The frequency with which they performed carotid endarterectomy in the 56 months studied varied from one to 219 operations. The mean was 31. All of the 24 surgeons were board certified. There were 12 thoracic surgeons, four neurosurgeons, and eight general vascular surgeons. All the general vascular surgeons had completed formal training programs in vascular surgery. All the surgeons were members of the division of vascular surgery and privileges to perform carotid endarterectomy were granted by the department of general surgery after reviewing the applicant's credentials.

Of the 743 procedures, 553 (74%) were performed for symptoms referable to the operated artery. There were 190 procedures performed on asymptomatic lesions. Of the latter group, 146 (77%) lesions were of hemodynamic consequence, as demonstrated by OPG. Thus, 94% of the carotid endarterectomies were performed for symptomatic disease or lesions of hemodynamic consequence. There was no morbidity or mortality associated with the 44 procedures on hemodynamically inconsequential asymptomatic lesions. These were usually lesions noted in patients who had undergone contralateral endarterectomy or were detected in patients prior to other major surgery.

A new neurologic deficit was noted postoperatively in 39 patients (5.3%). Deficits were temporary in 26 (3.5%) and permanent in 13 (1.8%). A deficit was considered temporary if the symptoms resolved within 30 days following surgery. There were 20 deaths in the series of 743 carotid endarterectomies (2.7%). Fifteen of these were attributed to neurologic causes and five were cardiac related. Thus, the permanent stroke/mortality rate was 33/743 (4.4%). Two of the cardiac related deaths occurred in the group of 59 patients who underwent combined coronary bypass grafting and carotid endarterectomy. None of the patients in this subgroup suffered either a temporary or permanent neurologic deficit. Of the 190 asymptomatic patients operated upon, five or 2.6% incurred stroke or death.

The sensitivity and specificity of the OPG-Gee in detecting hemodynamically significant lesions is well documented.[8] There were 42 patients in whom the OPG was considered equivocal. These 42 patients had preoperative OPG tests which suggested, but were not diagnostic of, unilateral carotid stenoses of pressure-significance (75% or greater, cross-sectional area), since the reduction of the ophthalmic systolic pressure on the side of the suspected stenosis was not at least 5 torr as required by the standard criteria for a positive OPG. All of the 42 patients were noted to have a reduction of calibrated ocular pulse amplitude on the side of the suspected stenosis to less than 30% of that noted on the opposite side. In all of these 42 patients arteriography and operative findings confirmed severe stenoses. This additional criterion has been formalized in a recent report.[9] By incorporating this new criterion with the standard criteria, the 42 tests were considered true-positive studies.

Ocular pneumoplethysmography was positive in 40/743 (5.4%) of the recovery room tests. On the fourth postoperative day 60/743 (8%) were positive and indicated thrombosis or persistence of a lesion of hemodynamic consequence. There were 15 strokes among these 60 patients, and ten of them were fatal.

The incidence of temporary neurologic deficit, permanent stroke, and death was examined with respect to the frequency with which the operation was performed by the surgeon. Figure 1 illustrates the relationship of postoperative permanent strokes plus mortality to the frequency with which the surgeon performed carotid endarterectomy. This relationship fits a straight line with a correlation coefficient of 0.93.

Table 1 tabulates the results when subdivided by the number of procedures the surgeon performed. Four of the 24 surgeons performed 456 of the procedures. There were 20 strokes (4.4%) and 11 of the 20 were fatal. There was one cardiac death, without associated brain injury. The nonfatal stroke was 9/456 (2.0%) and the mortality was 12/456 (2.6%). The combined stroke/mortality rate was 4.6%. Temporary postoperative neurologic deficit included those associated with operative manipulation of cranial nerves, transient exacerbation of preoperative neurologic deficits, and all new transient neurologic deficits. Transient symptoms or deficits were noted following 19 of the procedures (4.2%).

The remaining 20 surgeons performed 287 procedures. Temporary neurologic deficits were noted following seven procedures (2.4%). There were eight strokes (2.8%), and four of the eight were fatal. There were four cardiac deaths without associated brain injury. The nonfatal stroke rate was 4/287 (1.4%) and the mortality rate was 8/287 (2.8%). The combined stroke/mortality rate was 4.2%. There was no significant difference between the two groups in any of the measured parameters. Even if one compares the group of 13 surgeons who did 10 or fewer cases in the 56 months of the study to those 11 who did more than 10 carotid endarterectomies, no statistically significant differences could be demonstrated in morbidity or mortality.

Discussion

The age range and sex distribution of the 743 patients in this series is similar to that reported by others. Thompson noted a mean age in his series of 63.1 years and DeWeese reported an age range in 46–80 years.[2,3] A preponderance of males is noted by most authors being 65–67% of each of the above reports, respectively. The current series does differ somewhat in that it includes 59 patients who underwent coronary bypass grafting and carotid endarterectomy as a combination procedure. In this subgroup there were two deaths (3.4%) and no permanent neurologic deficits.

For the entire series the mortality rate (2.7%), the permanent stroke rate (1.8%), and the temporary neurologic deficit (3.5%) were similar to numerous other reports.[2,3] The overall permanent stroke/mortality rate in our series was 4.4%. This finding from a community hospital is markedly different from the 21.1% permanent stroke/death rate reported by Easton.[5] Part of this difference may be explained by the fact that of the 228 carotid operations reported by Easton only 25% were done for ipsilateral TIAs and only 56% were done for ipsilateral TIAs or mild strokes. In an abstract reviewing the more recent experience at that same community hospital, the combined stroke/mortality rate in 474 operations was 4.4%.[6] These dramatically improved results were attributed to better patient management. In a similar turnabout, West et al reported a decrease in the permanent stroke/mortality rate from 10% (1967–70) to 0.9% (1971–75). They felt their improved results were due to not only better patient management, but also to improved surgical technique, and recommended careful consideration of the surgeon as well as the institution before recommending surgery.[7]

Selection of patients for surgery followed an evaluation similar to that recommended by Sandok et al.[10] Symptoms (transient ischemic attack or stroke) were referable to the operated carotid artery in 74.4% of the patients. In the 190 asymptomatic patients, noninvasive studies (OPG-Gee) indicated a hemodynamically significant lesion in 76.8% and this was confirmed angiographically. Postoperatively, permanent stroke or death occurred in 2.6% of this subgroup. Other series report 10–46% of patients operated upon for asymptomatic lesions or symptoms not directly attributable to the operated carotid artery.[2,5] Long-term follow-up of the 743 operations was varied because of the large number of surgeons involved in the study. Most of the patients have been seen at six month intervals and non-invasive testing performed.

The OPG was positive in 5.4% of the recovery room tests and 8.1% of the tests performed in the fourth postoperative day. These results are similar to the data reported by Ortega et al.[11] In contrast to Ortega's data obtained from the experience of three surgeons in one group who accepted immediate reexploration when the OPG was abnormal in the recovery room, the data from the study included an additional 21 surgeons, a number of whom had not adopted this policy. This may be the reason for the increase in the fourth postoperative day positive OPG tests since asymptomatic occlusions were not diagnosed or treated immediately postoperatively. It is clearly a difficult decision to return the asymptomatic patient to the operating room following carotid endarterectomy.

If the OPG was found to be positive in the recovery room the result was communicated immediately to the surgeon. At the discretion of the surgeon the patient was returned immediately to the operating room and the endarterectomy site explored. Evaluation included digital palpation of a thrill or pulse gradient across the repair, Doppler ultrasound for the presence and quality of flow, operative angiography, and repeat arteriotomy to correct any defect (distal flap, thrombosis, narrowing) found. The results of this method of management are presented in detail elsewhere and are beyond the purpose of this presentation.[10]

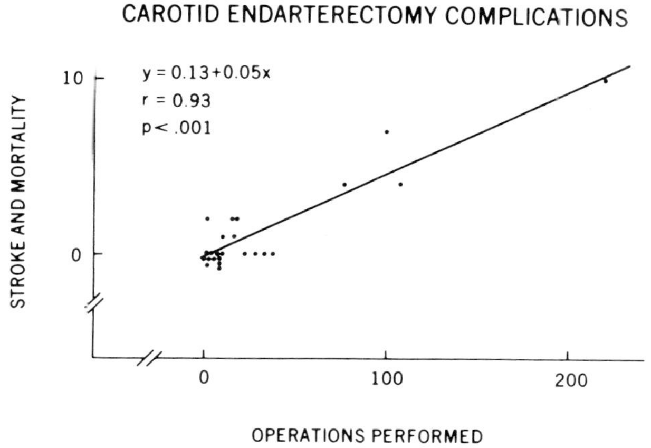

FIG. 1. Frequency of permanent stroke and mortality as a function of the number of carotid endarterectomies performed. Each point is the result for an individual surgeon's experience over a 56 month interval.

The current series was analyzed to determine the results of surgery based upon the frequency with which the individual surgeon performed the operation. The combined permanent stroke and mortality rate did not appear to change with the frequency with which the surgeon performed the operation (fig. 1). The linear relationship had an excellent correlation coefficient of 0.93 with a significant of $p < .001$. When the results of individual surgeons were segregated according to the number of operations performed per year, the above relationship was confirmed in that there was no statistically significant difference in the incidence of either neurologic deficit (temporary or permanent) or death (table 1). Although we expected to demonstrate a learning curve with regard to the results of operation, this was not the case. This may be explained by the fact that all 24 surgeons performing the procedures had reached the plateau phase of the curve and thus even in those who did the operation infrequently the results were as good as for those who performed endarterectomy more commonly Since all the surgeons were certified by their appropriate board and they had been granted privileges for performing carotid endarterectomy only after being approved by the division of vascular surgery in the department of general surgery, this explanation seems possible. An alternate explanation may be that calculation of an individual complication rate is suspect because of the large number of surgeons (13) who did so few carotid endarterectomies (<10) during the 56 months of the study (type two error). It should be noted that the four highest complications rates, calculated as a percentage from the raw data plotted in figure 1, were incurred by surgeons who did less than 20 procedures during the study period. Similar results have been reported by Robertson et al from Baptist Memorial Hospital in Memphis, Tennessee. In a retrospective study of a year interval, two experienced neurosurgeons performed 182 carotid endarterectomies while a group of eight "vascular surgeons" did 158 such operations. The morbidity and mortality were similar for both groups. However, the experience of the entire neurosurgical service for the same time interval was 385 carotid operations and the mortality and morbidity data for the 16 neuro-

TABLE 1. *Mortality and Morbidity Following Carotid Endarterectomy*

Frequency of procedure (per year)	>24	24 or Less
Number of surgeons	4	20
Temporary deficit	19 (4.2%)	7 (2.4%)
Permanent deficit	9 (2.0%)	4 (1.4%)
Mortality	12 (2.6%)	8 (2.8%)
Total procedures	456	287

There is no statistically significant difference in the parameters measured for the two groups.

surgeons performing the remaining 203 operations (average 12.6 each) was, "considerably higher", than for the more experienced neurosurgeons.[12]

It appears that carotid endarterectomy in a community hospital is a safe procedure, with a combined stroke/mortality rate of less than 5%. This safety is not predicated on frequency of performance of the operation, but it appears to be directly related to the adequacy of initial training, under a wide variety of circumstances. Careful assessment of this training will insure good surgical judgment and technical expertise.

ACKNOWLEDGMENT

The authors wish to express their gratitude to the surgeons of the Lehigh Valley Hospital Center for their participation in this study.

REFERENCES

1. Eastcott HHG, Pickering GW, Rob C. Reconstruction of internal carotid artery in a patient with intermittent attacks of hemiplegia. Lancet 1954;2:994.
2. Thompson JE, Austin DJ, Patman RD. Carotid endarterectomy for cerebrovascular insufficiency: Long-term results in 592 patients followed up to thirteen years. Ann Surg 1970;172:663–678.
3. DeWeese JA, Rob CG, Satran R, Norris FH, Lipchik EO, Zehl DN, Long JM. Surgical treatment for occlusive disease of the carotid artery. Ann Surg 1968;168:85–94.
4. Carmichael JD. Carotid surgery in the community hospital. 467 consecutive operations. Arch Surg 1980;115:937–939.
5. Easton JD, Sherman DG. Stroke and mortality rate in carotid endarterectomy: 228 consecutive operations. Stroke 1977;8:565–568.
6. Modi JR, Finch WT, Sumner DS. Update of carotid endarterectomy in two community hospitals. Springfield revisited. Stroke 1983;14:128.
7. West H, Burton R, Roon AJ, Malone JM, Goldstone J, Moore WS. Comparative risk of operation and expectant management for carotid artery disease. Stroke 1979;10:117–121.
8. Gee W. Carotid physiology with ocular pneumoplethysmography. Stroke 1982;13:666–673.
9. Gee W, Rhodes M, Denstman FJ, Jaeger RM, Tilly DA, Stephens HW, Morrow RA, Lin FZ. Ocular pneumoplethysmography in head-injured patients. J Neurosurg 1983;59:46–50.
10. Sandok BA, Furlan AJ, Whisnant JP, Sundt TM. Guidelines for the management of transient ischemic attacks. Mayo Clin Proc 1978;53:665–674.
11. Ortega G, Gee W, Kaupp HA, McDonald KM. Postendarterectomy carotid occlusion. Surg 1981;90:1093–1098.
12. Robertson JT, Auer NJ. Extracranial occlusive disease of the carotid artery. *In:* JR Yonmans, Neurological Surgery, WB Saunders, West Washington Square, Philadelphia, Pa., 19105.

Creativity in Neurosurgical Publications

RICHARD A. DAVIS, M.D.

> . . . the more original a discovery the more obvious it seems afterwards. The creative act is not an act of creation in the sense of the Old Testament. It does not create something out of nothing; it uncovers, selects, re-shuffles, combines, synthesizes already existing facts, ideas, faculties, skills. The more familiar the parts, the more striking the new whole. Arthur Koestler. *The Act of Creation*

THIS REPORT is an analysis of the scientific publications of 50 of the first American neurosurgeons. The analysis deals with the subject matter of these publications, the current interest in this subject matter, and the lasting influence of individual or aggregate publications as measured by high citation frequency. An attempt has been made to designate objectively which of these authors and their scientific contributions were creative.

The characteristics which distinguish a scientific work as creative are controversial. In this report, "creative" has been defined as an original or unique idea which conforms with the facts or reality either as an abstraction or application, and which becomes an addition to what can be referred to as "our cultural heritage."[1] The criteria previously used to designate a preeminent article in neurosurgery have include presumed educational importance, the generally accepted eminence of the author, a broad concensus on excellence of the report, and individual bias.[2–6] There have been no previous attempts at objective analysis of neurosurgical publications to differentiate between those which are lasting and eminent and those which are ephemeral and obscure.

Citation analysis, introduced by Garfield in 1955,[7] is a quantitative methodology which lends itself to statistical consideration of the literature. The rationale behind citation analysis is that reports which have remained influential will be cited more often in the current literature than those reports whose concepts and ideas have become obsolete. Under the assumption that the reports which proved to be most influential in changing the direction and scholarship in neurosurgery will be those that are most creative, it follows that frequency of citation will correlate directly with the creativity level of a particular author or publication.

Methods

The publications of 50 of the first American neurosurgeons in this study spanned the years 1896 to 1980. No living neurosurgeon was included in the analysis; all were affiliated with universities or other academic units. The individual bibliographies, which formed the basis of this study, were limited to only those articles, chapters, and books for which the neurosurgeon was listed as the first author. All such articles were tabulated from the Index Medicus, and if cited at least once between 1965 and 1979, were identified in the Science Citation Index (SCI). These bibliographies and entries in the SCI formed the statistical basis of this study. Only chapters and books which were listed in the SCI between 1965 and 1979 were considered in this investigation. The SCI has tabulated the author, journal volume, page, and year of all scientific publications which have been cited since 1955. The period of citation analysis was 1965 to 1979. "Cited articles" refers to the number of articles (first-authored) which received at least one citation during this 15-year period. "Citations for articles" refers to the total number of citations for all articles. "Citations for books and chapters" refers to the total number of citations in these categories. "Total citations" refers to the aggregate number of citations for articles, books, and chapters. The statistical methods included the Student's t test and the Pearson correlation coefficient.

From the Hospital and School of Medicine, University of Pennsylvania, Philadelphia, Pennsylvania.
Excerpted from: Davis RA. Creativity in neurosurgical publications. Neurosurgery 1987;20:652–663.

TABLE 1. *The 50 Neurosurgeons and Their Locations*

Name	Birth–death	Location
Adson	1887–1951	Rochester, MN
Bagley	1882–1957	Baltimore
Bailey	1892–1973	Chicago
Baldwin	1918–1970	Bethesda, MD
Browder	1894–1976	New York
Campbell	1901–1956	Albany, NY
Coleman	1879–1953	Richmond, VA
Craig	1892–1960	Rochester, MN
Crutchfield	1900–1972	Charlottesville, VA
Cushing	1869–1939	Boston
Dandy	1886–1946	Baltimore
Davidoff	1898–1975	New York
Davis	1896–1982	Chicago
Elsberg	1872–1948	New York
Fay	1895–1963	Philadelphia
Fincher	1900–1969	Atlanta, GA
Frazier	1870–1936	Philadelphia
Furlow	1902–1980	St. Louis, MO
German	1899–1981	New Haven, CT
Grant	1891–1967	Philadelphia
Heyl	1906–1975	Hanover, PA
Horrax	1887–1957	Boston
Ingraham	1898–1965	Boston
Jelsma	1900–1975	Louisville, KY
Keegan	1889–1978	Omaha, NB
Klemme	1896–1957	St. Louis, MO
Matson	1913–1969	Boston
Mixter	1880–1958	Boston
Munro	1889–1973	Boston
Naffziger	1884–1961	San Francisco
Peet	1885–1949	Ann Arbor, MI
Penfield	1891–1976	Montreal, Canada
Peyton	1892–1962	Minneapolis, MN
Pilcher	1904–1949	Nashville, TN
Poppen	1903–1978	Boston
Rand	1886–1979	Los Angeles
Sachs	1879–1958	St. Louis, MO
Scarff	1898–1978	New York
Scott	1906–1979	Philadelphia
Scoville	1906–1984	Hartford, CT
Semmes	1885–1982	Memphis, TN
Snodgrass	1906–1975	Galveston, TX
Spurling	1894–1968	Louisville, KY
Stookey	1887–1966	New York
Teachenor	1888–1953	Kansas City, KS
Van Wagenen	1897–1961	Rochester, NY
Voris	1902–1984	Chicago
White	1895–1981	Boston
Wilkins	1904–1985	Oklahoma City, OK
Wycis	1911–1972	Philadelphia

Results

Authors

The respective names of the neurosurgeons, dates of birth and death, and locations of their institutions are listed in Table 1. Figure 1 contains the data on journal articles, number of cited articles, percentage of articles cited, and citations for articles for each author. The group wrote 3792 first-authored reports, for which there was a total of 12,908 citations; 46% of these articles were cited at least once between 1965 and 1979. Approximately 50% of the articles were written by 12 authors or 24% (Adson, Bailey, Craig, Cushing, Dandy, Davis, Elsberg, Frazier, Grant, Penfield, Sachs, and White). Fifty percent of all citations for journal articles were for seven authors (14%): Cushing (1526), Penfield (1396), Dandy (1339), Bailey

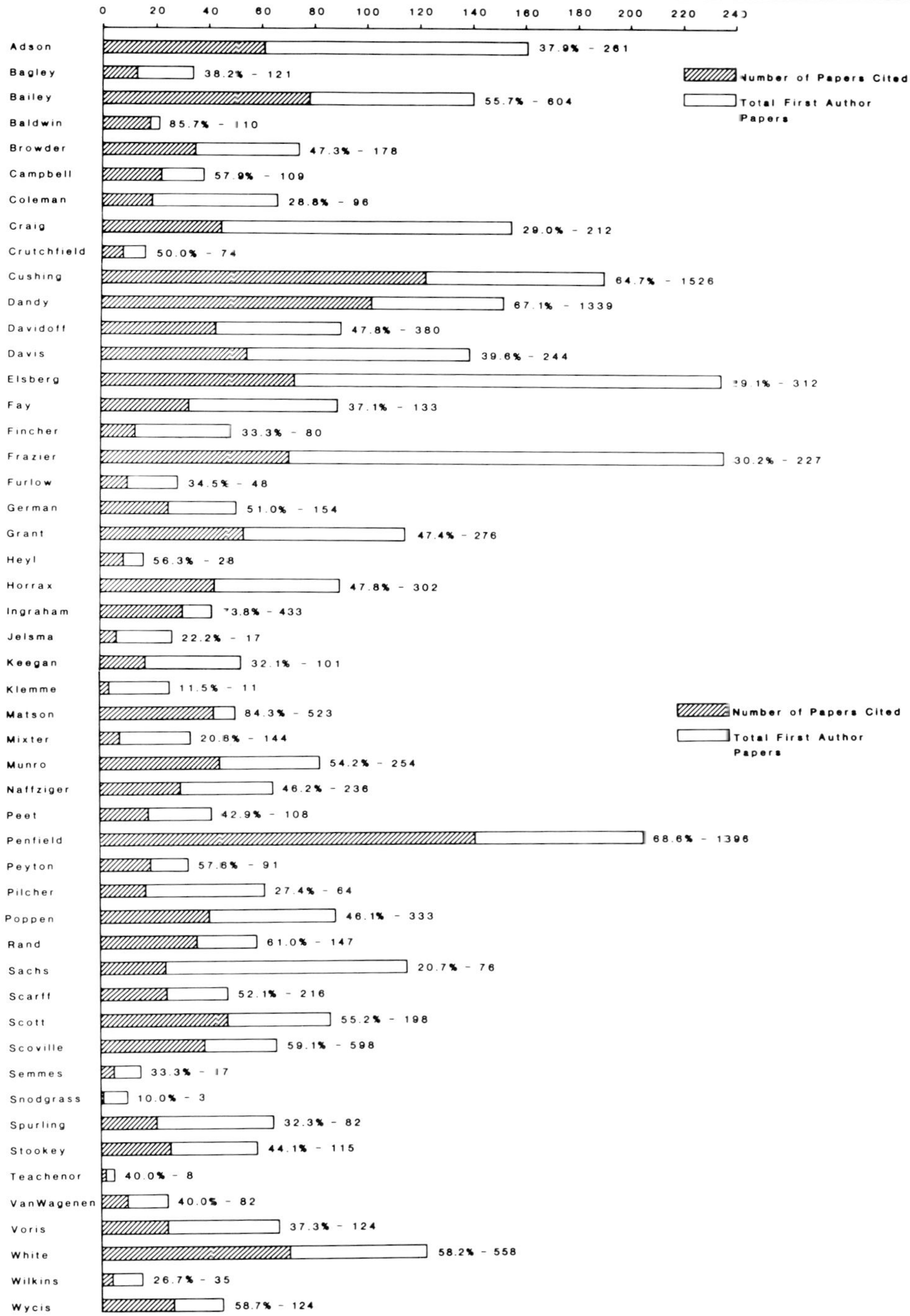

FIG. 1. The bar chart for each author depicts the relationship between the number of first-authored reports published and the number of those reports that were cited. The numbers above each bar chart are the percentages of an author's reports that were cited and the total number of citations for all published reports.

(604), Scoville (598), White (558), and Matson (523). The most prolific author was 47 times more productive than the least, and the author with the greatest number of citations for articles had 507 times as many as the author with the fewest citations for journal articles.

The number of articles written by an author was found to correlate with both cited articles ($r = 0.86$), citations for articles ($r = 0.62$), and total citations ($r = 0.59$).

Authors and Creative Peaks

The ten most creative authors were Bailey, Cushing, Dandy, Davidoff, Elsberg, Ingraham, Matson, Penfield, Scoville, and White. The respective careers of these ten authors were divided into 5-year periods beginning with the date of first publication, and citations for articles published during each of these periods were tallied, in order to determine the creative peaks of each author. Seven of the most creative neurosurgeons were older than 50 years when they reached their creative peaks; Cushing's most creative period was near the end of his surgical career. Bailey, Dandy and Davidoff were most creative during the early years of their professional lives.

Subjects and Citations

The subjects on which these 50 neurosurgeons wrote the most number of articles were central nervous system tumors (484 articles with 2332 citations) of which Bailey wrote 45 articles, but Cushing received 474 citations for 38 articles. There were 330 articles on neurophysiology which received 2319 citations; Penfield contributed more on this subject (53 articles) and also received the largest number of citations (705). A total of 282 journal articles were written on head injury with 556 citations; Munro wrote 21 articles on this subject, but Ingraham received 82 citations for fewer number of articles. There were 30 authors whose most frequently cited subject also was the subject on which the author wrote the most number of reports. There were more articles written, but fewer citations, on sympathectomy for the treatment of hypertension and vascular disorders than more specific and well-defined neurosurgical problems such as the management of pain, epilepsy, the intervertebral disc, peripheral nerve injuries, trigeminal neuralgia, and hydrocephalus. Despite the extensive clinical and laboratory interest in sympathectomy, this procedure became obsolete with introduction of effective medication, and subsequently neurosurgical operations for pain relief, epilepsy, trigeminal neuralgia, and Parkinson's Disease followed a similar, but less rapid, "decay pattern." Psychosurgery and stereotactic surgery for various extrapyramidal disorders also were the subjects of considerable interest in the literature, but largely have been abandoned because of pharmacological advances.

Era of Publication

The 3792 articles published between 1896 and 1980 had a normal distribution frequency which peaked in 1938. To determine whether the proximity of an author's career to the 15-year period (1965–1979) in which citations were tabulated, had an effect on citation frequency, the interval between 1896 and 1980 was divided into 5-year periods. The single 5-year period in which the largest number of first-authored reports was written was between 1936 and 1940; the most number of cited reports occurred between 1931 and 1935, and the largest number of total citations for articles was between 1926 and 1930. There was no statistical difference between the number of first-authored reports, cited reports, or total citations for articles written before 1925 and after 1950. During the 30-year interval after 1950, the percentage of publications cited (mean $\pm$ SE = 51.7% $\pm$ 6.7) was significantly greater ($P < 0.05$) than during the 30-year period before 1925 (mean $\pm$ SE = 34.9 $\pm$ 2.9). However, there was no statistical difference in the mean of average citation frequencies before 1925 or after 1950.

First Publication

The average age at the time of the first scientific publication was 29 years; the youngest to publish was Pilcher (age 23 years), and the oldest was Semmes (age 42). There was slight negative correlation between age at the time of first publication and the number of reports published by an author ($r = -0.34$), but no significant correlation between the author's age at first publication and citations for articles ($r = -0.22$). Nineteen (38%) of the authors' initial publications led to further investigation and expansion of the original topic. There were 16 authors whose first publications were basic research reports, and 12 of these authors made further contributions which were related to the initial field of interest. Authors whose first publication was a research report published significantly more articles than those whose first article was clinical. The authors in the former group each averaged 108 articles, whereas authors in the latter group averaged 61 articles (t test value = 2.90, $P < 0.006$). However, there was no significant difference in citations for articles, or total citations.

Research Reports

There were 418 research articles written by 39 of the 50 neurosurgeons, which comprised only 11% of all first-authored articles. More than one third (38%) of all research publications were written by three authors, Bailey (62 articles), Davis (52 articles), and Penfield (45 articles). The subject matter of neurosurgical laboratory investigation was predominantly neuropathology, but other areas of interest included experimental hydrocephalus and epilepsy, the relationship of cardiopulmonary physiology to cerebral blood flow, and neurophysiology. The percentage of an author's articles which were research publications did not correlate with the number of first-authored articles ($r = 0.08$), citations for articles ($r = 0.16$), or total citations ($r = 0.20$).

Military Publications

A total of 99 articles was written on various military topics, which represented 3% of all articles studied. These military medical articles were written by 27 of the 50 authors, only three of whom wrote more than nine or more articles. Craig, Spurling, and White were the most productive, and their interests included head and peripheral nerve injuries, and vascular disorders in chronic exposure to cold.

Chapters and Books

Citations for books constituted 29% of total citations, and the most-cited books received more citations than the most-cited articles. Penfield and Cushing together accounted for 50% of all citations for books, whereas Penfield wrote significantly more textbook chapters and had more citations for those chapters. There were significantly fewer citations for chapters in books than for either books or journal articles.

Medical History and Education

There were 116 journal articles on medical education, but these were not often cited. Penfield and Cushing wrote more and were cited more on these subjects than other authors. They were concerned with the philosophy, history, and development of medical education, whereas Furlow, Heyl, and Matson emphasized the educational and professional qualifications of neurosurgeons. The most frequently cited journal article, with a historical perspective, was Scarff's overview of the first 50 years of neurosurgery.[8]

Neurosurgical Classics

Garfield[7] arbitrarily ranked a scientific article to the "classic" status if there were more than four citations for that article each year. In this study the criteria were more stringent, and a "classic" article in neurosurgery averaged five or more citations each year for the 15-year period of analysis. A "classic" book had ten or more citations each year of the period of analysis. The most cited article was that of Scoville and Milner, "Loss of Recent Memory After Bilateral Hippocampal Lesions,"[9] and the most-cited book was *Epilepsy and the Functional Anatomy of the Human Brain* by Penfield and Jaspar.[10] Cushing wrote five of the ten most-cited articles, and Penfield wrote four of the ten most-cited books.

Discussion

The concept of creativity is both abstruse and controversial. It generally is agreed that creative thought involves ideas which have an enduring practical or theoretical relevance. Criteria which recognize creative ideas in a narrow discipline such as neurosurgery have remained, so far, undefined, vague, and singularly subjective. Citation analysis recognizes those articles which have influenced the course of a surgical discipline and are therefore creative. In addition, citation analysis, as demonstrated by the data in this study, is important for a contemplated publication. Use of the SCI identified individual authors and subjects of interest to the investigator. Similarly, other authors who have published and have been cited in a particular field, also can be identified. Citation analysis reveals that a variety of journals publish articles on a general range of titles, which suggests that a literature review should not be confined to the cumulative index of a single specialty journal. The SCI suggests which articles are appropriate for use in a collective review, historical treatise, or introduction to an article or book currently being written. Finally, citation analysis as a part of a thorough search of the literature, reveals whether a clinical report in progress or a proposed research project already has been completed.

Authors who wrote more articles had more cited articles and more citations for articles than their less-productive counterparts. The relationship between productivity and creativity, or quantity and quality, has been referred to by Simonton[11] as the constant-probability-of-success model of creative productivity. Simonton's model "clearly predicts that quality is a probabilistic consequence of quantity." The data in this study confirm this prediction as demonstrated by the absence of correlation between the number of articles written and both the percentage of articles cited and average citations per article. Another aspect of the importance of productivity and its relationship to creativity is a theorem formulated by Price[12] which states that 50% of all scientific contributions are made by the square root of all of the scientific contributors. This prediction was accurate in this study for total citations for articles, but not first-authored reports. Nevertheless, the single, if not the most important component in the constellation of factors which comprise creativity, is productivity.

The 5-year creative peak of seven of the ten authors with the largest total citations for articles, chapters, and books occurred after the age of 50 years. This shift of age distribution toward the end of their surgical careers suggested that factors such as astute observation, exercise of judgement, the wisdom of experience, as well as persistent motivation, rather than periods of exceptional productivity, brilliance and discovery, characterized this group of creative neurosurgeons. These data and conclusions are consistent with Simonton's assertion that creative scientists "do not cease their contributions once they have begun to shake up the foundations of normal science . . . their endeavors to reform scientific thought continue almost unabated into the last years of life."[11] Despite the current emphasis on research in the education and training of neurosurgeons, research experience had little effect upon creativity. Authors whose initial article was a research topic did not have significantly more citations for articles or total citations than authors whose first publication was clinical. However, if the first publication was a research project, authors were significantly more productive.

The journal articles, chapters, and books of 50 of the first American neurosurgeons have been identified and studied objectively by citation analysis. If an idea is creative, it will be influential and alter the scholarship and progress of a scientific discipline. Because unique concepts have had an impact on the direction, and influenced the course of neurosurgery, they have been recognized by citation analysis. It follows that high levels of citation correlate with creativity. Creativity and notable productivity have engendered not only a literature of imaginative research but also diverse clinical endeavors which have shaped the scientific foundation of American neurosurgery. As a result, these research and clinical achievements have established a surgical discipline which is characterized by a formidable tradition of excellence. All of these authors have contributed to the development and continuing progress of neurosurgery, but some of them have more brightly illuminated it by their creativity.

REFERENCES

1. Stent GS. Paradoxes of Progress. San Francisco: WH Freeman, 1978;105.
2. Troland CE, Otenasek FJ. Selected Writings of Walter E. Dandy. Springfield: CC Thomas, 1957.
3. Bucy PC. Neurosurgical Giants: Feet of Clay and Iron. New York: Elsevier, 1985.
4. Davis RA. Neurosurgical Contributions of Loyal Davis. Philadelphia: WB Saunders, 1973.
5. Matson DD, German WJ. Harvey Cushing: Selected Papers on Neurosurgery. New Haven: Yale University Press, 1969.
6. Wilkins RH. Neurosurgical Classics. New York: Johnson, 1965.
7. Garfield E. Citation indexes for science. Science 1955;122:108–111.
8. Scarff JE. Fifty years of neurosurgery, 1905–1955. Surg Gynecol Obstet 1955;101:417–513.
9. Scoville WB, Milner B. Loss of recent memory after bilateral hippocampal lesions. J Neurol Neurosurg Psychiatry 1957;20:11–21.
10. Penfield W, Jaspar H. Epilepsy and the Functional Anatomy of the Human Brain. Boston: Little, Brown, 1954.
11. Simonton DK. Genius, Creativity, and Leadership. Cambridge, MA: Harvard University Press, 1984.
12. Price D. Little Science, Big Science. New York: Columbia University Press, 1963.

Effect of Small Intestinal Resection on Fat Absorption

FRANK GUMP, M.D., ROBERT BEALS, M.D., AND HAROLD G. BARKER, M.D.

A NUMBER of clinical and experimental studies have reported segmental differences in the absorptive ability of the small intestine. The absorption of fat has received particular attention because steatorrhea is often observed following extensive small bowel resection. However, evidence regarding the relative importance of various segments of the small intestine in the absorption of fat is still conflicting, particularly when different methods of investigation are compared.

Jensenius[7] studied fecal fat loss in dogs following resections of either the proximal or distal two thirds of the small intestine and noted more fat loss following the distal resections. A similar study by Kremen, Linner and Nelson[8] confirmed these findings and led the authors to conclude that the ileum is the primary area of fat absorption. Other authors[3,14] have failed to demonstrate any nutritional differences following resection of comparable segments of proximal or distal small intestine.

The site of maximum fat absorption has been placed in the jejunum by some authors using other experimental approaches. Frazer[5] administered olive oil stained with Sudan IV to rats and noted that the upper jejunal mucosa was preferentially filled with fat globules. Benson, *et al.*[1] in a similar experiment placed the primary site of fat absorption in the third quarter of the small intestine. A different technic was employed by Borgstrom and his associates[2] when they studied absorption in humans by sampling intestinal contents at various levels with a long tube after feeding corn oil. These authors concluded that fat absorption takes place primarily in the proximal jejunum. Goldstein, Wirts and Kramer[6] instilled labeled fat through a Miller-Abbott tube placed at various small bowel levels and concluded that maximum fat absorption takes place from the midsegments.

In the present study labeled fat and fatty acid have been used in tolerance tests combined with partial small bowel bypassing operations in dogs.

Methods

Three groups of mongrel dogs were utilized. Group I consisted of three animals who had the proximal 50 per cent of the small bowel removed from intestinal continuity. Under aspetic conditions the small bowel was exposed and measured along its mesenteric border from the pylorous to the ileo cecal valve. The intestine was then divided just distal to the ampulla of Vater and pancreatic duct ostium and again at a point midway between the pylorus and cecum. The blood supply of the intervening defunctionalized segment was preserved and the ends were brought out as cutaneous fistulae. An end-to-end, one layer silk anastomosis was employed to re-establish intestinal continuity around the defunctionalized segment. This preparation was preferred to resection because it minimizes damage to the circulation of the remaining segments.

A second group of three dogs was prepared in a similar fashion but the defunctionalized portion consisted of the distal 50 per cent. Once again intestinal continuity was re-established by end-to-end anastomosis, this time between the mid point of the small bowel and a point a few centimeters proximal to the ileo cecal valve. Group III consisted of two dogs in whom the middle 50 per cent of the small intestine was removed from continuity with the

From the Department of Surgery, Columbia University, College of Physicians and Surgeons and the Surgical Service, Presbyterian Hospital, New York, New York.

Presented before the American Surgical Association, Boca Raton, Florida, March 21–23, 1961.
Supported in part by United States Public Health Service Grant RG-2926 (C9).
This article has been reproduced from *Annals of Surgery*, Vol. 154, No. 3, September 1961.

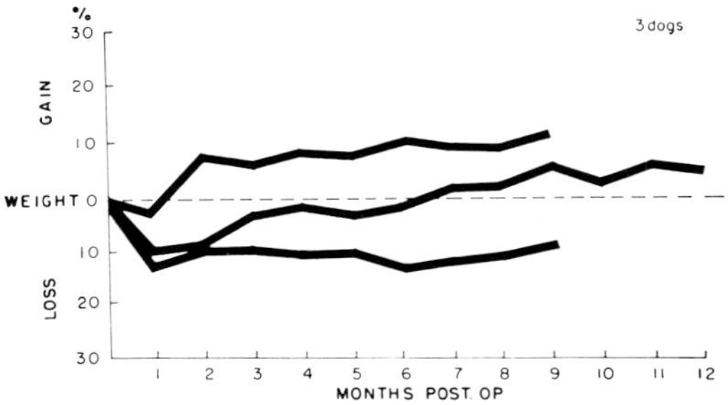

FIG. 1. Weight curve of dogs with proximal bypasses

gastrointestinal tract. In the remainder of this communication the term "resection" is sometimes used for brevity but the bypass operation was actually used in all cases.

The absorption of I^{131} labeled neutral fat was studied in all dogs prior to operation and the results compared with those of identical tests done after operation. Similar pre- and postoperative tests were also carried out using I^{131} labeled oleic acid. The neutral fat used was olive oil labeled with I^{131} in our own laboratory. Ten ml. containing about 20 microcuries of I^{131} were instilled into the stomach of unanesthetized fasting dogs by means of a tube. After a brief training period it was possible to pass the stomach tube without restraining the dogs. The animals were pretreated with Lugol's solution in order to block the selective uptake of I^{131} by the thyroid. Blood samples were drawn at one, two, three, four, six, eight and sometimes ten hours. Stools were collected for 72 hours taking care to avoid contamination by urine. This was possible because diarrhea did not follow the operative procedures and the dogs were trained to defecate during their twice a day outings on the dog run.

The blood specimens were centrifuged and the plasma pipetted into counting tubes and counted in a well type scintillation counter to an accuracy (±1.S.D.) of 2.0 per cent or better, proper decay factors being applied when necessary. The lipoproteins were then precipitated according to Turner's method[13] and the radioactivity of the precipitate determined.* Plasma radioactivity at each sampling time was expressed as the total activity present in the calculated plasma volume as percentage of the dose administered. The plasma volume was assumed to be 5.4 per cent of body weight. All stools were collected for 72 hours, combined, homogenized and the radioactivity determined. One fat and one fatty acid absorption test was carried out in each dog preoperatively. The postoperative tests were carried out two or more months after operation and again both fat and fatty acid tests were performed in all dogs. In the Groups I and II dogs the tests were repeated at least twice. All together 18 neutral fat and 19 fatty acid tests were performed postoperatively in the eight dogs. The postoperative value recorded at each sampling time for each dog was derived by averaging all the studies done postoperatively in that particular animal for fat and fatty acid respectively. In Groups I and II the "t" test was then applied at each sampling time to test for significance in the difference between these averages and the preoperative values.

The dogs were weighed at weekly intervals following operation for periods varying from eight to 14 months.

Results

Weight

All of the animals initially lost weight after the operation but six of the eight dogs subsequently completely regained their preoperative weight (Fig. 1–3). One dog required 22 weeks to regain the preoperative weight, but the other five did so by 12 weeks. One dog in the first group and one in the second failed to completely regain their preoperative weights. However, both of these dogs survived the operation and stabilized at new levels which were 81 and 88 per cent of their original weights, respectively. There was no discernible correla-

* The precipitation of lipoproteins was carried out in the first few experiments but was later discontinued since it did not yield any additional information.

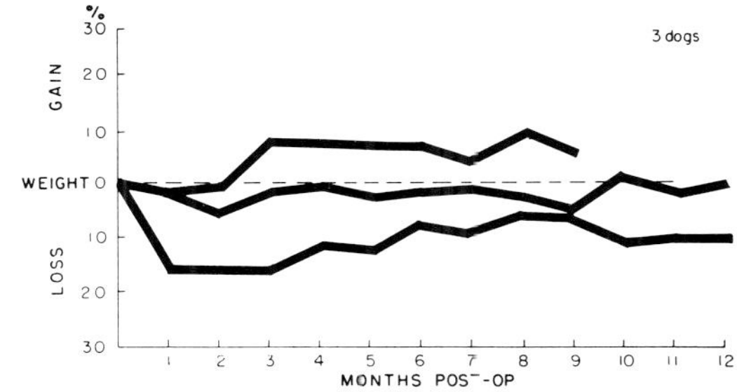

FIG. 2. Weight curve of dogs with distal bypasses.

tion between the level of intestinal resection and the rate of clinical recovery, rate of weight gain or eventual weight achieved.

Plasma Radioactivity

Pre- and postoperative plasma radioactivities were compared at each sampling time and the values are shown in Figure 4. With neutral fat as the test material, the removal of the distal small bowel had no significant effect on the plasma curves. The Group I dogs (proximal resection), however, showed statistically very significant reductions ($p < .01$) in plasma radioactivity at the two-three-four- and six-hour points and a significant reduction ($p = .03$) at 8 hours. With fatty acid as the test material again no apparent defect was produced by distal small bowel resection. In the Group I dogs (proximal resection), the data suggest that the operation may have impaired fatty acid absorption to some extent. The observed decrease in plasma radioactivity approached significance at two hours ($p = .08$) and three hours ($p = .07$). Thereafter, no significant difference was evident.

Stool (Table 1)

Preoperatively the radioactivity recovered in the stools after feeding neutral fat tagged with I^{131} averaged 9.0 per cent of the dose administered. This corresponded to the 11 per cent recorded after feeding fatty acid to the unoperated dogs. A modest and almost equal increase in these values was noted after resection of either proximal or distal half of the small bowel. In the Group I dogs, 15 per cent was found after feeding neutral fat while 17 per cent was noted when fatty acid was administered and the corresponding average values in the Group II dogs were 16 per cent for fat and 19 per cent for fatty acid. Stool studies were not performed on the Group II dogs where the mid 50 per cent had been resected. The postoperative increase in fecal fat following proximal or distal resection may be real but the range was wide and no statistically significant difference from the preoperative figures could be demonstrated.

Discussion

Dogs tolerate resection of half their small bowel very well and under the conditions of the present study are usually able to completely regain their preoperative weight regardless of

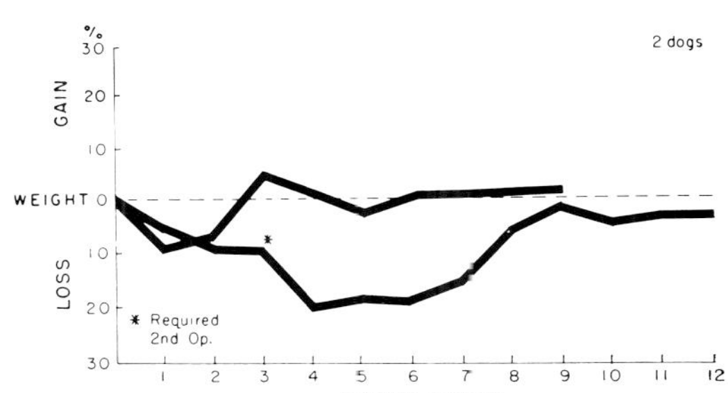

FIG. 3. Weight curve of dogs with middle bypasses. One dog prolapsed the bypassed segment and required reoperation for correction of the prolapse.

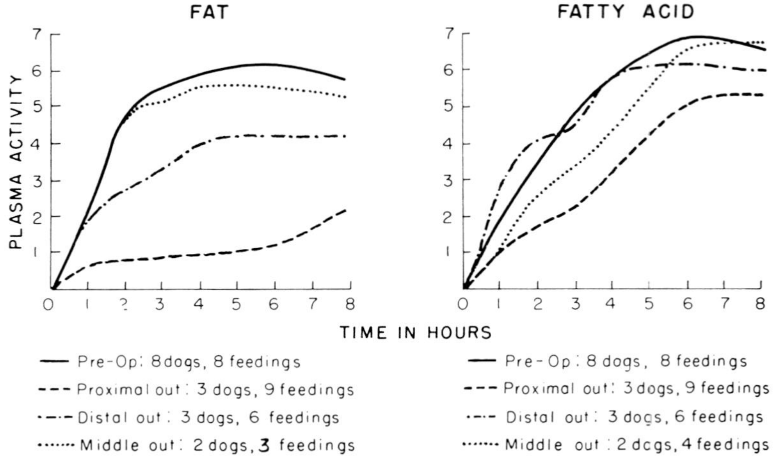

FIG. 4. Mean plasma radioactivity curves for all preoperative dogs and for all three groups of postoperative dogs.

which 50 per cent portion of the small intestine is removed. Greater resections frequently impair ability to regain preoperative weight.[4,8]

There are certain limitations to any conclusions drawn from weight loss data when used to evaluate absorption after resections. Such measurements actually assess ability to utilize a mixed diet rather than specific single elements of the diet. The extent of the resection required to produce a significant alteration in weight precludes studies of the function of shorter segments. Severe malnutrition in and of itself may alter absorption. It is with these considerations in mind that some investigators have felt that only studies in intact (or at least normally nourished) subjects or animals are meaningful as regards the physiology of normal absorption. This is not to say that information on subjects or animals with extensive resections and their effects is not equally valuable from other standpoints but such data may not justify inferences about normal absorptive patterns. In working with a preparation where the sacrifice of absorptive capacity was largely a loss of what might be called reserve capacity we were able to at least avoid overt malnutrition. However, some of the other limitations mentioned above are obviously encountered in the present study and in part these studies measure not only sites of maximum absorption but also the ability of remaining segments to take over for the removed ones.

Despite the fact that body weight and fecal radioactivity studies fail to distinguish between proximal, distal and middle resections when only 50 per cent of the small bowel is removed, definite differences between the groups are observed in the plasma radioactivity curves. Since there is no reason to suspect different rates of iodine disposal from the blood in the three groups of dogs it would seem clear that there is a difference in absorption from the intestine. It is evident from the Group I dogs that resection of the proximal small bowel prevents the *rapid* uptake of neutral fat seen in the intact dog. This amounts to a marked delay in absorption lasting for at least 6 hours. No such profound and prolonged alteration occurred in these dogs when fatty acid was given although there probably was a mild delay. The dogs in which the distal 50 per cent of the small intestine was bypassed did not exhibit any significant abnormality in their plasma radioactivity curves after feeding either fat or fatty acid. That the alterations described are only delays in absorption and not actual failure

TABLE 1. *Average Fecal Radioactivity*

	Neutral Fat		Fatty Acid	
Preoperative	9%		11%	
Postoperative	Group I 15%	Group II 16%	Group I 17%	Group II 19%

to absorb is evident from the fact that 72-hour stool radioactivity is essentially equal in both groups of dogs.

Fat absorption in dogs with proximal resections appears to be "catching up" at the eight-hour mark and it would be desirable to follow curves of plasma radioactivity beyond this point. Unfortunately, such attempts are unreliable because the late plasma radioactivity in the dog then begins to depend more on disposal factors and less on continuing intestinal absorption. Following a tagged fat meal the plasma level of radioactivity is more sustained in the dog than in the human. Lipid precipitation studies revealed that during the late hours there is persistance of a considerable amount of free I^{131} in the dog blood stream. Apparently under the conditions of the present experiments excretion of iodide in the urine was slower than in humans. It is known that in dogs, unlike humans, iodide clearance is related to chloride intake and iodide clearance is apt to be very low except in the presence of a high chloride intake.[11] Furthermore there is no advantage in plotting only the lipid bound iodine as advised by Turner[13] since the small amount of lipid bound radioactivity that can be measured after eight hours does not accurately reflect absorption at this time and actually neglects the portion already absorbed and converted to the free form. For these reasons efforts to carry plasma curves beyond eight hours were abandoned.

The unoperated dog exhibits an earlier and more rapid absorption of neutral fat than of fatty acid and this same phenomenon also holds in the human.[9] This must surely be due to the absorption of a certain amount of undigested fat without enzymatic alteration. The only other possible explanation would be that there is a faster gastric emptying time when giving fat than after fatty acid. It is unlikely that this could consistently be of sufficiently different duration to explain the findings. The jejunectomized dogs lost this early rapid uptake of neutral fat and it therefore seems likely that the normal mechanism or pathway for absorption of undigested fat has been interfered with or removed. Proximal resection did more however than just slow neutral fat absorption to equal that of normal fatty acid absorption. The plasma radioactivity curve after feeding neutral fat became much lower than the normal fatty acid curve. This additional slowing may or may not be due to interference with absorption of undigested fat. If sufficient fat is normally absorbed in this form then the entire alteration could be due to the same mechanism. However, it is possible that this additional portion* of the alteration could be due to interference with enzymatic digestion. Thus emulsification is necessary before digestion and the partial duodenectomy included in the proximal resections could disturb the churning motion which is thought to aid emulsification. It is further conceivable that the anastomoses were so close to the common duct and pancreatic duct ostea that free flow could have been disturbed although care was taken to avoid this. Stimulation to secretion of digestive enzymes may have been ill timed so that proper mixing did not occur.

Regardless of the presence or absence of altered digestion following jejunectomy it is apparent that neutral fat is normally absorbed to a large extent in the jejunum and fatty acid absorption is more evenly distributed throughout the small bowel with only a slightly larger share being localized in the jejunum. Thus both undigested fat and fatty acids are easily absorbed in the jejunum whereas only fatty acid is absorbable to any important extent in the ileum. The jejunectomized dogs were eventually able to absorb neutral fat from the ileum only after it had been digested and this is apparently a slow process, at least after jejunectomy.

It is now believed that not only the undigested fats but also most of the long chain fatty acids are absorbed via the lacteals.[12] If this is true it is necessary to conclude from our data that 1) the jejunal lacteals absorb both fat and fatty acid but they absorb undigested fat more rapidly and more completely; and 2) the ileal lacteals absorb fatty acid but little or no undigested fat.

Patients with pancreatic enzyme deficiency but normal intestines are observed to absorb fatty acids normally but neutral fat poorly.[10] This would seem to constitute evidence that the

* It would be inconsistent with our data to assume that the entire alteration could be due to a digestive defect. Thus as stated above there is evidence in the normal dog and human that at least a certain amount of fat is absorbed in an undigested form. Likewise the exclusive presence of a digestive defect would not explain the mild depression in fatty acid absorption which jejunectomy seems to produce.

amount of absorption of fat in the undigested form is small. Possibly there is a species difference involved but alternative explanations exist. Patients who lack pancreatic enzymes may also lack proper emulsification of the neutral fat which is necessary before its absorption. Some of these patients have also had resections of the duodenum and part of the jejunum so that critical absorbing surfaces for undigested fat may have been removed. The further possibility exists that fat traverses proximal bowel too rapidly for absorption; then with lack of enzymes, absorption cannot take place in the ileum.

This study illustrates the complexities involved in any effort to localize the site of fat absorption in the small intestine and explains some of the conflicting data reported previously. Adaptive abilities of remaining segments create difficulties in evaluating the function of any resected segment. Also, normal plasma radioactivity curves following a tagged fat meal do not necessarily rule out an absorptive defect that can become evident only over a long period of time. Fifty per cent resections were deliberately selected in order to avoid marked nutritional changes and therefore we are not able to shed any light on the weight loss that has been reported to follow distal but not proximal resections of greater magnitude. Quite possibly carbohydrate and protein absorption must be studied to fully evaluate such results.

Conclusions

1. Intestinal absorption of fat and fatty acid has been studied in dogs following resection of various 50 per cent segments of the small intestine.

2. Fifty per cent resection was well tolerated and no segmental differences in absorption could be shown by stool or body weight measurements.

3. Iodine^{131} tagged fat and fatty acid studies showed a marked *delay* in absorption of neutral fat in jejunectomized dogs. Fatty acid absorption was probably also affected but to a lesser degree.

4. It is postulated that a considerable part of neutral fat is absorbed in the form of undigested fat and that this process is largely localized in the proximal small bowel. When this area is removed absorption is slower but eventually takes place from lower segments following enzymatic digestion.

REFERENCES

1. Benson JA, Jr., Chandler GN, Vansteenhuyse FE, Gagnon JO. Studies concerning the site of fat absorption in small intestine of the rat. Gastroenterology 1956;30:53.
2. Borgstrom B, Dahlqvist A, Lundh G, Sjovall J. Studies of intestinal digestion and absorption in the human. J Clin Invest 1957;36:1521.
3. Clatworthy HW, Jr., Saleeby R, Lovingood C. Extensive small bowel resection in young dogs: Its effect on growth and development. Surgery 1952;32:341.
4. Flint JM. The effect of extensive resections of the small intestine. Bull Johns Hopkins Hosp 1912;23:127.
5. Frazer AC. Differentiation in the absorption of olive oil and oleic acid in the rat. J Physiol 1943;102:306.
6. Goldstein F, Wirts CW, Kramer S. Studies of I^{131} labeled triolein absorption from various levels of the small bowel in man. Clin Res 1959;7:261.
7. Jensenius H. Results of experimental resections of the small intestine on dogs. Universitetsforlaget, NYT Nordisk Forlog Copenhagen, Arnold Busch, 1945.
8. Kremen AJ, Linner JH, Nelsor CH. An experimental evaluation of the nutritional importance of proximal and distal small intestine. Ann Surg 1954;140:439.
9. Malm JR, Reemtsma K, Barker HG. Comparative fat and fatty acid intestinal absorption test utilizing radioiodine labeling-results in normal subjects. Proc Soc Exp Biol and Med 1956;92:471.
10. Reemtsma K, Malm JR, Barker HG. The comparative absorption of labeled fat and fatty acid in the study of pancreatic disease. Surgery 1957;42:22.
11. Riggs DS. Renal clearance of iodide in the dog. Federation Proc 1949;8:328.
12. Simmonds WJ. The intestinal absorption of fat, fatty acid and fat soluble dye into thoracic duct lymph in unanaesthetized rats. Aust J Exp Biol Med Sci 1955;33:25.
13. Turner DA. The absorption, transport, and deposition of fat. Am J of Dig Diseases 1958;3:594.
14. Weckesser EC, Ankeney JL, Portmann AF, Price JW, Cebul FA. Extensive resection of the small intestine followed by vagotomy. Surgery 1951;30:465.

DISCUSSION

DR. ARNOLD J. KREMEN: I am most happy to have seen this paper of Dr. Gump's and really to see that there is a renewed interest and additional work going on in this area. Unfortunately, it is a confusing area to work in, and to date many of the reports relating to various functions and various levels of function have been controversial.

I suspect that if as much study, effort and work had gone on in 20 feet of intestinal mucosa as has gone on in the comparatively smaller stomach and duodenum, the function of various levels of small bowel would be established, and I would not have to be up here discussing it.

Some six years ago, I reported to this group on a similar study with somewhat different results. At that time, we had also isolated varying segments of the small intestine in an effort to ascertain differences of function, if they existed, and our tests were essentially chemical on stool analysis of fats.

I believe a 50 percent resection of the smaller intestine at no matter what level rarely produces, in dogs, any measurable postoperative nutritional deficiencies. Chances are that this also applies to humans. However, when one gets into situations where it is necessary for whatever reason to resect larger amounts than this—and I am sure you can all imagine such situations, either vascular accidents or neoplastic diseases—then I think the situation becomes somewhat more crucial.

(Slide) There are some of the experimental preparations that we had made at the time of the previous study, and the one group of animals that did most poorly is Group 3, where 50 per cent of the distal small bowel is taken out of stream, and the ileocecal valve was bypassed. These animals, over a period of six months, lost almost 50 percent of their weight, and did not tend to regain it.

It has also seemed to us from clinical experiences that, when it is possible to save a small amount of terminal ileum, such patients have done considerably better postoperatively, particularly when the ileocecal valve has been preserved. This may well be of importance in doing colectomies with ileoproctoscopies. If one can save the very terminal portion of the ileum, it has been our belief that the patients have much less postoperative diarrhea.

DR. JONATHAN E. RHOADS: The data which Dr. Gump has presented are reassuring to the clinical surgeon confronted with the need to resect long segments of intestine, though extended clinical experience alone has shown that resection of much more than 50 per cent of the small bowel is well tolerated, and segments including all of the small bowel, except the duodenum plus perhaps 18 inches, have been compatible with life in some patients.

The fact that the dog can suffer 50 per cent loss of ileum without impairment of fat absorption quantitatively measured, whereas loss of the lower duodenum and jejunum does impair the rate of absorption of neutral fat, but not of fatty acids, is interesting.

There appear to be two plausible explanations for the findings. First, that neutral fat is absorbed as such through the jejunum, but not so well through the ileum. The other explanation is that the jejunum and lower duodenum contribute more to the hydrolysis of the neutral fat to fatty acids than in the case of the ileum.

Limitations of time prevented a full discussion of these alternatives in the oral presentation, but such a discussion is included in the manuscript.

The authors favor the first explanation and concede that the jejunum in the dog has a specialized ability to absorb the neutral fat. Further experiments will be necessary to determine the extent to which each of these mechanisms plays a role.

DR. FRANK GUMP: [Closing] We selected 50 per cent resections because we wanted to work with dogs that were in an almost normal nutritional state. We believed these animals might be preferable in studying the normal mechanisms of fat absorption.

I did not have a chance to say that the ileocecal valve was in place in all of our animals. We did not study any dogs where this was bypassed.

Exterioriization Without Colostomy for Perforative Sigmoid Diverticulitis

JAMES W. KNECHT, M.D., F.A.C.S.

AN ALTERNATE METHOD of treating perforative sigmoid diverticulitis is exteriorization of the loop over a bar without subsequent opening of the bowel to create a colostomy. Exteriorized perforations close and heal spontaneously and bowel movements occur normally per rectum despite an exteriorized sigmoid loop. The septic focus is removed from the peritoneal cavity. Once the colostomy bar is removed, the exteriorized loop slowly recedes into the abdomen and wound contraction closes the wound completely, leaving a ventral hernia. The procedure is rapid, simple, and effective. A functioning colostomy is avoided and hospitalization time is shortened. The operative technique, postoperative care, and results of treatment in five patients are described.

There is a reluctance to operate on patients with a clinical diagnosis of acute diverticulitis. Conservative treatment with antibiotics, nasogastric suction, and intravenous fluids is recommended. However, the clinical diagnosis may be uncertain, or the patient may fail to respond to medical treatment. Exploration is then indicated, and drainage plus diverting colostomy, or resection and proximal colostomy, is usually performed. The reluctance to operate earlier for acute diverticulitis stems from the fear of committing the patient to a colostomy and several additional operative procedures. Most surgeons still would not perform a primary resection and anastomosis on an unprepared left colon in the presence of pus and peritonitis. Colostomy and resection can be avoided, and yet, the diseased bowel segment removed from the peritoneal cavity by exteriorization without subsequent colostomy. This procedure has been performed in five cases.

Operating Technique

The operative procedure is performed through a lower midline incision. After exploration to rule out appendicitis, perforated carcinoma, perforations elsewhere in the bowel, and gangrenous bowel, the diseased segment of sigmoid colon is simply exteriorized over a bar, if it's mobile, or the left colon is mobilized sufficiently to allow for exteriorization. The incision is closed around the exteriorized loop leaving room for one finger between slightly compressed bowel and approximated fascia. Prior to closure, the peritoneal cavity is lavaged with cephalothin in saline. The exteriorized loop serves as a generous drain, and no additional drainage is required.

Postoperative Care

Dressing changes are instituted until the perforation has sealed. Purulent drainage is absorbed by gauze dressings which are changed as often as necessary. The suppurative infection in the exteriorized bowel clears just as infection clears when a wound is widely opened and drained. Once the postoperative ileus subsides, bowel function resumes through the exteriorized loop, and the patient has normal bowel movements. The exteriorized perforated sigmoid usually heals in one to two weeks. Once the perforation has closed, the supporting rod is removed, and the patient can be discharged with a gauze dressing over the bowel. The exteriorized bowel recedes gradually into the peritoneal cavity within 12 weeks. Concomitantly, the wound contracts and skin completely covers the bowel. An incisional hernia usually remains. Wound care is simple. The patient removes his dressing and cleanses his operative site with soap and water in the shower daily, and then reapplies a

From the Department of Surgery, Jersey Shore Medical Center, Neptune, New Jersey.
This article has been reproduced with permission from the *American Journal of Proctology, Gastroenterology & Colon & Rectal Surgery,* Vol. 31, No. 12, December 1980.

gauze dressing. An elastic support belt can be worn. He can continue in his normal activities, but should avoid heavy lifting.

Results

Exteriorization has been performed in five patients with acute sigmoid diverticulitis (Table 1). None of these patients had prior bowel symptoms or previous attacks of diverticulitis. An unequivocal preoperative diagnosis of acute diverticulitis was made in only one of the five patients. Exteriorization was easily performed in three. In two patients, mobilization of the left colon was required to effect exteriorization. Frank anterior perforations closed spontaneously within two weeks in two patients. One mesenteric perforation healed within a similar time span. One large perforation began functioning as a colostomy postoperatively and failed to heal before the patient expired. In all of the four surviving patients, normal bowel movements occurred despite an exteriorized sigmoid colon.

The hospitalization time ranged from 12 to 17 days. Four patients were discharged with exteriorized sigmoid colons. All four patients had complete spontaneous regression of the exteriorized bowel to beneath the level of the skin, and spontaneous closure of the skin over the regressed bowel, within a 3 month time period. Two patients had subsequent elective sigmoid resections, and repair of ventral hernias. One patient was 87 at the time of his exteriorization, and chose to live with his incisional hernia. He was last seen 3½ years later without bowel problems.

The last patient operated upon requires further discussion. This was the only case of acute diverticulitis without frank perforation. A preoperative diagnosis of appendicitis or diverticulitis was made. He was treated medically for 24 hours without improvement. Subsequent operation disclosed an inflamed indurated sigmoid colon segment about 3 inches long. There was no frank perforation or pus. The segment was exteriorized after first mobilizing the left colon. Some surgeons would consider leaving a nonperforated acute diverticulitis alone, and close the abdomen, and continue with medical management rather than commit this patient to colostomy and multistaged procedures. If the patient failed to improve, or suddenly deteriorated due to perforation, another operation would be required, with the patient worse off than before. Exteriorization without colostomy in this type of case is of obvious benefit.

Discussion

The clinical diagnosis of diverticulitis is often uncertain. Out of seven cases of perforative sigmoid diverticulitis operated on by Watkins, two were diagnosed preoperatively as acute appendicitis, and one as acute pelvic inflammatory disease.[1] In Miller's series of fourteen free perforations, seven were diagnosed as diverticulitis, three as appendicitis, and four as perforated viscus.[2] Few surgeons would advocate the medical treatment of acute appendicitis. Yet, acute sigmoid diverticulitis, not infrequently, presents as mid or right sided abdominal pain and tenderness, due to a mobile sigmoid loop. The differential diagnosis of acute diverticulitis includes appendicitis, perforated carcinomas of the colon, mesenteric vascular occlusions, strangulated bowel obstructions, pelvic inflammatory disease, and left ureteral calculus. Barium enema examination may be diagnostic, but there is a reluctance to request barium enema examination on patients with clinically acute abdominal signs for fear of spillage of barium through a perforated diverticulum. The definitive diagnosis is made only at the time of surgery.

Acute diverticulitis presenting as an acute surgical abdomen frequently means perforation. Byrne reported 40% perforations in 106 cases operated upon.[3] Peritonitis was present in 14%, and abscess formation in 26% of the 106 cases. The mortality rate in those cases were 26 and 39%, respectively. Localio states that "If there is evidence of a spreading peritonitis or if a previously stabilized and subsiding abscess shows evidence of enlargement with spread in peritoneal signs, then urgent operation is indicated. To persist with conservative management is to court disaster."[4]

The most popular operation for perforative sigmoid diverticulitis is drainage plus diverting colostomy, followed by resection and anastomosis as a later elective procedure, and finally colostomy closure (three-stage procedure). The major criticism of this operative approach, is

TABLE 1. *Clinical Data on Five Cases of Exteriorization*

Patient	Age	Onset	Prior bowel symptoms	WBC	Preoperative diagnosis	Preoperative Medical therapy (hr.)	Operative findings	Hospital stay (days)	Complications	Mortality
1	59	24 hours	0	19,000	Appendicitis vs. divertic- ulitis	Several	Pus in pelvis. Mesenteric perforation.	17 (Elective resection and anastomosis 3 months later. 15 day stay)	Minor wound infection	0
2	48	5 days	0	11,300	Acute divertic- ulitis	24	Pus in pelvis. One cm. free perforation.	17 (Elective resection 4 months later. 16 day stay)	Pneumonitis	0
3	87	2–3 days	0	1,900	Perforated viscus	Several	Generalized peritonitis. Free perforation in sigmoid.	17	Pneumonitis	0
4	67	8 hours	0	2,800	Perforated viscus	Several	Fecal peritonitis, Large free perforation in sigmoid.	13	Preoperative septic shock BP 60 Postoperative respiratory renal failure	Yes 13 days
5	51	2 days	0	19,000	Appendicitis vs. divertic- ulitis	24	Inflamed ulcerated sigmoid segment with adematous mesentery. No perforation identified. No pus.	12	0	0

TABLE 2. *Summary of Exteriorizations for Perforative Diverticulitis*

	Cases	Mortality
Bacon	6	0
Black	1	0
Knecht	5	1
Linder	1	0
Localio	3	0
Miller, Wichern	1	1
Rodkey, Welch	2	0
Smiley	1	0
Staunton	5	0
Watkins, Oliver	6	0
Total	31	2

that the septic focus remains in the peritoneal cavity, and continues to leak and further contaminate.

Smiley reported 19 cases of perforated sigmoid diverticulitis.[5] Nine out of 16 patients treated by proximal colostomy and drainage died.[5] In Byrne's series, the traditional three-stage procedure resulted in a 28% mortality among 32 cases.[3] Classen, however, reported a combined three-stage mortality of only 11% in 211 cases.[6]

A second criticism of the three-stage procedure is the prolonged period of morbidity and hospitalization required. In Levy's series of 28 three-stage operations, the average time from initial surgery to colostomy closure and normal bowel function was 32 weeks.[7]

The next most popular operation is resection of the perforated segment, bringing out the proximal end as a end colostomy, and either bringing out the distal end as a mucus fistula, or closing it and leaving it in situ. In recent years this two-stage procedure has been performed more frequently, as it gets rid of the septic focus, preventing continued peritoneal soilage. However, it does result in a colostomy. At a later date, reexploration is performed with resection of the colostomy, mobilization of the colon, and reanastomosis of the proximal and distal ends of bowel.

Nahrwold reported one death among ten cases of perforated sigmoid diverticulitis treated by resection without anastomosis.[8] Hospitalization time averaged 21 days for the first stage. Reanastomosis (second stage) was performed 16 weeks later.

Resection and primary anastomosis is a third operative method of treating this disease. Localio found in the literature 39 patients treated by primary resection and anastomosis with three deaths, (a mortality of 7.7%) but felt its usage in the patient with perforation and spreading peritonitis "overly venturesome."[4] If an anastomatic leak occurs, the results can be disastrous!

A fourth alternative, exteriorization, has been performed infrequently for perforative diverticulitis (Table 2). Exteriorization has the advantage of removing the septic focus from the peritoneal cavity, and can be performed more rapidly than resection with or without anastomosis. The major criticism is that exteriorization cannot be performed in most cases. I do not believe this criticism is valid.

Stanton reported five exteriorizations with subsequent colostomies in 14 cases of perforative diverticulitis.[9] However, in retrospect, he felt he could have exteriorized 12 out of the 14 cases. In seven personal consecutive cases of perforative sigmoid diverticulitis, I was able to exteriorize five. Exteriorization was not possible in one extremely obese patient with a shortened mesentery, and in one patient with a very low perforation.

Exteriorizations usually have been followed by resection of the exteriorized segment and colostomy, or the exteriorized perforation has simply been opened so it functions as a colostomy. In either case, the patient has a colostomy, and this remains until an elective operation can be performed to resect the colostomy or reanastomose the previously resected bowel. Bacon, Localio, Miller, Rodkey, Smiley, Stanton and Watkins all exteriorized with colostomy.[1,2,4,5,9–11] Exteriorization without subsequent resection or colostomy has been rare.

In 1930, Black reported spontaneous closure of an exteriorized sigmoid perforation and complete healing over the wound in one patient.[12] He intended to remove the exteriorized segment later, but did not, because of the "rapidity with which the extruded bowel became covered over." Linder, in 1962, reported exteriorization without colostomy.[13] He observed that exteriorized perforations heal, and that the bowel recedes into the abdomen in 8 to 12 weeks, during which time the bowel functions normally.

The five cases described, further illustrate that sigmoid diverticular perforations can heal when exteriorized. Colostomy with an abdominal anus can be avoided. Exteriorized sigmoid colon recedes spontaneously, and the wound contracts, providing complete wound closure. Multiple operations are not always necessary. If a later elective resection and anastomosis is planned, at least the patient does not have to spend this interim caring for a colostomy. Patients don't like colostomies. Perhaps by utilizing exteriorization without colostomy, there will be less reluctance to operate for sigmoid diverticulitis. It is hoped that early operation, as has been the case for acute appendicitis, can lead to a reduction in the mortality and morbidity still associated with diverticular perforation.

REFERENCES

1. Watkins GL, Oliver GA. Management of perforative sigmoid diverticulitis with diffusing peritonitis. Arch Surg 1966;92:928–933.
2. Miller DW, Wichern WA. Perforated sigmoid diverticulitis. Am J Surg 1971;121:536–540.
3. Byrne JJ, Garick EI. Surgical treatment of diverticulitis. Am J Surg 1971;121:379–382.
4. Localio SA, Stahl WM. Diverticular disease of the alimentary tract. Part 1. The colon. Curr Probl Surg, 1967.
5. Smiley DF. Perforated sigmoid diverticulitis with spreading peritonitis. Am J Surg 1966;111:431–434.
6. Classen JN, Bonardi R, O'Mara CS, Finney DCW, Sterioff S. Surgical treatment of acute diverticulitis by staged procedures. Ann Surg 1976;184:582–585.
7. Levy SB, Fitts MD, Lench JB. Surgical treatment of diverticulor disease of the colon. Ann Surg 1967;166:947–953.
8. Nahrwold DL, DeMuth WE. Diverticulitis with perforations into the peritoneal cavity. Ann Surg 1977;185:80–85.
9. Staunton MDM. Treatment of perforated diverticulitis coli. Br Med J 1962;1:916–918.
10. Bacon HE, McKay ER. Surgical management of diverticulitis of the sigmoid. J Int Coll Surg 1948;11:560–569.
11. Rodkey GV, Welch CE. Surgical management of colonic diverticulitis with free perforation or abscess formation. Am J Surg 1969;117:265–269.
12. Black JM. Perforative diverticulitis of the colon. Br Med J 1931;1:180.
13. Linder JM, Hoffman S. Exteriorization in the surgical management of acute free perforations in diverticulitis of the sigmoid colon. Surg Gynecol Obstet 1962;114:755–757.

Voiding Function and Dysfunction: A Coordinated Overview

ALAN J. WEIN, M.D.

DURING THE TENURE of Jonathan Rhoads at the University of Pennsylvania, Philadelphia, the greatest strides in urologic research and their clinical correlation have been made in the physiology and pharmacology of lower urinary tract function and the evaluation, classification, and management of voiding dysfunction. Our basic research has concentrated primarily on the correlation of neuromorphology, neurophysiology, and neuropharmacology in normal function and various states of dysfunction, on the relationship between the metabolic and functional characteristics of bladder smooth muscle, and on the mechanisms of action of various drugs on the bladder and outlet.

The hallmark of our clinical achievements has been accurate and expandable simplification, brief and logical enough for the clinician to remember and use in daily practice, but embodying all the concepts necessary for expansion and inclusion of all pertinent details in those situations which require it. It seems particularly appropriate for this volume to briefly summarize our current views on voiding function and integrate these with an approach to voiding dysfunction which begins with a tabularized simplification of lower urinary tract function emphasizing the "target points" for evaluation, classification and management of all types of voiding dysfunction.

Relevant Anatomy, Physiology, and Pharmacology of the Lower Urinary Tract

Anatomically and embryologically the bladder has traditionally been divided into detrusor and trigone regions. Neuromorphologically and neuropharmacologically, it is more appropriately divided into "body" and "base," a distinction made on the basis of distinct differences between the smooth muscle lying circumferentially above (body) and below (base) the level of the ureterovesical junction. Bladder smooth muscle bundles are, to a greater or lesser extent, loosely organized in the area of the bladder base into an outer longitudinal, middle circular, and inner longitudinal layer. There is significant disagreement regarding the continuity of some longitudinal smooth muscle from the bladder into the urethra. The entire urethral length in the female and proximal portion (down to the urogenital diaphragm) in the male contains smooth muscle which is capable of affecting urethral resistance. The "smooth sphincter" refers to the smooth muscle of the bladder neck and proximal urethra. This is not an anatomic sphincter, but a physiologic one. Normally, resistance increases in the smooth sphincter during bladder filling and urine storage, and decreases in this area during an emptying bladder contraction. The classical view of the "external sphincter" is that of a striated muscle within the leaves of the urogenital diaphragm which, on contraction, is capable of stopping the urinary stream. This concept has been expanded to include an intramural and extramural portion. The extramural portion corresponds roughly to the classical external urethral sphincter and the urogenital diaphragm. The intramural portion denotes skeletal muscle intimately associated with the urethra in both sexes above the urogenital diaphragm, continuous from that level for a variable distance to the bladder neck, and forming an integral part of the outer muscular layer of the urethra. In the male, although some striated muscle is seen in the prostatic capsule and parenchyma, this intramural portion is primarily located between the verumontanum and the urogenital diaphragm. Activity increases in the striated sphincter during the filling/storage phase of micturition, and virtually disappears during normal emptying.

The classical view of the peripheral autonomic nervous system involves a two-neuron

From the Division of Urology, University of Pennsylvania School of Medicine, Philadelphia, Pennsylvania.

system: preganglionic neurons emanating from the central nervous system and making synaptic contact with cells within ganglia, from which postganglionic neurons emerge to innervate peripheral organs. This relatively simple concept, although still useful for the purposes of discussion, has undergone much contemporary expansion and modification.

Most innervation of the lower urinary tract actually emanates from peripheral ganglia which are at a short distance from, adjacent to, or within the organs they innervate (the "urogenital short neuron system"). Additionally, the efferent autonomic pathways do not necessarily conform to the classical two-neuron model, as they are often interrupted by more than one synaptic relay. For many years the only autonomic neurotransmitters recognized were acetylcholine and norepinephrine. It has become obvious that further transmitters are involved in various components of the autonomic nervous system, and a once relatively simple concept of chemical neurotransmission has been expanded to include synaptic systems which involve modulator transmitter mechanisms, prejunctional inhibition or enhancement of transmitter release, postjunctional modulation of transmitter action, co-transmitter release, and the secondary involvement of locally synthesized hormones and other substances such as prostaglandins. All of these are subject to neuronal and hormonal regulation, desensitization and hypersensitization. Finally, these relationships may be altered by changes which occur secondary to disease or destruction in the neural axis, obstruction of the lower urinary tract, aging, hormonal status, and chronic drug administration.

The pelvic and hypogastric nerves supply the bladder and urethra with efferent parasympathetic and sympathetic innervation, respectively, and both convey afferent sensory impulses from these organs to the spinal cord. The parasympathetic efferent supply is classically described as originating in the grey matter of sacral spinal cord segments S_2 to S_4. This preganglionic supply ultimately is conveyed by the pelvic nerve. Efferent sympathetic fibers to the bladder and urethra are thought to originate in spinal cord segments T_{11} to L_2, and are carried within the hypogastric nerves. Bilaterally, at a variable distance from the bladder and urethra the hypogastric pelvic nerves meet and branch to form the pelvic plexus. Divergent brances of this pelvic plexus innervate the pelvic organs. Efferent innervation of the striated sphincter is classically thought to be somatic, and to emanate from sacral spinal cord segments S_2 to S_4 *via* the pudendal nerve. Some believe that the striated sphincter also is innervated by branches of the autonomic nervous system as well.

Cholinergic innervation is abundant to all areas of the bladder of animals and of man. Although most authorities agree about the existence of a cholinergic innervation at least of the proximal urethra in animals, there is considerable disagreement regarding the extent (and in some cases existence) of a similar innervation in man. It is generally agreed that abundant muscarinic cholinergic receptor sites exist throughout the bladder body and base of various animal species and of man. A sustained bladder contraction is produced by stimulation of the pelvic nerves, and it is generally agreed that reflex activation of this pelvic nerve excitatory tract is responsible for the emptying bladder contraction of normal micturition, and for the involuntary bladder contractions seen with various diseases of the neural axis and response to lower urinary tract obstruction. Whether acetylcholine is the sole neurotransmitter released during such stimulation is highly controversial. Atropine resistance refers to the only partial antagonism exhibited by atropine of the bladder response to pelvic nerve stimulation or isolated bladder strips to electrical field stimulation. Atropine resistance is generally agreed to occur in various experimental animal models, and the most logical explanation seems to be release of additional neurotransmitter(s) besides acetylcholine in response to nerve stimulation. Whether atropine resistance actually occurs in normal man is a matter of controversy. However, one should not ignore the possibility that different types of atropine resistance may exist in various types of bladder hyperactivity, regardless of the normal state of affairs.

Adrenergic innervation of the bladder and urethral smooth musculature has been extensively demonstrated in animals. These studies have shown that the smooth musculature of the bladder base and proximal urethra possesses a rich adrenergic innervation, whereas the bladder body has a sparse but definite such innervation. The density of innervation seems in all areas to be less than that of the cholinergic systems. However, there is considerable disagreement as to even the presence of postganglionic sympathetic innervation in the bladder and proximal urethra of man. There is general agreement that the smooth muscle of

TABLE 1. *Functional Classification of Voiding Dysfunction*

- Failure to store
  - Because of the bladder
  - Because of the outlet
- Failure to empty
  - Because of the bladder
  - Because of the outlet

the human male bladder neck possesses a dense adrenergic innervation, but little consensus otherwise. Even those authorities who ascribe a significant influence of the sympathetic nervous system on the micturition cycle have difficulty demonstrating more than a sparse adrenergic innervation in other areas of the bladder and urethra. There is general agreement, however, that the smooth muscle of the bladder and proximal urethra in a variety of animals and in man contains both alpha and beta-adrenergic receptors. Alpha-adrenergic responses predominate in the bladder base and proximal urethra, whereas beta-adrenergic responses predominate in the bladder body. Additionally, there is general agreement that there is a significant inhibitory influence exerted on parasympathetic ganglionic transmission by postganglionic sympathetic fibers.

Other peripheral neurotransmitters doubtless exist in the lower urinary tract, and this is the object of much contemporary investigation. Adenosine triphosphate (ATP) has been postulated as the "other" excitatory neurotransmitter in cases of atropine resistance. Pharmacologic evidence for a role for prostaglandins in bladder contractility also exists. VIP generally has been shown to have an inhibitory effect on bladder muscle contractility, and has been postulated to act as a modifier of bladder activity during filling.

TABLE 2. *Expanded Functional Classification*

- Failure to store
  - Because of the bladder
    - Detrusor hyperactivity
      - Involuntary contractions
        - Suprasacral neurologic disease
        - Bladder outlet obstruction
        - Idiopathic
      - Decreased compliance
        - Fibrosis
        - Idiopathic
    - Sensory urgency
      - Inflammatory
      - Infectious
      - Neurologic
      - Psychologic
      - Idiopathic
  - Because of the outlet
    - Stress incontinence
    - Nonfunctional bladder neck/proximal urethra
- Failure to empty
  - Because of the bladder
    - Neurologic
    - Myogenic
    - Psychogenic
    - Idiopathic
  - Because of the outlet
    - Anatomic
      - Prostatic obstruction
      - Bladder neck contracture
      - Urethral stricture
    - Functional
      - Smooth sphincter dyssynergia
      - Striated sphincter dyssynergia

TABLE 3. *Urodynamics Simplified*

	Bladder	Outlet
Filling/storage	P_{Det} (FCMG)*	P_{Ureth}† Fluoro‡
Emptying	P_{Det} (VCMG)§	P_{Ureth}† Fluoro‡ EMG‖
	Flow¶ RU#	

* Filling cystometrogram (recording of detrusor pressure during filling).
† Urethral pressure(s).
‡ Fluoroscopy.
§ Voiding cystometry (recording of detrusor pressure during voluntary or involuntary emptying).
‖ EMG of periurethral striated muscle.
¶ Flowmetry.
\# Residual urine determination.

Micturition basically is a function of the peripheral autonomic nervous system. However, the ultimate control of lower urinary tract function obviously resides at higher neurologic levels. There is general consensus that the micturition "center" in the spinal cord is primarily localized to segments S_2 to S_4, with the major portion at S_3. However, there is little question that the brain stem, specifically the neurons of the pontine-mesencephalic grey matter, contains the nuclei which are the origin of the final common pathway to bladder motor neurons. Input to this area is derived from the cerebellum, basal ganglia, thalamus and hypothalamus, and cerebral cortex. Bladder contraction elicited by stimulation at or above this area seems to occur with a decrease in activity of the periurethral striated musculature, as in normal micturition. The region of the cerebral hemispheres primarily concerned with bladder function consists of the superomedial portion of the frontal lobes and the genu of the corpus callosum. Transection experiments indicate that the net effect of these areas is inhibitory. Strong evidence is accumulating that endogenous opioid peptides influence micturition by a tonic inhibitory effect on detrusor reflex pathways. These inhibitory effects could be mediated at several levels, including the peripheral bladder ganglia, the sacral spinal cord, and the brain stem micturition center. Different types of opioid receptors may be responsible, at different sites, for different types of effects on bladder contractility.

What follows is a concise and simplified description of the normal processes involved in lower urinary tract function which seems consistent with existent data and opinions. The two functions of the lower urinary tract are the storage and active expulsion of urine. During bladder filling at physiological rates, intravesical pressure initially rises slowly despite large increases in volume. This phenomenon is due primarily to the passive elastic and viscoelastic properties of the smooth muscle and connective tissue of the bladder wall. There is little neural efferent activity until a certain critical intravesical pressure is reached, after which there is a gradual reflex increase in pudendal nerve activity which causes increased activity in the striated sphincter.

In animals, and perhaps in humans as well, an additional spinal sympathetic reflex also results. The efferent limb of this reflex is through the hypogastric nerve, resulting in inhibition of bladder contractile activity through an effect on parasympathetic ganglionic transmission and also in an increase in outlet resistance because of active stimulation of the adrenergic receptors in the smooth sphincter.

A decrease in bladder body contractility mediated through beta adrenergic receptors also may play a role. A tonic inhibitory influence exerted by endogenous opioids very likely plays a contributory role in maintaining bladder stability during filling. Intraurethral pressure normally is greater than intravesical pressure, and this relationship is maintained during increases in intra-abdominal pressure because of the anatomic localization of the sphincter unit and the normally positive pressure transmission ratio to this area with respect to intravesical contents.

TABLE 4. *Therapy to Facilitate Bladder Filling/Urine Storage*

Inhibiting bladder contractility/decreasing sensory input
Timed bladder emptying
Pharmacologic therapy
Anticholinergic agents
Musculotropic relaxants
Polysynaptic inhibitors
Calcium antagonists
Beta-adrenergic agonists
Alpha-adrenergic antagonists
Prostaglandin inhibitors
Tricyclic antidepressants
DMSO
Bromocriptine
Biofeedback, bladder retraining
Bladder overdistention
Electrical stimulation (reflex inhibition)
Interruption of innervation
Subarachnoid block
Selective sacral rhizotomy
Peripheral bladder denervation
Cystoplasty (augmentation)
Increasing outlet resistance
Physiotherapy
Electrical stimulation of the pelvic floor
Pharmacologic therapy
Alpha-adrenergic agonists
Tricyclic antidepressants
Beta-adrenergic antagonists
Nonsurgical mechanical compression
Surgical mechanical compression
Vesicourethral suspension (SUI)
Circumventing problem
Antidiuretic hormone-like agents
External collecting device
Intermittent catheterization
Continuous catheterization
Urinary diversion

DMSO: dimethyl sulfoxide.

Although many factors are involved in the micturition reflex, it is intravesical pressure producing the sensation of distention that is primarily responsible for the initiation of voluntarily induced emptying of the lower urinary tract. The origin of the parasympathetic neural outflow to the bladder is in the sacral spinal cord. However, the actual organizational center for the micturition reflex in an intact neural axis is in the brain stem.

The final step in voluntarily induced micturition involves inhibition of the somatic neural efferent activity to the striated sphincter and an inhibition of all aspects of the spinal sympathetic reflex evoked during filling. Efferent parasympathetic pelvic nerve activity is ultimately what is responsible for a highly coordinated contraction of the bulk of the bladder smooth musculature. A decrease in outlet resistance occurs, with adaptive shaping or funneling of the relaxed bladder outlet. This involves reflex inhibition of striated and smooth sphincter tone, and may involve an active mechanism of beta adrenergic mediated smooth muscle relaxation in this area as well. Superimposed on these autonomic and somatic reflexes and modifying factors are complex peripheral and central inputs, both facilitory and inhibitory, which allow for the full conscious control of micturition.

Summary

Whatever disagreements exist, all "experts" would agree on certain points. The micturition cycle involves two relatively discrete processes: bladder filling and urine storage, and bladder emptying. Bladder filling and urine storage requires the following: (1) accommodation of increasing volumes of urine at a low intravesical pressure and with appropriate sensation; (2) a closed bladder outlet at rest which remains so during increases in intra-ab-

TABLE 5. *Therapy to Facilitate Bladder Emptying*

- Increasing intravesical pressure
  - External compression, valsalva
  - Promotion or initiation of reflex contractions
    - Trigger zones or maneuvers
    - Bladder training, tidal drainage
  - Pharmacologic therapy
    - Parasympathomimetic agents
    - Prostaglandins
    - Blockers of inhibition
      - Alpha-adrenergic antagonists
      - Opioid antagonists
  - Electrical stimulation
    - Directly to the bladder
    - To the spinal cord or nerve roots
- Decreasing outlet resistance
  - At a site of anatomic obstruction
    - Prostatectomy
    - Urethral stricture repair/dilation
  - At the level of the smooth sphincter
    - Transurethral resection or incision of the bladder neck
    - Y-V plasty of the bladder neck
    - Pharmacologic therapy
      - Alpha-adrenergic antagonists
      - Beta-adrenergic agonists
  - At the level of the striated sphincter
    - External sphincterotomy
    - Urethral overdilation
    - Pudendal nerve interruption
    - Pharmacologic therapy
      - Skeletal muscle relaxants
        - Benzodiazepines
        - Baclofen
        - Dantrolene
      - Alpha-adrenergic antagonists
    - Psychotherapy, biofeedback
- Circumventing problem
  - Intermittent catheterization
  - Continuous catheterization
  - Urinary diversion

dominal pressure; and (3) absence of involuntary bladder contractions. Bladder emptying requires the following: (1) a coordinated contraction of adequate magnitude of the bladder smooth musculature; (2) a concomitant lowering of resistance at the level of the smooth sphincter and the striated sphincter; and (3) absence of anatomic obstruction.

Each component of the two processes represents a "target point." Each target point is a focus for understanding relevant neuromorphology, neurophysiology, and neuropharmacology (as much or as little as desired or necessary) for classification of voiding dysfunction, for urodynamic evaluation, and for treatment.

Any type of voiding dysfunction must result from an abnormality of one or more of the factors listed as involved in the two phases of the micturition cycle. This division, with its implied subdivisions under each category into causes related to the bladder and causes related to the outlet, provides a perfect rationale for the classification of all types of voiding dysfunction into disorders related to bladder filling or urine storage, and disorders related to bladder emptying (Tables 1 and 2). There are indeed some types of voiding dysfunction which represent a combination of filling/storage and emptying disorders. Within this scheme, these combined disorders become readily understandable. Furthermore, one may take all aspects of urodynamic and video urodynamic evaluation and classify the individual component studies as to exactly what they evaluate in terms of either bladder or outlet activity during filling/storage or emptying (Table 3). Finally, one can then easily classify all known treatments for voiding dysfunction under the broad categories of whether they facilitate filling/storage or emptying, and whether they do so by an action primarily on the bladder or on the components of the bladder outlet and construct an easily understood but accurate "menu" for treatment (Tables 4 and 5).

BIBLIOGRAPHY

Barrett DM, Wein AJ. Controversies in Neuro-Urology. London, New York: Churchill-Livingstone, 1984.

Barrett DM, Wein AJ. Voiding dysfunction: Diagnosis, classification, and management. In: Gillenwater J, Grayhack J, Duckett J, Howards S, eds. Textbook of Urology. Chicago: Yearbook Medical Publishers, 1987;863–962.

Mundy AR, Stephenson TP, Wein AJ. Urodynamics: Principles, Practice and Application. London, New York: Churchill Livingstone, 1984.

Wein AJ. Classification of neurogenic voiding dysfunction: A review. J Urol 1981;125:605.

Wein AJ. Classification of voiding dysfunction. American Urological Association UPDATE Series, vol. 6, no. 4, 1986;1–8.

Wein AJ. Pharmacology of bladder and urethra. In: Stanton SL, Tanagho EA, eds. Surgery of Female Incontinence. Berlin, New York: Springer Verlag, 1986;229–250.

Wein AJ, Levin RM, Barrett DM. Voiding function: Relevant anatomy, physiology, pharmacology. In: Gillenwater J, Grayhack J, Duckett J, Howards S, eds. Textbook of Urology. New York: Yearbook Medical Publishers, 1987;800–862.

Wein AJ, Raezer DM. Physiology of micturition. In: Krane RJ, Siroky MB, eds. Clinical Neurourology. Boston: Little Brown, 1979;1–33.

The Mitrofanoff Principle in Continent Urinary Reservoirs

JOHN W. DUCKETT AND HOWARD M. SNYDER III

THE CONTINENT URINARY RESERVOIR has been a challenge for many years in urology. The ureterosigmoidostomy, as the oldest urinary diversion, garnered an unfavorable reputation in the mid 1950s that has carried through to the present. At the time it was being condemned by Ferris and Odel[1] and Stamey,[2] Leadbetter[3] was contributing his effective ureterosigmoid anastomosis that prevented reflux. Goodwin et al[4] and Hohenfellner[5] also reported an effective ureterocolonic anastomosis that prevented reflux and the ravages of pyelonephritis and stone formation. Simultaneous with these reports was Bricker's[6] ileal conduit that took over as the "ideal urinary diversion."

Except for a few sporadic reports over the past 20 years, the continent urinary reservoir received little impetus until the concept of clean intermittent catheterization (CIC) became widely accepted.[7] Intermittent catheterization of patients with spinal cord injuries and congenital neuropathic bladders has revolutionized the management of these problems and avoided the common need for permanent urinary diversions. It is CIC that has made possible the breakthroughs in continent urinary reservoirs in the last decade.

In 1969, Kock[8] created an intraabdominal catheterizable bowel reservoir entirely of ileum in patients after colectomy in order to avoid an ileostomy and its appliance. This met with varied success and acceptance. However, when he created the same type of reservoir for urine,[9,10] the continent reservoir gained popularity with patients with cancer of the bladder as an alternative to permanent urinary drainage into a collecting device.[11]

Gilchrist et al[12] proposed using the ileocecal segment as a reservoir, connecting the ureters into the cecum in an antirefluxing manner, and using the natural ileocecal valve for continence. This was not as successful as desired. Gil-Vernet[13] also contributed to the construction of a functioning artificial bladder.

Hendren,[14] in his undiversion experience, worked for many years developing a continent ileocecal intussusception to prevent reflux in order to place large ureters into the ileum.[15–17] These same principles have been used to create a cutaneous continent stoma for a urinary reservoir using ileum into colon.[18] However, the continent ileal stoma, through which to catheterize and drain the reservoir, is burdened by a considerable revision rate.

We intend to present the case for the Mitrofanoff principle as the most reliable and simplistic flap valve concept for continence and catheterization of the reservoir.[19,20]

Mitrofanoff Procedure

Mitrofanoff's original objective was a "cystostomy with a continent opening easy to catheterize and associated with the closure of the vesical neck using the tip of the appendix opening into the bladder at the end of an antirefluxing submucosal tunnel and the other end hemmed to the skin" (Fig 1). Such an appendicovesicostomy was performed in 16 children with encouraging success when first reported in 1980.[21] In 1985, Mitrofanoff[22] reviewed an additional eight patients, making a total of 16 males and eight females. The appendix was used in 21 cases and the ureter was used in two cases. In one case, a bladder tube was fashioned that was kinked back on itself to create a successful antirefluxing valve. Good results were achieved in 11 patients with follow-up continuing from 2 to 10 years. Five cases developed hydronephrosis and were converted to cutaneous diversion early; in retrospect, they should have had a bladder augmentation. In four other cases, bladder augmentation

From the Department of Urology, Children's Hospital of Philadelphia, Philadelphia, Pennsylvania.
This article has been reproduced with permission from *Seminars in Urology,* Vol. 5, No. 1, 1987.

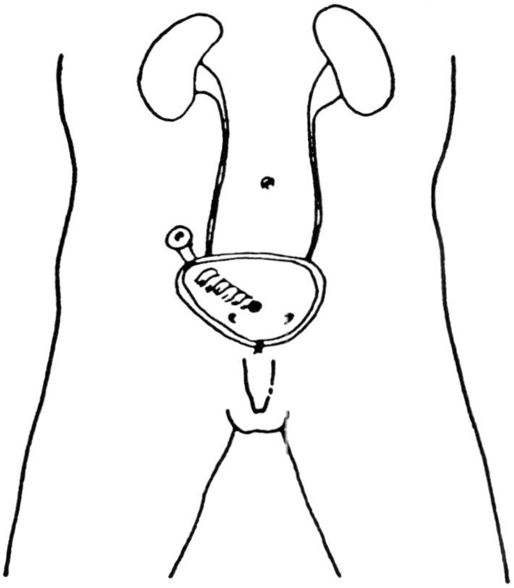

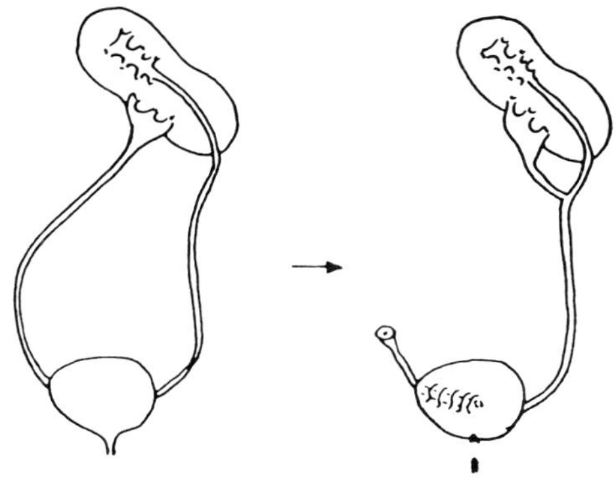

FIG. 1 (*left*). Mitrofanoff's original figure for continent cystostomy using transappendicular access to the bladder. (Reprinted with permission from Mitrofanoff P. Cystostomie continente trans-appendiculaire dans le traitement des vessies neurologiques. Chir Pediatr 1980;21:297–305.)

FIG. 2 (*right*). Original Mitrofanoff figure using the distal ureter as an access to the bladder for catheterization. (Reprinted with permission from Mitrofanoff P. Cystostomie continente trans-appendicularie dans le traitement des vessies neurologiques. Chir Pediatr 1980;21:297–305.)

was performed and the successful result was preserved. In two patients with an appendiceal implant, partial incontinence resulted and successful continence was achieved with the Benchekroun ileal nipple.[23,24] Another appendix kinked after 5 years when obesity became a problem; this was straightened surgically. One patient was lost to follow-up. Other Frenchmen also had successful experiences with this technique.[25–27]

In his original paper, Mitrofanoff described the successful use of a distal ureter brought to the skin as a catheterizable stoma to empty the bladder (Fig 2).[21] The lower ureter of the kidney brought to the skin was drained by high transureteroureterostomy (TUU). This technique has proved useful when the appendix is unsuitable or has been previously removed, and is possible even with a nondilated ureter.

Mitrofanoff Principle

The Mitrofanoff principle may be summarized as follows: (1) use of a narrow supple conduit (most frequently appendix or ureter) brought to the skin as a catheterizable stoma, (2) an antirefluxing connection of this conduit to a reservoir to provide continence (flap valve techniques are more satisfactory than nipple techniques), (3) a large low-pressure urine-storage reservoir (bladder, augmented bladder, bowel segment), (4) creation of an antirefluxing connection of the upper urinary tract to the reservoir to prevent reflux to the kidneys, and (5) intermittent catheterization to produce regular low-pressure complete emptying of the reservoir. We believe that the Mitrofanoff principle is a significant contribution and we will review our up-to-date experience in a variety of clinical settings.

Clinical Experience

Our experience at Children's Hospital of Philadelphia began in 1982. We studied 17 cases at Children's Hospital and five additional cases at an adult hospital (Hospital of the University of Pennsylvania, Philadelphia) or as a visiting professor elsewhere. The various clinical conditions are listed in Table 1.

Five of the 22 cases were prepubertal at the time of surgery. This group, predominantly adolescent to young adult, reflects the usual age when patients with urinary diversions request conversion to a continent urinary reservoir. We suspect more candidates for the Mitrofanoff procedure will come from the pool of adult myelomeningocele patients and paraplegias who will find it more convenient to catheterize an abdominal stoma rather than their urethras.

TABLE 1. *Primary Diagnoses*

Diagnosis	No. of Patients	Age (yrs)
Paraplegia	2	23, 30
Myelomeningocele	6	13, 14, 16, 16, 19, 19
Motor paralysis	1	22
Exstrophy/cloaca	5	7, 11, 16, 22, 23
Urethral absence/stricture	2	12, 19
Prune belly	3	7, 8, 15
Dysfunctional voider	1	17
Transplant	2	17, 22
Urethral valves		
Cloacal anomaly		

There are a variety of techniques in which we have used the Mitrofanoff principle. The classic Mitrofanoff, an appendicovesicostomy with closure of the bladder neck,[28] was performed in only five cases (Fig 3).[29] As it was continent, the bladder neck was preserved in the other six cases in which we used the appendix into the bladder. We augmented bladder capacity with a patch of ileum or sigmoid in nine of the 11 cases.

The next most common arrangement was to use an already established end ureterostomy as the catheterizing channel in five cases (Fig 4). The ureter was divided mid-way with an upper TUU and a lower ureterocystomy, leaving the skin ureterostomy blood supply to the distal ureter. A Leadbetter[3] ureteral implant into the tenia will prevent reflux into the upper

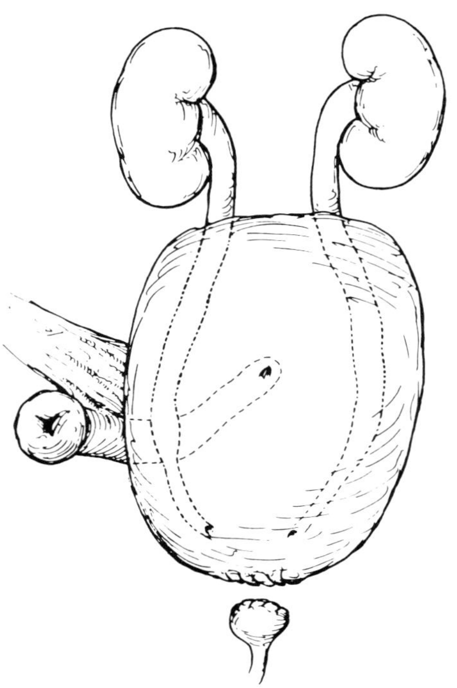

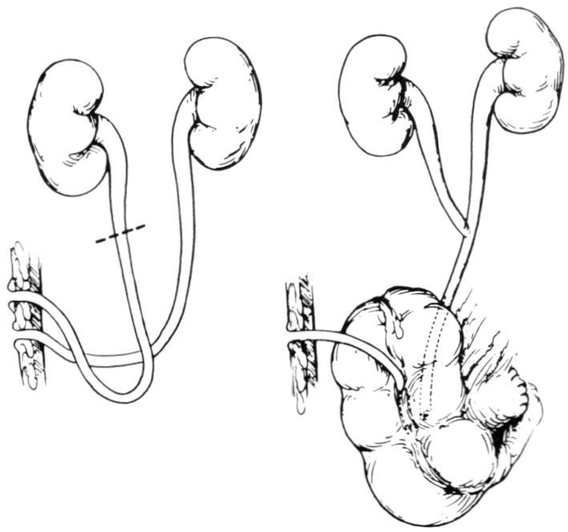

FIG. 3 (*left*). Classic Mitrofanoff. The isolated appendix is implanted with an antirefluxing submucosal tunnel into the posterior bladder wall; the bladder neck is closed to prevent urethral incontinence; the colonic end of the appendix is used as a stoma for catheterization. (Reprinted with permission from Duckett JW, Snyder HM: Continent urinary diversion: Variations on the Mitrofanoff principle. J Urol 136:58–62, © by Williams & Wilkins, 1986.)

FIG. 4 (*right*). End ureterostomies without bladder or urethra. The distal right ureter remains as a ureterostomy for catheterization; a right to left transureteroureterostomy is performed; both ureters are implanted into the cecal pouch in an antirefluxing submucosal trough. (Reprinted with permission from Duckett JW, Snyder HM: Continent urinary diversion: Variations on the Mitrofanoff principle. J Urol 136:58–62, © by Williams & Wilkins, 1986.)

tracts. In three cases, a bladder remnant supplied the vascularity to the distal ureter. In one, a solitary system, the small exstrophic bladder remnant was mobilized to the perineum, after removing the bladder mucosa. The ureteral orifice became the urethra catheterized into a cecal reservoir (Fig 5). Two other patients had small remnants of bladder with ureteral stumps. The ureteral orifice was mobilized to the skin, while the delicate stump produced a continent catheter port into an ileocecal reservoir.

In one case, a continent catheterizable stoma was produced by a tapered ileal segment implanted into the cecal wall. An appendicocecostomy, the Penn pouch, (Fig 6) was used in one case. The Penn pouch consists of the isolated appendix implanted into the colon for continence with the cecal end of the appendix as a small skin stoma for catheterization. Finally, one case was managed with an ileocecal pouch with the tapered ileum as the catheterized continent tract.[30]

Results

The variety of techniques used is listed in Table 2. Eighteen of the 22 patients had successful results with one procedure only. Success is measured by total continence, ease of catheterization with intervals greater than four hours, normal or stable upper tracts, and no pyelonephritis. Four patients had complications (18%). In one, a TUU developed an obstruction that required an operative revision. At the same time, a mild ureterostomy stomal leakage was controlled by imbricating the dilated ureter in the cecal pouch The same patient had three episodes of pyelonephritis due to contaminated catheterizations. Another patient sustained a renal leak that required placement of a stent with drainage. A third patient had urethral leakage that required a perineal revision of the bladder neck closure, which was unsatisfactory at the first procedure. The final complication was our only failure. This was an attempt at preserving the distal ureter attached to an ileal conduit as the catheterizable segment. We based the blood supply on a segment of bowel muscle and mesentery from the old ileal conduit. The mesentery was draped over the urinary reservoir, and as the reservoir filled, it must have compressed the mesentery and lead to devascularization of the ureter. This case has been managed successfully with a secondary tapered ileal segment implanted into the cecum with a submucosal course. This patient still has a slight problem with catheterization and uses a Conde tip to traverse a slight kink.

We used a complete bowel replacement of the bladder in ten cases; four of these were with cecum alone and six were with the ileum placed into the divided cecal wall in order to disrupt peristaltic waves and ensure low storage pressure.[31] The four cecal segments have

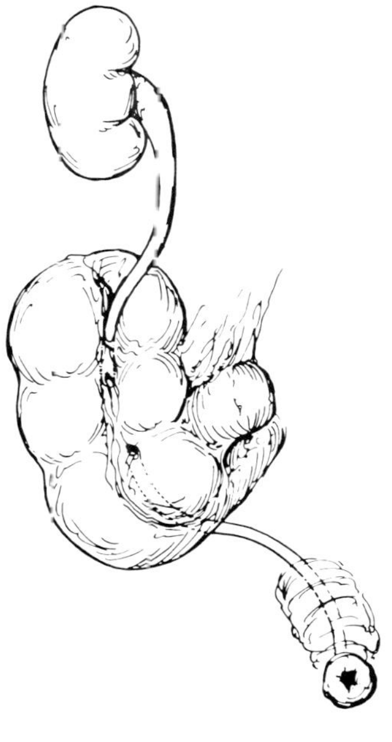

FIG. 5. Cloacal exstrophy variant. A solitary kidney with a ureteral orifice is placed into a small exstrophy bladder plate; the bladder muscle is mobilized to the perineum with the mucosa removed; the ureteral orifice becomes the urethra; both are divided into midureteral ends and implanted submucosally into the cecal reservoir for continence and antireflux. (Reprinted with permission from Duckett JW, Snyder HM: Continent urinary diversion: Variations on the Mitrofanoff principle. J Urol 136:58–62, © by Williams & Wilkins, 1986.)

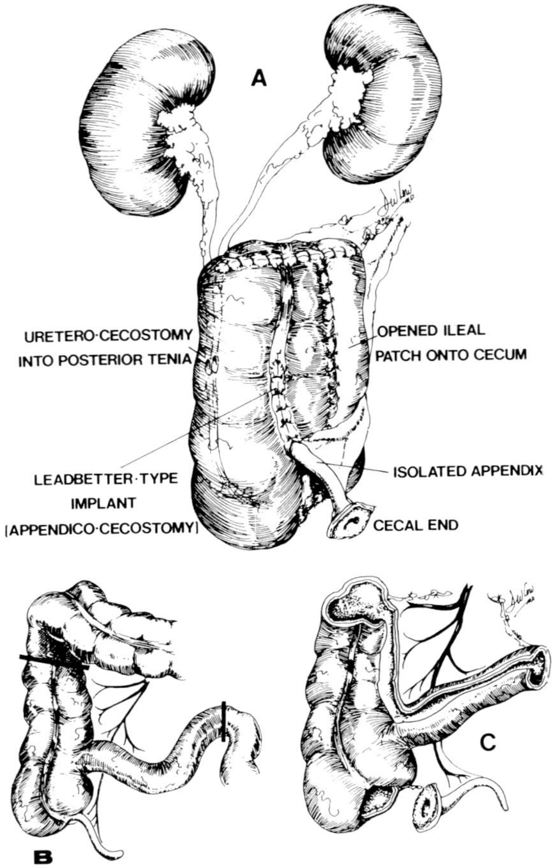

FIG. 6. Penn pouch. (A) Appendicocecostomy into the ileocecal pouch. (B and C) Preparation of the ileocecal pouch and the isolated appendix.

not had problems with high pressure waves, probably because they were long segments with a large capacity that damped the pressure rises produced by peristalsis.

Discussion

The basic elements of the Mitrofanoff principle will be discussed. Special credit should be given to the concept of CIC without which the continent urinary reservoir could not have developed. Lapides et al[7] deserve further praise for this seminal contribution to urology. The

TABLE 2. *Mitrofanoff Techniques*

Technique	No. of Patients
Appendicovesicostomy	11
Bladder neck closure	5
Ureterostomy and TUU	5
Bladder remnant and ureter	3
Ileal conduit*	1
Tapered ileum*	1
Imbricated ileum	1
Appendicocecostomy	1
Total	22

* Same patient.

general acceptance of self-catheterization as a way of life in patients who would otherwise be incontinent or who would require an external appliance for urine collection is testimony to the merit of the Lapides contribution. It also opened the door for innovative ways to construct continent urinary reservoirs.

A Large Low-Pressure Urine Storage Reservoir

This is achieved by using the bladder either alone or with a patch of ileum or sigmoid to augment the capacity. A wide "clam shell" sagittal opening of a small bladder effectively disrupts the ability of the detrusor to generate a high pressure and prevents the bowel patch from turning into a diverticulum. The opened bladder provides a large detrusor plate onto which the opened-out bowel patch may be added and into which the appendix or ureter(s) may be implanted. We have not excised any detrusor muscle. A generous augmentation is advised, and usually 20 to 30 cm of bowel is used.

In addition, the bladder neck may need to be closed if it is unable to prevent urethral leakage. This is a difficult procedure and a variety of methods have been reported.[21,28,32] If the bladder neck is competent, we would suggest it be left untouched (majority of our cases). Continuity of the bladder and urethra may be maintained as a "pop-off" element.

When no bladder is present, we currently prefer a long segment of cecum with the ileum incorporated into a longitudinal cecal split as a reservoir ("Le Bag").[33] The Mainz pouch is very similar, using two bends of ileum into a shorter cecal segment.[34,35] We have not had problems with our four cecal pouches due to high-pressure contractions of the intact bowel; perhaps the generous size of these segments has avoided this by damping the effect of peristaltic waves. We now ensure a low pressure by opening the cecum and incorporating an ileal patch, making impossible an effective peristaltic wave.

Another major concern, particularly in the myelomeningocele population, is bowel dysfunction related to removal of the distal ileum and cecum from bowel continuity. Several cases of intractable diarrhea are known in myelomeningocele patients; this may be due to lack of proper bile salt resorption in the distal ileum. Although this complication is rare and can be treated in most cases, the patients should be warned of the possibility. This may make the sigmoid an attractive alternative in children with a neurogenic rectum.

Antirefluxing Ureteroreservoir Connection

The colon will receive a ureterocolonic anastomosis with predictable success. A Leadbetter[3] reimplantation into a tenia trough with a mucosal closure of ureter to bowel will prevent reflux and avoid obstruction, especially with near-normal caliber ureters. Although we have not used it, the transcolonic tunneling of the ureters under the mucosa is equally effective.[4,5] The imbrication of bowel wall burying the ureter may also be effective in preventing reflux.[36] When we used the distal ureter for the Mitrofanoff (catheterizable) with a high TUU channel, there was only one antirefluxing bowel connection for the other ureter. We failed to stent one of these and paid for it with a renal urine leak, ascites, and a second surgical procedure.

A successful antirefluxing ureteroileal anastomosis has been reported by LeDuc et al.[37] This method lays the ureter into a mucosal slit of 3- to 4-cm length with fixation along the seromuscular wall. No attempt is made to cover the ureter with a mucosal tunnel. We have not yet tried this, but have successfully fixed the appendix into a mucosal trough in the trabeculated bladder with uneventful secondary epithelialization.

A Narrow Well-Vascularized Catheterized Conduit Made Continent by the Flap Valve Concept

The Mitrofanoff procedure initially used the isolated appendix with the cecal cuff brought to the skin as a stoma. The distal appendix with the tip amputated was implanted into the bladder like a ureter. Because of the excellent blood supply to the appendix, there is little concern for long-term harm to this mucosa-lined muscular conduit, even though it must withstand 1,500 to 2,500 catheter passages per year. Its small diameter actually facilitates catheterization (usually 10F to 14F catheter) by helping to avoid coiling of the catheter.

Using the ureter as the catheter conduit has many applications. The midureter may be divided and the upper part of the distal segment brought to the skin as an end ureterostomy. The distal attachment to the bladder must be continent, however, and violation of the blood supply to the vesicoureteral junction must be avoided. A detached ureteral reimplant would not seem wise unless it is done as an earlier separate procedure.[38] Three options to improve or assure continence of the distal ureter are available. First, a modified Lich-Gregoir-type[39] extravesical muscular trough reimplant should avoid injury to the distal ureteral blood supply. Second, a Hutch I-type[40] reimplant, which is essentially a transvesical Lich-Gregoir procedure, will work.[41] Proximal to the ureteral orifice, the ureter is dissected through the bladder wall and pulled into a submucosal position closing the bladder muscle beneath. Third, a Gil-Vernet[42] midline fixation of trigonal muscle may help to insure continence with no vesicoureteral reflux.

Use of the ureter as the Mitrofanoff channel into the bowel segment also provides much variety. Even if the ureters are dilated, an imbrication of the wall into the lumen[43] will narrow the ureteral diameter to permit implantation into a bowel tenia to secure an effective flap valve configuration.

Vascularity of the catheterizable ureter into the reservoir must be assured. If a pre-established end ureterostomy exists, the distal ureter will be well supplied through the stoma and the midureter will be safely divided without devascularization. Creation of a fresh end ureterostomy, while dividing the midureter and implanting into the bowel, would be most precarious.

We would also suggest an arrangement we have not yet tried, but which may be applicable to a moderately dilated system into a sclerotic unusable bladder. The distal end of the ureter could be brought to the skin for a catheterizable stoma, while the intact midportion of the ureter is tunneled into a colon segment for a long distance. A slit opening would then be made into the midureter into the lumen of bowel, preserving the ureteral blood supply but allowing two ureteral openings into the bowel, ie, one for catheterization and the other for urine from the kidney.[44]

In one bladder exstrophy patient, the capacity was so low that an augmentation could not be accomplished and still tubularize the bladder for continence. We narrowed the bladder into a 6-cm tube that was implanted into the cecum in a muscular tunnel for continence. This has been successful. A similar case was reported by Lobe et al.[45] Kropp and Angwafo[46] also describe a method of tubularizing a bladder flap that is then tunneled into the remaining bladder for continence.

The ileum itself or an old ileal conduit is too wide and bulky to place into the colon as a flap valve continent segment. Tapering of the ileal lumen by longitudinal excision also has limitations; the ileal mesentery may be quite fatty. Although the tapered ileum can be tunneled nicely, the mesentery is difficult to incorporate. Irregularities of the tapered lumen may make catheterization difficult due to diverticular formation or kinks.[47]

Rowland et al[30] used an imbricated ileal segment as the continence channel through which to catheterize. No intussusception of the ileocecal area is required and intraluminal irregularities are not present. With the cecal pouch and ileal patch on the right side, the imbricated ileal stoma may lie best in the left lower abdomen. Imbrication of the ileum should be performed with a permanent suture through the seromuscular coat only. Two layers of sutures will suffice. We have done this once with success.

A long tongue of cecum, eg, a Boari bladder flap, that could be narrowly tubularized would seem to have a precarious blood supply. However, a wider based flap tubularized *and* imbricated might be successful.

We were originally intrigued with the concept of the Benchekroun[23,24] nipple as a continence device. An ileal segment is intussuscepted in a reverse fashion with the seromuscular side on the inside. The outside lumen of ileal mucosa would be in continuity with the reservoir and fill with urine to compress the inner catheterizable lumen for continence. Although Benchekroun reported success with this in 25 cases,[24] we have not tried it.

Much has been written of the various ileal intussusception methods for the continent stoma.[10,11,17,18,48] We remain unconvinced that this concept will ultimately survive. We feel that the Mitrofanoff principle of a narrow lumen flap valve continence device is less complex and more dependable. The considerable variety of application of this principle makes it our preferred procedure.

Penn Pouch

Since the predominance of patients requesting a continent urinary reservoir will come from the bladder cancer population, we offer the Penn pouch as a rapidly accomplished and dependable alternative (Fig 6). Most of these patients will have their appendix intact and will have normal ureters. A pouch constructed from 20 cm of cecum and 20 cm of ileum, incorporated together after splitting the antimesenteric side of each, will provide a large-volume reservoir of low pressure. The ureters are implanted into the opened cecum as an antirefluxing anastomosis. The isolated appendix is placed into a seromuscular trough. The cecal end of the appendix is brought to the right inguinal area for the catheterizing port.

REFERENCES

1. Ferris DO, O'Dell HM. Electrolyte pattern of the blood after bilateral ureterosigmoidostomy. JAMA 1950;142:634–640.
2. Stamey TA. Pathogenesis and implications of electrolyte imbalance in ureterosigmoidostomy. Surg Gynecol Obstet 1956;103:736–758.
3. Leadbetter WF. Considerations of problems incident to performance of ureterosigmoidostomy: Report of a technique. J Urol 1952;65:8–18.
4. Goodwin WE, Harris AP, Kaufman JJ, et al. Open, transcolonic ureterointestinal anastomosis. Surg Gynecol Obstet 1953;97:295–300.
5. Hohenfellner R. Ureterosigmoidostomie, in Eckstein H, Hohenfellner R, Williams DI (eds): Surgical Pediatric Urology. Philadelphia, Saunders, 1977.
6. Bricker EM. Bladder substitution after pelvic evisceration. Surg Clin North Am 1950;30:1511–1521.
7. Lapides J, Diokno AC, Gould FR, et al. Further observations on self-catheterization. J Urol 1976;116:169–173.
8. Kock NG. Intra-abdominal "reservoir" in patients with permanent ileostomy. Preliminary observations on a procedure resulting in fecal "continence" in five ileostomy patients. Arch Surg 1969;99:223–231.
9. Kock NG, Nilson AE, Norle NL, et al. Urinary diversion by a continent ileum reservoir. Scand J Urol Nephrol 1978;49:23–31 (suppl).
10. Kock NG, Nilson AE, Nilsson LO, et al. Urinary diversion via a continent ileal reservoir: Clinical results in 12 patients. J Urol 1982;128:469–475.
11. Skinner DG, Lieskowsky G, Boyd SD. Technique of creation of a continent internal ileal reservoir (Kock pouch) for urinary diversion. Urol Clin North Am 1984;11:741–749.
12. Gilchrist RK, Merricks JW, Hamlin HH, et al. Construction of a substitute bladder and urethra. Surg Gynecol Obstet 1950;90:752–760.
13. Gil-Vernet JN. Technique for construction of a functioning artificial bladder. J Urol 1960;83:39–50.
14. Hendren WH. Some alternatives to urinary diversion in children. J Urol 1978;119:652–660.
15. Hendren WH. Reconstruction of previously diverted urinary tracts in children. J Pediatr Surg 1973;8:135–150.
16. Hendren WH. Nonrefluxing colon conduit for temporary or permanent urinary diversion in children. J Pediatr Surg 1975;10:381–398.
17. Hendren WH. Ureterocolic diversion of urine: Management of some difficult problems. J Urol 1983;129:719–729.
18. Månsson W, Sundin T. Experience with a continent caecal reservoir in urinary diversion. Scand J Urol Nephrol 1978;48:4 (suppl).
19. Duckett JW, Snyder HM. Use of the Motrofanoff principle in urinary reconstruction. World J Urol 1985;3:191–193.
20. Duckett JW, Snyder HM. Use of the Mitrofanoff principle in urinary reconstruction. Urol Clin North Am 1986;3:271–274.
21. Mitrofanoff P. Cystostomie continente trans-appendiculaire dans le traitement des vessies neurologiques. Chir Pediatr 1980;21:297–305.
22. Mitrofanoff P. Personal communication, August, 1985.
23. Benchekroun A. Continent caecal bladder. Eur Urol 1977;3:248–250.
24. Benchekroun A. Continent caecal bladder. Br J Urol 1982;54:505–506.
25. Weisgerber B. Colocystoplastie d'agrandissement a abouchement cutane temporaire. Chir Pediatr 1982;23:417–419.
26. Mollard P, Jourda R, Valla JS, et al. Colocystoplastie d'agrandissement et de substitution pour vessie neurologique congenitale de l'enfant. Chir Pediatr 1983;24:54–60.
27. Monfort G, Guys JM, Lacombe GM. Appendicovesicostomy: An alternative urinary diversion in the child. Eur Urol 1984;10:361–363.
28. Schneider KM, Reid RE, Fruchtman B. Closure of the bladder neck in patients undergoing continent vesicostomy. J Urol 1978;120:40–42.
29. Duckett JW, Snyder HM. Continent urinary diversion: Variations on the Mitrofanoff principle. J Urol 1986;136:58–62.
30. Rowland RG, Mitchell ME, Bihrle R. The cecoileal continent urinary reservoir. World J Urol 1985;3:185–190.

31. Light JK, Engelmann UH. Reconstruction of the lower urinary tract: Observations on bowel dynamics and the artificial urinary sphincter. J Urol 1985;133:594–597.
32. Turner-Warwick RT, Ashken MH. The functional results of partial, subtotal and total cystoplasty with special reference to ureterocaecocystoplasty, selective sphincterotomy and cystocystoplasty. Br J Urol 1967;39:3–12.
33. Light JK, Engelmann UH. Le Bag: Total replacement of the bladder using an ileocolonic pouch. J Urol 1986;136:27–31.
34. Thuroff JW, Alken P, Engelmann U, et al. The Mainz-pouch (mixed augmentation ileum'n coecum) applicable for bladder augmentation/substitution and continent urinary diversion). Presented at the 20th International Congress of the Society Internationale d'Urologie, San Francisco, September 6, 1982 (abstr 915).
35. Thuroff JW, Alken P, Engelmann U, et al. The Mainz-pouch (mixed augmentation ileum'n coecum) applicable for bladder augmentation/substitution and continent urinary diversion). J Urol 1986;136:17–26.
36. Kelalis PP. Urinary diversion in children by the sigmoid conduit: Its advantages and limitations. J Urol 1974;112:666–672.
37. LeDuc A, Camey M, Teillac P. Antireflux ureter implantation in an ileal loop. Presented at the 20th International Congress of the Societe Internationale D'Urologie, Vienna, 1985 (abstr 855).
38. Ashcraft KW, Dennis PA. The reimplanted ureter as a catheterizing stoma. American Pediatric Surgical Association meeting, Toronto, May 14, 1986 (abstr 6).
39. Gregoir W. Lich-Gregoir operation, in Eckstein H, Hohenfellner R, Williams DI (eds): Surgical Pediatric Urology. Philadelphia, Saunders, 1977.
40. Hutch JA. Vesico-ureteral reflux in the paraplegic: Cause and correction. J Urol 1952;69:457–463.
41. Hackler RN. Modified Hutch I vesicoureteroplasty in paraplegia. J Urol 1977;118:953–954.
42. Gil-Vernet JH. A new technique for surgical correction of vesicoureteral reflux. J Urol 1984;131:456–457.
43. Starr A. Ureteral plication: A new concept in ureteral tailoring for megaureter. Invest Urol 1979;17:153–156.
44. Young B, Mallen PR. Transvesical-ureteral transposition: A new operation for ureteral replacement. J Urol 1968;100:498–503.
45. Lobe TE, Smey P, Anderson GF. A neourethral enteroplication for urinary continence in a case of cloacal exstrophy. J Pediatr Surg 1985;206:616–618.
46. Kropp KA, Angwafo FF. Urethral lengthening and reimplantation for neurogenic incontinence in children. J Urol 1986;135:533–536.
47. Lobe TE. Conversion of an ileal-conduit into a neo-urethral enteroplication for urinary continence: Tips in its proper construction. American Pediatric Surgical Association Meeting, Toronto, May 14, 1986 (abstr 4).
48. King L. Protection of upper tracts in undiversion, in King LR (ed): Continent Reconstruction of the Lower Urinary Tract. Chicago, Yearbook Medical, 1987 (in press).

Effect of Biliary Decompression on Morbidity and Mortality of Pancreatoduodenectomy

JAMES H. THOMAS, M.D.

To evaluate the effect of levels of serum bilirubin on morbidity and mortality after pancreatoduodenectomy, a prospective study was designed to compare patients who underwent preoperative biliary decompression to those who did not. Preoperative biliary decompression decreased the mean serum bilirubin level from 15.8 to 5.8 mg/dl in one group of ten patients (Group A). The only statistical differences between this group and the two other groups of patients (Group B and C) who were not treated with preoperative biliary decompression was the level of serum bilirubin before pancreatoduodenectomy (5.8, 22, and 1.3 mg/dl in Groups A, B, and C, respectively). Only one death occurred in each group of patients. The numbers of nonfatal complications were comparable. These results suggest that there is no decrease in morbidity or mortality after pancreatoduodenectomy when the serum bilirubin level is decreased by preoperative biliary drainage.

IN SOME SERIES, hyperbilirubinemia has been associated with an increase in morbidity and mortality after pancreatoduodenectomy.[1,2] As a result, several authors have suggested routine preoperative decompression of the biliary tract.[1] Whipple, in 1935, originally described biliary decompression as the first part of a two-stage pancreatoduodenectomy, not only to decrease serum bilirubin, but also to minimize intraoperative and postoperative bleeding.[3] Currently, most surgeons perform pancreatoduodenectomy without previous biliary decompression. Howard,[4] in 1968, reported a series of 41 consecutive one-stage pancreatoduodenectomies with no mortality. Three prospective randomized studies have been conducted evaluating the effect of percutaneous transhepatic biliary decompression on postoperative morbidity and mortality.[5–7] However, the majority of patients in these reports had extrahepatic biliary obstruction secondary to metastatic cancer or benign disorders. The current prospective analysis was designed to evaluate the effect of preoperative biliary decompression by operative and nonoperative techniques on morbidity and mortality in patients undergoing pancreatoduodenectomy.

Materials and Methods

Thirty-four consecutive patients with periampullary cancer were evaluated. Ten patients (Group A) with an admission serum bilirubin level of equal to or greater than 10 mg/dl underwent decompression before pancreatoduodenectomy. In contrast, 13 patients (Group B) with an admission serum bilirubin level of equal to or greater than 10 mg/dl and 11 patients (Group C) with an admission serum bilirubin level of equal to or less than 4 mg/dl underwent pancreatoduodenectomy without biliary decompression.

Clinical, laboratory, operative, and pathologic factors shown to affect morbidity and mortality were recorded.[8] These factors included the following: age, weight loss, associated disease (cardiac, pulmonary, renal, and hepatic), serum bilirubin, albumin and alkaline phosphatase values, tumor size, operative time, blood loss, type of pancreatic anastomosis, experience of operator, pathologic diagnosis, extension of tumor to other organs, metastasis to regional lymph nodes, and residual tumor at the pancreatic, common bile duct or duodenal margins. Postoperative complications and deaths were recorded for all patients.

From the Department of Surgery, University of Kansas Medical Center, Kansas City, Kansas.
This article has been reproduced with permission from the *American Journal of Surgery*, Vol. 148, 1984.

Differences in clinical, laboratory, operative, and pathologic factors between groups were tested by standard statistical methods including analysis of variance, Student's t test, and chi-square contingency coefficients.

Results

Cholecystostomy was the most common method of biliary decompression (four patients). Cholecystojejunostomy (two patients), choledochostomy (two patients), and percutaneous transhepatic biliary decompression (two patients) also were performed. The duration of drainage before pancreatoduodenectomy varied from 9 to 50 days (mean, 24 days). Preoperative biliary decompression was successful in decreasing the serum bilirubin to less than 10 mg/dl in nine of ten patients. The mean serum bilirubin level in patients in Group A decreased from 15.8 to 5.8 mg/dl and the mean alkaline phosphatase decreased from 680 to 227 IU/l. There was no change in the serum albumin levels (3.4–3.3 g/dl) as a result of biliary decompression.

Group Comparison

A comparison of the risk factors for Groups A, B, and C is presented in Table 1. The mean ages of the patients were comparable. There was no difference in the occurrence of associated diseases. Although only three of 11 patients in Group C had experienced a 6.75-kg weight loss in contrast to eight of ten patients in Group A and seven of 13 patients in Group B, these differences were not significant. Although no patient in Group C underwent a total pancreatectomy, there was no difference in the methods of managing the pancreas between groups A, B, and C. The most common method of reconstruction after pancreatoduodenectomy was pancreatojejunostomy in 18 patients and pancreatogastrostomy in 17 patients. The mean operative time was comparable for all groups. Evaluation of the surgeons responsible for the operative procedure revealed each to have had greater than 5 years of experi-

TABLE 1. *Risk Factors, Morbidity, and Mortality in Patients Who Underwent Pancreatoduodenectomy*

	Group A	Group B	Group C	*P* value
No. of patients	10	13	11	NS
Mean age (yr)	66	62	62	NS
Patients with associated disease	5	7	4	NS
Patients with more than 6.75 kg weight loss	8	7	3	NS
Blood loss during operation (ml)	2707	2138	2072	NS
Pancreatic reconstruction				
Pancreatogastrostomy	7	4	6	NS
Pancreatojejunostomy	2	6	5	NS
Total pancreatectomy	1	3	0	NS
Mean duration of operation (h)	5.8	5	4.5	NS
Experience of surgeon (yr)	>5	>5	>5	
Final diagnosis				
Pancreatic cancer	10	12	1	<0.001
Ampullary cancer	0	1	6	<0.003
Duodenal cancer	0	0	6	<0.01
Mean tumor size (cm)	3.1	2.4	2.73	NS
Patients with metastatic lymphadenopathy	5	7	2	NS
Patients with tumor at resection margin	3	4	0	NS
Mean bilirubin level before decompression (mg/dl)	15.8	22	1.3	<0.0001
Mean bilirubin level after decompression (mg/dl)	5.75*	—	—	
Mean alkaline phosphatase level before decompression (IU/l)	680	497	244	<0.01
Mean alkaline phosphatase level after decompression (IU/l)	227†	—	—	
Mean albumin level before pancreatoduodenectomy (g/dl)	3.4	3.8	3.6	NS
Patients with nonfatal complications	4	8	4	NS
No. of deaths	1	1	1	NS

* $P < 0.001$ when compared with mean bilirubin level before decompression.
† $P < 0.01$ when compared with mean alkaline phosphatase level before decompression.
NS: not significant.

ence. Ampullary and duodenal cancers were more common in Group C and pancreatic carcinoma was more common in Groups A and B. These differences were significant. Tumor size was comparable for all groups. No differences were found in the number of patients with metastatic lymphadenopathy or the number of patients with tumor at the resection margins. There were no differences in mean albumin levels between patient groups.

The mean bilirubin level before decompression in Group A (15.8 mg/dl) was comparable to that in Group B (22 mg/dl). After decompression the bilirubin level in Group A decreased to 5.75 mg/dl. This decrease was significantly less than the bilirubin level in patients who did not undergo preoperative biliary decompression (Group B). Thus, the major difference between Groups A, B, and C was the level of serum bilirubin before operation. The incidence of complications and mortality rates also are recorded in Table 1. There was only one death in each group. Four nonfatal complications occurred in Groups A and C. These included urinary tract infections in two patients, pneumonia in two patients, one biliary fistula, and one colorectal fistula. Eight nonfatal complications occurred in Group B, including one enterocutaneous fistula and two wound abscesses. Although the number of complications was greater in Group B, the difference between groups was not significant.

Discussion

One of the major criticisms of pancreatoduodenectomy in the treatment of periampullary cancer is the high postoperative morbidity and mortality. In some series, the level of serum bilirubin has been identified as a major risk factor for the development of complications and death.[8] In contrast, other investigators, most notably Moosa *et al.*[9] and van Heerden *et al.*,[10] have reported mortality rates of 8% and 4%, respectively, in patients with hyperbilirubinemia. Thus, routine preoperative biliary decompression in patients with periampullary cancer and hyperbilirubinemia (serum bilirubin level 10 mg/dl or greater) remains controversial.

Nakayama *et al.*[11] described a postoperative mortality rate of 8.2% in 49 patients with malignant disease after preoperative biliary decompression compared with a postoperative mortality rate of 23% in 148 patients with malignant obstruction who underwent operation without biliary decompression. However, radical pancreatoduodenectomies were performed in only seven of the 49 patients. Denning *et al.*[1] found no difference in postoperative mortality but a significant increase in complications (56%) in 26 patients without preoperative biliary decompression as compared with 22 patients with preoperative biliary decompression (28%). However, as in the report of Nakayama and associates,[11] only a small number, nine patients, underwent pancreatoduodenectomy either after biliary decompression (three patients) or without decompression (six patients).

Two of the prospective studies comparing morbidity and mortality after preoperative transhepatic biliary decompression have found no significant decrease in morbidity and mortality associated with use of this technique. However, both reports, that of Pitt *et al.*[7] and McPhearson *et al.*,[6] describe only a total of 14 patients who underwent pancreatoduodenectomy. The majority of the patients in these two studies had other causes for extrahepatic biliary obstruction.

Hatfield *et al.*[5] compared morbidity and mortality in 28 patients with obstructive jaundice after preoperative external biliary drainage to 27 patients who had not undergone preoperative external biliary drainage. These authors described no improvement in postoperative morbidity or mortality as a result of decreasing the bilirubin to a mean of 134 μmol/l. Although the majority of patients in these authors' reports had pancreatic cancer only five patients underwent pancreatoduodenectomy. Our study is the first prospective study to determine the value of preoperative biliary decompression in patients undergoing pancreatoduodenectomy for periampullary carcinoma. The three groups described herein were identical with respect to major risk factors with the exception of preoperative bilirubin levels. There was no decrease in morbidity or mortality associated with decreasing serum bilirubin to less than 10 mg/dl before pancreatoduodenectomy.

Although the number of patients was small (with a large number of patients a slight, but significant difference might have been documented), from the available data we can only conclude that no marked or dramatic decrease in morbidity or mortality after pancreatoduodenectomy occurs in the presence of a decreasing serum bilirubin level caused by preoperative biliary drainage.

REFERENCES

1. Denning DA, Ellison EC, Carey LC. Preoperative percutaneous transhepatic biliary decompression lowers operative morbidity in patients with obstructive jaundice. Am J Surg 1981;141:61–63.
2. Braasch JW, Gray BN. Considerations that lower pancreatoduodenectomy mortality. Am J Surg 1977;133:480–484.
3. Warren KW, Cattell RB, Blackburn JD, Nora P. A long term appraisal of pancreatico-duodenal resection for periampullary carcinoma. Ann Surg 1962;155:653–662.
4. Howard JM. Pancreatico-duodenectomy: Forty-one consecutive Whipple resections without an operative mortality. Ann Surg 1968;168:629–637.
5. Hatfield ARW, Terblanche J, Fataar S *et al.* Preoperative external biliary drainage in obstructive jaundice: A prospective controlled clinical trial. Lancet 1982;2:896–899.
6. McPherson GAD, Benjamin IS, Hodgson HJF *et al.* Pre-operative percutaneous transhepatic biliary drainage: The results of a controlled trial. Br J Surg 1984;71:371–375.
7. Pitt HA, Gomes AS, Lois JF *et al.* Does preoperative percutaneous biliary drainage reduce operative risk or increase hospital cost? Ann Surg 1985;201:545–551.
8. Gilsdorf RB, Spanos P. Factors influencing morbidity and mortality in pancreaticoduodenectomy. Ann Surg 1973;177:322–327.
9. Moossa AR, Lewis MH, Mackie CR. Surgical treatment of pancreatic cancer. Mayo Clin Proc 1979;54:468–474.
10. van Heerden JA, McIlrath DC, Dozois RR, Adson MA. Radical pancreatoduodenectomy: A procedure to be abandoned? Mayo Clin Proc 1981;56:601–606.
11. Nakayama T, Ikeda A, Okuda K. Percutaneous transhepatic drainage of the biliary tract. Technique and results in 104 cases. Gastroenterology 1978;74:554–559.

Self-Experimentation and Our Rich Surgical Heritage

JOHN E. GATTI, M.D.

THE IMPORTANCE AND justification of human experimentation have seldom been questioned. Most of our medical and surgical advances were possible only through basic research with humans as the experimental subjects. Medical science had progressed for centuries with relatively little established control on human experimentation. The abuses of human rights in the name of medical science during World War II so shocked the world's sense of humanity that in the late 1940s directives governing the conduct of medical research were organized.

Unethical individuals are capable of dastardly crimes under the guise of medical research. Overzealous or misguided experimentors have shown through history that research can assume an all-consuming importance that concern for safety and comfort of patients is subjugated. It is obvious to all that limits placed on physicians by their Hippocratic Oath or reliance on a researcher's sense of moral propriety are not always sufficient to guide medical experimentation.

The Nuremberg Trials were a series of trials in which former Nazi leaders were indicted and tried as war criminals by an International Military Tribunal.[1,2] Among the war crimes explored by the tribunal were crimes against humanity, *i.e.*, exterminations, genocide, and experimentations.

Following the trial of the United States *vs.* Karl Brandt in 1948, ten principles governing human experimentation were drafted. These ten principles are often referred to as the Nuremberg Rules or Codes.[2]

An interesting and perplexing statement concludes Nuremberg Rule #5. The Rule reads:

> No experiment should be conducted where there is an 'a priori' reason to believe that death or disabling injury will occur; except, perhaps, in those experiments where the experimental physicians also serve as the subjects.

This statement recognizes the historical presence and importance of self-experimentation. There are many instances of well-conceived and executed self-experiments that have furthered medical science. However, many proved ill-founded or were based on incomplete medical knowledge or naiveté. The results were often predictable or readily obtainable with animal research; yet, all are interesting and engrossing examples of brave individuals who so believed in themselves and their work that they did not hesitate to subject themselves to self-experiments.

Surgeons have contributed greatly to the advancement of medical science. The contributions by these men of surgery will remain an inspiration to those of us who have chosen surgery as a vocation. Moreover, we should be proud of the legacy of surgeons that have tested their hypotheses on themselves. Our recent infatuation with the prospective, randomized clinical investigation should not make us lose sight of the brave surgeons that have given us a rich surgical heritage of daring, selfless, and enlightening self-experiments.

John Hunter (Fig. 1) in 1767 at the age of 37 attempted to determine the mechanism of gonorrhea transmission. He innoculated his own penis with a urethral discharge from a prisoner with documented gonorrhea. He did this after he scarified his glans with a surgical knife. The prisoner apparently had contracted both gonorrhea and syphilis as Hunter developed both diseases. Understandably, Hunter erroneously concluded that both syphilis and

From the West Jersey Health System and Our Lady of Lourdes Hospital, Camden, New Jersey.

Figures 1 through 8 were published courtesy of the Historical Collections of the Library, College of Physicians of Philadelphia.

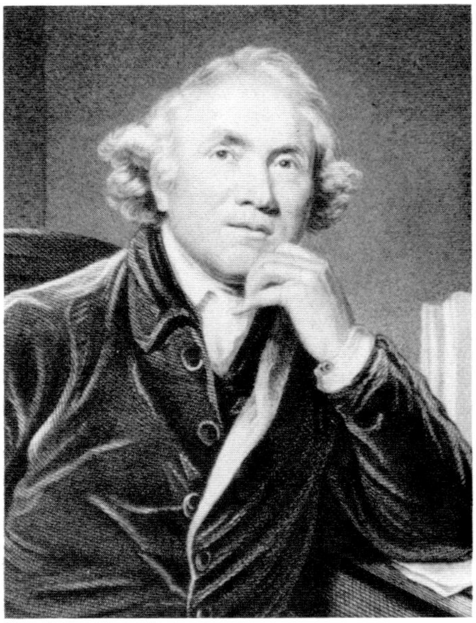

FIG. 1. John Hunter, M.D.

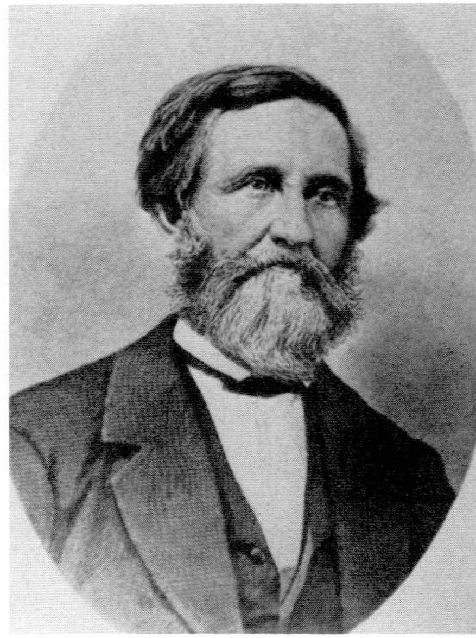

FIG. 2. Crawford Long, M.D.

gonorrhea were different expressions of the same disease. The raging controversies involving these maladies were only further muddied after Hunter published his self-experiment.[3]

Hunter decided to postpone his marriage for 4 years until he was satisfied that he had cured the syphilis with mercury therapy. There has been speculation that he died of a dissecting aneurysm because of his sudden, painful death and the observation that differential pulses were identified. The suggestion has been made that his aneursym was syphilic in nature.[3]

There are many examples of surgeons that have experimented with anesthetic gases prior

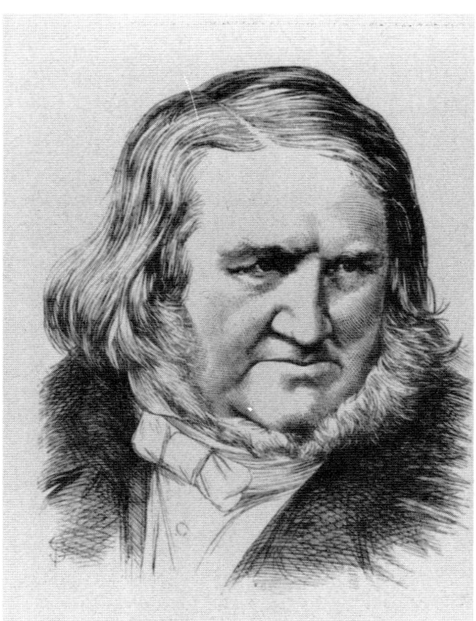

FIG. 3. James Simpson, M.D.

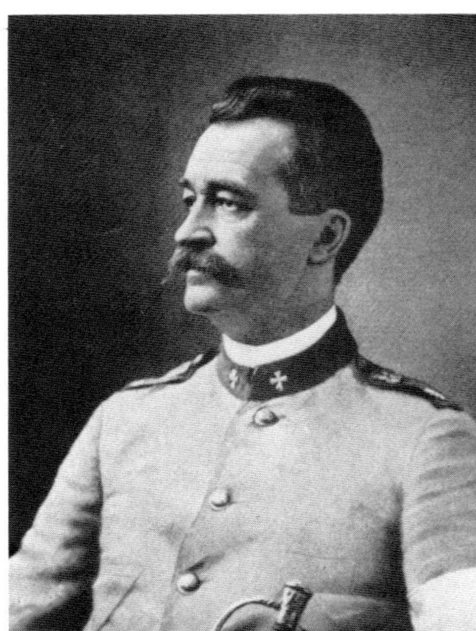

FIG. 4. Nicholas Senn, M.D.

to the general acceptance of surgical anesthesia. Mention of the pioneers in the use of anesthesia for surgery is appropriate. In 1842, Crawford Long (Fig. 2) of Jefferson, Georgia, first used ether on himself before adopting it as a regular adjunct to his surgery practice. Long was a graduate of the University of Pennsylvania Medical School (1839) and was only 27 years old when he first began using ether as an anesthetic. For unknown reasons, he did not publish his significant discovery until 1849.[4] Horace Wells in 1844 allowed himself to be anesthetized with nitrous oxide and had his abscessed tooth extracted by another oral surgeon of Hartford, Connecticut.[4] James Simpson (Fig. 3), an Obstetrician and General Surgeon of Edinburgh, Scotland, self-experimented with chloroform in 1847 and later used it in his practice.[4]

Referred to as the "Billroth of America," Nicholas Senn (Fig. 4) had a distinguished career as a surgeon in Milwaukee and Chicago. His interest in medical research was evident in his early years as a medical student at the Chicago Medical College. In 1866, at the age of 22, he ingested a large quantity of digitalis to evaluate its cardiac effect. As a surgeon in Milwaukee, he self-experimented with hydrogen gas insufflation of the colon as a means of evaluating the integrity of the bowel. Senn is a past president of the American Medical Association and is credited with many of the early advances in intestinal surgery, anal surgery, fractures, and plastic surgery.[5,6]

Johann Nussbaum, a German surgeon, participated in many self-experiments with morphine. In 1872, he submitted a paper to the German Surgical College that detailed his many experiments with oral, subcutaneous, and intravenous administration of morphine. He was a known morphine addict, but his addiction did not prevent him from making many contributions to surgery in the area of antisepsis and hospital-acquired infections.[4]

Carl Koller, (Fig. 5) often called the "Father of Ophthalmology," published the results of his self-experiments with cocaine in 1884. While a surgeon at New York University (age 27), he uncovered the anesthetic properties of topical cocaine when applied to the cornea. Initially, using animals in his experiments, he later tested the effect on the human eye by exposing his own corneas to the generous application of cocaine. His experiments greatly expanded the number of procedures that could be employed to treat various ophthalmologic disorders. The publication of his self-experiments generated a great deal of interest in the medical community.[4]

William Halsted (Figs. 6 and 7) was quick to recognize the potential of a drug such as

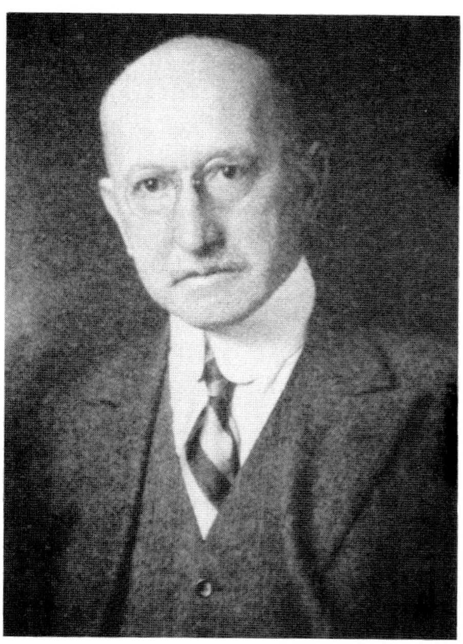

FIG. 5. Carl Koller, M.D.

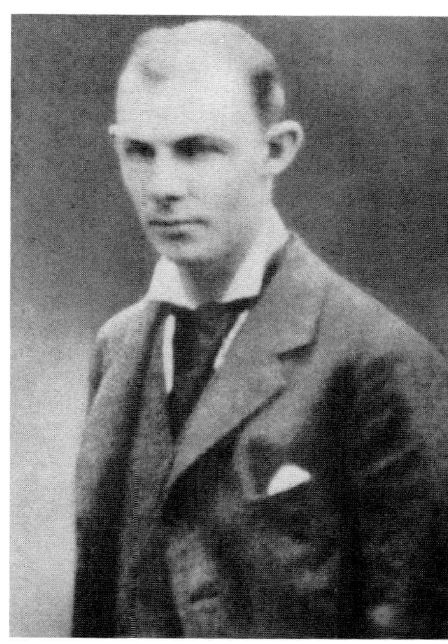

FIG. 6. William Halsted, M.D.

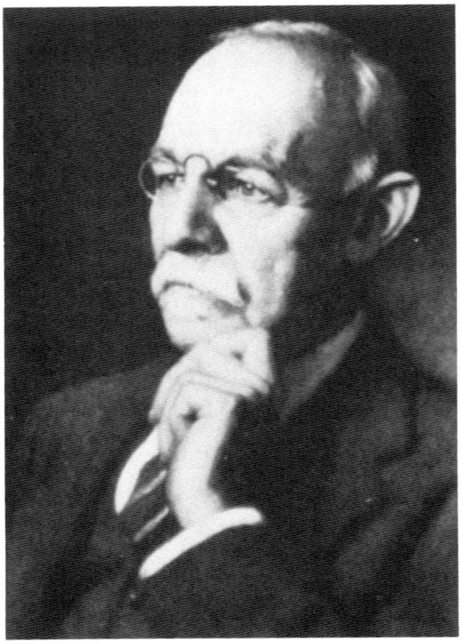

FIG. 7. William Halsted, M.D.

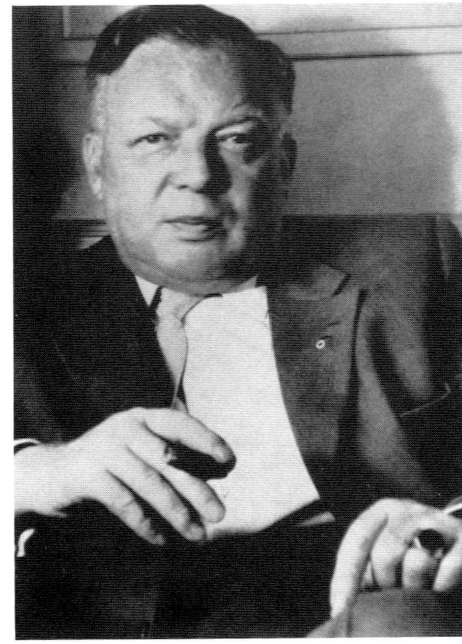

FIG. 8. Werner Forssman, M.D.

cocaine. Shortly after Koller's experiments, Halsted initiated self-experimentation with cocaine. At age 33, while a surgeon at Bellevue and Presbyterian Hospitals in New York, he began injecting cocaine subcutaneously. He soon adopted the use of cocaine to his practice and performed a large number of surgical procedures with cocaine as a local anesthetic. In 1889, he moved to Baltimore, and despite his well-known addiction to cocaine, his truly distinguished career advanced the science and practice of surgery as did that of no other American surgeon. His techniques and innovations improved the surgical treatment of breast, thyroid, vascular, and gastrointestinal diseases.[4,7]

While a surgical intern in Berlin, Germany, Werner Forssman (Fig. 8) acted on his intuition that cardiac catheterization from a peripheral vein was possible. In 1929 at the age of 25, he experimented with catheterization techniques; first on cadavers, and then on himself. He performed a cut-down on his own brachial vein and threaded a crude catheter up his arm and into his right ventricle. He had to walk from his lab and go up two flights of stairs to the x-ray department so that he could document the position of the catheter in his heart. He served in the German Army in World War II and was captured early in the war. He spent time in an allied prison camp but returned to practice urology in Germany at the end of the war. In 1956, he shared the Nobel Prize for his innovative research in cardiac physiology and catheterization.[8,9]

John H. Crandon (Fig. 9) made himself the subject of an experiment documenting the physical and physiologic effects of Vitamin C deficiency. In 1939, while a surgical resident in Boston, he removed Vitamin C from his diet. The first 2 months of his 6-month diet allowed only cheese, bread, eggs, boiled chicken, and meat. The remaining 4 months of the diet prohibited all meat. Blood samples were taken, often daily for months at a time, to evaluate his serum proteins and vitamin levels. He allowed a large skin incision to be made on his back to test wound healing. The wound exhibited poor healing and serial biopsies were taken to study the progress of wound healing during the period of Vitamin C deficiency. He reported symptoms of lethargy toward the latter part of the experiment; however, he continued to work normally as a surgical resident at the Boston City Hospital in the Harvard Program while the study was in progress.[10] Dr. Crandon recently retired after many active years as a General Surgeon in Winthrop, Massachusetts.

While a surgical resident in Glasgow in 1942, Thomas Gibson began experimenting with skin allografts. He was treating a 2-year-old girl with burns and placed pinch grafts from her

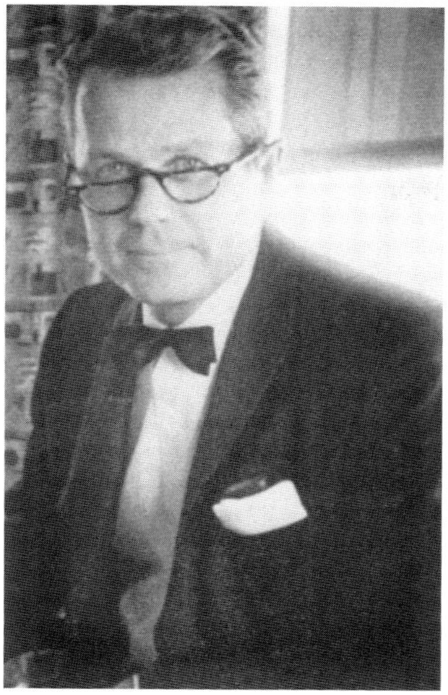

FIG. 9. John H. Crandon, M.D.

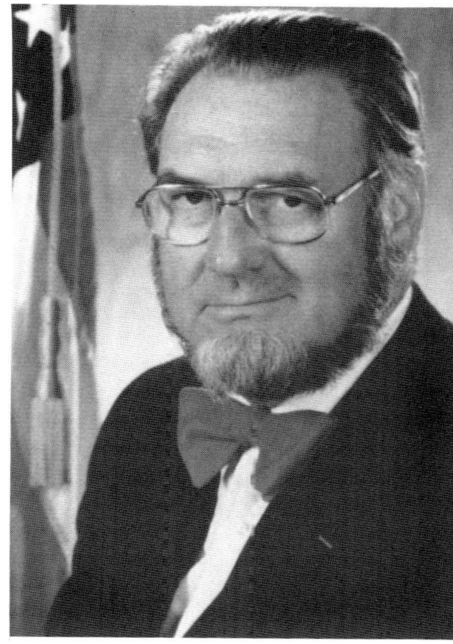

FIG. 10. C. Everett Koop, M.D.

father onto the patient's burn only to observe their dissolution. He took similar grafts from another patient and injected them, on several occasions, into his own buttock. He was conscripted into the Royal Army Medical Corps and abandoned his research. Medawar continued the skin grafting experiments in Oxford and shortly thereafter defined the immunologic phenomenon of graft rejection. Mr. Gibson only recently reported his self-experiments in 1986 in the *British Journal of Plastic Surgery.*[11] He is a Professor of Plastic Surgery in Glasgow, Scotland.

C. Everett Koop (Fig. 10) participated in intravenous gelatin infusions studies in 1944 while a young surgeon at the Hospital of the University of Pennsylvania. Serum nitrogen exchanges and serum proteins were examined during the many months of these experiments.[12] Archibald Fletcher shared the authorship of these hyperalimentation experiments with Dr. Koop and also was part of the study group. Dr. Koop is the present Surgeon General of the United States, and Dr. Fletcher is a general surgeon in Africa.

Also in 1944 during World War II, James D. Hardy (Fig. 11) participated in a hemodilution experiment. While a medical resident at the Hospital of the University of Pennsylvania, he allowed 1115 cc of blood to be removed during a 24-hour period. The physiologic effects of this blood loss was carefully documented. He did not show clinical signs of hypovolemia until more than 750 cc of blood had been removed. After removal of the 1115 cc, his article related that "to the observer, he looked and acted like a sick man."[13] The blood was ultimately returned to him after the observation period. This study clearly demonstrated that recumbent patients may show no signs of hemorrhage until large volumes of blood have been lost. Dr. Hardy began his surgical training in 1946, and he has had many productive years in surgery. He is presently the Chief of Surgery at the University of Mississippi.

Nicholas S. Gimbel (Fig. 12) has participated in numerous self-experiments. In 1949, while a surgical resident at the Hospital of the University of Pennsylvania, he became part of the experimental group to study the fate of infused albumin. He and his collaborators found that the positive nitrogen balance observed was due to retained albumin and that the albumin caused signs of cardiac decompensation. Later, as a surgeon on the Wayne State University staff, he studied the epithelization of experimental burns and skin graft donor sites on his own skin. His observations on the epithelization of wounds are carefully described in numerous articles on the subject.[14,15] Dr. Gimbel is retired and presently resides in Washington, D.C.

In 1966, an interesting article appeared in the plastic surgery literature that was authored

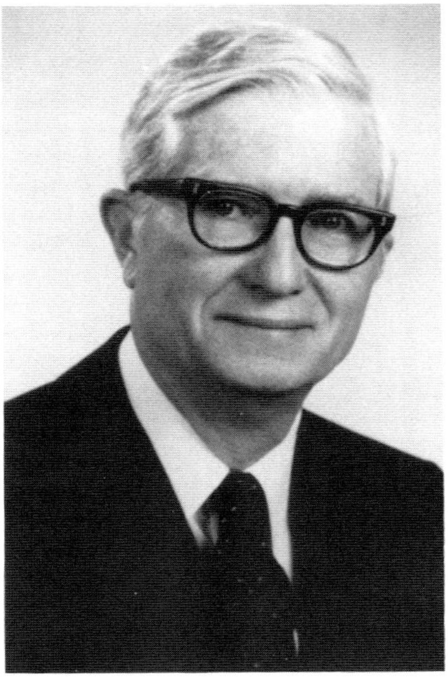

FIG. 11. James D. Hardy, M.D.

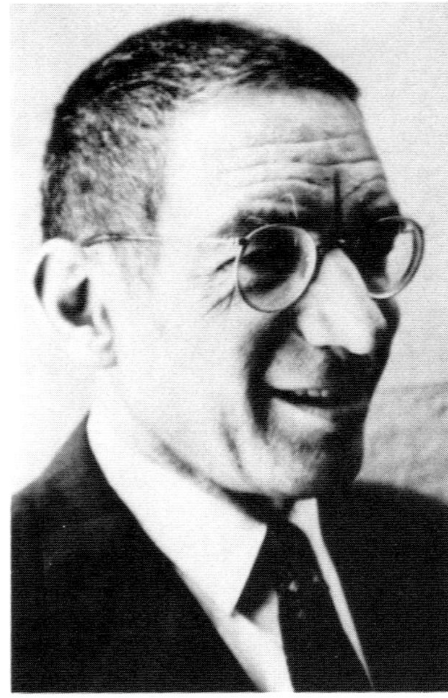

FIG. 12. Nicholas S. Gimbel, M.D.

by two Swedish surgeons. Per Klingenström and Bengt Nylen described an experiment in which Dr. Klingenström had a tubed-pedicle flap raised on his medial arm and then transferred to his chest wall by Dr. Nylen. The flap was "walked down" the chest to the abdomen and back again, with the pedicles being divided at 7-day intervals.[16] The experiment was performed to prove that pedicled flaps could be transferred in shorter periods of time than the generally accepted interval of 3 weeks. Dr. Klingenström apparently continued his usual daily schedule with the tubed-flap in its various stages of readiness during the many months of the experiment. He recently related that his wife was happy when the experiment ended and the tube was sent to the pathologist. Dr. Nylen died unexpectedly in an accident, and Dr. Klingenström is an active surgeon in Stockholm.

Certainly, there are many more instances of self-experimentation by surgeons. Our legacy in surgical research has included a rich assortment of daring, intelligent, and unusual individuals. It is not possible to estimate the number of authors who have failed to mention in their articles that they were included in the experimental group of human subjects. This report is an attempt to draw attention to the indomitable spirit of adventure and courage that researchers may possess.

While we must admire those early doctors who advanced the seemingly ancient art of medicine in the face of unfathomable odds and poor initial results, we must reserve a special reverence for those who have participated in self-experimentation. The surgeons mentioned in this report are representative of the individuals who possessed such an intensity of dedication and spirit of adventure that they did not hesitate to subject themselves to experimentation in the testing of their hypotheses. Those individuals who engage in human experimentation should be mindful of these surgeons and their selflessness and courage. Before we ask a patient to undergo an experimental protocol, it may be appropriate for us to examine what our own response and tolerance would be. H. G. Wells said it succintly: "It is not reasonable that those who gamble with men's lives should not stake their own."

ACKNOWLEDGEMENT

I wish to thank Jonathan E. Rhoads, M.D., for his assistance in the preparation of this manuscript.

BIBLIOGRAPHY

1. Goetz PW (Ed). The New Encyclopaedia Britannica. Chicago: Encyclopaedia Britannica, Inc. 1986;8:834.
2. Beecher HK. Experimentation in man. JAMA 1959;169:461–478.
3. Lasky II. John Hunter, The Shakespeare of Medicine. Surg Gynecol Obstet 1983;156:511–518.

4. Wangensteen OH, Wangensteen SD. The Rise of Surgery. University of Minnesota Press, 1981;167–176, 277, 279–281, 283, 293–294.
5. Natvig P. Nicholas Senn of Milwaukee and Chicago. Plast Reconstr Surg 1978;61:167–176.
6. Romm S. Nicholas Senn. Contemp Surg 1984;24:100–104.
7. Martyrs of Medicine (Editorial). JAMA 1921;90:1712–1713.
8. Altman LK. Auto-experimentation, an unappreciated tradition in medical science. N Engl J Med 1972;286:346–352.
9. The Doctor as the Guinea-Pig (Editorial). Med J Aust 1969;2:65–66.
10. Crandon JH, Lund CC, Dill DB. Experimental human scurvy. N Engl J Med 1940;223:353–370.
11. Gibson T. The second set phenomenon as first shown in skin allografts. Br J Plast Surg 1986;39:96–102.
12. Koop CE, Fletcher AG, Riegel C, Lockwood JS. Gelatin as a plasma expander. Surgery 1944;15:839–858.
13. Shenkin HA, Cheney RH, Govons SR, Hardy JD, Fletcher AG, Starr I. On the diagnosis of hemorrhage in man. Am J Med Sci 1946;208:421–436.
14. Gimbel NS, Farris W, Leveen HH, Marshall E. A technique for studying epithelization in man, with evidence for its acceleration by certain fatty acids. Surgery 1964;56:678–684.
15. Mikhail GR, Farris W, Gimbel NS. The pattern of superficial blood vessels in healing skin donor sites. J Invest Dermatol 1965;44:75–82.
16. Klingenstrom P, Nylen B. Timing of transfer of tubed pedicles and cross-flaps. Plast Reconstr Surg 1966;37:1–12.

A System Approach to Trauma Care in Pennsylvania

WILLIAM E. DEMUTH, JR., M.D.

MORE THAN 40 YEARS have passed since surgeons returning to civilian life from World War II came to realize that the care given the injured civilian was markedly inferior to that provided our military personnel in combat. This observation led to a nationwide movement to study the problems and to implement change. The effort was joined by the National Academy of Sciences and the National Research Council which called together recognized experts, military and civilian, and a landmark document, *Accidental Death and Disability: The Neglected Disease of Modern Society*[1] was published in 1966. The perceived requirements for the development of a satisfactory system of trauma care were outlined. Many of these requirements have been met; many are yet to be addressed. Local, state and regional attempts were made to develop a system and some of them such as San Francisco, San Diego, and Maryland are quite successful.

The painfully slow process in Pennsylvania finally has led to the far-from-completed system which is acknowledged by many authorities to be the most advanced in the United States. Our prescribed standards for trauma center designation are undeniably the most stringent and the mandated goal is the development of a state-wide, not regional, system.

Background

The most visible impetus to the development of a system of trauma care was the passage of Act 45, signed into law by Governor Thornburgh in July 1985 after being given broad support by both House and Senate. The law mandated that the private sector develop a designation process for hospitals within 2 years. Lacking this, the Department of Health would be required to do so, a concept deemed by some to be a threatening intrusion into our traditional approach to health care. Government intervention was specifically resisted by the Hospital Association of Pennsylvania, without whose support the process would have stalled.

It would be impossible to describe in detail all of the events which made our current situation possible, but a few highlights might be of interest because so many individuals identified with the University of Pennsylvania played vital roles.

The return of the Twentieth General Hospital from Burma in 1945 brought with it the military experience with obvious emphasis on traumatic injury. Drs. Julian Johnson, Henry Royster, Robert Groff, William Fitts, Cletus Schwegman, James Donald, Charles Kirby, and James Maxwell appeared on the scene. All were greatly supported by their former Commander and new chairman of the Department of Surgery, Dr. I. S. Ravdin. Dr. Fitts had developed a special interest in fractures, largely because of his association with Dr. Ernest Brav (Mayo Clinic) in Burma. General surgical residents at Penn were afforded an excellent opportunity to care for fractures and other injuries, and some excellent work in the field of trauma was done in the Harrison Department of Surgical Research during that time.

It seemed this group had just returned when the Korean War began. With great foresight, the military seized the opportunity to get first rate scientific research done on the battlefield, and the United States Army Surgical Research Team in Korea was deployed in 1951 under the direction of Captain John Howard, a well known name at the University of Pennsylvania. Many believed this was the most significant step taken up to that time to establish

From the College of Medicine, Pennsylvania State University, Hershey, Pennsylvania, and the Pennsylvania Trauma Systems Foundation.

TABLE 1. *Partial List of Current and Past Pennsylvanians in the American Association for the Surgery of Trauma*

Blakemore	Gurd	Rhoads
Cayten	Hardy	Roberts
Corriere	Heppenstall	Sugerman
Cram	Holst	Thompson
Curreri	Howard	Waldhausen
Dudrick	Mackie	Wein
Fitts	Miller	Wilmore
Gennarelli	Nance	Wolferth
Gimbel	O'Neill	Zintel
Goodwin	Peskin	
Graham	Ralston	

trauma care as a speciality. Excellent clinical research was done, and the concept of the general surgeon being the captain of the team was promoted.

The translation of institutional commitment into the broader scope of trauma care might have remained stagnant had not Drs. Rhoads and Fitts pursued the development of a voluntary health agency, an element thought by the National Research Council to be vital to a viable system. A meeting was called in Philadelphia in 1969 and was attended by a wide variety of specialists in trauma care from across the nation. This effort was to result in Pennsylvania becoming the first Division of the American Trauma Society to be chartered in 1973. Drs. Fitts and Howard later became presidents of the national organization and Dr. Rhoads currently is Chairman of the Board of Directors. Hundreds of professional and lay people donated funds to mount a program for public education by the American Trauma Society (ATS), and for the first time the public would be taught what trauma meant. Pennsylvania talent was exported as well. When Dr. Howard moved to the Medical College of Ohio at Toledo he developed the North West Ohio Unit of the ATS with the great support of Dr. William Blakmore, then Chairman of the Department of Surgery of that institution. Many others moved from Pennsylvania to make very significant contributions on the national scene and the membership roster of the American Association for the Surgery of Trauma reflects this interest. Table 1 contains a partial list of names of current and past Pennsylvanians. These and others not named here have contributed greatly to the base upon which modern trauma care now stands.

In the 1960s and 1970s the American College of Surgeons (ACS) Committee on Trauma cautiously also moved along the course suggested by the 1966 study and pursued the establishment of standards of care to be applied to prehospital and hospital care. In 1976, *Optimal Care of the Seriously Injured*[2] was published. These standards are accepted worldwide. They constantly are being updated and in 1987 a revised, more inclusive document was released. The Advanced Trauma Life Support course for physicians was established. All physicians participating in the trauma center system in Pennsylvania must complete this course and recertification is required every 3 years.

During this span of years Dr. Fitts and Dr. Fraser Gurd, known to us for his tenure in the Harrison Department in the 1950s, became highly influential in this ACS activity, and Dr. Gurd still is Senior Consultant to the Committee on Trauma.

Meanwhile, the Pennsylvania Committee on Trauma of the ACS and Council on Education and Science of the Pennsylvania Medical Society (PMS) labored for nearly two decades addressing the Commonwealth's deficient status. Progress seemed imperceptible but a "White Paper"[3] was published in 1971. Many were involved, among them Drs. William Bouzarth and John Howard. The terribly inadequate ambulance "system" (mostly in the domain of morticians), and the absence of any apparent desire to differentiate between the capabilities of more than 200 hospitals, left no problems in identifying goals. By 1978 we were encouraged by a survey done by the PMS which showed that substantial improvement had occurred, but nothing as sophisticated as trauma center designation then was in sight.

As might be imagined, the individuals responsible for the activity in the ACS, PMS, and ATS often were one and the same and their zeal gradually caught the attention of people influential in government. Lt. Governor Ernest Kline gave early support to the ATS and we were aided greatly by his influence. As in Maryland, it took a few unfortunate clinical experiences involving important constituents to spark the legislative fire.

In the fall of 1983, a group of legislative sponsors was recruited following hearings held in Harrisburg and other localities by Senator Roy Wilt. A bill, SB 1177, was drafted and after careful consultation it was passed to become Act 45 of 1985. In 1984 the Legislative Budget and Finance Committee had issued a report to the General Assembly recommending enactment of a new emergency medical services law, and Act 45 contains many of the features suggested. Also, HB 1627 which established the voluntary trauma center accreditation program, was introduced by Representatives Gladeck and Greenwood, unanimously endorsed by the Legislature and was signed into law in 1984. These pieces of enabling legislation cleared the way for the process to begin.

The Hospital Designation Process

Act 45 provides for no government funding, one apparent reason for its easy passage. The PMS and the Hospital Association of Pennsylvania (HAP) contributed the seed money to start the operation, and the Pennsylvania Trauma Systems Foundation was formed to develop and implement the program.

The Pennsylvania Trauma Systems Foundation is a nonprofit 19-member body representing professional, government, hospital, and organizational interests. The PMS and HAP each appoint four members chosen on the basis of interest and expertise and the usual committee structure is in place with heavy emphasis on Standards and Policies and Procedures. Carol Forrester, RN, was selected to be director, which was a most fortunate choice. The office of president is to be alternately held by PMS and HAP appointees and board membership terms are staggered. Dr. Charles Wolferth's expertise as a member of the Committee on Trauma of the ACS and as President of the Pennsylvania Emergency Health Services Council made him the natural choice to head the Committee on Standards. His diligence and commitment were indispensable. Dr. James O'Neill chaired the Subcommittee on Pediatric Standards. Legal mandates required of the Foundation included the following: (1) the development of standards with ACS guidelines being the minimal acceptable standard; (2) designation of Level I (Regional Resource) and Level II (Regional) trauma centers within 2 years of passage; and (3) trauma center designation to be based on a voluntary initiative arising within hospitals desiring designation; recurrent inspection and verification at intervals is required and designation is to be withdrawn if standards are not maintained.

In the fall of 1985 the Foundation circulated the Standards to all hospitals in the Commonwealth and invited the submission of applications from those seeking Regional Resource or Regional Trauma Center designation. A separate set of standards was developed for pediatric trauma center designation and offered to both children's and general hospitals. Applicants were required to complete a detailed application which would reflect institutional commitment, physical characteristics, and staffing and equipment capabilities. Extensive written and telephone communications between applicants and Foundation staff ensued.

Initially, 52 hospitals indicated interest, and after completing the initial process 36 elected to pursue designation. Surveys of these institutions were to be conducted by six teams of five members each: a trauma surgeon, a neurosurgeon, an emergency medical specialist, a trauma nurse coordinator, and a hospital administrator were selected. All members of the survey teams were chosen because of expertise and experience, and all were chosen from outside the state. All were carefully screened for conflict of interest issues. Elaborate review mechanisms which assured anonymity of the applicant hospitals to the Foundation were developed and executed, and at the end of the first year's process ten Regional Resource, eight Regional, and two Pediatric Trauma Centers were designated.

The Future

Although we are encouraged by progress to date, some obvious hurdles must yet be cleared. Act 45 does not convey responsibility for the development of standards for a third larger category of hospital which seems vital in planning for a comprehensive system for all of our 12,000,000 population. Many of our 67 counties clearly will not in the forseeable future support trauma centers such as those already designated and existing hospitals must be identified in which adequate resuscitation and speedy transport to designated centers can be assured. Transfer protocols must be developed and surface and air transport implemented. As stated, the Pennsylvania Trauma Systems Foundation has no authority to proceed with this process so a legislative amendment will be required. Without question, this integration of the many hospitals not currently designated as trauma centers into a system will be infinitely more difficult than what has been done to date. Competition among hospitals is an established fact, and cooperation, crucial in a system approach, may be difficult to come by, but parochial interests must yield to the public good for it to succeed.

Since any hospital may apply for trauma center designation under the prescribed voluntary system, the potential exists for having too many for the available patient load. All trauma centers must submit data into a trauma registry under Foundation auspices and outcome results will be thereby made known within constraints of confidentiality. The ACS Committee on Trauma has consistently required a minimum number of trauma patients to be treated in trauma centers and the Foundation will abide by these guidelines. Furthermore, the expense of sustaining a designated center in the absence of sufficient revenue may lead hospitals to have second thoughts about the desirability of continuing in the system. The opportunity for entry into the designation process is ongoing on an annual basis, and the ultimate number to be designated is not known.

The optimal geographic distribution of trauma centers probably can never be achieved in Pennsylvania or anywhere else where a broad land area with uneven population must be served. The northern two thirds of the Commonwealth, an area of about 30,000 sq mi, is distinctly underserved whereas the distribution in the large metropolitan areas in the south clearly have too many trauma centers. As previously stated, the obvious remedy in the north is the designation of hospitals (Level III, resuscitation, or whatever) with careful integration into the system depending upon availability, transport capability, *etc.* Over time, fiscal reality and patient flow patterns may clarify the problem of distribution, if one exists, in the south.

Possibly the most important deficit yet to be addressed is the current status of prehospital care and triage policy. Great advances have been made over the last two decades: licensing, prescribed configurations for ambulances, medical evacuation, communications, *etc.* However, the "Golden Hour" concept becomes a vain hope if seriously injured patients are initially moved to hospitals incapable of providing the level of care required. Current law does not delegate authority to the Pennsylvania Trauma Systems Foundation for the solution to this aspect of care. Whether "by-pass" can ever be mandated is open to question but without it an optimal system will not become a reality. At this time it is anticipated that the Department of Health will develop regulations requiring collection of data from ambulance services in an effort to improve prehospital care. Act 45 confers this authority; when it will happen is uncertain.

Is all of this justified? Accumulating evidence suggests that the designation of truly competent trauma centers and the establishment of satisfactory triage may avoid a third or more of the deaths which now occur after traumatic injury. One of the earliest observations was that of Fitts and associates, published in 1964.[4] Data gathered from the Medical Examiner's Office of Philadelphia showed many missed opportunities for salvage among 950 deaths. More recently, other studies[5–8] which measured surgeon response times, time to operation, and appropriate resuscitative measures all have demonstrated marked improvement in mortality statistics when patients are taken to trauma centers initially. Although our registry contains too few cases to date for us to statistically validate the success of the system so far, we are encouraged by the early data.

Conclusion

This brief account of recent history cannot give credit to every individual or event which has brought us to the threshold of a system of trauma care in Pennsylvania. It is clear that the University of Pennsylvania Department of Surgery has been the fountain-head from which it has sprung and all who have been part of it may be justly proud.

REFERENCES

1. National Academy of Sciences, National Research Council. Accidental death and disability: The neglected disease of modern society. Washington, D.C.: National Academy of Sciences, National Research Council, 1966.

2. Bulletin, American College of Surgeons. Optimal resources for care of the seriously injured. Chicago: American College of Surgeons, 1976.
3. Pennsylvania Medical Society. 1970 Commission on Emergency Medical Services. Pa Med 1971;June:43–70.
4. Fitts WT, Lehr HB, Bitner RL, Spelman JW. An analysis of 950 fatal injuries. Surgery 1964;56:663.
5. Mullner R, Goldberg MA. An evaluation of the Illinois trauma system. Med Care 1978;16:140.
6. Systems of trauma care: A study of two counties. Arch Surg 1979;114:455.
7. Cales RH. Trauma system profile Orange County California. Trauma Center Newsletter, Vol. 1, issue 2. October 1980.
8. Lowe DK, Gately HL, Goss JR, Frey CL, Peterson CG. Patterns of death, complication and error in the management of motor vehicle accidents: Implications for a regional system of trauma care. J Trauma 1983;23:503.

Secondary Treatment of Craniofacial Trauma

LINTON A. WHITAKER, M.D.

Experience with 101 patients in the last 14 years, followed for a minimum of 1 year, and all treated 3 months or longer from the time of the initial injury with secondary craniofacial reconstruction is described. The bulk of the patients were in the age group 20 to 39 years, and had extensive craniofacial trauma 1 to 5 years before the secondary craniofacial procedure. Eighty percent required multiple smaller operations in addition to the extensive secondary procedure. There was near equal distribution between males and females. In only five instances were segmental shifts of bone carried out. In the remainder, the principle of onlay bone grafts, with cranial bone as the preferred material was used for restoration of contour defects. Extensive stripping of soft tissue with over correction to counteract the pull of scarring in the opposite direction is an essential component of the corrections. Three-dimensional imaging has demonstrated the necessity for good bone to bone contact to achieve maximum maintenance of bone graft volume. If there is only partial contact, there will be resorption of the bone grafts to varying degrees. Whereas multiple operations are almost invariably the rule, true complications are rare, with virtually none occurring in the series. The most frequent one has been irritation around the eye after treatment of enophthalmus. When possible, acute restoration of the craniofacial structure is desirable, using principles described here for secondary craniofacial reconstruction. When that is not possible, successful secondary reconstruction usually can be carried out.

CRANIOFACIAL TRAUMA centers on the orbit. Its treatment involves an extensive reconstructive procedure which at a minimum requires bone grafting, and the use of a coronal incision, thus distinguishing it from maxillofacial trauma.[1,2] A fundamental truth of craniofacial trauma is that when treated acutely, one has the best chance for a total restoration of the face to its previous structural relations. The acute phase approach is generally possible up to about 3 weeks after trauma. After that, there is a gray zone time of several weeks before bone fragments become solidly fixed into position, so that they are moved only with difficulty. In addition, scarring begins to be a dominant factor after 3 weeks, thus resisting shifts in the direction of correction to normal. The reconstructions thus become secondary ones.

Secondary treatment of craniofacial trauma is possible based on principles of cranio-orbital surgery, with highly predictable improvements, but in general with the results falling short of what would have been possible with primary treatment. Our experience has been with 101 patients having secondary treatment of cranio-orbital traumatic deformity, contrasting these patients with ten having acute reconstruction for similar problems, since March 1972.

The principles of secondary craniofacial reconstruction evolved from this experience include the following:

1. Use of the coronal incision with extensive subperiosteal dissection, and mobilization of the soft tissue of the involved orbit or orbits from all bony structures involved with the trauma.

2. Segmental osteotomies where possible, to reposition large bony segments such as possibly the frontal bone, and the zygoma; but especially the maxilla and mandible. Rarely is this step possible in the orbit, or over the maxillary sinus, and infrequently, in the upper face.

From the Department of Surgery (Plastic) and the Craniofacial Program, University of Pennsylvania, the Hospital of the University of Pennsylvania, and the Department of Plastic Surgery, Children's Hospital of Philadelphia, Philadelphia, Pennsylvania.

3. Liberal use of onlay bone grafts for filling in contour defects, often in preference to segmental shifts of bone. This is especially true when bone is comminuted, and stripping soft tissue would result in multiple free segments. Cranial bone is preferable to rib which is in turn preferable to iliac.

4. Slight over corrections are advisable, especially in treating enophthalmus or on any occasion when attempting to restore soft tissue contours by means of bone correction.

5. Reattachment of the medial and lateral canthi in an over corrected position, attempting to overcome the contracture and directional changes of scar are important.[3,4]

6. Doing as much as possible at any one procedure, especially the first, is fundamental, since most will involve multiple operations for further refinements.[5–8]

7. Multiple operations are almost axiomatic.

Our experience clinically, and new studies with three dimensional imaging confirm the superiority of cranial bone (to that of endochondral bone) as a graft material, both in maintenance of volume, and in terms of donor site morbidity.

Materials

In the period 1972 through June 1986, 101 patients have had secondary treatment of craniofacial trauma. This contrasts with ten patients having acute craniofacial trauma treated over the same period of time, allowing some comparison of what can be achieved using this philosophical and technical approach.

All patients grouped in the secondary craniofacial trauma category had had trauma at least 3 months before treatment. Delay of treatment at our center was because of initial treatment having been done elsewhere, and in those instances, sometimes was delayed because of other injuries leaving the details of craniofacial reconstruction as a secondary consideration with life support efforts coming first. Only one patient was younger than 1 year of age, a forceps injury at birth causing a fracture of the right frontal bone and supraorbital ridge. Seven patients were older than 40 years of age, and the biggest bulk of patients were in the decade of 20 to 29 years of age. Ninety percent of the patients treated were between 10 and 39 years of age. The majority had had their initial treatment in the time frame 1 to 2 years before surgery, and the next greatest bulk in the time frame 2 to 5 years before the cranio-orbital reconstructive procedure. These two groups comprise 67% of those treated. Only three were treated at 3 to 6 months after trauma. Fifty-two of the patients were males, and 49 were females. Starting with the extensive secondary cranio-orbital reconstructive procedure as the first step, there was an average of two additional operative procedures done on each patient. Eighty patients had one or more operations after the major secondary craniofacial reconstructive procedure, and very likely all 101 could have benefited from additional revisional procedures. However, because their result was considered adequate, even though virtually always short of total restoration to normal, the additional 21 patients elected not to have further surgery.

The major procedure was done on an elective basis after seeing the patient in the office for evaluation. The evaluation included complete craniofacial physical examination, x-rays in the earlier part of the series, and in the last 4 years, three-dimensional imaging in addition to Quint x-rays, 8-inch by 10-inch photographs, and examination by ophthamologists, neurosurgeons, and orthodontists when the eye, calvarium or occlusion were in question. On detailed craniofacial physical examination inferior or retrodisplacement of bone fragments was the most frequent finding, typically unilaterally, but occasionally bilaterally. Bilateral involvement most often occurred in midface or mandibular fractures, and only rarely in frontal bone or orbital problems. After those evaluations, the procedures were scheduled, and the first procedure was done as extensively and completely as possible.

Most often revisions included more soft tissue work, including scar revisions, secondary revisions around the eyelids, further treatment of enophthalmus or canthal malpositon, septoplasty, and the like. Patients had as many as five additional more minor procedures after the major secondary cranioorbital procedure. Average time for the major secondary cranio-orbital procedure was 4 hours, and length of stay averaged initially 5 days after surgery, and more recently 3 days.

The focal point of the problems in this experience has been the orbit. Canthal displacement, enophthalmus, and malunited fractures about the orbit and midface have constituted the bulk of the problems. The second largest number of patients involved malunited fractures of frontal bone, and the least most frequent group had involvement of the maxilla and mandible with malposition. Only three patients in the entire series had repositioning of the mandible, all by sagital split, and two patients had maxillary repositioning with osteotomies. Decisions to do this were based only on the patient's orthognathic need. Otherwise, if malocclusion was not present, onlay bone grafts or synthetic material were invariably used to augment and provide contour restoration of areas where fractures had occurred. In general, the more complex and extensive the injury, the less likelihood that everything could be corrected in one operation or indeed at all.

Methods of Treatment

The procedures were done almost invariably under hypotensive general anesthesia, with the patients initially going to the intensive care unit, but in more recent years, avoiding that step. The procedures involved a coronal incision with extensive subperiosteal dissection of the frontal bone area, and the involved orbit or orbits. The dissection was sufficiently extensive to release all soft tissue except at the optic foramen, and infraorbital fissure. The lacrimal sac was left intact where that was possible, although there was a high incidence of nasolacrimal obstruction as a result of trauma, usually requiring reconstructive procedures. Dissection of the zygomatic arch, and malar midface structures was done for exposure, and to aid in repositioning the palpebral fissure. Lateral canthopexies were done according to principles previously described, attempting to overcorrect the position of the lateral canthus, since scar invariably pulls the canthus into an inferiorly placed position, and tends to return it to that position even after extensive freeing and over correction. Since the detail of the operation has been worked out, the repositioning procedures have been highly successful. The same is true of the medial canthus, where transnasal medial canthopexy is essential to the success of repositioning that aspect of the palpebral fissure.

Enophthalmus has been a major problem, but now is usually treated successfully. Sixty-five patients were treated specifically for enophthalmus. Measurements were initially with the Luedde exophthalmometer, often producing an inaccurate reading. More recently, computed tomography (CT) scans to note the position of the globes in relation to one another have been done. The finding of enophthalmus is, however, basically a clinical one.

Initially in the series, camouflage of the deep supratarsal sulcus was done by filling in with dermis grafts, or by pericranial flaps. Subsequently, increasing amounts of endochondrial bone which had initially been used in the orbit to reposition the eye were used behind the globe to try to give it anterior projection. As resorption of bone was a frequent difficulty, cranial bone has since been used in 48 patients, with more consistently reproducible results. The bone is placed behind the globe, circumferentially, but more in general inferiorly, since vertical displacement of the eye is also usually a problem in enophthalmus. Consequently reconstruction of the floor of the orbit with cranial bone grafts, using split calvarium, without penetrating the inner table of the skull is the procedure of choice. These bone grafts are used to augment and restore contours of the zygoma, infraorbital rim, floor of the orbit, and behind the eye. In addition, they are used in the frontal bone and supraorbital region, as well as on the mandible.

In no instance were upper face, orbital, or midface structures repositioned with segmental osteotomies. In every case observed in our experience, there were comminutions of bone in these areas that made evaluation and fixation of the bone structures an unnecessarily complicated procedure when it was believed that restoration of contours could be equally achieved by addition of bone onto the underlying retrodisplaced and comminuted segments. As previously noted, osteotomies of the mandible and maxilla were done in five patients. In these instances, the tooth-bearing segment, all involving total maxilla or mandible were moved, and provided a point of fixation, using orthodontic bands and intermaxillary fixation to restore normal occlusion. If the occlusion was normal, and contour disturbances only were present, the principal of onlay bone grafting again was used.

Onlay bone grafting frequently was used to restore retrodisplaced comminuted nasal fractures. In the last 6 years, where there has been adequate soft tissue cover, Proplast has been used in the malar-midface area in 23 patients, to fill out the retrodisplaced side. This is only possible where there is good soft tissue cover, which generally exists in the malar-midface area.

More recent procedures have involved reduction osteoplasty of the laterally bowed zygo-

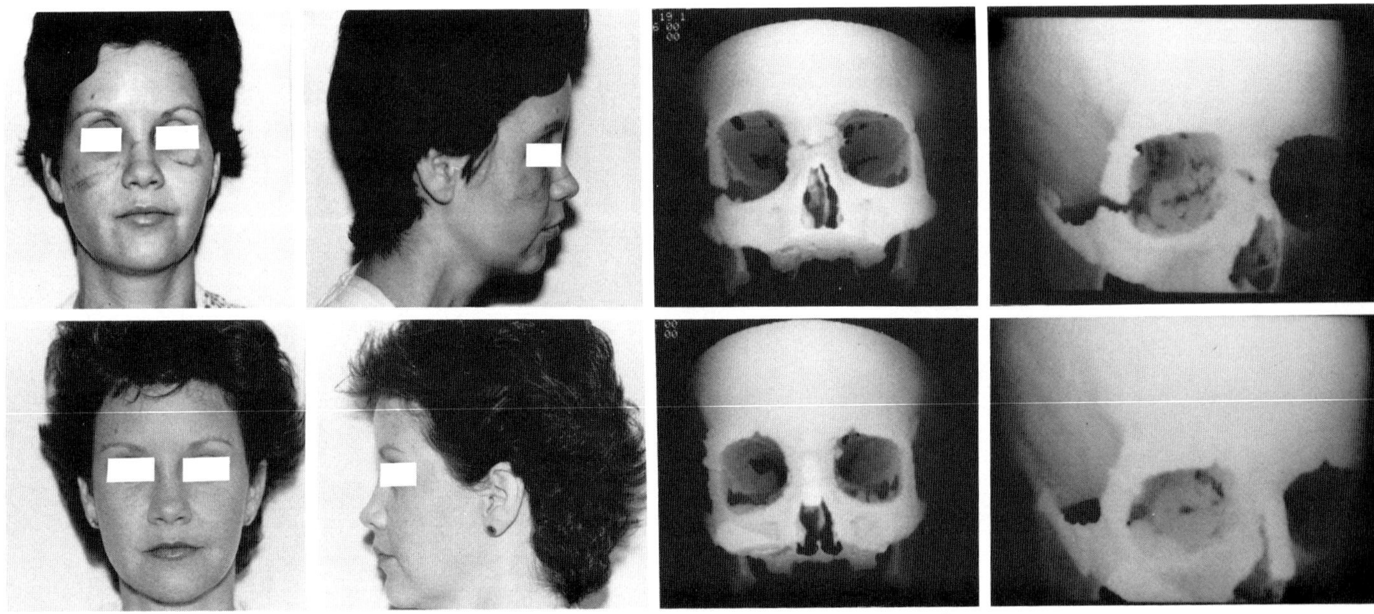

FIGS. 1A–1H. (A, top left) A patient with a LeFort III fracture, including extensive nasoethmoid complex fractures. Notice the widening in the medial canthal region, and the excessively deep supratarsal sulci, as well as the midface flatness seen in the acute phase. (B, top left center) The patient is seen in profile. (C, top right center) A three-dimensional image of the LeFort III, including nasoethmoid complex fractures with craniofacial dysjunction and an inferior displacement of both orbits, especially the right one. (D, top right) A 45° angle three-dimensional image of the same patient. (E, bottom left) The patient is seen 3 months after extensive craniofacial reconstruction, acutely. The procedure involved a coronal incision, repositioning of the medial and lateral canthi, intermaxillary fixation, reduction of nasoethmoid complex fractures, cranial bone grafting of the dorsum of the nose and floor of the orbit on the right, and internal fixation of multiple fracture sites. (F, bottom left center) A profile view 3 months after the reconstructive procedures. (G, bottom right center) Postoperative three-dimensional images showing the cranial bone grafts of the nose, right anterior zygoma, right lateral orbital rim, floor of the orbit on the right, and fracture reductions. (H, bottom right) A 45° angle three-dimensional image view of the same patient.

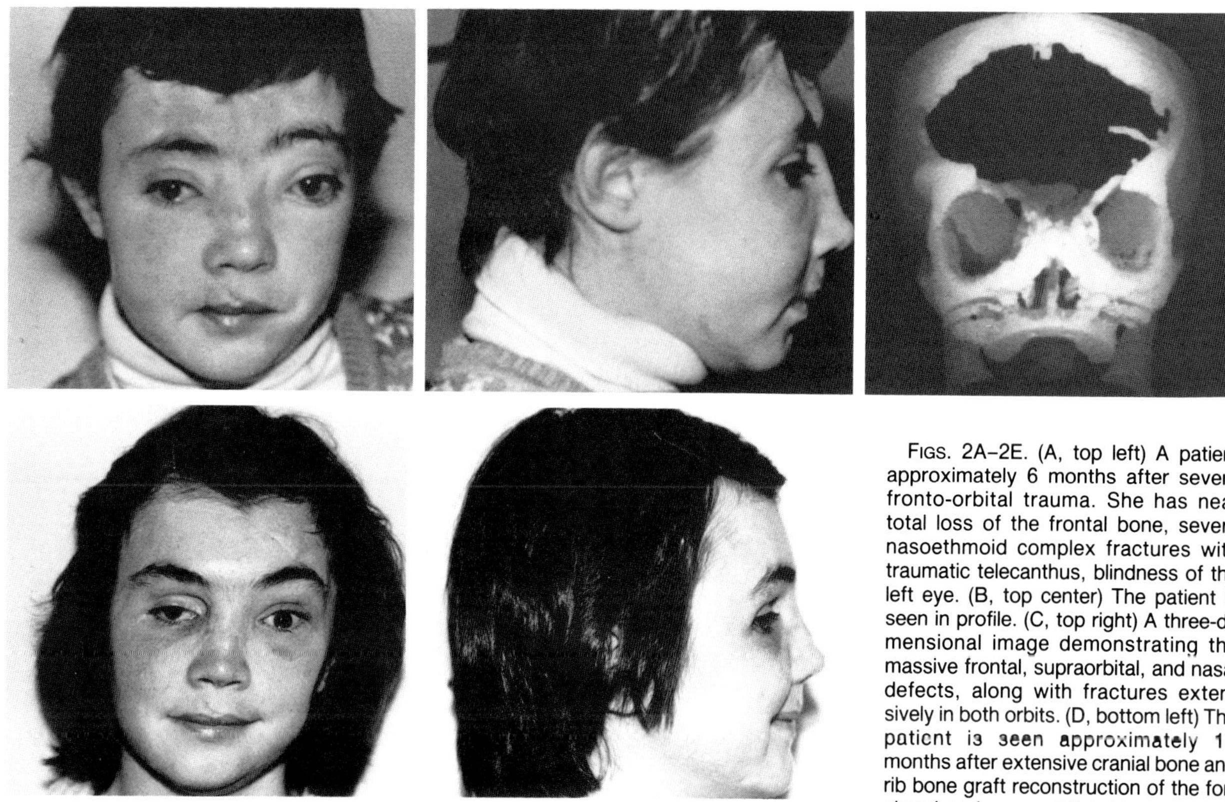

FIGS. 2A–2E. (A, top left) A patient approximately 6 months after severe fronto-orbital trauma. She has near total loss of the frontal bone, severe nasoethmoid complex fractures with traumatic telecanthus, blindness of the left eye. (B, top center) The patient is seen in profile. (C, top right) A three-dimensional image demonstrating the massive frontal, supraorbital, and nasal defects, along with fractures extensively in both orbits. (D, bottom left) The patient is seen approximately 15 months after extensive cranial bone and rib bone graft reconstruction of the forehead and supraorbital ridges, as well the nasoethmoid region, and repositioning of the orbits. (E, bottom right) A profile view of the same patient about 15 months after the reconstructive procedure.

matic arch that typically occurs with a tripod fracture of the zygoma by exposure beneath the temporalis fascia. In addition, filling out sunken or hollowed temporal regions has been done with the use of Proplast beneath the temporal muscle. Synthetic material including Silastic and Proplast have been used in contour distortions along the mandible, but with less success.

Scar revisions were done where possible at the initial procedure, including the use of scar excision and layered closure, z-plasties, w-plasties, and dermabrasion. Subsequent dermabrasion, dermis grafts, pericranial flaps, and muscle flaps have been used to fill in contour defects.

Three-dimensional imaging has demonstrated the dynamics of what happens with grafted bone. It has been clearly demonstrated in our studies that cranial bone in contact with cranial bone maintains its volume quite well. If there is incomplete contact, there will be resorption of bone. This varies in amounts depending on the degree of contact. In general, the biological boundaries of the patient's initial and genetically determined original contour of the face could be restored with grafting when attempts were made to restore the contour beyond that of the original one, there tended to be more reabsorption of bone.

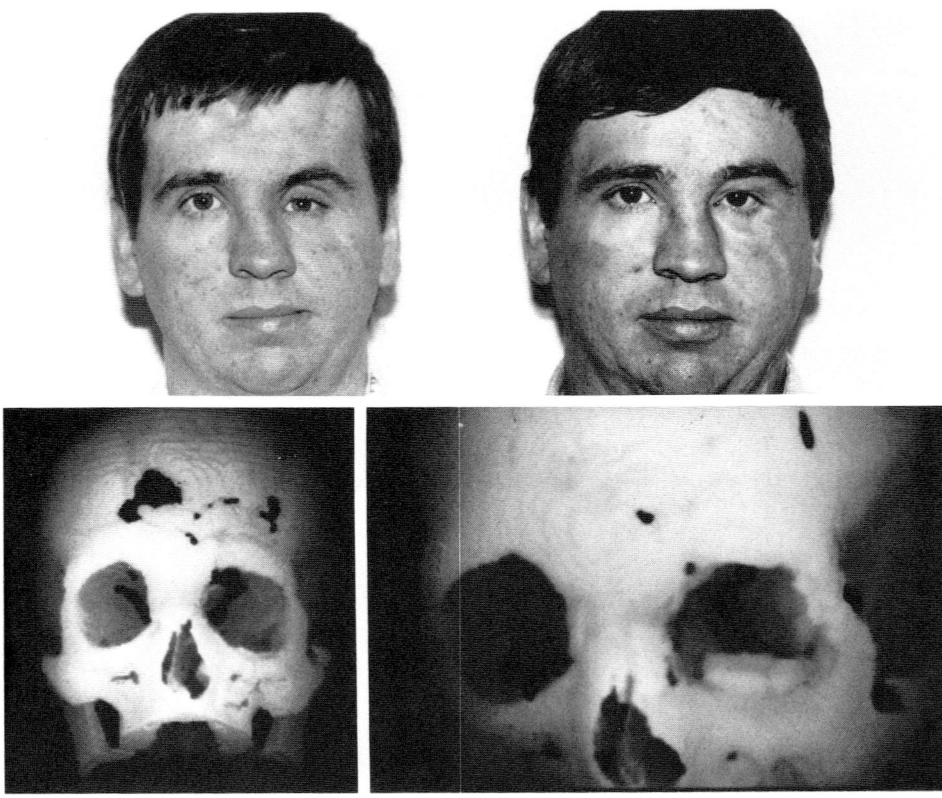

FIGS. 3A–3D. (A, top left) A patient approximately 3 years after multiple operations elsewhere after extensive left fronto-orbital and zygomatic trauma in a motor vehicle accident. The left frontal bone is almost entirely missing. He has inferior displacement of the left brow, lateral displacement of the medial canthus, inferior displacement of the entire left orbit, left enophthalmus, and retrodisplacement of the left zygoma. (B, top right) The patient is seen approximately 2 years after reconstruction of the left forehead with extensive cranial bone grafting, cranial bone graft reconstruction of the left orbital floor, left medial and lateral canthopexy, elevation of the left eye, and correction of enophthalmos with cranial bone grafts. (C, bottom left) The three-dimensional image demonstrates some of the forehead defects present before the secondary reconstruction was done. There is also the extensive inferior displacement of the floor of the left orbit, and disruption of the zygoma on the left. (D, bottom right) The bone grafts for reconstruction of the left orbital floor are seen, and the continuity of the frontal bone that has been reestablished with bone grafts is demonstrated.

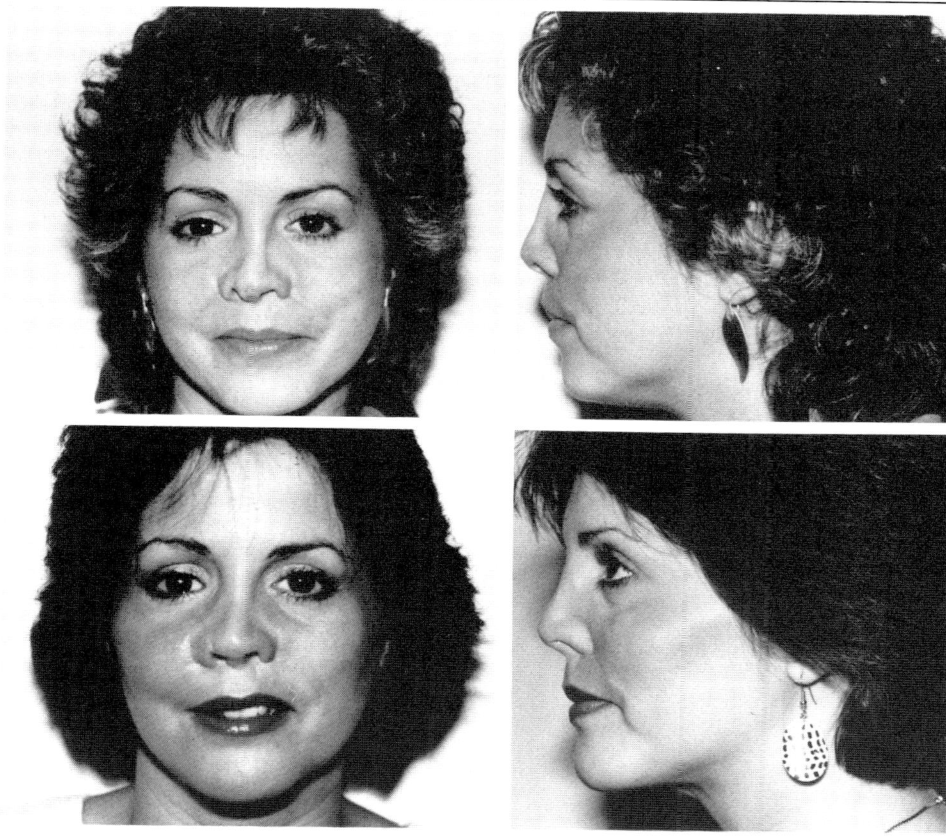

FIGS. 4A–4D. (A, top left) A patient after extensive motor vehicle trauma, and multiple operations done elsewhere. The patient is seen with distortions of the nasal bone, medial canthi, lateral canthi, and midface with retrodisplacement. She also has retrodisplacement of her mandible. (B, top right) The patient is seen in profile particularly demonstrating the retrodisplacement of the chin. (C, bottom left) The patient is seen 2 years after reconstruction of the nasal bone with cranial bone grafts, right medial and lateral canthopexies, cranial bone and Proplast reconstruction of both zygomas, and a sliding genioplasty. (D, bottom right) The patient is seen in profile. (Reprinted with permission from Whitaker LA. Aesthetic augmentation of the malar-midface structures. Plast Reconstr Surg 1987;80:342.)

Results

Our experience is a 14-year one, with a minimum 1-year follow-up on patients treated by secondary reconstruction of craniofacial deformities. The evolution of principles has involved increasingly extensive freeing of soft tissue and the use of bone grafts which were initially predominantly rib or iliac, and more recently cranial bone. Synthetic material has been refined, so that Proplast for malar-midface and temporal as well as some frontal bone contouring is now done consistently successfully.

The procedures have resulted in consistent success with minimal problems except that the total restoration to previous normal contour is rarely entirely possible. Without question, the optimum time is in the acute phase for treatment of contour problems resulting from trauma (Figs. 1A–1H). After that, multiple operations are the norm. This occurred in 80% of our patients where multiple operations were necessary to restore the contours to results that were satisfactory for the patients. In some, this was never achieved, and the patients simply decided that they had had enough surgery without continuing with more operations. Specifically in enophthalmus, the problems were persistent, as they were generally in soft tissue deficit problems. Scarring remained the dominant problem, with the scar contracture process creating pulls that sometimes resulted in recurrent enophthalmus, canthal distortions,

distortions of the nose, and scarring of the face that sometimes were extremely difficult or impossible to overcome. With the use of cranial bone in the orbital cavity, and the extremely extensive dissection that has been done in recent years, this has been less of a problem, and in two instances, enophthalmus has even been over corrected.

The fact that membranous bone in the craniofacial skeleton heals often without bony union, unless there is precise edge to edge apposition, has made it important to use the principle of onlay bone grafts or synthetic material for repositioning or restructuring of contour deformity. It is rare that segments of bone (unless they are extremely large ones) can be shifted after the acute phase to restore the contour. In our experience this never occurred, except in the mandible and maxilla where use of the teeth for fixation provided large stable segments that were possible to move in five patients. Three were mandibular sagital split osteotomies, and two were maxillary LeForte I osteotomies. In all other instances in the nose, malar-midface, orbit, and frontal bones, onlay bone grafts were used.

The principle of counteracting the pull of scar in an adverse direction with extensive dissection, mobilization, and firm fixation in the opposite or normal direction is one that has been used. The more aggressively this is done, the more likely the soft tissue is to stay in a corrected position. It was consistently observed that the more simple the fracture displacements, with fewer structures involved, the more the likelihood of success. That is, if a fracture of the orbital floor and tripod complex only was involved, without lateral orbital wall, supraorbit, medial orbit, and forehead–frontal bone, and without extensive full thickness soft tissue scarring, there was a greater likelihood of success.

The only times that bone graft absorption was a dominant problem were in two instances where patients had gunshot wounds of the midface, with scarring sufficiently extensive to result in inadequate vascularity, and the need for free flaps after resorption of bone. After well-vascularized free flaps were set in place, bone graft take was assured.

Using the principles described, the procedures are successful to a point, restoring faces to normal or near normal in most instances. The limitations are primarily those of soft tissue deficits, and scar pulls in the direction away from the norm. These can be overcome to a large extent by extensive dissection, freeing, and overcorrection of soft tissue as well as bone (Figs. 2A–2E, 3A–3D, and 4A–4).

REFERENCES

1. Converse JM, Smith B, Wood-Smith D. Orbit and naso-orbital fractures. In: Converse JM, ed. Reconstructive Plastic Surgery vol. 2. Philadelphia: WB Saunders 1977.
2. Jones WD III, Whitaker LA, Murtagh F. Applications of reconstructive craniofacial techniques to acute upper facial trauma. J Trauma 1977;17:339.
3. Fox SA. Downward displacement of medial canthus. Ann Ophthalmol 1971;3:1082.
4. Jackson I, Munro I, Salyer K, Whitaker LA. In: Atlas of Craniomaxillofacial Surgery. St. Louis: CV Mosby, 1982.
5. Tessier P. Total osteotomy of the middle third of the face for faciostenosis or for sequellae of LeFort III fractures. Plast Reconstr Surg 1971;48:533.
6. Whitaker LA. Severe traumatic oculo-orbital displacement. In: Transactions of the Sixth International Congress of Plastic and Reconstructive Surgery, August 1975. Paris: Masson Press, 1975;377.
7. Whitaker LA, Schaffer D. Severe traumatic oculo-orbital displacement: Diagnosis and treatment. Plast Reconstr Surg 1977;59:353.
8. Whitaker L. Traumatic craniofacial deformity: Late Treatment. Scand J Plast Reconstr Surg 1981;15:307.
9. Spira M, Gerow FJ, Hardy SB. Correction of post-traumatic enophthalmus. Acta Chir Plast (Prague) 1974;16:2.

A Team Approach to Drool Control in Cerebral Palsy

ARTHUR S. BROWN, M.D., JOY SILVERMAN, M.S., CCC-SP, SALLY GREENBERG, M.ED., DANIEL F. MALAMUD, PH.D., MANUEL ALBUM, D.D.S., ROBERT W. LLOYD, D.M.D., AND MILTON SARSHIK, M.D.

An analysis of the surgical reduction of drooling in children with cerebral palsy is presented, describing a team approach to the problem. All children were housed in a residential facility. The criteria for selection and evaluation of these patients by speech therapists, dentists, plastic surgeons, pediatricians, and teachers are also presented. Results show this approach to be successful: there were minimal post-operative complications; the amount of drool was significantly reduced; and the overall performance of the patients was improved.

CEREBRAL PALSY is a disorder of neuromuscular function due to a malfunctioning of the brain.[8] The origin of this nonprogressive brain dysfunction may be either prenatal, perinatal, or postnatal.[5] The degree of involvement may vary and the accompanying salivary incontinence may be present to a lesser or greater degree. The lack of full orofacial motor control, along with decreased head and neck control, contributes to the problem of increased drooling.

It is estimated that as many as one in 330 children is born with cerebral palsy. Many of these children are considered mildly affected according to the criteria of Minear.[9] A functional capacity classification as well as a therapeutic classification has been described (Table 1). The children in our study are moderately to severely affected; they are nonambulatory and have diminished ability to function independently.

There are many reasons to justify eliminating or decreasing the drooling of these children. Drooling requires children either to wear bibs or have frequent clothing changes, so that they can stay relatively dry. The drooling also interferes with their use of books, toys, and other materials in home, school, and therapy sessions. Communication boards and electronic communication devices allow a degree of communication for nonverbal children and those with poor degrees of verbal intelligibility. Drooling can interfere with the child's ability to communicate by means of these adjunctive devices. Furthermore, children who drool tend to receive less physical affection and contact because of their wetness and occasional malodor associated with the drool.

If diminished salivary incontinence is realized without associated side effects or morbidity, then the technique is worthy of recommendation. Many approaches to diminish the amount of drooling have been used, including behavior modification, tympanic neurectomy, radiation of the salivary glands, and direct surgical intervention Because the former three methods have not been successful on a permanent basis, a different surgical approach has been advocated[1,12,13] for the moderately or severely involved patient.

A modification of the original operation described in 1967 by Wilkie[12] has been used to decrease the morbidity inherent in retropositioning the ducts of the parotid glands. This

From the Division of Plastic and Reconstructive Surgery, UMDNJ/Rutgers Medical School at Camden and Cooper Hospital/University Medical Center, Camden, New Jersey; the Home of the Merciful Saviour for Crippled Children, Philadelphia, Pennsylvania; and the University of Pennsylvania School of Dental Medicine, Philadelphia, Pennsylvania.

Supported in part by NIH grant #DE 05462.

This article has been reproduced with permission from *Annals of Plastic Surgery*, Vol. 15, No. 5, November 1985.

TABLE 1. *Classification of Cerebral Palsy*

	Classification and definition	Clinical involvement
	Functional capacity	
Class I	Patients with cerebral palsy with no practical limitation of activity	None
Class II	Patients with cerebral palsy with slight to moderate limitation of activity	Minimal
Class III	Patients with cerebral palsy with moderate to great limitation of activity	Moderate
Class IV	Patients with cerebral palsy unable to carry on any useful physical activity	Severe
	Therapeutic	
Class A	Patients with cerebral palsy not requiring treatment	None
Class B	Patients with cerebral palsy who need minimal bracing and minimal therapy	Minimal
Class C	Patients with cerebral palsy who need bracing and apparatus, and the services of a cerebral palsy treatment team	Moderate
Class D	Patients with cerebral palsy limited to such a degree that they require long-term institutionalization and treatment	Severe

* Modified from Minear [9]

modified procedure in which both submandibular glands are excised and the ducts of the parotid glands ligated bilaterally is our choice for surgical treatment.[2,3]

Since there is scant literature addressing the consequences following surgical diminution of salivary flow, a study was designed to evaluate a select patient population in a protected environment. The patients in this study are residents of a domiciliary institution for children with cerebral palsy, where close observation can be assured. Among the specific areas of interest are the overall functioning of the children postoperatively; changes in incidence of pharyngitis, otitis media, or dental caries; changes in feeding patterns and taste; articulatory differences; classroom performance; social interaction with peers, family, therapists, teachers, and housemothers; and surgical morbidity.

Methods

The Home of the Merciful Savior is a residential facility for children with cerebral palsy, ranging in age from 3 to 13 years. From this group, 10 children (6 boys and 4 girls, ages 6 to 11) were selected as candidates for surgical drool control by their speech therapists with input from house care staff, nurses, teachers, and other therapists. The selection of these 10 children was based on the following criteria: quantity of drool, results of questionnaires (Fig. 1) distributed to the staff, child's feelings about his drooling, parental concern, general condition, and age.

After the initial selection of proposed candidates, the clinical impression of excessive drooling was confirmed by a quantitative analysis of the amount of saliva lost while the child was doing a specified task, such as using his language board. The task was repeated during the same time of day on ten different occasions for 20-minute periods while measuring the total amount of drool. One child was eliminated from the study because the amount of saliva collected was not substantial. It should be noted that all 10 children in the study had some degree of oral-motor involvement; 2 were judged to be mildly involved, while 8 had moderate to severe oral-motor disability according to the classification of Minear (Table 2).

Additional preoperative assessment was done utilizing video-fluoroscopy to record barium-enhanced swallowing function studies with the child in an upright position. Attention was paid to the synchrony of tongue movements, dyskinetic movements of the oral muscu-

TABLE 2. *Results of Surgical Reduction of Drooling in 10 Patients*

Patient	Overall oral-motor disability*	Quantity of drool†		Interference with activities‡	
		Preoperatively	Postoperatively	Preoperatively	Postoperatively
J. L.	Severe	Severe	Moderate	Marked	Mild
T. W.	Severe	Severe	None	Marked	None
A. W.	Mild-moderate	Moderate	Mild	Moderate	Mild
M. M.	Moderate-severe	Severe	Mild	Moderate	Mild
R. K.	Severe	Severe	None	Marked	None
V. K.	Severe	Severe	None	Moderate	None
A. S.	Severe	Severe	Mild	Marked	Mild
B. R.	Severe	Severe	None	Marked	None
Z. E.	Mild	Severe	Mild	Marked	Mild
J. G.	Mild	Moderate	None	Moderate	None

* According to Minear [9]
† Mild = less than 1 g/collection; moderate = 1-3 g/collection, severe = greater than 3 g/collection
‡ Activites monitored included speech therapy, classroom performance, eating, etc. (subjective evaluation)

Drooling Questionnaire

Date: | Filled out by:

Key: 1 Yes Always Usually; 2; 3; 4; 5 No Never Rarely; 6 I don't know

Patient name	Trunk and head control	Lip closure*	Feeding difficulties	Interacts with others	Child's awareness of drooling	Interference with activities*	Awareness of drooling by others	Parental concern	Child drools*

*Most consistent results

FIG. 1. Questionnaire on drooling.

lature, and whether aspiration occurred. In addition, all children were evaluated by the team pedodontists for routine dental care and prophylaxis. Dental impressions were taken of the patients for fabrication of individual fluoride gel trays to help maintain dental integrity after salivary reduction.

At the conclusion of the above assessment, an in-depth discussion between the plastic surgeon and the parents was conducted. The operative procedure with its potential complications, hospitalization, and general anesthesia were discussed. All parents or responsible guardians agreed that these children would be given topical fluoride to prevent the dental caries production that might possibly be enhanced by a diminution in saliva.

Hospitalization averaging five days was required. A general anesthetic utilizing nasotracheal intubation was used for all patients. Upper neck incisions in a skin fold were used for the submandibular gland excision, along with a subcapsular resection of the gland. Suction catheters using a "butterfly" catheter and vacuum tube were employed for 48 to 72 hours. Catgut sutures were used intraorally after submucosal ligation of Stensen's duct, and sub-

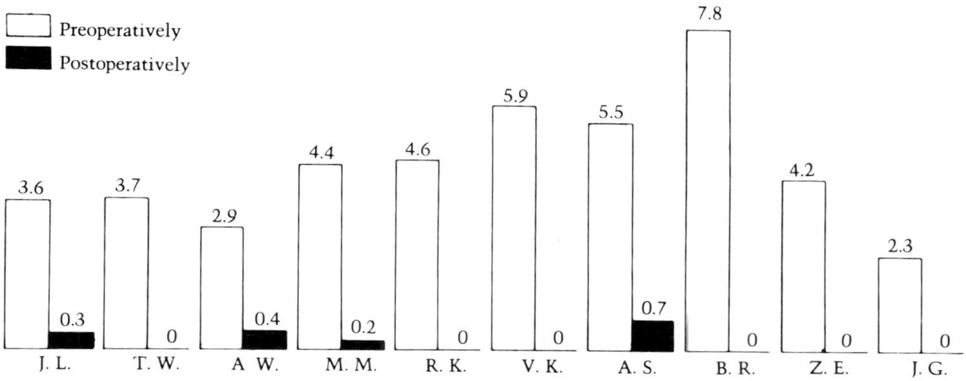

FIG. 2. Amount of decrease of drool after surgery compared with preoperative levels (grams) during 20-minute collection.

cuticular sutures of a monofilament material were used for the skin approximation. Antibiotics were not used routinely.

Results

Plastic Surgery

There was mild to moderate swelling postoperatively about the cheeks, which resolved by the time of discharge from the hospital. This did not create any compromise in swallowing or airway exchange. All skin incisions healed primarily and were of little concern to the patients. There was marked diminution in the amount of drooling in all children studied (Fig. 2). Although the character of the saliva has become thicker and less viscid than preoperatively, the need for frequent clothing changes has been eliminated. Decreased drooling has also resulted in less irritation around the lips and commissures of the mouth.

The only negative effect of the operation has been occasional dry and/or cracked lips. This problem was made more difficult because of the child's inability to moisten his own lips, due to severe oral motor involvement. Application of petroleum jelly easily eliminated this problem. One child developed a cutaneous abscess of his left cheek ten days after discharge from the hospital. This was treated with antibiotics and local drainage, with complete resolution.

Comparison between the preoperative and postoperative quantitative assessment of the drool produced revealed meaningful reduction in all children (Table 3). Questionnaires used for the preoperative and postoperative assessment were compared with objective data. The evaluators' opinions postoperatively closely paralleled the objective findings from measuring the amount of drool produced.

TABLE 3. *Quantification of Drooling in Operated Patients*

Patient	Age (yr, mo)	Sex	Mean grams of drool per 20 minutes	
			Preoperatively	Postoperatively
J. L.	7, 9	F	3.63	0.27
T. W.	8, 10	F	3.67	0.00
A. W.	8, 10	F	2.95	0.04
M. M.	6, 10	F	4.40	0.02
R. K.	9, 10	M	4.62	0.00
V. K.	10, 11	M	5.90	0.00
A. S.	6, 6	M	5.50	0.74
B. R.	7, 8	M	7.85	0.00
Z. E.	9, 2	M	4.16	0.05
J. G.	9, 1	M	2.30	0.00

Biochemistry

Salivary proteins involved in anticaries activity include secretory IgA and a large number of nonimmunological factors such as lysozyme, lactoferrin, lactoperoxidase, and bacterial agglutinins[7,9]. Agglutinins involved in the aggregation of *Streptococcus sanguis* and *Streptococcus mutans* display a normal distribution in the general population.[6] These agglutinins are distinct from the adhesive proteins that bind bacteria to the tooth surface[10] and thus form part of a clearance-adherence system in the mouth. We have recently demonstrated that caries-resistant individuals display an increased bacterial aggregating activity and a decreased bacterial adhesion, thus promoting bacterial clearance.[11] It was possible, therefore, that reduced salivary flow might decrease the quantity of these antibacterial proteins.

Accordingly, samples of whole saliva were collected and tested at several concentrations for aggregating activity against *S. sanguis* M5 or *S. mutans* KPSK2, as described elsewhere.[4] *S. sanguis* is one of the earliest organisms involved in plaque formation, while *S. mutans* is thought to be a major contributor to dental caries.

As shown in Table 4 there is a wide range of bacterial aggregating activity for both *S. sanguis* and *S. mutans* within the study population. Activity is greater for *S. mutans* than for *S. sanguis,* as has been previously reported.[10] Agglutinin activity for *S. mutans* stayed the same or increased in 7 of 9 patients and decreased approximately 50% in 2 patients (V. K. and M. M.). Thus, despite the lack of parotid and submandibular gland saliva in this patient population following operation, considerable agglutinin activity was found to remain in the mouth, presumably of sublingual and minor gland origin. It appears, therefore, at least in terms of bacterial agglutination, that removal of parotid function and the submandibular glands has not compromised the patients.

Dentistry

Dentistry for children who are profuse droolers often becomes tedious. Visits become prolonged to enable the dentist to provide effective treatment. Decreasing salivary flow enables dental examinations and treatment to be performed quickly, efficiently, and much more easily for both the dentist and the patient.

The patients in the study were followed for a period of three years by two pedodontists who alternately examined the children three times a year. The incidence of dental caries did not increase. In fact, these children were more cooperative when they underwent routine dental care. This may be because of the frequent examinations and resultant densensitization.

The water supply in Philadelphia, where these children reside, is fluoridated. Initially, fluoride gel was used topically in a tray system daily for all children. This regimen later was done every other day. Evidence to date from this controlled group of patients does not indicate whether or not the topical application of fluoride gel was necessary to control any further caries. Currently, no children are receiving topical fluoride and all are caries-free.

Pediatrics

These children experienced no delay in growth or development following the operation. Growth curves were not adversely affected and showed no change following the operation.

TABLE 4. *Saliva-Mediated Bacterial Aggregation*

	Percent aggregation			
	Preoperatively		Postoperatively	
Patient	*S. sanguis*	*S. mutans*	*S. snaguis*	*S. mutans*
J. L.	4	0	1	64
T. W.	40	46	20	68
R. K.	1	1	0	44
V. K.	3	66	3	32
M. M.	0	56	8	30
A. W.	5	57	10	48
A. S.	0	45	0	49
Z. E.	0	10	15	55
J. G.	2	57	18	69

Their nutritional status was maintained. In fact, these children showed better food intake following the surgical procedure. One explanation might be that they had better tactile sensibility following reduction of their salivary flow and were also able to taste food that was not appreciated prior to their drool reduction.

No increase in upper respiratory infections or otitis media was noted in this group following operation. Even though a reduced rate of otitis media is expected with increasing age, no adverse effects can be attributed to the operative procedure with regard to infectious processes of the upper respiratory tract or middle ear.

Discussion

We have substantially reduced the amount of drooling in all patients following their operations. Psychologically, all the children seemed to benefit. They received many positive comments about their appearance. The children seemed less apprehensive about interactions with people outside of their home and school environment. Other children were eager to undergo this surgical procedure with the hope of eliminating or reducing their drooling.

Adverse comments from people in the child's environment about his or her drooling were eliminated. The children received much more physical affection. They were no longer given bibs to wear and were allowed to play with additional toys and handle more books and materials than previously. One 7-year-old boy, who had seemed relatively unaware of his drooling problem but in fact was quite concerned about it, told his mother that he wanted to go to the shopping mall without a bib and that she could now throw out all his bibs. Another child asked the surgeon if he could please have the operation soon to get rid of his messy, smelly drool, having seen others successfully treated. It appears that subjective opinions of persons working closely with these children regarding the severity of the drool are consistent and accurate. Therefore, choosing candidates for future operations could be based on this subjective assessment with confidence.

Improved feeding patterns and/or improved articulatory patterns could prove to be additional benefits following the operation. Dryer contact points available for the articulators used in both eating and speech could provide the child with additional sensory information necessary for improvement in these areas. A closer look at this problem with a subsequent group of children might be helpful in planning therapeutic intervention and prognosticating potential gains expected with intensive therapy. Also, aberrant swallowing patterns as seen on barium-enhanced swallowing function tests utilizing video-fluoroscopy will form the basis of another paper. In addition, periodic examination of these children who underwent the drool control operation will be continued.

REFERENCES

1. Brody GS, Wilkie TF. Surgical treatment of drooling. In Fredricks S, Brody GS (eds), Symposium on the Neurologic Aspects of Plastic Surgery, Vol 17. St Louis, CV Mosby, 1978, p 18.
2. Dundas DF, Peterson RA. Surgical treatment of drooling by bilateral parotid duct ligation and submandibular gland resection. Plast Reconstr Surg 1979;64:47.
3. Glass LW, Nobel GL, Vecchione TR. Treatment of uncontrolled drooling by bilateral excision of submaxillary glands and parotid duct ligations. Plast Reconstr Surg 1978;62:523.
4. Golub EE, Thaler M, Davis C, Malamud D. Bacterial aggregating activity in human saliva: simultaneous determination of free and bound cells. Infect Immun 1979;26:1028.
5. Holm VA. The causes of cerebral palsy. JAMA 1982;247:473.
6. Malamud D, Appelbaum B, Kline R, Golub EE. Bacterial aggregating activity in human saliva: comparisons of bacterial species and strains. Infect Immun 1981;31:1003.
7. Mandel ES. Salivary factors in caries prediction. In Bibbey, Shern (eds), Methods of Caries Prediction. Special Supplement of Microbiology Abstracts. 1978, pp 147–158.
8. McDonald ET, Chance B Jr. Cerebral Palsy. Englewood Cliffs, NJ, Prentice Hall, 1964, p 12.
9. Minear WL. A classification of cerebral palsy. Pediatrics 1956;18:841.
10. Rosan B, Malamud D, Appelbaum B, Golub E. Characteristic differences between saliva-dependent aggregation and adhesion of streptococci. Infect Immun 1982;35:86.
11. Rosan B, Appelbaum B, Golub E, et al. Enhanced saliva-mediated bacterial aggregation and decreased bacterial adhesion in caries-resistant vs. caries-susceptible individuals. Infect Immun 1982;38:1056.
12. Wilkie TF. The problem of drooling in cerebral palsy: a surgical approach. Can J Surg 1967:10:60.
13. Wilkie TF, Brody GS. The surgical treatment of drooling—a ten year review. Plast Reconstr Surg 1977;58:791.

Personal Computer-Assisted Planning of Craniofacial Surgery

LAWRENCE P. KERR, WAYNE KASHINSKY, AND SAMUEL P. PEJO

BOTH SKILL AND COMMUNICATION are paramount to the plastic and reconstructive surgeon. Among the many requisite skills are the analysis of form, the choosing of technique, and the anticipation of change. Frequently, measurements are compared against norms; subjective judgements are formed according to aesthetic values.

The surgeon must plan well. Information should be accurately, clearly, and efficiently communicated to patient and colleagues. Accurate record keeping furthers advances in the field.

History

This research began with the exploration of two- and three-dimensional graphic representation and record keeping in planning in 1975. While the results were encouraging, they were not formally published[1,2] as a clinical tool because of several limitations. These included high cost and limited availability of unique sophisticated equipment, limited availability of computer time on that equipment, and the immense investment of surgeons' time that would have been needed. More recent work, such as that presented at this symposium,[3,4] while promising and inspiring, is also limited by similar overwhelming complexity.

Other planning tools, such as cephalometry, photographic montage, plaster moulage, and artistic sketching, are likewise cumbersome and time consuming. Although less expensive, the representations obtained by these methods have been inadequate and awkward.

Instead, a system of easily modified computer images is proposed. The purpose of this paper is to describe the use of the personal computer as an aid to planning, evaluation, communication, and recording in the field of craniofacial surgery.

The personal computer is rapidly becoming familiar as an aid to the productivity of an individual. Such familiarity recalls its accounting and business functions, laboratory use, and most commonly, word processing strengths. Except for video games, its graphics capabilities have been largely unexplored.

The recent introduction of inexpensive, universally available computer systems and peripherals, with standard software support, allows the commonly available personal computer to be used in extensive and sophisticated preoperative planning and postoperative analyses. These computers are always available on the surgeon's desktop (or even in the operating suite), can be used actively with the patient, and are portable and efficient.

Methods

A computer, software, and peripheral system was assembled from commercially available sources. An image—patient, slide, photograph, CAT scan, or X-ray—is created by a video camera and copied into the computer. It, then, is translated by a digitizer into an electronic form acceptable to the computer. The personal computer is used to process and manipulate the image. Finally, it is viewed on the computer video display screen, saved, or printed.

The following hardware and software are used:

Apple MacIntosh Computer, 512K, and Imagewriter, MacPaint, Apple Computer Corporation, 20525 Mariani Avenue, Cupertino, CA 95014

From the Proceedings of the First International Congress of The International Society of Cranio-Maxillo-Facial Surgery, Cannes-La Napoule, 1985.

This article has been reprinted with permission from *Craniofacial Surgery*, Springer-Verlag, Heidelberg, 1987.

MAGIC video camera, interface, and software system. New Image Technologies, Inc., Suite 104, 10300 Greenbelt Rd., Seabrook, MD 20706

Accessory Pak 1, Silicon Beach Software, P.O. Box 261430, San Diego, CA 92126

Digitizing electronically divides the picture into many small sections (512 by 342). These small sections are called pixels. Each pixel is either dark or white. In a manner reminiscent of a pen-and-ink sketch, patterns of dark and light points substitute for the full gray scale. Thus a pattern is formed of pixels. Each pixel is given a unique place in the memory of the computer. The image is said to be bit mapped. It is the manipulation of this memory which allows the image to be changed, redisplayed, and evaluated.

Results

Cephalometrograms can be measured directly on the screen by scaling rulers to size. Preoperative tracings can be electronically retraced and moved.

Film prints of computerized axial tomographic (CAT) scans can be similarly measured and analyzed. Sections can be traced and overlapped.

Manipulation of the images is done using various electronic maneuvers presented in a simple manner as tools. Sections of the image can be delimited and moved. Patterns can be erased or added. This is done with both aesthetic evaluation and as a response to measurements. Changes and reformulations are seen on the video screen in an instant and are just as quickly reformulated.

Limitations of the effect of surgery on the final result can be anticipated. A case of orbital dystopia with orbital advancement, elevation, and rotation illustrates the anticipated bony correction. The simulation allows the surgeon to prognosticate the soft tissue deficiency and ptosis that require secondary reconstruction.

Soft tissue reconstruction, such as lateral canthopexy performed with maxillary resection, can be simulated. The aesthetic impact of the choice of maxillary osteotomies can be evaluated.

Limitations

The limitations of the technique are two. First, some resolution is lost because patterns of the white and dark pixels are used instead of full gray scale representation.

Secondly, the correction made in one dimension cannot be reformulated and viewed in another dimension. The image of the patient from an anterior-posterior view cannot be changed and then turned through 90° to revisualize it from a lateral view. While this is theoretically possible, no standard programming now exists to achieve it, and it is the purpose of this paper describe only hardware and software that are universally available without modification or custom programming.

Discussion

These examples illustrate some of the power of the personal computer as an aid to the planning of craniofacial surgery. It has equal utility in the practice of general plastic surgery.

Patients enthusiastically accept the technological intrusion into the patient-doctor relationship and seem to find the warmth and confidence of increased understanding and communication rather than coldness and fear of mechanization. The issue of implied guarantee is that of the display of another patients' slides. The image shown to the patient is only an approximation; it does not constitute and should not be interpreted as an exact representation of the postsurgical results. Intended results are not guaranteed. Probably, the increased understanding gained from the technique outweighs the issue of implied guarantee.

The limitations of this two-dimensional analysis are real, but universal availability, low cost, ease of use, and the quickly interactive nature of the personal computer will allow all plastic surgeons to benefit from modern technology.

The inexperienced computer user can learn to use the system quickly. No programming or previous computer experience is necessary. No special vocabulary or programming language needs to be learned. Familiarity with the use of light and photography in arranging the video camera is more helpful.

The system is only one part of the increased productivity uniquely afforded by the personal computer. Writing of reports, patient education, accounting, numerical analysis, preparation of slides, time, financial and resource management, and information retrieval are all part of the same system.

Early product announcements forecast equipment which will allow higher resolution, greater speed, and color, further improving the utility of the method. Three-dimensional analyis is conceivable and is dependent only on software development.

Further, the technique is an interesting blend of computer technology and art, of quantitative analysis and aesthetics. Neither sort of analysis excludes the other, but rather the whole is coordinated. The facility and rapidity of the personal computer as part of this relationship create richer understanding, creativity, and communication.

ACKNOWLEDGEMENT

Support from the American Association of Plastic Surgeons is gratefully acknowledged.

REFERENCES

1. Kerr LP (1977) Report to the American Association of Plastic Surgeons. (unpublished)
2. Bourne DA (1978) Three-dimensional picture processing and its bio-medical applications. Image understanding systems and industrial applications. Proc SPIE 155:91–102.
3. Marsh JL, Vannier HH (1983) The "third" dimension in craniofacial surgery. Plast Reconstr Surg 71:759–767.
4. Hemmy DC, David DJ, Herman GT (1983) Three-dimensional reconstruction of craniofacial deformity using computed tomography. Neurosurgery 13:534–541.

Management of the Chronic Radiation Wound

DENNIS J. LYNCH, M.D. AND RALEIGH R. WHITE IV, M.D.

IN THE PAST 50 YEARS radiation therapists have gradually enhanced their ability to deliver photons at higher energy and to deeper tissue levels. The result is clearly demonstrated in improved survival rates for patients with seminoma, Hodgkin's disease, and laryngeal and cervical cancer. Older concepts of single modality treatment with either surgery or radiation alone have become outdated, and for the more advanced cancers, combinations of x-ray treatment and surgery have become commonplace.

Early methods of radiation therapy delivered low voltage radiation that was classed as orthovoltage (300,000 volts). Orthovoltage radiation concentrated the dosage at the skin level and the amount of treatment could be gauged by the degree of skin erythema. Skin erythema helped to prevent overdosage, but low voltage radiation also had limited potential to cure deeply situated cancers.[7]

The modern radiotherapist now has megavoltage[16] therapy (1 to 35 million volts) that can be delivered with a variety of devices that include cobalt units and linear accelerators. These larger x-ray units have the capability of delivering the photon energy to the deeper tissue planes while sparing the skin. The skin cannot be used as an indicator, and the quality of treatment very much depends on the skill of the radiotherapist and his or her ability to calculate and effectively apply a safe yet therapeutic dosage.

In the application of x-ray treatment the risk-benefit curve must be kept in mind. Rapidly proliferating cancer cells are destroyed at lower dosage levels than normal tissues. As the dose is increased, the probability of damage to normal tissue also rapidly increases, and the slope of each curve overlaps at the higher dose levels.[9] In order to avoid damage to the normal tissues, there are a variety of maneuvers that the radiotherapist may utilize, but in order to have the best chance for tumor control, tissue tolerance levels must frequently be approached for effective treatment.

The tissue effects of radiation[3] can be classified according to their time of onset after the treatment dose has been delivered. Acute injury occurs during the course of radiation treatment and the effects are observed in the more rapidly proliferating tissue such as skin, bone marrow, intestine, and bladder. Skin erythema is a good example of the acute reaction and like most acute effects of radiation it is self-limited and completely reversible.

The chronic radiation effect usually presents as a wound complication a number of years after the course of treatment. The injury occurs in the slowly proliferating vasculo-connective tissues. Progressive fibrosis and proliferative endarteritis develop within the portals of treatment and produce chronically indurated tissues. The degree of induration and ischemia is directly related to the total dose of radiation delivered to the area. When this type of damage occurs proximally in an extremity it is not unusual for distal lymphedema to be a problem. Evidence of this effect is apparent in the patient with lymphedema after axillary radiation for breast cancer. The ischemic soft tissue and bone within the treatment portal have little resistance and are vunerable to trauma, spontaneous necrosis, mixed bacterial invasion, and osteoradionecrosis, often resulting in a chronic wound that does not heal. This type of wound is frequently extensive and even life threatening in patients compromised by other major disease processes.

From the Texas A & M University College of Medicine and Division of Plastic Surgery, Scott and White Clinic, Temple, Texas.

This article has been reproduced with permission from *Surgical Clinics of North America*, Vol. 62, No. 2, April 1982.

The radionecrotic wound is chronic and does not heal, and the patient often requires narcotics for analgesia. Hypoproteinemia, anemia, and malnutrition are commonly associated problems. Heavy pelvic radiation can be associated with obstructive urinary tract and intestinal complications. In order to manage the wound problem it is necessary to correct the systemic problems with such measures as transfusion, enteral or parenteral hyperalimentation, and specific antibiotics.

Wound Excision

The key to successful management of these patients lies in achieving a healed wound. To accomplish this result it is necessary to excise the necrotic and ischemic tissue and control heavy bacterial contamination.[15]

Marino applied the term "biologic excision" to the management of the radiation wound.[10] This refers to the fact that within most radiation portals there are critical structures such as bone, nerve, tendon, and major blood vessels, that cannot be sacrificed. The excision of the radionecrotic wound almost always falls short of complete debridement of the damaged tissue. Wound coverage must then be achieved in an adverse environment in which some dead tissue remains. Parasitic types of tissue cover such as skin grafts and tubed pedicle flaps are not reliable answers. "Biologic excision" refers to the application of a well-vascularized pedicle flap that brings new blood supply to the wound environment and eventually leads to healing. Long-term drainage must be provided beneath such a flap to allow escape of the separating debris. It is not unusual for such a flap to have drainage from beneath it for one to two months before healing is complete.

In planning the excision of these wounds it is very helpful to obtain the size and position of the previous radiation treatment portals. When the dosage has been applied homogeneously to a portal of radiation, the excision must include most of the same portal. When information about the portal size is not available, the entire area of indurated soft tissue should be included. These indurated tissues cannot be reliably used as part of the skin flap coverage and must be discarded.

When the wound has undergone deep necrosis and heavy bacterial invasion with inadequate drainage, it is reasonable to plan an initial debridement that unroofs the wound and falls short of final excision. Aerobic and anaerobic bacterial cultures should be obtained to direct antibiotic treatment to specific bacterial sensitivities. Topical antimicrobials such as mafenide acetate, silver sulfadiazine, or povidone iodine should be used in the wound to reduce the local bacterial growth. However, after one to two weeks of local wond care, definitive excision and wound coverage must be accomplished utilizing the concept of biologic excision.

Wound Coverage

Brown established the principle of well-vascularized skin flap coverage for the chronic radiation wound.[5] In areas of deep necrosis that develop long after megavoltage treatment there is no other effective method of wound closure. Occasional exceptions occur after orthovoltage for more superficial lesions. When the entire area of injury can be excised and a well-vascularized bed of soft tissue provided, a skin graft can be used instead of a pedicle flap.

In the past 30 years the armamentarium of the plastic surgeon has expanded so that there are many new options to exercise in choosing well-vascularized pedicle tissue for permanent coverage of these wounds. Brown utilized the random skin flap, which did not have a specific anatomic vascular pedicle on which the flap was built.[5] By necessity these flaps were short (2 to 1 ratio of length to width) to insure tissue perfusion at the tip of the flap. A one-stage transfer was not always possible and "delaying" incisions were frequently necessary. These awkward tools have now been largely replaced by pedicle flaps that are built on anatomically well-identified vascular pedicles.

The axial pattern skin flap[14] is built on a specific arterial pedicle. By adding a random flap to the end of an axial flap, a significant increase in the ratio of length to width can be designed (4 to 1) without compromising reliability. The increased length and mobility makes this tool much more versatile. The standard examples of this group are the deltopectoral flap[6] and groin flap.[13] The deltopectoral flap is built upon the perforating branches of the internal mammary artery. It has been very useful in reconstruction of defects after treatment of osteoradionecrosis of the mandible and other problems related to head and neck cancer. The groin flap is built on the femoral triangle and the superficial circumflex iliac artery. Variations of this flap can be utilized to rotate over lower abdominal defects after radiation treatment of bladder carcinoma.

The myocutaneous flap is a more recent innovation that utilizes the vascular pedicle of major muscles to carry the muscle and the overlying skin to an adjacent site as an island pedicle or even to a distant site as a free flap utilizing microvascular anastomosis.[11] The classic example in this group is the gracilis myocutaneous flap.[12] It is built on the medial circumflex branch of the deep femoral artery and it can be tunneled proximally to reconstruct the groin, perineum, penis, and vagina.

The latissimus dorsi myocutaneous flap is built on the axillary origin of the thoraco-acromial artery.[4] It provides a long leash for transfer of skin and muscle from the low back to the head and neck, breast, and upper extremity. It has become a routine method of reconstruction of the breast and can be utilized even in the patient whose chest wall has been heavily irradiated. The pectoralis major can also be moved on its vascular pedicle originating in the axilla.[2] Skin, muscle, and rib can be transferred, potentially providing a well-vascularized bone graft to a previously radiated site of oral carcinoma and jaw resection.

The omentum provides a very long vascular leash. Skin cannot be transferred with it, but a skin graft can vascularize and grow on its surface. The technique of omental lengthening has been well described, and a long vascular pedicle is built on the right gastroepiploic artery. It can be transferred[8] upward to repair defects of the chest wall after radiation for breast cancer. It is an alternative to the latissimus dorsi and pectoralis major myocutaneous flaps, which can also be utilized for this purpose. It can be transferred beneath the inguinal ligament to gain coverage of the femoral triangle in cases of radiation necrosis in this critical area. Femoral hernia is an expected complication and requires a second operation to divide the pedicle and close the hernia defect.

Free pedicle flaps[11] transferred by microvascular anastomosis should potentially be the most versatile tool in managing the radiation necrotic wound. Particularly advantageous should be the potential to transfer a vascularized bone graft. The difficulty lies in the vessels of the recipient site, which have also been damaged by the radiation. This reduces the reliability of the free flap, and in most circumstances a permanent vascular pedicle would be preferred.

Prevention

Just as the state of the art of pedicle flap surgery has changed dramatically in the past 30 years, so has the technique of radiation therapy.[9] With the back-up of support of physicists and computerized dose calculations, treatment has become more sophisticated and safety has improved. Computerized tomographic scanning and ultrasonography give more accurate estimates of tumor size and location so that the dose can be delivered to the tumor volume with less exposure of the surrounding normal tissue. Rotational fields of treatment, variations of field size, and combinations of external radiation beam with implantation devices are all strategies that improve safety. It appears that effectiveness is also increased by combining radiation with drugs such as dactinomycin, doxorubicin, and bleomycin. Research with hyperbaric oxygen, particle irradiation, and hypoxic cell sensitizers (metronidazole) is leading to improved safety and effectiveness.

Because of the delayed appearance of wound complications after radiation therapy, it is difficult to evaluate the morbidity related to this type of treatment. The trend at this time, however, seems to be clearly toward few complications, and it is the plastic surgeon's expectation and hope that fewer of the complex wound problems will present for treatment in the future.

ACKNOWLEDGMENT

The authors are grateful to Dr. Odis D. Skinner for his technical advice regarding radiation therapy.

REFERENCES

1. Alday ES, Goldsmith HS. Surgical technique for omental lengthening based on arterial anatomy. Surg Gynecol Obstet 1972;135:103.
2. Ariyan S. Pectoralis major, sternomastoid, and other musculocutaneous flaps for head and neck reconstruction. Clin Plas Surg 1980;7:89.

3. Bloomer WD, Hellman S. Normal tissue responses to radiation therapy. New Engl J Med 1975;293:80.
4. Bostwick J. Sixty latissimus dorsi flaps. Plast Reconstr Surg 1979;63:31.
5. Brown JP, Freyer M, McDowell F. Permanent pedicle carrying flaps for repairing defects in avascular areas. Ann Surg 1951;134:486.
6. Daniel RP, Cunningham D, Taylor G. The deltopectoral flap: Anatomical and hemodynamic approach. Plast Reconstr Surg 1975;55:275.
7. Fletcher G. The evolution of the basic concepts underlying the practice of radiotherapy from 1949 to 1977. Radiology 1978;127:3.
8. Jurkiewicz M, Arnold P. The omentum: An account of its use in the reconstruction of the chest wall. Ann Surg 1977;185:548.
9. Kinsella T, Bloomer WD. New therapeutic strategies in radiation therapy. J.A.M.A. 1981;245:1669.
10. Marino H. Biological excision: Its value in the treatment of radionecrotic lesions. Plast Reconstr Surg 1967;40:180.
11. Maxwell G. Musculocutaneous free flaps. Clin Plast Surg 1980;7:111.
12. McCraw J et al. Vaginal reconstruction with the gracilis myocutaneous flap. Plast Reconstr Surg 1976;58:176.
13. McGregor I, Jackson I. The groin flap. Br J Plast Surg 1972;25:3.
14. McGregor I, Morgan G. Axial and random pattern flaps. Br J Plast Surg 1973;26:202.
15. Robinson D. Surgical problems in the excision and repair of radiated tissue. Plast Reconstr Surg 1975;55:41.
16. Slazman F, Smedal M. Indications for supervoltage radiotherapy. N Engl J Med 1967;277:1295.

Porcine Pancreaticoduodenal Allotransplantation With Inclusion of the Spleen (Irradiated and Nonirradiated) to Prevent Thrombosis

DONALD C. DAFOE, M.D., DARRELL A. CAMPBELL, JR., M.D., ROBERT M. MERION, M.D., RICARDO V. LLOYD, M.D., ALLEN S. LICHTER, M.D., AND JEREMIAH G. TURCOTTE, M.D.

THE SUCCESS RATE for transplantation of the pancreas as treatment of insulin dependent diabetes mellitus has been increasing. The recent Pancreas Transplant Registry report showed a 1-year graft survival (independence from exogenous insulin) of 46% with a 1-year patient survival rate of 85%.[1] This graft survival lags behind the approximate 70% to 80% 1-year graft survival achieved with transplantation of other organs such as the kidney, liver, and heart. A major contributor to decreased pancreas graft survival is technical failure which has accounted for 26% of pancreas graft losses.[1] Thrombosis is a common cause of technical failure.

In 1982, Starzl and colleagues reported the successful clinical transplantation of composite pancreas allografts which included the duodenum, a length of jejunum, in some cases, and the spleen.[2] The primary rationale behind this technique was the maintenance of the normal vascular anatomy and the prevention of thrombosis. In particular, the spleen may provide a physiologic arteriovenous fistula and maintain patency of the graft splenic and portal vein. Despite the antithetical nature of the intentional transplantation of immunocompetent tissue, it was hypothesized that inclusion of the spleen may have an immunologic advantage regarding allograft acceptance as supported by experimental work. After the report by Starzl *et al.* several pancreas transplant programs, including the University of Michigan, began to transplant the donor spleen with the whole-organ pancreas graft and a periampullary "button" or segment of duodenum.[3–5]

After clinical use of the pancreaticoduodenal allograft (PDA) with the donor spleen (PDA + S) technique, reports of life-threatening graft *versus* host disease (GVHD) appeared and continued use of PDA + S was discouraged.[3,4] However, if the immunocompetent cells in the donor spleen could be eradicated with lethal irradiation (PDA + S*) then the immunologic disadvantages might be eliminated and hemodynamic advantages preserved.

This report describes our laboratory investigation with pancreas allografts which included the donor spleen. Using a porcine model, we compared graft survival in three groups: PDA recipients; PDA + S recipients; and PDA + S* recipients.

Materials and Methods

Animals

Farm-bred pigs, 10 to 12 weeks of age (20–25 kg) were recipients of PDA grafts. Nonlittermate pigs were used as PDA donors.

After transplantation animals were allowed free access to water. A single morning meal of Purina Chow Animal Feed (Ralston-Purina Co., St. Louis, MO) was given. Pancreatic enzyme replacement was provided with Viokase (Viobin Corp., Monticello, IL), 1 Tbsp with each feed. Pigs surviving beyond 28 days after transplantation were killed using a method

From the Departments of Surgery, Pathology, and Radiation Therapy, University of Michigan Hospitals, Ann Arbor, Michigan.

Supported by a Michigan Diabetes Research and Training Center Pilot/Feasibility grant and an American Diabetes Association Research and Development Award

TABLE 1. *Results of Pancreaticoduodenal Allograft Transplantation in Pancreatectomized Pigs*

Graft	n	Rejection (d after transplantation)		Mean glucose ± SD*	K value†
PDA	10	0/10	$P < 0.01$‡	95 ± 8	−2.40
PDA (no immunosuppression)	3	3/3 (8, 12, 15)		—	—
PDA + S	8	5/8 (7, 11, 15, 15, 16)		95 ± 13	−2.24
PDA + S*	5	0/5		92 ± 23	−2.45

PDA: pancreaticoduodenal allograft; PDA + S: PDA with the donor spleen; PDA + S*: PDA with the irradiated donor spleen; IV GTT: intravenous glucose tolerance tests.

* Mean glucose values determined in normoglycemic animals over the 28 days after transplantation.

† K values were generated from IV GTT carried out in surviving hormoglycemic animals on the twenty-eighth day after transplantation; normal K value, −2.50.

‡ Fisher's exact test.

which was in accordance with the policies of the University Laboratory Animal Medicine Department.

Surgical Technique

The recipient animal was placed under general anesthesia, the native pancreas removed to produce diabetes and PDA, PDA + S or PDA + S* transplanted. The anesthetic and surgical technique has been described in detail.[6] Anticoagulation was not given.

Irradiation Technique

In the PDA + S* group, the donor spleen was irradiated with 1000 rad—a dose which has been shown to destroy splenocytes[7]—while the pancreas was shielded. The irradiation technique has been described.[8]

Immunosuppressive Medications

Immunosuppression consisted of cyclosporine (Sandoz Co., East Hanover, NJ), 6 mg/kg/day intravenously (IV), and prednisolone, 1.5 mg/kg/day IV tapered to a maintenance dose of 0.5 mg/kg/day by 7 days after transplantation. Immunosuppression was discontinued after 28 days.

Studies

Daily blood glucose levels were determined using the glucose oxidase method with the Beckman Glucose Analyzer (Smith, Kline and French, Philadelphia, PA). Rejection was defined as a blood glucose > 150 mg/dl for 3 consecutive days or hyperglycemia and histologic findings at autopsy consistent with severe rejection. Twenty-eight days after transplantation, IV glucose tolerance tests (IV GTT) were performed on pigs which had been fasted overnight. Awake and unrestrained pigs received 0.5 g/kg of glucose as an IV bolus. Samples for blood glucose were drawn before glucose challange and 3, 5, 10, 20, 30, 45, 50, and 90 minutes after.

Data Analysis

Mean daily glucose values are expressed ± SD. Data from IV GTT were used to calculate K values, the slope of the linear regression of glucose on time, from 3 to 90 minutes after glucose bolus. A comparison of the incidence of rejection in the groups was done with the Fisher's exact test. Glucose values between the groups were compared using the Wilcoxon Rank Sum test.

Experimental Design

The study was a comparison of graft survival in recipients of technically successful PDA, PDA + S, and PDA + S* transplants.

Experimental groups consisted of the following: (1) PDA recipients, n = 10; (2) PDA + S recipients, n = 8; and (3) PDA + S* recipients, n = 5. A group of three nonimmunosuppressed whole-pancreas allograft recipients (two PDA, one open duct) acted as a control group for alloreactivity.

Results

In the nonimmunosuppressed control group, rejection occurred in each case. Hyperglycemia was present beginning on 8, 12, and 15 days after transplantation. The mean daily glucose increased from 83 ± 22 mg/dl to 282 ± 79 mg/dl ($P < 0.001$) (Table 1).

Of PDA recipients, none became hyperglycemic with the 28-day immunosuppressive regimen of cyclosporine and prednisone. The mean daily glucose for PDA recipients was 95 ± 8 mg/dl.

With the same immunosuppressive regimen, 5 of 8 PDA + S recipients developed rejection an average of 13 days after transplantation (range, 7–16 days). This difference between rejection incidence in the PDA (zero of ten) and PDA + S (five of eight) groups was statistically significant ($P < 0.01$). The mean daily glucose before the declaration of rejection or death in PDA + S recipients was 88 ± 21 mg/dl but rose to 275 ± 59 mg/dl ($P < 0.0001$). Two PDA + S recipients developed hyperglycemia and died acutely. Histologic study of the pancreas in these two cases and each of the other three cases of hyperglycemia in the PDA + S group confirmed the existence of rejection with findings of fibrosis, acinar cell loss, perivascular round cell infiltrate, intimal proliferation, and endothelial "foam" cells. Islet cell numbers were reduced. Changes in the duodenum of rejected grafts included slough of mucosa and lack of muscle with submucosal inflammatory cell infiltrate. Histologic examination of the spleen showed intimal proliferation and fibrosis.

In the PDA + S* group, there was no rejection during the 28 days after transplantation. The mean daily blood glucose was 92 ± 23 mg/dl. At autopsy, the irradiated spleen was fibrotic.

Using IV GTT data generated from surviving pigs on the twenty-eighth day after transplantation, the K values in the three experimental groups were as follows: −2.40 in the ten PDA recipients; −2.24 in three PDA + S recipients; and −2.45 in the five PDA + S* recipients. The K value in normal pigs (n = 17) determined in earlier studies was −2.50.[9]

Signs of GVHD, such as massive diarrhea, were not seen in any of animals in the experimental groups. In one normoglycemic animal with a skin rash, a full-thickness skin biopsy did not show changes of GVHD. No grafts were lost due to thrombosis.

Discussion

Thrombosis of the transplanted pancreas has been a major cause of graft loss. According to Pancreas Transplant Registry data, thrombosis claimed 12% of all pancreas allografts transplanted during 1983 to 1986.[1] The pathogenesis of thrombosis in pancreas transplantation has not been studied thoroughly. However, one study demonstrated a drop in blood flow to the pancreas to about 70% of control values when the splenic vessels were ligated.[10] Superimposed upon decreased flow is inflammation of the allograft from manipulation of the pancreas during retrieval and transplantation. Additional insults due to warm ischemia, cold ischemia during preservation, and reperfusion injury may contribute to low flow and thrombosis. Thrombosis frequently has occurred despite patent vascular anastomoses and has originated on the venous side of the allograft in the portal vein.

One attempt at prevention of thrombosis was the creation of a distal arteriovenous fistula (AVF) between the splenic artery and vein.[11] However, venous hypertension or "steal" of blood from the pancreatic parenchyma could occur with the AVF technique. In fact, when pancreas grafts with AVF were transplanted in primates, hemorrhagic pancreatitis uniformly resulted.[12] To address the thrombosis problem, Starzl and colleagues[2] suggested the use of a composite graft which included the whole pancreas, spleen, jejunum, and duodenum. It was reasoned that such a graft would preserve the normal vascular arcades and maintain blood flow.

The immunologic consequences of transplantation of the pancreas with the donor spleen are uncertain. Islet cell transplantation studies have demonstrated that depletion of sensitizing cells, such as splenocytes, resulted in prolonged graft survival.[13] Therefore, transplantation of the pancreas with the donor spleen is contrary to laboratory work in islet cell transplantation. On the other hand, all classical methods of induction of tolerance require exposure of the immunologically modulated host to allogeneic hemopoietic cells.[14] Bitter-Suermann *et al.* found evidence for a beneficial effect on transplantation of the pancreas when "conditioned" by donor strain spleen allografts in rats.[15] Other investigators, however, found this phenomenon to be specific for certain inbred strains of rats.[16] In rats, auxiliary splenic transplants were accompanied by improved skin and renal graft acceptance.[17] In guinea pigs, splenic transplants from a high-responder strain to a low-responder strain resulted in tolerance of recipient-to-donor strain skin grafts and suppression of antidonor mixed leukocyte reactivity.[18] Kountz and Cohn showed extended survival of kidney transplants in dogs which received a donor spleen transplant if recipient splenectomy also was done.[19] In this canine study, acceptance frequently followed an initial episode of GVHD suggesting surviving donor cells in the recipient (chimerism) were responsible for induction and/or maintenance of a tolerant state.

Indeed, we have documented chimerism in a patient who accepted a pancreaticoduodenal allograft which included the nonirradiated donor spleen.[5] A death due to GVHD in PDA + S recipient has been reported.[3] Another PDA + S recipient developed GVHD but *in vivo* irradiation of the transplanted donor spleen was successfully used to destroy the germinative cells responsible for GVHD.[4] Laboratory work in rodents also has demonstrated avoidance of GVHD by irradiation of parental strain donor pancreaticosplenic grafts transplanted into streptozotocin diabetic F1 hybrids (a GVHD model) without affecting pancreas graft function.[20]

Kootstra *et al.* first applied *ex vivo* irradiation of the donor spleen before PDA transplantation in three patients.[21] In his report, he underscored the apparent value of donor spleen inclusion by noting only one case of pancreas transplant thrombosis had occurred in the 25 cases reported.

At the University of Michigan, we have transplanted 21 PDA.[22] In three cases the nonirradiated donor spleen was transplanted with the PDA and in five cases the donor spleen was irradiated with 1000 rad *ex vivo*. Thirty-one percent (four of 13) of PDA without the donor spleen thrombosed in the absence of an apparent technical cause. In the eight recipients of PDA + S or PDA + S* grafts, one early thrombosis was clearly due to torsion of the graft portal vein. When the donor spleen was removed in a PDA + S* recipient because of thrombocytopenia, thrombosis resulted within 24 hours. Recipients of PDA + S or PDA + S* grafts had transient leukopenia and thrombocytopenia. No GVHD was seen.

In the porcine study presented herein, five of eight recipients of PDA + S grafts experienced rejection while maintained on a regimen of immunosuppression which prevented rejection in ten PDA recipients during a 28-day period after transplantation. The inclusion of the spleen in the pancreas graft had a clear detrimental effect on graft survival. The mechanism by which the donor spleen induces rejection is not well defined. The donor spleen provides a constant source of immunocompetent cells which express donor antigens and Ia antigens possibly stimulating a rejection response. However, the detrimental effect of donor spleen inclusion on PDA survival was abrogated by irradiation before transplantation.

Since the main impetus for inclusion of the donor spleen in the PDA is hemodynamic—prevention of thrombosis—the differences in blood flow in the various experimental groups, recipients of PDA, PDA + S and PDA + S*, would be important to document. If hemodynamic studies confirm that inclusion of the irradiated spleen significantly improves blood flow to the pancreas graft and prevents thrombosis, then this technique may be valuable in pancreatic transplantation.

REFERENCES

1. Sutherland DER, Moudry KC. Pancreas Transplant Registry Report. Clin Transplant 1987;1:3.
2. Starzl TE, Iwatsuki S, Shaw BW Jr *et al.* Pancreaticoduodenal transplantation in humans. Surg Gynecol Obstet 1984;159:265.
3. Sollinger HW, Kalayoglu M, Hoffman RM *et al.* Experience with pancreatcocystostomy in 24 consecutive pancreas transplants. Transplant Proc 1985;(Suppl 2)17:141–143.
4. Gonwa TA, Goeken NE, Schulak JA *et al.* Failure of cyclosporine to prevent *in vivo* T cell priming in man: Studies in allogeneic spleen transplantation. Transplantation 1985;40:299.
5. Dafoe DC, Campbell DA Jr, Marks WH *et al.* Karyotypic chimerism and rejection in a pancreaticoduodenosplenic transplant. Transplantation 1985;40:572.
6. Dafoe DC, Campbell DA Jr, Marks WH *et al.* Association of inclusion of the donor spleen in pancreaticoduodenal transplantation with rejection. Transplantation 1985;40:579.
7. Thomas ED, Storb R, Buckner CD. Total-body irradiation in preparation for marrow engraftment. Transplant Proc 1976;8:591.
8. Dafoe DC, Campbell DA Jr, Marks WH *et al.* The effect of irradiation of the donor spleen on rejection of porcine pancreaticoduodenosplenic allografts. Transplantation 1986;42:686.

9. Dafoe DC, Campbell DA Jr, Marks WH *et al.* Detrimental effects of 4 hours of cold storage on porcine pancreaticoduodenal transplantation. Surgery 1986;99:170.
10. Garvin PJ, Castaneda MA, Niehoff ML *et al.* An *in-situ* evaluation of distal splenic arteriovenous fistula on pancreas function in an isolated pancreas segment. Arch Surg 1985;120:1148.
11. Calne RY, McMaster P, Rolles K. Technical observations in equential pancreas allografting: Observations on pancreatic blood flow. Transplant Proc 1980;12:51.
12. DuToit DF, Heydenrych JJ, Louw G *et al.* Intraperitoneal transplantation of vascularized segmental pancreatic autografts without duct ligation in the primate. Surgery 1983;94:471.
13. Lacy PE. Experimental immuno-alteration. World J Surg 1984;8:198.
14. Steinmuller D. Methods for induction of permanent graft survival. Transplant Proc 1979;11:1198.
15. Bitter-Suermann H, Save-Soderbergh J. The course of pancreas allografts in rats conditioned by spleen allografts. Transplantation 1978;26:28.
16. Squifflet J, Sutherland DER, Florack G. The course of combined pancreas and spleen allografts in rats. Transplantation 1982;34:302.
17. Bramis JP, Schauzer H, Sloane C. Specific impairment of humoral and cellular allograft immunity after splenic allotransplantation in rats. Transplant Proc 1978;9:341.
18. Bitter-Suermann H, Shevach EM. Induction of transplantation tolerance in guinea pigs by spleen allografts: I. Operative techniques and clinical results. Transplantation 1982;33:45.
19. Kountz SL, Cohn R. Prolonged survival of a renal homograft by simultaneous splenectomy and splenic homotransplantation. Surg Forum 1962;13:59.
20. Schulak JA, Sharp WJ. Graft irradiation abrogates graft-*versus*-host disease in combined pancreas–spleen transplantation. J Surg Res 1986;40:326.
21. Kootstra G, van Hooff JR, Jorning PJG *et al.* A new variant for whole pancreas grafting. Transplant Proc 1987;19:2314.
22. Dafoe DC, Rosenberg L, Campbell DA Jr *et al.* Clinical pancreaticoduodenal allotransplantation with inclusion of the donor spleen (irradiated and nonirradiated) to prevent thrombosis. Transplant Proc 1988;(Suppl 1)20:876.

The Role of Afferent Lymphatics in the Rejection of Skin Homografts

CLYDE F. BARKER, M.D. AND R. E. BILLINGHAM, F.R.S.

BOTH CYTOLOGICAL STUDIES and those concerned with the adoptive transfer of transplantation immunity have demonstrated that the principal seats of specific reactivity to orthotopic skin homografts are the regional lymph nodes.[1] On this basis it has been widely assumed that the lymphatic vessels draining the graft bed carry antigenic material to the nodes, thus constituting the afferent path of the immunologic reflex. An observation which has been widely construed as sustaining this premise is the partial or complete exemption from rejection enjoyed by small homografts implanted into vascularized sites, such as the brain, or the cheek pouch of the Syrian hamster, which lack a conventional lymphatic drainage.[2] However, anatomical differences in the vascular beds of such grafts, as compared with those of orthotopic skin grafts, combined with the impossibility of serially inspecting intracranial grafts, render this sort of evidence inconclusive and it has recently been questioned by Lance.[3] More compelling is Lambert et al.'s[4] evidence that temporary lymphatic discontinuity, established in rabbits' ears bearing skin homografts, both delays regional node response and prolongs graft survival by the time required—about 4 days—for demonstrable alternative lymphatic channels to develop.

It may also be pointed out that there is no evidence that afferent lymph draining a recently transplanted orthotopic skin homograft contains effective antigenic material. However, Hall[5] has shown that the lymph, draining areas bearing recently transplanted skin homografts, contains much cellular debris though both the origin and the antigenic status of this material is uncertain.

In the case of renal homografts, on the other hand, there is cogent evidence that the establishment of lymphatic connections with the host is *not* essential for evocation of sensitivity[6–9]. Particularly telling is Strober and Gowans'[10] demonstration that if a homologous kidney is coupled extracorporeally to a rat's femoral artery and vein for a period of 5–12 hr, the animal subsequently develops a state of specific sensitivity. This occurs despite the absence of any direct contact or lymphatic connections between the host tissues and the alien organ. This finding has lent considerable strength to Medawar's[11,12] concept of "peripheral sensitization" according to which immunologically competent small lymphocytes in the blood stream engage with fixed antigens in the graft itself, possibly at the level of its vascular endothelium, and then return to the host, probably via the regional lymphatics. On reaching the nodes, or other lymphoid tissues, they settle out and, by cytologic transformation and mitotic activity, generate the effector cell population that mediates the immune response.

The experiments described in this communication make use of vascularized, skin pedicles, whose draining lymphatics can be preserved, interrupted, and restored at will, as beds for "orthotopic" skin homografts[13]. It will be shown that an intact lymphatic drainage in the graft bed is an essential prerequisite for sensitization of the host. Evidence bearing upon the manner in which sensitivity to skin homografts is evoked and put into effect will also be presented.

This work was supported in part by United States Public Health Service Grant AI-07001.

From the Departments of Medical Genetics and Surgery, University of Pennsylvania School of Medicine, Philadelphia, Pennsylvania.

This article has been reproduced with permission from the *Journal of Experimental Medicine*, Vol. 128, No. 1, July 1, 1968.

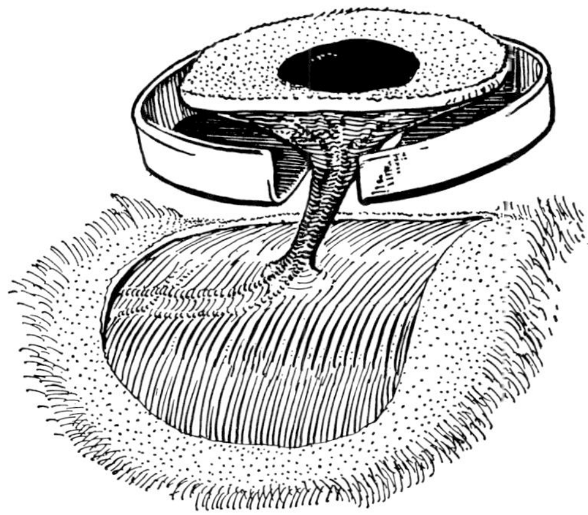

FIG. 1. Showing a freshly prepared isolated skin flap with its vascular umbilical cord and inlaid skin homograft. After closure of the skin defect with interrupted sutures the plastic dish housing the flap will be glued to the underlying skin.

Materials and Methods

The experimental animals were adult guinea pigs derived from domestically maintained sublines of the isogenic strains 2 and 13. These strains are known to differ by seven or eight transplantation antigens and reject mutually exchanged skin homografts within 10 days[14,15].

Principle of the Experiments and Preparation of the Isolated Skin Flaps

To evaluate the importance of lymphatic drainage for the rejection of orthotopic skin homografts it is essential to be able to observe the latter for long periods after transplantation to vascularized skin beds experimentally deprived of their draining lymphatic vessels. The procedure employed is a modification of that devised by Frey and Wenk[16].

Circular, full-thickness skin flaps, 3–4 cm in diameter and including the panniculus carnosus muscle, were cut from the shaved right flanks of guinea pigs anesthetized with Nembutal. A single vascular bundle or "umbilical cord" about 2–3 mm in diameter and containing an artery, a vein, and some nerves was left intact connecting the isolated flap with its host to maintain viability (Figs. 1 and 5). The circular skin defect was closed with interrupted sutures, leaving a small central gap for the emergent nourishing umbilical cord of the flap. The latter was then placed in a small (35 × 10 mm) plastic Petri dish in the bottom of which a radial slit had been cut out to accommodate the umbilical cord (see Fig. 1). The dish was glued firmly to the underlying skin with Eastman 910 adhesive. After placing the lid on the Petri dish it was secured in place and protected from displacement by winding many turns of 1 inch wide plain gauze bandage round the animal's trunk, the under layers

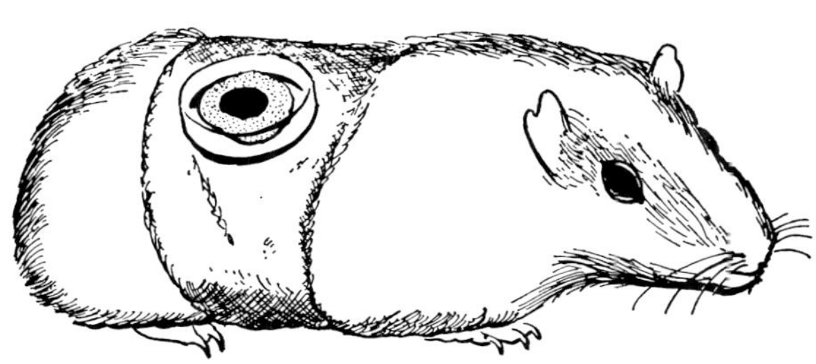

FIG. 2. A guinea pig bearing an intra-flap skin homograft in a plastic dish. Note the protective dressing applied around the animal's trunk.

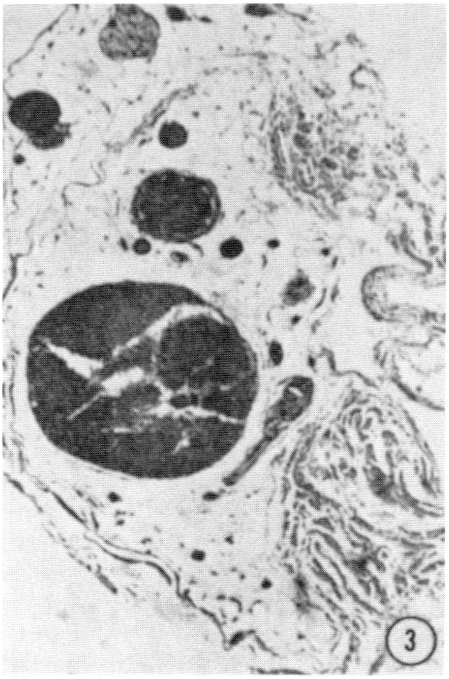

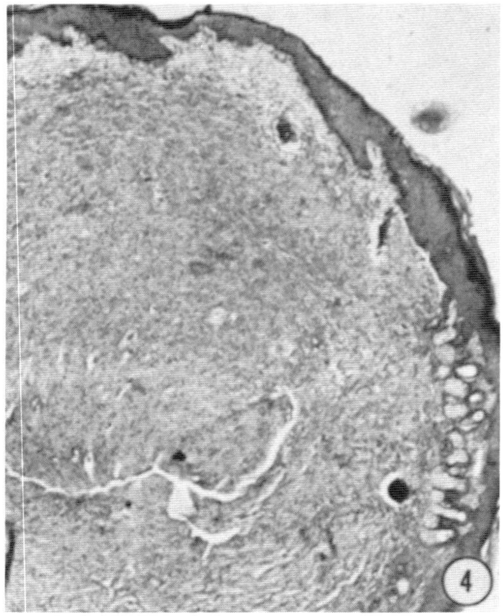

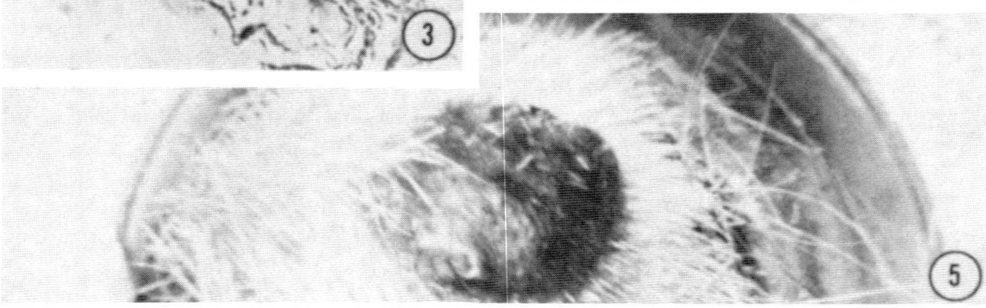

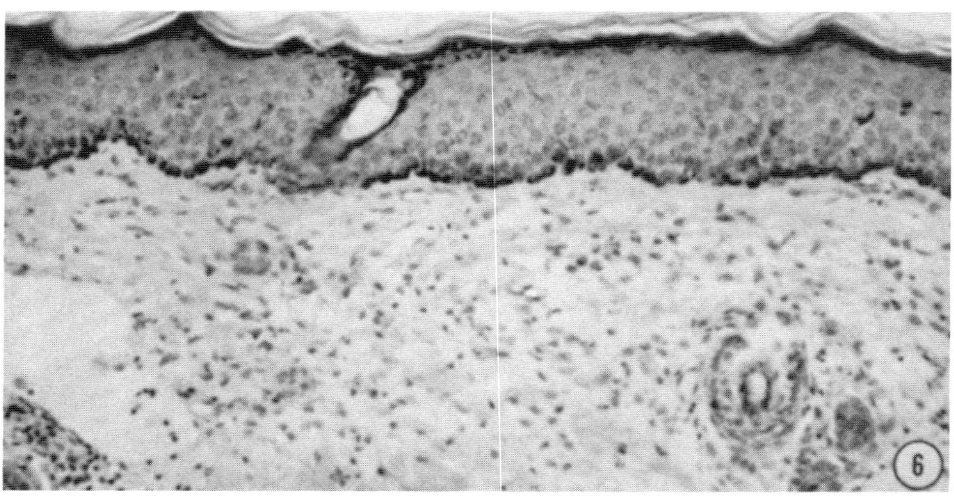

All histological specimens stained with hematoxylin and eosin.

FIG. 3. Transverse section through freshly prepared vascular "umbilical cord" uniting a skin flap to the site from which it was excised. Note the prominent blood vessels and nerve and the loosely knit connective tissue matrix that supports them. ×70.

FIG. 4. Section through vascular umbilical cord or pedicle sustaining a healthy, partially isolated skin flap preparation of 40 days' standing. This pedicle has become greatly thickened through the laying down of new fibrous connective tissue and it is completely epithelialized. Note the cluster of sebaceous glands of apparently de novo formation. ×35.

being affixed to the skin by means of Mastisol[17]. Such a dressing allowed the animal normal mobility and the layer of bandage overlying the lid of the dish could easily be removed for periodic inspections without anesthetizing the animal (Fig. 2).

Immediately after their dissection, circular, shallow, partial thickness beds 1 cm in diameter were cut in the centers of the flaps. Thin, full-thickness skin grafts, removed from the donors' ears and freed from all adherent cartilage and fat, were then carefully fitted into these beds. The spotted coloration of the guinea pigs enabled pigmented skin grafts to be transplanted to white host skin flaps in all experiments so that epidermal melanocytes[18] could be used as donor epidermal markers to help follow the fate of grafts subjected to chronic reactions of low-grade intensity.

Revelation of lymphatic vessels was accomplished by very superficial intradermal injections of a 2% aqueous solution of Patent Blue V, via a No. 30 gauge syringe needle[19]. When injected into intact flank skin this dye promptly and consistently revealed the complex plexus of fine lymphatic vessels and the major afferent lymphatic channels leading to the prominent regional nodes which also became stained.

Skin grafting entailed the transfer of standard, full-thickness discs of ear skin, 1 cm in diameter and cut with the aid of a trephine, to partial thickness beds of appropriate size prepared in the skin flaps or on the sides of the hosts' chests. The operative technique has been described in full elsewhere[17].

Inspection and scoring of grafts: Primary inspection of all grafts was carried out on the 6th postoperative day. Subsequent inspections were made daily for the first 6–8 days and at less frequent intervals thereafter. The survival times of the grafts were determined on the basis of the outward appearance of their epidermis[17] and the median survival times estimated by Litchfield's[20] nomographic method. Representative grafts were excised at various intervals after transplantation, fixed in formol-mercuric chloride and embedded in paraffin wax. Transverse sections were cut at 8–10 μ and stained with Ehrlich's hematoxylin and eosin.

Sensitization of guinea pigs for transfer experiments was accomplished by grafting the animals bilaterally with 2.0–2.5-cm discs of the relatively thin skin from the donors' abdomens. This grafting was followed, 10–14 days later, by the intraperitoneal and subcutaneous administration of a coarse cell suspension in 4 ml of Hanks' solution corresponding to ¼ of a donor equivalent of splenic and lymph node tissue. Animals were used for transfer experiments 8 days after receipt of the booster inoculations.

Suspensions of lymphoid cells were prepared by removing the donors' spleens, and axillary, brachial, cervical, inguinal, and mesenteric nodes aseptically, cutting them up into small fragments with scissors, and then lightly pressing them through a 50-mesh stainless steel screen. The expressed coarse fragments were taken up in Hanks' solution and gently sucked in and out of a pipette to effect further dissociation of the tissue. The resultant fine suspension was washed and resuspended in Hanks' solution.

Lymph node cell suspensions appropriate for intravenous injection were prepared according to our standard procedure[17].

Leukocytes were prepared by withdrawing blood from the heart into 20-ml syringes containing 5 IU of heparin and 2 ml of a 10% solution in normal saline of high molecular weight dextran. Erythrocytes were removed by sedimentation in the inverted syringe, with the needle up. The leukocyte-rich plasma was taken off and washed once in chilled Hanks' solution containing heparin (1 IU/ml). Leukocyte counts were made with the aid of a hemocytometer.

Results

Base Line Data: Survival Times of Single Orthotopic Skin Homografts Exchanged Between Guinea Pigs of Strains 2 and 13

To provide controls for the work to be described, single ear skin grafts 1 cm in diameter were exchanged between 20 guinea pigs of strains 2 and 13, each graft being carefully fitted

FIG. 5. An intra-flap pigmented ear skin homograft of 30 days' standing. The host flap has undergone some contraction and thickening so that it is now a fully epithelialized, mushroom-shaped structure. ×3.

FIG. 6. Section through pigmented ear skin homograft which has been in residence in a standard skin flap on an unsensitized guinea pig's trunk for 22 days. The healthy epidermis displays the characteristic stratigraphy of ear skin. There is a barely distinguishable mononuclear cell infiltration and two perivascular concentrations of mononuclear cells. ×220.

into a partial thickness bed of appropriate size prepared in the shaved skin of the lateral thoracic wall. With both the 13 → 2, donor/recipient strain combination and the converse one, all the grafts were rejected within 8–10 days (Table 1). Because of the close similarity between the survival times of the two series of grafts (median survival times 8.7 ± 0.2 days and 9.2 ± 0.2 days, respectively), animals of both strains were used as donors or recipients, depending upon their availability.

Six animals which had rejected "first-set" grafts were rechallenged with donor strain skin 2–8 wk later. In all cases destruction of these grafts was complete on the 6th postoperative day.

The Fate of the Skin Flaps

The pediculated skin flaps used to provide beds for the experimental skin homografts remained healthy and well vascularized as evidenced by the *uninterrupted* postoperative growth of their fur. It may be pointed out that in free skin grafts, by contrast, all the original hairs of the graft are shed in association with a phase of migratory and mitotic activity of the follicular epithelium which leads to cystic dilatation of the pilo-sebaceous units and total disruption of their normal structure. Follicular regeneration ensues and, usually after the 2nd postoperative week, new hairs begin to pierce the skin surface[21]. The present finding therefore affords formal proof that it is temporary disruption of the skin's blood supply rather than massive trauma which is responsible for the phoenix-like activity of the follicles in free skin grafts.

On the 6th postoperative day the flaps were swollen by edema and there was build-up of granulation tissue on the cut surfaces. Subsequently, epithelium migrated down from the upper surface of the flap resurfacing its edges and underside. The vascular pedicle slowly increased in thickness and ultimately became epithelialized, so that by about the 30th postoperative day the flap had assumed a somewhat mushroom-like shape with a pedicle of 5 mm or more in diameter. Although the rate of blood flow through these flaps is not known it was found that on severance of the umbilical cord a fine stream of blood under arterial pressure spurted out immediately.

Repeated tests in which Patent Blue V dye was injected intradermally into freshly prepared skin flaps or those prepared 6–30 or more days beforehand revealed a rich lymphatic network *within* the flap. However, they consistently failed to reveal the existence of any lymphatic connections between flap and the host's trunk, and the regional nodes were never stained. Likewise no lymphatics were observed in histological sections of established vascular umbilical cords. Additional testimony of the absence of a lymphatic drainage in the flaps was the observation that a clear, lymp-like fluid containing about 500 lymphocytes/mm^3 usually exuded from the cut surfaces of flaps transected to obtain specimens for histology.

In most instances the viability of the flaps terminated abruptly after 20–30 days through

TABLE 1. *Survival Times of First- and Second-Set Ear Skin Homografts Transplanted Orthotopically to Partial Thickness Beds Prepared in Intact Flank Skin, and of First-Set Skin Grafts Transplanted to Similar Beds Prepared in Standard Partially Isolated Skin Flaps in Guinea Pigs*

Location of graft bed	Type of graft	No. of animals tested	Survival times of grafts (days)	Median survival time (days)
Intact flank skin	First-set	10 (strain 13 → strain 2) 10 (strain 2 → strain 13)	8 × 8; 2 × 9 6 × 8; 2 × 9; 2 × 10	8.7 ± 0.2 9.2 ± 0.2
	Second-set	6	6 × <6	<6
Isolated skin flap	First-set	25	4 × 20; 21; 6 × 22 2 × 23; 24; 25; 26 27; 28; 32; 2 × 33* 52; 54*; >57‡; 100‡	

Survival times without superscripts indicate grafts that died as a consequence of nonspecific necrosis of their host flaps.

* Indicates grafts that were rejected as a consequence of a specific reaction.

‡ Indicates surviving homografts in flaps that were removed from their protective dishes and sewn back into place on the day indicated.

TABLE 2. *Effect of Sensitization of the Host on the Survival of Skin Homografts in Standard Skin Flaps*

Means of sensitization	Day of administration of sensitizing material ± day of intra-flap grafting	No. of animals tested	Survival times of intra-flap skin homografts (days)
Single orthotopic skin homograft	−20–30 days	6	6 × <6
Single orthotopic skin homograft	0	4	7, 3 × 8
150 × 10^6 homologous lymph node cells, intravenously	+7–10	3	8, 2 × 9
10–20 × 10^6 (strain 2 × strain 13) F_1 hybrid lymph node cells intradermally	0	5	7, 8, 9, 16, 24

ischemic necrosis caused by torsion, shearing, or strangulation of their umbilical cords. Occasionally it was possible to preserve flap viability for as long as 50 days or more. Loosening of the attachment of the plastic capsule containing the flap to the host's skin was frequently responsible for its demise.

The Fate of Skin Homografts in Isolated Skin Flaps

Skin homografts transplanted to beds in freshly prepared skin flaps healed in just as rapidly and as well as grafts transplanted to intact skin. At the primary inspection a cuticular "ghost" could be picked off the graft surface to reveal a hyperplastic superficial epidermis displaying pigment dilution. Within a few days the grafts reassumed their intense black color and a sparse crop of hairs, typical of ear skin, was usually regenerated by about the 20th day. Of 25 skin homografts transplanted to flap beds, 22 remained in a perfectly healthy, autograft-like condition (Figs. 5 and 6) either until they were removed electively for histological examination, or they succumbed as a consequence of flap necrosis taking place 20–100 days postoperatively (see Table 1). Although most of the grafts in this series were 1 cm in diameter, grafts 2 cm in diameter gave equally good results, indicating that graft size is not critical.

Histological examination of excised grafts of 22 days' duration confirmed their healthy status. It did, however, reveal the existence of some diffuse and perivascularly concentrated mononuclear cells beneath the graft dermis (see Fig. 6).

Three of the 25 grafts studied did appear to succumb to specific chronic, low-grade reactions, manifested by loss of hair, dilution of pigmentation, contracture, and weakness of epithelial attachment, at 33, 33, and 54 days respectively. In these cases epithelialization of the vascular umbilical cord had taken place to produce a rather robust-looking pedicle of attachment (see Fig. 4) so that the possibility existed that lymphatic connections had been reestablished between the isolated skin flap and the host.

It need hardly be stressed that the survival times of all the homografts in the present series represent highly significant prolongations of the life expectancy of similar grafts transplanted to sites prepared in intact skin—by a factor of more than two.

Since 3/25 grafts were *specifically* rejected after more than 30 days, in subsequent experiments in which homografts in isolated flaps were used as indicators of sensitization, rejections taking place after 30 days could not be interpreted as reliable evidence of sensitization of the host by the particular procedure under investigation. This assumption follows since the lymphatic isolation of the flaps could not be absolutely relied upon after this time.

The Susceptibility of Skin Homografts in Skin Flaps to Transplantation Immunity

Since the efferent pathway of the immunologic reflex is provided by the vasculature of the graft, it was anticipated that specific active sensitization of the host would curtail the survival of skin homografts transplanted to skin flaps. Confirmatory evidence for this has been forthcoming. Skin homografts placed in isolated flaps prepared in the flank skin of guinea pigs that had previously rejected orthotopic skin grafts from the donor strain were consistently rejected just as swiftly as if they had been transplanted orthotopically (Table 2). Furthermore, when normal guinea pigs received two skin homografts on the same occasion, one transplanted to intact skin on the thoracic wall and the other transplanted to a skin flap, *both* grafts underwent simultaneous rejection 7–8 days after operation.

Likewise the intradermal inoculation of as few as 10–20 million homologous leukocytes, distributed over five different sites, in the intact trunk skin of hosts which received intra-flap test skin homografts at the same time also procured the rejection of the grafts. Well-established intra-flap homografts were only slightly less vulnerable than recently transplanted grafts to the sensitization elicited in their hosts by proxy. Thus grafts of 7–10 days' standing were rejected in 8–9 days when their hosts were injected intravenously with a suspension of 150 million donor lymphoid cells in Hanks' solution (see Table 2).

More compelling evidence that the afferent arc of the immunologic reflex is interrupted in the skin flaps was forthcoming from the following experiment. Four guinea pigs which had borne healthy intra-flap skin homografts for 18–28 days, and whose grafts had succumbed as a consequence of flap necrosis, were rechallenged with skin homografts from the original donor strain, the challenge grafts being placed in newly created flaps on the *left* (i.e. previously unoperated) sides of their trunks. All the secondary grafts healed in and survived in a perfectly healthy condition for as long as their host flaps remained viable, 18–28 days, again indicating the inability on the part of the previous intra-flap grafts to sensitize the recipients (Table 3).

The observation that skin homografts transplanted orthotopically to animals bearing long-established intra-flap grafts from the same strain were rejected in a nonimmune manner (see Table 3) also indicated that the chronic presence of the intra-flap grafts had failed to sensitize their hosts.

Evidence that Interruption of Lymphatic Vessels Constitutes the Break in the Afferent Pathway of the Immunological Reflex

As already mentioned, all attempts to demonstrate the presence of patent lymphatics in the vascular pedicles of flaps were unsuccessful[16]. However, if a bridge of undivided skin, 1–3 cm wide, was left at one place on the perimeter of an isolated flap to maintain continuity with the host's trunk skin, lymphatic communication between the flap and host skin across the bridge was consistently demonstrable by dye injection. Skin homografts placed in such flaps were consistently rejected within 8–11 days if the bridges were located caudally (Table 4).

However, if the bridges were located *dorsally* on the flap perimeter, the survival times of the grafts ranged from 10–17 days (Table 4). This significant disparity in the survival times of the two series of grafts correlates with anatomical evidence that on the flank the predominant lymphatic channels are in the cephalo-caudad axis rather than dorso-ventral[22]. This correlation suggests that the lymphatic drainage from flaps with caudally located skin bridges is superior to that of flaps with dorsally located skin bridges.

Keller's[22] careful anatomical studies of the guinea pig's lymphatic system suggested that if skin flaps were raised from skin sites near to the axilla, instead of the flank, a large lymphatic vessel would accompany the group of blood vessels in the umbilical cord and lead directly to the axillary lymph node. Dye injection tests confirmed that this was indeed the case. When homografts were placed in flaps located in the axillary region, and in which the lymphatic drainage had purposefully been preserved, they were rejected within 9–17 days. However, if a ligature was tied around the lymphatic vessels in a pedicle (revealed by dye injection of the flap) the usual anomalous longevity of intra-flap skin homografts obtained.

Lymphatic continuity between isolated skin flaps bearing healthy skin homografts of long

TABLE 3. *Evidence of the Failure of Intra-Flap Skin Homografts to Sensitize Their Hosts*

Location of second-set test skin homografts transplanted to animals which had previously born intra-flap skin homografts for 20 days	No. of animals tested	Survival times of second-set test grafts (days)
Orthotopic	8	3 × 8; 4 × 9; 10
Intra-flap, on left flank	4	18*; 20*; 26*; 28*

* Survival of these grafts terminated by flap necrosis and not by specific rejection.

TABLE 4. *Effect of Preservation or Restoration of Lymphatic Drainage on Fate of Freshly Transplanted or Established Skin Homografts in Skin Flaps, and Effect of Regional Lymphadenectomy on Fate of Orthotopic Skin Homografts*

Location and type of host flap	Location of intact skin bridge on flap perimeter	No of animals tested	Survival times of intra-flap skin homografts (days)
Flank, with skin bridge, 1–3 cm wide, housed in plastic dish	Caudally	5	8, 9, 2 × 10, 11
Flank, with skin bridge 1–3 cm wide, housed in plastic dish	Dorsally	6	10, 2 × 13, 15, 16, 17
Axilla, individual lymphatic channel identified and preserved; flap housed in plastic dish	None	6	2 × 9, 10, 11, 12, 17
Axilla, individual lymphatic channel identified and ligated; flap housed in plastic dish	None	2	28, 28
*Flank, isolated flap of 22–25 days' duration bearing healthy skin homografts removed from plastic dish and sewn back into fresh wound to restore lymphatic continuity	None	4	14, 16, 19, 23
*Flank, isolated flap of 100 days' duration bearing healthy graft removed from dish and sewn back into fresh wound to restore lymphatic continuity	None	1	28
Flank, isolated flap dissected and immediately sewn back into wound, instead of being placed in plastic dish	None	6	13, 3 × 18, 19, 20
Excision of cervical, axillary, brachial and inguinal nodes, followed by transplantation of orthotopic skin homograft ipsilaterally	—	4	13, 3 × 14

* In these experiments the survival times indicate the number of days the established intra-flap homografts lived *after* the flaps were sewn back into freshly prepared wounds.

standing (22–25 days) and their hosts could easily be restored simply by removal of the protective Petri dishes, trimming off a very thin layer of skin from the margins and undersides of the flaps, and then suturing them back in place in freshly cut full-thickness wounds, in the hosts' flank skin, leaving the vascular pedicles intact. Subsequent dye injections confirmed the reestablishment of lymphatic continuity. Such "replaced" flaps soon lost their initial privileged status as indicated by the rejection within 14–23 days of skin homografts which had hitherto survived for periods from 22 to 100 days (in one case).

To determine whether this belated rejection, after reincorporation of the host flap in trunk skin, is simply a function of the time required for restoration of a lymphatic drainage rather than a manifestation of incomplete graft adaptation[23] or some other phenomenon, the following experiment was carried out on six guinea pigs. A skin flap with its intact vascular pedicle was raised in the usual manner and a skin homograft inserted in a shallow bed at its center. However, instead of placing the flap in a protective plastic dish it was *immediately* sutured back into the wound from which it was taken. Although both the flaps and their grafts healed in with normal promptitude, five of the six grafts survived for at least 18 days, instead of the 9–10 day expectation of survival of similar grafts transplanted to beds prepared in intact flank skin (see Table 4). This significant prolongation of graft survival suggested that reestablishment of lymphatic continuity between flap skin and its bed, or perhaps with host skin at its edges, may require as long as 3–10 days. It also suggests that neither antigenic material nor activated lymphocytes from the homografts escape in the material that exudes from the undersurface of the flaps.

Influence of Lymphadenectomy and the Length of the Afferent Lymphatic Pathway on Skin Homograft Survival Times

Surgical excision of the regional nodes that normally drain the skin of the side of the trunk—the cervical, axillary, brachial, and inguinal nodes—did not impair the healing-in of orthotopic skin homografts transplanted immediately after lymphadenectomy but did prolong their survival times by 3–4 days (see Table 4). This is in accord with the findings of similar experiments carried out on mice and rabbits[24,25]. The failure of regional lymphadenectomy to have a more striking influence on the longevity of skin homografts is probably related to the speed with which a collateral lymphatic drainage opens up. These findings certainly emphasize that lymphatic interruption must be *complete* if the afferent arc of the immunologic reflex is to be broken[4].

Although it has been suggested that the anomalous longevity of homografts placed in the testes is a consequence of the remoteness of this organ from its nearest draining lymph node near the kidney[26], we have been unable to show that the length of the afferent lymphatic path affects the survival of orthotopic homografts of skin. Ear skin homografts of DA rat skin transplanted to beds prepared near to the ends of the tails of Lewis hosts were rejected just as rapidly as similar grafts transplanted to the lateral thoracic wall.[1]

Influence of Attracting Host Mononuclear Cells into Graft-Bearing, Isolated Skin Flaps

If sensitization to homografts does occur peripherally and the anomalous survival of the intra-flap grafts is attributable to the inability of locally "activated" small lymphocytes to return to the host, any artifice that would increase the number of mononuclear cells entering the graft might procure graft destruction. The latter might be accomplished either (*a*) by a local graft-versus-host type reaction[27] or (*b*) as a consequence of an effective number of the immunologically "primed" lymphocytes returning to the host by the intravenous route after peregrination through the parenchyma.

As a means of procuring the infiltration of intra-flap skin homografts by a "nonspecific" population of mononuclear cells, delayed hypersensitivity to dinitrochlorobenzene was induced in three guinea pigs. Skin homografts were then transplanted to standard skin flaps on these animals. On the 7th and again on the 15th postoperative day the entire flap surface, including that of the inlaid skin homografts, was challenged with a 0.1% solution of dinitrochlorobenzene in acetone. Although both challenges incited typical delayed inflammatory reactions, the associated infiltration of the grafts by mononuclear cells did not prejudice their survival, since the grafts lived for 33, 34, and 86 days.

Ability of Isolated Skin Flaps to Sustain Skin Heterografts

Small scale trials were carried out to determine whether the skin flaps would provide a favorable environment for heterografts and, by implication, indicate the importance of lymphatic drainage for sensitization to grafts of this type. It was found that ear skin heterografts from AU strain mice, BN rats, and CB hamsters were all rejected within 8–10 days after transplantation to flap sites, whereas similar grafts transplanted to beds prepared in intact guinea pig's skin were invariably completely necrotic within 6 days. Evidently the flaps do provide a minor degree of protection to heterografts, though greatly inferior to that afforded to homografts. A similar state of affairs applies to the hamster's cheek pouch and probably to the brain. It may be that the release of powerful, soluble, species-specific antigenic material into the host's blood stream is largely responsible for inciting a host's rejection of heterografts.

Attempts to Extend the Isolated Flap Technique to Animals of Other Species

Isolated, vascularized skin flaps without demonstrable lymphatic continuity with the host have been constructed in adult rats and shown to be capable of prolonging the survival of

[1] Barker, C. F., and R. E. Billingham. 1968. Unpublished observations.

skin homografts to a significant degree. With the Lewis → DA donor/host strain combination, where the median survival time of skin homografts transplanted to conventional orthotopic sites is 7.3 ± 0.72 days, intra-flap skin homografts have lived for 14–20 days. However because of the rat's great propensity to chew its dressings, reinforcement of the plain bandage securing the flap-containing Petri dishes to the flank with plaster impregnated bandage was obligatory. Even this artifice proved only partially satisfactory, insofar as most of the flaps and their grafts were lost through the host's gnawing.

Mice were unsatisfactory for flap experiments on the grounds that only the main cephalo-caudad blood vessels are large enough for use in umbilical cord construction to sustain isolated skin flaps and these are accompanied by lymphatics. With the CBA → A combination homografts inlaid in such flaps were rejected almost as rapidly as those transplanted to conventional sites in the integument.

Donawick[2] has raised relatively large skin flaps on the flanks of calves and maintained them in 100 × 15 mm diameter plastic Petri dishes. However, because of edema and infection they proved unsatisfactory as graft sites.

Among the laboratory mammals the guinea pig seems to be the animal of choice for these preparations on account of its relatively large size, shape, and docile behavior.

Some Applications of the Isolated Flap Technique

The fact that skin homografts sustained in skin flaps are easily accessible for inspection under conditions which preclude their sensitizing the hosts and yet leave them fully susceptible to a state of preexisting or subsequently incited sensitivity suggested their possible utility as a sensitive tool in transplantation immunology. In the sections that follow experiments are described which indicate some of the possible applications of this tool.

Use of Intra-Flap Skin Homografts as Indicators of Adoptive Immunization

The capacity of lymphoid cells from specifically sensitized animals to transfer transplantation immunity adoptively between members of an inbred strain is demonstrable in two ways: (*a*) in terms of their ability to enable normal, isologous recipients to reject, in an accelerated manner, test skin homografts from donors of the alien strain in respect of which the donors of the transferred lymphoid cells have been sensitized[24] or (*b*) by their ability to procure the destruction of healthy, well-established skin homografts on hosts previously rendered specifically tolerant of the tissue antigens of the alien donor strain more rapidly than a similar number of lymphoid cells from a *normal*, isologous donor[28]. Analysis of the immunological performance of the transferred cells in their new host is complicated in procedure (*a*) by the fact that the host itself soon responds to the antigens of the challenge graft, so that weak levels of sensitivity of transfer origin may escape detection. In procedure (*b*), which is exceedingly sensitive in terms of the small number of sensitized cells required to abolish tolerance, the chimeric status of the host seems to be important. Persisting donor-type cells—descendants of the original tolerance-conferring inoculum—provide an antigenic stimulus for the transferred sensitized cells additional to that furnished by the tolerated skin homograft and probably contribute to the sensitivity of the method. The intra-flap skin homograft in the guinea pig suggested itself as a useful challenge tissue for adoptive transfer experiments on the grounds that it was sustained by a completely normal host which was normally incapable of developing sensitivity against it—at least during a 30 day observation period.

When relatively large numbers of isologous lymphoid cells or peripheral blood leukocytes (1–2 donor equivalents or 140–325 × 10^6 cells respectively) from sensitized animals were transferred intraperitoneally, destruction of intra-flap test skin homografts transplanted within the range 3 days before to 7 days after cell transfer was consistently complete within 10 days or less. There ws no evidence that adoptive immunization of hosts prior to or concomitant with test skin grafting was more effective than when transfer of the sensitized cells was delayed until the 5th or even the 7th day after grafting. Indeed, the data (Table 5)

[2] Donawick, W. J. 1968. Personal communication.

TABLE 5. *Survival Times of Test Skin Homografts in Skin Flaps on Guinea Pigs That Received Isologous Lymphoid Cells, Peripheral Blood Leukocytes, or Serum From Specifically Sensitized Donors*

Material transferred from specifically sensitized isologous donors	Day of transfer ± day of test grafting	No. of hosts tested	Survival times of test skin grafts in flaps (days)	Interval between lymphoid cell transfer and destruction of test skin homograft (days)
1–2 donor lymphoid equivalents	−3	2	7, 7	7
1 donor lymphoid equivalent	0	2	6, 6	6
or 200 × 10⁶ leukocytes		2	6, 6	
1 donor lymphoid equivalent		3	8, 8, 9	~6
2 donor lymphoid equivalents	+2	3	7, 8, 8	
150 × 10⁶ leukocytes		2	7, 8	
1 donor lymphoid equivalent	+5	4	8, 9, 9, 10	~4
or 325 × 10⁶ leukocytes		2	9, 9	
1 donor lymphoid equivalent	+7	3	10, 10, 11	~3
200 × 10⁶ leukocytes		1	10	
75 × 10⁶ leukocytes	0	5	7, 2 × 8, 13, 14	~10
50 × 10⁶ leukocytes	0	6	7, 12, 13, 16, 30, 34*	
30 × 10⁶ leukocytes	0	2	28*, 30	
20 × 10⁶ leukocytes	0	3	30, 32, 60	
Serum 2.5 ml i.p. on days 0, +2, and +4	—	4	23*, 36*, 55, 67*	
Serum 2.5 ml i.p. on days +7, +9, and +11	—	2	24, 43	

* Indicates grafts that succumbed as a consequence of ischemic necrosis of their host flaps.

suggest that the transferred cells accomplished more rapidly the destruction of grafts that were already healed-in at the time of transfer than grafts that were freshly transplanted.

To define the lower limit of the number of sensitized cells that must be transferred to procure graft rejection, peripheral blood leukocytes from sensitized animals were transferred, in dosages ranging from 20–75 million, to isologous hosts which received intra-flap test grafts on the *same* day. It was found that whereas 75 million cells consistently brought about rejection in 7–14 days and 50 million cells resulted in the rejection of four out of six intra-flap grafts within 16 days, dosages of 30 or 20 million leukocytes were ineffective, in the sense that they allowed graft survival for 30 days or more in animals whose flaps survived for this length of time (see Table 5).

It must be conceded that, as in all adoptive transfer experiments using normal, as opposed to specifically tolerant hosts, the remote possibility exists that the sensitivity recorded by the intra-flap homografts was due to active immunization of the host by antigenic material, originating from the homografts used to sensitize the primary hosts and unavoidably carried over into the secondary hosts with the transferred lymphoid cells[24]. To minimize this risk many experiments were carried out with peripheral blood leukocytes, predominantly lymphocytes, since antigenic material is less likely to be associated with them than with lymph node or splenic cell suspensions.

A small scale test was carried out to appraise the capacity of immune serum to prejudice the well-being of intra-flap skin homografts. One group of four animals received three intraperitoneal injections of 2.5 ml of antiserum on alternate days commencing on the day of test skin grafting. Two other guinea pigs were similarly treated except that administration of the antiserum was delayed until the 7th day *after* skin grafting. In the first series of tests all grafts had conspicuously weak surfaces at the first postoperative inspection and in some there appeared to be progressive deterioration to the point of complete necrosis. However, all the grafts subsequently made a full recovery, as evidenced by the regeneration of an

TABLE 6. *Concomitant Transplantation of an Orthotopic Skin Homograft and Intra-Flap Indicator Skin Homograft Followed by Excision of the Sensitizing Grafts at Intervals to Determine Duration of Residence Necessary for Sensitization*

Time sensitizing grafts in place before excision (days)	No. of animals tested	Survival times of "indicator" skin grafts in flaps
2	4	36, 42, 59, 93
3	5	17*, 18, 36, 54*, 69*
4	6	9, 9, 17, 40*, 42*, 50
5	2	20, 25
6	4	3 × 10, 17
Not excised	4	7, 3 × 8

* Indicates grafts which were destroyed nonspecifically as a consequence of host flap necrosis.

intensely black superficial epidermis, and enjoyed long survival times before flap necrosis occurred. Nevertheless, prolongation of serum treatment might well have brought about the complete destruction of these grafts. Even in those animals whose grafts had healed-in *before* initiation of antiserum treatment there were indications that the latter exerted a definite though transient adverse effect, for their epidermis too underwent a phase of weakness of attachment to the underlying dermis.

The findings of these serum experiments show very clearly that in guinea pigs as in certain other species[29,30], humoral factors, under some conditions, exert a demonstrable adverse effect on skin homografts. It need hardly be emphasized that the effect of immune serum in the present study was trivial compared with that of sensitized cells.

Determination of the Period of Residence Required for an Orthotopic Skin Homograft to Sensitize its Host

Each of a series of guinea pigs received two ear skin homografts from the same donor. One of these grafts, the "indicator," was transplanted to a standard flap raised on the host's right flank; the other (the "sensitizing" graft) was transplanted to a shallow bed cut in intact skin on its left flank. After the sensitizing grafts had been in residence for periods of 2–6 days they were excised, together with generous amounts of contiguous host tissue, and the indicator grafts observed for signs of the development of sensitivity on the part of the host.

The results, summarized in Table 6, show that when the sensitizing grafts were in place for 3 days or less only one of the indicator grafts was rejected within 30 days. 4 days' residence of the sensitizing grafts caused definite "rejection crises" at 6–10 days in the indicator grafts as evidenced by epithelial weakness and 50% of them succumbed. However, the remainder recovered and enjoyed long survival times.

The presence of the sensitizing grafts for a minimum of 5–6 days seemed mandatory for the indicator grafts to be rejected within 30 days. Indeed, only when the sensitizing grafts had been in place for 6 days did the majority of the animals reject their indicator grafts as rapidly as ordinary orthotopic skin homografts. Other studies indicate that a skin homograft must be in residence for a minimum of 4 days in order to sensitize the host[31,32].

The relatively long period for which an orthotopic skin homograft must remain in residence on a guinea pig to evoke sensitivity is surprising since nearly all guinea pigs develop sensitivity to topically applied simple chemicals, such as oxazolone, even if the painted skin sites are excised within 24 hr of the application of the sensitizer[33]. This finding implies that either a sufficient amount of contact allergen becomes fixed to epidermal tissue and enough of the resultant complex finds its way into the lymphatic drainage[33], or a sufficient number of host lymphocytes undergo peripheral sensitization and return to the host within this time[34] for delayed hypersensitivity to develop. The disparity with respect to the time taken for sensitivity to develop in response to skin grafts on the one hand and the chemical sensitizers on the other hand might, of course, be more apparent than real, depending upon the sensitivity of the system used to detect altered host reactivity.

Significance of Reestablishment of Direct Lymphatic or Vascular Channels Between a Skin Graft and its Bed for Sensitization of Host

Some evidence suggests that the presence of a skin homograft on a freshly prepared bed may lead to sensitization of the host even if steps are taken to prevent healing-in of the graft. McKhann and Berrian[32] found that, in mice, if skin homografts were removed from their beds and replaced by fresh grafts from the same donor strain every 24 hr for 4 days, and then removed permanently, the hosts could later be shown to be sensitized.

Confirmation of this interesting observation has been obtained with the aid of the intra-flap grafting system. An intra-flap indicator skin homograft was placed on one side of a guinea pig's body and, at the same time, an orthotopic skin homograft from the same donor strain was transplanted to a bed prepared in intact skin on the opposite side of its body. These sensitizing grafts were subsequently removed daily from their beds and replaced with fresh ear skin homografts for a 4 day period after which no further homografts were applied. Of the three animals treated in this way two rejected their intra-flap grafts after 9 and 23 days, respectively, indicating the development of a weak level of sensitivity on the part of the host. The remaining animal's graft survived for 90 days, its demise resulting from trauma. A weakness of both the present as well as McKhann and Berrian's[32] experimental design is that it fails to exclude the possibility that the sensitivity induced by the transiently applied skin homografts was actually caused by donor leukocytes unavoidably carried over in the graft vasculature.

Encouraged by this small-scale confirmation of Berrian and McKhann's observation, we sought evidence whether the copious lymph or tissue exudate that normally escapes from the cut surfaces of recently prepared skin flaps bearing skin homografts contains antigenic material capable of sensitizing the host if allowed to seep into an open wound.

It is pertinent to mention here that, unlike blood vessels, severed lymphatics in a cutaneous wound may remain open for as long as 48 hr, and materials introduced into the wound pass directly into the lymphatics through their gaping ends[35].

Standard flaps were cut from flank skin in the usual manner and skin homografts fitted into shallow beds at their centers. However, instead of closing the donor wounds around the bases of the vascular pedicles, the skin flaps were replaced directly into the defects from which they had been cut. Protective dressings were then applied and removed daily when the skin flaps were carefully lifted up from their beds and replaced to prevent healing and establishment of direct lymphatic continuity with the host. This maneuver was repeated daily for 5 days. The flap was again lifted, and, after closure of the wound beneath it, inserted into a plastic Petri dish in the standard manner. That the fluid which seeped from the flap into the wound beneath did not contain antigenic material was suggested by the observation that in only one out of five such preparations was the intra-flap graft rejected within 30 days.

The negative results of this experiment suggested that the skin flaps either prevented the escape of antigenic material from the grafts, or, alternatively, did not allow the return to the host of peripherally sensitized lymphocytes, as a consequence of the lymphatic interruption. To investigate these possibilities, we transplanted skin homografts to standard flaps housed in plastic dishes. Then, after 1 or 2 wk, the intra-flap homografts were carefully excised, together with a narrow margin of host tissue. At the same time the flaps were removed from their protective capsules and sewn into freshly prepared wounds in the flanks, care being taken not to injure the vascular umbilical cords. To determine whether this artifice resulted in sensitization of the host, and therefore obtain evidence whether there had been residual antigenic material and (or) peripherally sensitized lymphocytes trapped within the connective tissue of the flap, we prepared a second flap on the hitherto unoperated left flank of each animal and transplanted an "indicator" skin homograft to it. This operation was carried out 3 wk after the original flap had been resutured into the host skin. In none of six animals treated in this way did rejection occur within 30 days.

The present findings are consistent with previous failures to sensitize rats by means of orthotopic split-skin homografts prevented from making direct contact with host tissue by a cell-impermeable Millipore membrane[36], or to sensitize mice by means of suspensions of homologous cells sequestered in Millipore diffusion chambers inserted intraperitoneally or subcutaneously.

Discussion

On the basis of studies employing as graft sites partially isolated, vascularized skin flaps deprived of lymphatic connections with the host, it has been shown that, for elicitation of hypersensitivity to orthotopic skin homografts, as for the induction of hypersensitivity to simple chemicals[16], an intact afferent lymphatic drainage in the host skin is mandatory—i.e., lymphatics constitute the afferent pathway of the immunologic reflex. The susceptibility of intra-flap skin homografts to specific sensitization, acquired either actively or adoptively, is consistent with the well-founded belief that blood vessels constitute the efferent pathway of the immunological reflex.

Immunologically, the status of skin grafts transplanted to alymphatic skin flaps is comparable to that of small homografts implanted into the brain, the hamster's cheek pouch and possibly the anterior chamber of the eye, in the sense that none of these sites have demonstrable lymphatic connections with regional nodes. In the hamster, isografts of cheek pouch "skin" survive and maintain their tissue-specific characteristics if transplanted to the animal's trunk[2]. If thin grafts of ordinary skin are transplanted to very shallow beds cut in the centers of well-established pouch skin grafts, they are usually exempted from the normal rejection process despite their vascularized status. This situation closely resembles that obtaining in the partially isolated skin flaps in guinea pigs since the host cheek pouch skin connective tissue seems to be devoid of lymphatics[2].[1] In these various privileged sites specific sensitivity on the part of the host is immediately effective. Other sites in which the reactivity of an unsensitized host to orthotopic skin homografts is diminished are the integument of limbs affected by Milroy's disease in the dog[37] [3]—a congenital anomaly due to anatomical shortcomings of the lymphatic drainage; and areas of the integument of cattle from which the lymph is drained off through a thoracic duct cannula, irradiated extracorporeally, and then returned to the circulation[38].

Various experiments have been described emphasizing the need for *complete* interruption of the lymphatic drainage in its bed to obtain a significant prolongation of survival of an orthotopic skin homograft. Indicative that the richness of the lymphatic drainage in its bed may affect the life expectancy of a skin homograft was the finding that retention of small skin bridges uniting skin flaps to host skin resulted in a normal rate of rejection of intra-flap homografts when the bridges were located caudally, whereas homograft survival was prolonged when the bridges were sited dorsally. These observations correlate with the anatomy of the lymphatic vessels draining the guinea pig's flank[22].

The rate of reestablishment of lymphatic drainage in skin grafts has been repeatedly investigated by various means[39–41]. The results of two different experiments in the present study bear upon this problem. Firstly, when skin flaps bearing healthy, long-established skin homografts were surgically replaced in appropriate beds to allow restoration of lymphatic drainage, the mean subsequent survival time of the grafts was 18 days—compared with the 9 day median survival time of a primary orthotopic skin homograft. This finding indicates that the time required for reestablishment of a functional lymphatic drainage in a free skin graft cannot exceed about 9 days. An independent confirmation of this estimate derived from the observation that the mean survival time of skin homografts transplanted to skin flaps which were *immediately* replaced in their donor sites after preparation was also 18 days. On the basis of India ink injection studies Scothorne[41] estimated that the lymphatic drainage of full thickness grafts of ear skin on guinea pigs' ears was restored on the 5th postoperative day by anastomosis of host lymphatics in the graft bed with preexisting *intrinsic* lymphatics of the graft. The richer vascularity of ear skin as compared with that of the trunk may account, in part, for the difference between the two estimates.

So far as orthotopic homografts of skin are concerned, one of the most important unresolved questions is the identity of the putative agent(s), transmitted by the lymphatics of the bed, which initiates the formation of "effector" cells, and probably the synthesis of humoral

[3] Barker, C. F., R. E. Billingham, and D. Patterson. 1968. Unpublished observations.

isoantibodies, in the regional nodes. Until recently it was almost axiomatic that antigenic material was involved. Hall's[5] studies on the afferent lymph draining skin graft sites on the limbs of sheep indicated that cellular debris passes along this route. However, the alternative possibility that the inductive phase of the response to homografts may occur peripherally, as a result of some kind of interaction between blood-borne immunologically competent cells (small lymphocytes) and fixed antigen, possibly at the surfaces of vascular endothelial and other cells[11,12], merits serious consideration. Indeed, Strober and Gowans'[10] experiments show that extracorporeal circulation of a rat's arterial blood through the vascular bed of an ex vivo renal homograft and its return via the venous circulation for as short a time as 5 hr result in sensitization of the animal.

The exemption from rejection enjoyed by homografts in partially isolated skin flaps, or in other privileged sites, is not necessarily inconsistent with the concept of peripheral sensitization or difficult to reconcile with Strober and Gowans'[10] observations. Firstly, in the case of a free skin graft, peripheral activation of host lymphocytes may take place principally in the graft *bed*, or in its parenchyma, rather than within its vasculature, and the activated cells pass down the draining lymphatics. Secondly, differences in the amount of endothelium in the skin graft's vasculature as compared with that of a whole organ graft and the effective "contact time" available for interaction of host lymphocytes with graft antigen may be important factors[10].

If peripheral sensitization at the intravascular level is assumed to be less efficient in the case of small grafts, with limited endothelial surfaces available for lymphocyte contact, the well-established sensitizing potency of small orthotopic skin homografts[42] is difficult to explain. Facts pertinent to this question are (*a*) that although vascular connection between a graft and its bed is not mandatory, the presence of a patent lymphatic drainage in the bed is essential for sensitization[4], and (*b*) that a minimum period of about 4 days' contact between a homograft and its bed is required. One possibility is that antigenic material of graft origin, or immunologically "primed" lymphocytes, promotes sensitization more effectively if allowed to travel in high concentration along a lymphatic channel impinging upon a *single* draining node system, rather than being diluted in the systemic venous circulation befor reaching lymphoid tissue. The well-known relative inefficiency of the intravenous route for eliciting transplantation immunity and the finding that regional lymphadenectomy prolonged the survival of skin homografts by 4–5 days lend some support to this interpretation.

Another factor to be taken into consideration is the extent of the tissue trauma associated with free skin grafting—which entails approximation of two cut surfaces. This situation is likely to be highly effective in attracting macrophages to the site. Since these cells play an important intermediary role in processing some kinds of antigen[1,43] and they are abundant in the afferent lymph draining from skin grafted sites[4,5], they may be important in the inductive phase of sensitivity to homografts.

If endocrine homografts survive in immunologically privileged sites for prolonged periods of time[23], or if renal homografts are chronically maintained in conventional sites by immunosuppressive procedures[44], they may progressively become less vulnerable to immunological attack. After a certain "critical" period they may be capable of surviving a degree of resistance to which they would have succumbed at an earlier stage. One explanation of this phenomenon of graft "adaptation" turns upon the possibility that a progressive, surreptitious replacement of stromal or vascular endothelial cells takes place in the graft[23]. The present finding that skin homografts which had been protected in skin flaps for up to 100 days were rejected after restoration of lymphatic connections between the flaps and the host's trunk hints that skin homografts do not undergo adaptation.

On the basis of various experimental findings[45] it was conceivable that, during its residence in a skin flap, a skin homograft might continuously release antigenic material into the host's venous circulation leading to a state of tolerance. That this did not occur in this experimental situation was evidenced by the fact that animals bearing intra-flap homografts of 2–43 days' standing reacted with normal vigor against second-set grafts transplanted to conventional sites.

Summary

Experiments have been carried out on guinea pigs of two isogenic strains to elucidate the role of afferent lymphatic vessels in the rejection of orthotopic skin homografts. Graft beds were prepared in partially isolated skin flaps with an intact sustaining vascular "umbilical cord" in which a lymphatic connection with the host could be retained or abolished at will.

In the absence of demonstrable lymphatic connections between flap and host, intra-flap homografts long outlived similar grafts transplanted to conventional sites in intact skin and, rather than being specifically rejected, died as a consequence of ischemic necrosis of the flap. When lymphatic drainage was retained, intra-flap homografts were rejected in the usual manner. Hosts of long-term intra-flap homografts did not develop sensitivity, as evidenced by the "first set" type rejection of subsequent test grafts, or by the long-term survival of a second skin graft transplanted to a new flap raised on the opposite side of the host's body.

Intra-flap skin homografts were rejected if (*a*) the hosts had been presensitized, (*b*) they were grafted concomitantly with skin homograft placed in a conventional site, or inoculated with a suspension of donor lymphoid cells, or (*c*) if the lymphatic drainage was restored by reimplantation of the hitherto partially isolated flap to an appropriate vascular bed. These findings and others indicate that an intact lymphatic drainage in its bed is essential for an orthotopic skin homograft to sensitize its host.

Various experiments were carried out in which intra-flap homografts were used as "indicators" for the acquisition of specific active or adoptive immunity by their hosts.

By transplanting skin homografts to conventional beds concomitantly with intra-flap grafts and then excising the former at various intervals, it has been found that a graft must be in residence for a minimum period of 4 days to evoke the development of a detectable level of sensitivity in the host. Furthermore, by replacing either freshly prepared or long-term skin flaps bearing skin homografts in vascular beds on the trunk and determining the subsequent survival times of the homografts, evidence has been obtained suggesting that reestablishment of a functional lymphatic system in a free skin graft may take as long as 9 days.

Using intra-flap homografts as indicators of adoptive immunization of the host, we found that as few as 50×10^6 isologous peripheral blood leukocytes from a specifically sensitized animal will transfer an effective level of sensitivity. We also found that hyperimmune serum, in relatively large amount, exerts a weak but definite adverse effect upon either freshly or recently transplanted intra-flap grafts.

ACKNOWLEDGMENTS

We are deeply indebted to Dr. Willys K. Silvers for his invaluable criticism of the manuscript and to Mr. George H. Sawchuck for expert technical assistance.

BIBLIOGRAPHY

1. Wilson DB, and Billingham RE. 1967. Lymphocytes and transplantation immunity. *Advan. in Immunol.* 7:189.
2. Billingham RE, and Silvers WK. 1962. Studies on cheek pouch skin homografts in the Syrian hamster. *In* Transplantation, Ciba Foundation Symposium. J. & A. Churchill, Ltd., London. 90.
3. Lance EM. 1967. A functional and morphologic study of intracranial thyroid allografts in the dog. *Surg. Gynecol. Obstet.* 125:529.
4. Lambert PB, Frank HA, Bellman S, and Farnsworth D. 1965. The role of the lymph trunks in the response to allogeneic skin transplants. *Transplantation.* 3:62.
5. Hall JG. 1967. Studies of the cells in the afferent and efferent lymph of lymph nodes draining the site of skin homografts. *J. Exptl. Med.* 125:737.
6. Hume DM, and Egdahl RH. 1955. Progressive destruction of renal homografts isolated from the regional lymphatics of the host. *Surgery.* 38:194.
7. Nathan P. 1964. Antigen release from the transplanted dog kidney. *Ann. N.Y. Acad. Sci.* 120:458.
8. Vetto RM, and Lawson RK. 1967. The role of vascular endothelium in the afferent pathway as suggested by the alymphatic renal homotransplant. *Transplantation.* 5:1537.
9. Lavender AR, Forland M, Rams JJ, Thompson JS, Russe HP, and Spargo BH. 1968. Extracorporeal renal transplantation in man. *J. Am. Med. Assoc.* 203:103.
10. Strober S, and Gowans JL. 1965. The role of lymphocytes in the sensitization of rats to renal homografts. *J. Exptl. Med.* 122:347.
11. Medawar PB. 1957 The homograft reaction. *Proc. Roy. Soc. (London), Ser. B.* 149:145.
12. Brent L, and Medawar PB. 1967. Cellular immunity and the homograft reaction. *Brit. Med. Bull.* 23:55.
13. Barker CF, and Billingham RE. 1967. The role of regional lymphatics in the skin homograft response. *Transplantation.* 5:962.
14. Bauer JA. 1957. Histocompatibility in inbred strains of guinea pigs. *Ann. N.Y. Acad. Sci.* 73:663.

15. Billingham RE, and Silvers WK. 1965. Re-investigation of the possible occurrence of maternally induced tolerance in guinea pigs. *J. Exptl. Zool.* 160:221.
16. Frey JR, and Wenk P. 1957. Experimental studies on the pathogenesis of contact eczema in the guinea pig. *Intern. Arch. Allergy Appl. Immunol.* 11:81.
17. Transplantation of Tissues and Cells. 1961. Billingham RE, and Silvers WK, editors. The Wistar Institute Press, Philadelphia.
18. Billingham RE, and Silvers WK. 1960. The melanocytes of mammals. *Quart. Rev. Biol.* 35:1.
19. Hudack SS, and McMaster P. 1933. The lymphatic participation in human cutaneous phenomena. *J. Exptl. Med.* 57:751.
20. Litchfield JT. 1949. A method for rapid graphic solution of time-percent effect curves. *J. Pharmacol. Exptl. Therap.* 97:399.
21. Billingham RE. 1958. A re-consideration of the phenomenon of hair neogenesis, with particular reference to the healing of cutaneous wounds in adult mammals. *In* The Biology of Hair Growth. Montagna W, and Ellis RA, editors. Academic Press Inc., New York. 451.
22. Keller G. 1937. Die Lymphgefäsze der Haut des Meerschweinchens. (II Beitrag). *Z. Infektionskrankh. Parasitar. Krankh. Hyg. Haustiere.* 52:250.
23. Woodruff MFA. 1959. Evidence of adaptation in homografts of normal tissue. *In* Biological Problems of Grafting. Albert F, and Medawar PB, editors. Blackwell, Oxford. 83.
24. Billingham RE, Brent L, and Medawar PB. 1954. Quantitative studies on tissue transplantation immunity II. The origin, strength and duration of actively and adoptively acquired immunity. *Proc. Roy Soc. (London), Ser. B.* 143:58.
25. Stark RB, Dwyer EM, and De Forest M. 1960. Effect of surgical ablation of regional lymph nodes on survival of skin homografts. *Ann. N.Y. Acad. Sci.* 87:140.
26. Russell PS, and Monaco AP. 1965. The Biology of Tissue Transplantation. Little, Brown and Co., Boston.
27. Billingham RE. 1968. The Biology of Graft-Versus-Host Reactions. Harvey Lectures, 1966/1967. Academic Press Inc., New York.
28. Billingham RE, Silvers WK, and Wilson DB. 1963. Further studies on adoptive transfer of sensitivity to skin homografts. *J. Exptl. Med.* 118:397.
29. Stetson, CA. 1963. The role of humoral antibody in the homograft reaction. *Advan. in Immunol.* 3:97.
30. Scott Clark D, Foker JE, Good RA, and Varco RL. 1968. Humoral factors in canine renal allograft rejection. *Lancet.* I:8.
31. Henry L, and Dammin GJ. 1962. Time and dose relationships in the developments of immunity to skin homografts in mice. *J. Immunol.* 89:841.
32. McKhann CF, and Berrian JH. 1959. Transplantation immunity: some properties of induction and expression. *Ann. Surg.* 150:1025.
33. Turk JL, and Stone SH. 1963. Implications of the cellular changes in lymph nodes during the development and inhibition of delayed type hypersensitivity. *In* Cell-Bound Antibodies. Amos B, and Koprowski H, editors. Wistar Institute Press, Philadelphia.
34. Turk JL. 1967. Response of lymphocytes to antigens. *Transplantation.* 5:952.
35. McMaster PD, and Hudack SS. 1934. The participation of skin lymphatics in repair of the lesions due to incisions and burns. *J. Exptl. Med.* 60:479.
36. Woodruff MFA. 1957. Cellular and humoral factors in the immunity to skin homografts: experiments with a porous membrane. *Ann. N.Y. Acad. Sci.* 64:1014.
37. Patterson DF, Medway W, Luginbuhl H, and Chacko S. 1967. Congenital hereditary lymphoedema in the dog. Part I. Clinical and genetic studies. *J. Med. Genet.* 4:145.
38. Chanana AD, Brecher G, Cronkite EP, Joel D, and Schnappauf H. 1966. The influence of extracorporeal irradiation of blood and lymph on skin graft rejection. *Radiation Res.* 27:330.
39. Egdahl RH, and Varco RL. 1956. Intradermal fluorescein test for homograft rejection period. *Transplantation.* 3:152.
40. McGregor IA, and Conway H. 1956. Development of lymphatic flow from autografts and homografts of skin. *Transplant. Bull.* 3:46.
41. Scothorne RJ. 1958. Lymphatic repair and the genesis of homograft immunity. *Ann. N.Y. Acad. Sci.* 73:673.
42. Billingham RE, Brent L, Brown JB, and Medawar PB. 1959. Time of onset and duration of transplantation immunity. *Transplant. Bull.* 6:410.
43. Mitchison NA. 1967. Immunological tolerance. *J. Clin. Pathol.* 20:451. (Suppl.)
44. Murray JE, Ross Sheil AG, Mosely R, Knight P, McGavic JD, and Dammin GJ. 1964. Analysis of mechanism of immunosuppressive drugs in renal homotransplantation. *Ann. Surg.* 160:449.
45. Billingham RE, and Silvers WK. 1964. Studies on homografts of foetal and infant skin and further observations on the anomalous properties of pouch skin homografts in hamsters. *Proc. Roy. Soc. (London), Ser. B.* 161:168.

Spontaneous Diabetes in Rats: Destruction of Islets Is Prevented by Immunological Tolerance

ALI NAJI, WILLYS K. SILVERS, DON BELLGRAU, AND CLYDE F. BARKER

Spontaneous diabetes occurring in "BB" rats (derived from a colony of outbred Wistar rats) is the result of destruction of pancreatic islets by infiltrating mononuclear cells (insulitis) and may be a disease very similar to human juvenile onset diabetes. Both diseases probably have an autoimmune etiology. Evidence is presented that islets transplanted to diabetic BB rats are destroyed by the original disease process. Inoculation of bone marrow from normal (nondiabetes-susceptible) rat donors into neonatal BB recipients usually prevents the development of hyperglycemia.

THE SPONTANEOUS development of diabetes mellitus was observed in 1977 in several members of a colony of outbred Wistar rats[1]. Selective breeding of these diabetic "BB" rats in our colony has resulted in an increase in incidence of the disease to about 30 percent. The onset of severe hyperglycemia (3 to 7 mg/ml) in affected animals is sudden and usually occurs between 60 and 180 days of age in previously normal animals and with equal frequency in both sexes. Nonaffected animals remain permanently normoglycemic. Pathophysiologic characteristics of the syndrome include hypoinsulinemia, hyperglucagonemia, and if insulin therapy is not provided, ketoacidosis and death. Morphologically the pancreas from newly diabetic rats shows a striking mononuclear infiltration (insulitis) with selective β-cell destruction. Both the metabolic and histologic abnormalities closely resemble those of insulin-dependent juvenile onset diabetes of humans. As in the case of the human disease, the etiology is unknown. However, in both BB rats and human diabetics a cell-mediated, organ-specific autoimmune pathogenesis seems possible, based on the characteristic lymphocytic infiltration of the islets. In BB rats an autoimmune mechanism is also implicated by the finding that reversal of the insulitis and return of normoglycemia occurs in 36 to 60 percent of acutely diabetic rats treated with rabbit anti-rat lymphocyte serum (ALS)[2].

Since the BB rat may provide an animal model of human insulin-dependent diabetes, it was important to determine whether the pathogenetic process responsible for the disease was also capable of destroying the islets of a transplanted pancreas, an issue of utmost importance in the outcome of this therapy in humans. We previously reported that transplantation of allogeneic islets from Wistar Furth (WF) donors results in long-term correction of the hyperglycemia of BB recipients treated with ALS[3]. However, when immunosuppression was stopped, hyperglycemia returned within a few days and transplanted islets were noted to be infiltrated by lymphocytes, a histological finding that can be indicative of either rejection or recurrence of the original disease. We have now conducted islet transplantation experiments in diabetic BB rats using procedures designed to exclude the possibly confusing influence of rejection or immunosuppression.

Although BB rats are not genetically uniform, serological lymphocyte typing, mixed lymphocyte culture reactions, and skin graft assays all indicate that inbreeding has significantly minimized the histoincompatibilities in our colony. Thus, not only do all these rats appear to have the same major histocompatibility genotype (RTI^u)[4] but 11 of 16 skin grafts exchanged between members of the colony survived for more than 100 days[5]. We therefore reasoned

From the Departments of Surgery and Human Genetics and Immunobiology Research Unit, University of Pennsylvania, Philadelphia, Pennsylvania.

that islets transplanted among BB rats would also frequently escape early rejection, especially if we used multiple donors so that, on the basis of chance, some islets would be compatible with the recipient. Indeed, this appeared to be the case when we transplanted islet allografts from BB donors to BB recipients that had reached adulthood without becoming spontaneously diabetic. We observed that BB rats with no diabetes in their ancestry for two generations show a less than 5 percent incidence of spontaneous diabetes. We induced hyperglycemia (plasma glucose > 3.5 mg/ml) in such rats by injecting them intravenously with streptozotocin (65 mg/kg), a specific β-cell toxin. Four to seven days later each recipient received islets from eight normoglycemic BB donors. The isolated islets were transplanted by embolization via the portal vein to the liver[6]. Although no immunosuppressive agent was given, islet transplant survival was prolonged, with 6 of the 11 recipients remaining normoglycemic for 60 to 300 days before they were killed (Table 1). Histological examination of the rats revealed healthy islets in the liver but few if any viable β cells in the native pancreas. The remaining five animals also became normoglycemic after islet transplantation, but suffered recurrent hyperglycemia in 2, 12, 13, 14, and 17 days, apparently because the islets were rejected.

In a second series of experiments we used eight BB recipients with naturally occurring diabetes of recent onset (<30 days). In these recipients of BB islets (also from eight normoglycemic BB donors) the normoglycemic period after transplantation did not exceed 4 days (Table 1). Histological examination of the liver showed islets heavily infiltrated by mononuclear cells. These results suggested that the β cells transplanted to naturally diabetic recipients were destroyed by the original disease process rather than by rejection.

To provide further evidence for this contention, we transplanted allogeneic, but RT1 compatible, WF islets to diabetic BB rats made immunologically tolerant by exposure at birth to WF bone marrow cells[7]. Islet transplantation in six such rats that developed spontaneous diabetes resulted in normoglycemia which persisted for only 2 to 11 days prior to recurrence of diabetes. The islet failure could not be attributed to rejection since these rats were tolerant of WF antigens as confirmed by their acceptance of WF skin grafts. Biopsy revealed that the lymphocytic infiltration of the transplanted islets was similar to that of the islets in the native pancreas[8]. In contrast, the same islet transplantation procedure permanently cured six other tolerant BB animals in which hyperglycemia was induced with streptozotocin[9] (see Table 1).

A serendipitous finding in the BB rats rendered immunologically tolerant of WF cells is also important. These rats proved to have a much lower than expected incidence of diabetes. Of 239 untreated (nontolerant) offspring of nondiabetic BB parents, 13 developed the disease (5.44 percent), whereas of 91 tolerant rats of similar parentage only one became diabetic (1.09 percent) ($P < .05$)[10]. Of 151 nontolerant rats with one diabetic parent, 29 developed diabetes (19.2 percent); and of 58 tolerant animals, only four (6.89 percent) developed the disease ($P < .05$). To confirm this finding we undertook a controlled prospective study in which half of the newborn pups of seven BB litters were selected at random and rendered tolerant of WF (see Table 2)[11]. The remaining pups were left untreated as controls. The incidence of diabetes was expected to be especially high in these litters since both parents were diabetic. The tolerant and nontolerant rats were raised together and cared for in an identical fashion, and blood samples were examined for glucose content at weekly intervals. Eighteen of 28 nontolerant rats (64.3 percent) became diabetic, whereas only 4 of 27 (14.8 percent) of the tolerant rats developed hyperglycemia ($P < .001$). Thus, there was a strikingly reduced incidence of diabetes in diabetes-prone BB rats tolerant of WF antigens.

The studies reported here may be pertinent to the therapy or prophylaxis of diabetes as well as to our understanding of its pathogenesis. Inasmuch as the hyperglycemic syndrome in BB rats seems remarkably similar to human diabetes, the finding that the disease recurs in transplanted pancreatic tissue, independently of rejection, could portend badly for the success of human pancreatic transplantation. However, since we have previously demonstrated that islet allografts can survive and function in ALS-treated BB rats, and since a few human pancreas allografts have been successful for more than a year[12], recurrent disease seems unlikely to occur in heavily immunosuppressed patients. Nevertheless, the results of our experiments, which strengthen the evidence of autoimmune factors in diabetes, indicate that recurrent disease could be a potential problem, especially if optimal histocompatibility, improved drugs, or other protocols in the future allow avoidance of rejection with no or minimal immunosuppression. A precedent for such a problem is provided by the results of renal transplantation in victims of another, probably autoimmune, disease, glomerulone-

TABLE 1. *Outcome of Islet Transplantation in BB Rats*

Islet donor	Recipient	Type of diabetes*	Number of recipients	Cured	Rejecting transplants or with recurrent diabetes	Time showing normoglycemia after islet transplantation (days)‡
BB†	BB	Streptozotocin	11	6	5 (rejecting)	Cured: >60, >60, >120, >150, >180, >300; rejecting: 2, 12, 13, 14, 17
BB†	BB	Spontaneous	8	0	8 (recurrent diabetes)	1, 1, 2, 2, 2, 3, 3, 4
WF	BB tolerant of WF	Streptozotocin	6	6		>30, >75, >90, >90, >90, >120
WF	BB tolerant of WF	Spontaneous	6	0	6 (recurrent diabetes)	2, 2, 6, 6, 8, 11

* Both spontaneous and streptozotocin-induced diabetics had plasma glucose values of >3 mg/ml prior to transplantation.

† All donors were normoglycemic animals with histologically normal islets and were from the nondiabetes-prone BB stock.

‡ The day of rejection or recurrent diabetes was defined as that day on which the plasma glucose increased to >2 mg/ml, but in both types of islet failure the plasma glucose subsequently increased to pretransplantation levels within a few days.

TABLE 2. *Prospective Study of Incidence of Diabetes in Seven Litters of BB Rats in Which Half of the Members of Each Litter Were Inoculated With 50 × 10^6 Bone Marrow Cells From Normal WF Donors*

Group	Number of rats	Diabetics*	Percentage
Tolerant	27	4	14.8†
Nontolerant littermates	28	18	64.3†

* All diabetic rats had plasma glucose values of >3 mg/ml; normoglycemic rats had plasma glucose values of <1.5 mg/ml.
† $P < .001$.

phritis. Recurrence of the original disease occurred in normal kidneys taken from identical twins in 11 of 17 instances[13].

The finding that neonatal BB rats inoculated with WF bone marrow cells failed to develop the expected incidence of diabetes in later life suggests an entirely new approach to therapy or prophylaxis of diabetes. The mechanism by which allogeneic bone marrow protected these rats from diabetes is not obvious; it seems unlikely to be tolerance of WF histocompatibility antigens per se, since a few tolerant rats did become diabetic and their disease was capable of destroying transplanted WF islet tisue, despite the fact that transplanted WF skin was accepted. Another possibility is destruction by the WF cells of a "forbidden clone" of BB cells responsible for autoimmune diabetes in unmodified BB rats. Perturbations in the immunological network may be the underlying cause of diabetes if autoimmunity is involved. In this regard there is experimental evidence that T cell immunoregulatory malfunction is a dominant factor in the etiology of autoimmune disease[14]. Persistence in BB rats of a population of lymphohematopoietic cells from normal nondiabetes-prone WF donors could play a role in keeping an autoimmune process in abeyance. The chimeric cells might, for example, correct possible deficiencies in BB lymphocyte subpopulations—such as suppressor cells. Alternatively, if the syndrome is triggered by a yet to be detected virus, the chimeric cells could reequip the BB hosts with competent antiviral clones which they may lack. Study of these possible mechanisms in this animal model should provide fruitful avenues for future investigations of etiology and therapy of diabetes.

REFERENCES AND NOTES

1. Nakhooda AF, Like AA, Chappel CI, Murray FT, Marliss EB. Diabetes 26, 100 (1977). Our animals were derived from a breeding nucleus of nine litters of rats received from Bio Breeding Laboratories (thus BB) of Ottawa, Canada, and from the Banting Research Center in Ottawa.
2. Like AA, Rossini AA, Guberski DL, Appel MC, Williams RM. Science 206, 1421 (1979); Naji A, Silvers WK, Barker CF. Transplant. Proc. 1981;13:826.
3. Naji A, Silvers WK, Plotkin SA, Dafoe DC, Barker CF. Surgery 1979;86:218.
4. Lymphocytes from 22 BB rats (members of 14 different litters) all were RTI^{u} when serologically typed. Moreover, in 20 instances no proliferative response occurred when WF (RTI^{u}) lymphocytes were exposed in vitro to irradiated BB lymphocytes (one-way mixed lymphocyte culture).
5. In the remaining five rats the grafts were rejected between 12 and 19 days.
6. Ziegler MM, Reckard CR, Barker CF. J. Surg. Res. 1974;16:575.
7. To induce tolerance we inoculated BB rats intravenously within 24 hours of birth with 50 × 10^6 bone marrow cells from WF donors [RE Billingham, in Transplantation of Tissues and Cells (Wistar, Philadelphia, 1971), p. 87]. In young adulthood these rats were grafted with WF skin to assess their putatively tolerant state (ibid., p. 1). All these grafts were accepted for the remainder of the lifetime of the animals.
8. Two of these recipients that suffered recurrent diabetes were challenged with a second WF skin graft which they permanently (more than 100 days) accepted, again confirming the persistence of the tolerant state.
9. All of these rats remained normoglycemic through a 1- to 4-month observation period after which they were killed and found histologically to have healthy transplanted WF islets.
10. Statistical analysis was performed by a chi-square test.
11. All of these rats accepted WF skin for more than 200 days when challenged with such transplants at 4 to 5 weeks of age.
12. Sutherland DER, Goetz FC, Najarian JS. Transplant. Proc. 1981;13:291.
13. Glassock RJ, Feldman D, Reynolds ES, Dammin GJ. Medicine (Baltimore) 1968;47:411.
14. Cantor H, and Gershon RK. Fed. Proc. Fed. Am. Soc. Exp. Biol. 1979;38:2058.
15. We thank P. Thibert for providing our breeding nucleus of BB rats. Sawchuck G, Naji M, Markmann J, Black G, and Koberlein B provided excellent technical assistance. The work was supported by PHS grants AM26007, AM19525, and CA18640 and by the Thomas McCabe Fund and Reynolds Foundation.

Physiological and Immunological Consequences of Transplanting Isolated Pancreatic Islets

CRAIG R. RECKARD, M.D., MORITZ M. ZIEGLER, M.D., AND CLYDE F. BARKER, M.D.

Transplantation of isolated islets of Langerhans has been suggested as a treatment for diabetes which would not only minimize technical complications but also perhaps avoid rejection. An intraperitoneal injection of 600 to 1,200 isologous islets, which were isolated by collagenase digestion, into streptozotocin-induced diabetic rats, rendered their hosts normoglycemic for as long as 11 months. Homologous islets initially fared as well as isografts but were rejected within 12 days, sensitizing their hosts to subsequent donor-strain skin grafts. A brief period of treatment with antilymphocyte serum (ALS) greatly extended homograft survival, but no more so than skin or heart transplants of identical genetic makeup. Islets appear to be at least as vulnerable to rejection as other tissues.

PANCREATIC TRANSPLANTATION has been attempted by several groups[1,12] in the hope that the rapid progression of vascular complications associated with diabetes might thus be prevented or retarded. If, as suggested by Siperstein,[18] diabetes is caused by a generalized thickening in capillary basement membranes which only secondarily damages pancreatic islets, transplantation affords no advantage over insulin therapy. If, on the other hand, the diabetic patient's fundamental defect is an inadequate beta cell, replacement with normal pancreatic tissue might be indicated in many patients. Whether the pancreas is primarily or secondarily involved in diabetes has not been answered by clinical experience in transplantation because only one of the thirty patients receiving such grafts has survived as long as a year.[1] Many of the failures have resulted either from technical difficulties or from rejection of the duodenal segment usually transplanted along with the pancreas as a conduit for exocrine secretions. Gold and associates[7] have recently described a technique which obviates use of donor duodenum by implanting the pancreatic duct into the ureter. Still, approximately 98 percent of the tissue mass in a whole pancreatic transplant is extraneous since the islets comprise only one to two percent of the organ.

Since the islets have often appeared relatively undamaged in rejected whole organs,[12] they may be less susceptible to the homograft reaction than the acinar tissue. A free transplant of isolated islets of Langerhans therefore has the attractive possibilities of avoiding difficult technical problems and lessening the chance of rejection on the basis of minimal antigenicity and immunologic vulnerability. Several investigators have described some degree of success with isolated islet preparations. Moskalewski[14] described the recovery of isolated guinea pig islets several weeks after transplantation. Reemtsma[17] found that piscine islet tissue would briefly decrease the blood sugar in diabetic rats. Strautz[20] improved the diabetic state of obese mice by placing islets from normal mice, protected in Millipore chambers, into their peritoneal cavities. Ballinger and Lacy[2] reported an impressive amelioration of diabetes in rats (indicated by weight gain and decreased glycosuria) by islet transplantation to intramuscular and intraperitoneal sites. The present study indicates that nor-

From the Department of Surgery and Medical Genetics, and the Harrison Department of Surgical Research, University of Pennsylvania, Philadelphia, Pennsylvania.

Supported in part by United States Public Health Service Grant No. AI09275.

Presented at the Thirty-fourth Annual Meeting of the Society of University Surgeons, New Orleans, La., Feb. 8–10, 1973.

This article has been reproduced from *Surgery*, Vol. 74, No. 1, July 1973, with permission from the C. V. Mosby Company.

moglycemia may be achieved in previously diabetic rats for as long as 11 months after transplantation of *isologous* pancreatic islets. Islet *homografts,* however, proved vulnerable to rejection, in fact more so than either skin or vascularized whole organ transplants.

Materials and Methods

Adult rats of the isogenic strains ACI (AgB^4), DA (AgB^4), Fischer (AgB^1), and Lewis (AgB^1), which weighed anywhere from 150 to 250 grams, were used without regard to sex. They were fed standard rat diet and allowed free access to food and water. Metabolic cages allowed measurements of urine outputs.

Diabetes was induced by the intravenous injection of 55 to 65 mg per kilogram of streptozotocin, a specific beta cell toxin[9] obtained through the courtesy of Dr. William Dulin, Upjohn Laboratories. Plasma glucose and insulin determinations were done by amputating small portions of the tails of ether-anesthetized rats and collecting blood in heparinized capillary tubes. The Beckman autoanalyzer was used for plasma and urine glucose determinations, and immunoreactive insulin values were obtained with the use of an immunosorbent technique (Phadebas insulin test kit). Blood for serial glucose determinations was taken from unfasted animals during morning hours. Intravenous glucose tolerance tests were done by injecting 1 mg per gram of body weight of a 50 percent glucose solution into a peripheral vein of ether-anesthetized animals.

Pancreatic islets were isolated by a modification of Lacy and Kostianovsky's[10] method. While the animals were under ether anesthesia, the common bile duct was occluded as it entered the duodenum, catheterized proximally with a polyethylene catheter and injected with 10 cc of Hanks solution, thus distending the pancreatic ducts and disrupting acinar tissue. The pancreas was removed, placed in cold Hanks solution, diced into 1 to 2 mm pieces, and incubated for 20 minutes with a 0.6 percent solution of collagenase at 37°C while being continually agitated. Then a pinch of desoxyribonuclease was added, and the preparation was washed four times with 40 cc of cold Hanks solution containing 200 U of aprotinin (Trasylol) per cubic centimeter. The supernatant of each wash, containing only acinar tissue, was decanted after settling for two minutes. The islets settled more rapidly and were thus concentrated, though some acinar tissue remained, contaminating the islet preparation. Sometimes 100 cc of neutral red (6 mg per 100 cc of saline) was injected into the aorta prior to excising the pancreas to stain the islets for easy recognition under a dissecting microscope at a magnification of $\times 25$. About 200 islets could be isolated from a single pancreas, 60 minutes being required for the entire process.

The resultant islet preparation was administered intraperitoneally (I.P.) via a small incision in anesthetized rats. Approximately 600 islets (three pancreas equivalents) were usually given at once with some animals receiving several doses.

Antilymphocyte serum (ALS) was prepared by three biweekly intravenous injections of 7 to 8×10^9 lymphocytes from outbred rats into a horse which was exsanguinated one week after the third injection. The decomplemented serum had a lymphoagglutinin titer of 1:20,000.

Full-thickness skin grafts were carried out by standard methods. Auxiliary hearts were transplanted by the technique of Ono and associates.[15]

Median survival times (MST) were calculated by Litchfield's[13] nomographic method. The end-point of skin graft survival was epidermal necrosis; of heart survival, it was the cessation of a palpable beat; and of islet survival, it was the return of the plasma glucose to over 200 mg percent.

Results

Effects of Streptozotocin

In 125 normal unfasted rats, the plasma glucose was 50 to 210 mg percent (mean 132 $\pm$ 5.84) (S.D. 20.2). Plasma glucose levels up to 200 mg percent were considered normal. After intravenous streptozotocin (55 to 65 mg per kilogram) was administered, hyperglycemia occurred within 24 hours. In two of fifty streptozotocin-treated animals, spontaneous reversion to normoglycemia was seen during the first week, but this never occurred if the blood sugar was over 400 mg percent one week after treatment. Only rats with plasma glucose over 400 mg percent for at least one week and more often for two to 12 weeks were used as islet recipients. A group of 11 diabetic animals had polyuria (98.1 cc per 24 hours versus a normal value of 4.0 cc); polyphagia (eating 40.6 Gm versus a normal intake of 17.1 Gm of rat pellets per day), and glycosuria (7.50 Gm glucose per 24 hours versus the normal value of 0.36 Gm). Most lost weight though this varied somewhat with the dose of streptozotocin and the strain of rat. Of 24 diabetic rats studied, the mean weight loss per 30 days was 7.03 percent of body weight. Mortality figures also depended upon the strain of rat employed and the dose of streptozotocin given, but of 24 ACI rats receiving 55 mg per kilogram, nine (37.5 percent) died within one month. Table 1 summarizes these parameters in diabetic rats and compares them to those in the normal state and after islet transplantation.

Histological study of tissues from diabetic rats confirmed destruction of beta cells after streptozotocin treatment. Small distorted islets of very abnormal appearance remained.

Suitability of Recipient Site

Attempts were made to locate a site at which large numbers of isologous islets would become rapidly vascularized and later identifiable histologically. Several whole pancreata of fetal origin or aliquots of 200 isolated adult islets were transplanted under the splenic or renal capsule, under the serosa of the stomach, intradermally, intramuscularly, or into the testicle. Small numbers of islets were identified microscopically one to two weeks later, but it appeared that autodigestion had destroyed much of the tissue in these confined spaces. No remission of diabetes was seen in these animals.

The intraperitoneal site was then evaluated, since it allowed injection of larger numbers of islets, provided a large absorptive surface to reduce chances of autodigestion and because Ballinger and Lacy[2] had used it with success, although their rats had not consistently achieved normoglycemia.

Intraperitoneal (I.P.) Isologous Islet Transplants

A total of 800 to 1,800 islets were injected intraperitoneally, usually in divided doses of three pancreas equivalents (600 islets) on consecutive days. Although this was well tolerated by most animals, a few rats developed ascites, peritonitis, and subsequently died. Approximately a twofold increase in the serum amylase was seen in most rats the day after islet treatment. Later inspection at laparotomy revealed little if any sign of inflammation, nor could the transplanted islets ever be visualized. There was, however, almost immediate physiological evidence of their survival. Of 16 diabetic rats treated with I.P. isologous islets, 12 (75 percent) became normoglycemic (plasma glucose < 200 mg percent) within twenty-four hours and because blood sugars remained normal for at least two months, these were considered successful transplants. Fig. 1 shows the plasma glucose values of these animals after islet treatment. Eight currently have remained normoglycemic from two to eleven months after treatment. However, three gradually reverted to the diabetic state between five and six months after their islet transplants. One animal died of a respiratory infection while still normoglycemic three months postoperatively.

During the period of normoglycemia all of the rats seemed healthier than in their diabetic state, and all resumed the continuous pattern of weight gain which characterized the normal rat (16.1 percent increase in body weight during the first month postoperatively and 8.9 percent during the second month). Polyphagia, polydipsia, polyuria, and glycosuria also disappeared. The mean daily food and water consumption were 17.4 Gm and 29.7 ml, respectively, after treatment versus 46.6 Gm and 143.1 ml, respectively, in the diabetic state. Urine volume fell from 98.1 cc a day to 6.7 cc per day and 24 hour urine glucose values from 7.56 to 0.38 Gm per day immediately after the islet treatment. Table I summarizes these values.

Pancreatic biopsies taken during the period of normoglycemia showed distortion of islets and no regeneration of beta cells, helping to exclude the possibility that the hosts' native islets had recovered and were maintaining normoglycemia.

Fate of Islet Homografts

Islet homografts from donors differing from the recipients by a strong histoincompatibility (Fischer → ACI) functioned only evanescently, ranging from one to three days (Fig. 2).

TABLE 1. *Metabolic Studies on Normal, Diabetic, and Islet-transplanted Rats**

	Normal rats		Unmodified diabetics		Rats with functioning islet isografts	
	Value	No. of rats	Value	No. of rats	Value	No. of rats
Plasma glucose (mg./100 ml.)	132	125	572 ± 28.3	24	130.0 ± 9.97	12
Food eaten (Gm./24 hr.)	17.1	5	46.6 ± 2.46	11	17.38 ± 0.57	9
Water consumed (ml./24 hr.)	25.6	5	143.1 ± 13.1	11	29.7 ± 5.3	9
Urine volume (c.c./24 hr.)	4.0	5	98.1 ± 10.6	11	6.77 ± 1.78	9
Urine glucose (Gm./24 hr.)	0.36	5	7.50 ± 0.71	11	0.38 ± 0.97	9
Percent weight lost (−) or gained (+) per 30 days	(+) 5	5	(−) 7.03 ± 1.94	24	(+) 16.9 ± 2.17 (1st mo.) (+) 8.91 ± 2.1 (2nd mo.)	9 8
Percent mortality per 30 days	0	25	37.5	24	8.33	12†

* Results are expressed as mean values for the group ± S.E.M. for the number of animals studied.
† One death, three months after transplantation.

When donor and host were compatible at the AgB locus (ACI → DA) blood sugars in ten previously diabetic recipients remained normal for seven to 12 days (MST, 8.1 days) before hyperglycemia returned, presumably as a result of rejection.

Whether the recipients of homologous islets had become sensitized was determined by challenging six Fischer recipients of 800 to 1,200 AgB compatible Lewis islets with donor strain skin grafts two to 12 weeks after the islets were injected. These grafts were rejected in an accelerated manner (<7 days versus the normal 10.0 ± 0.8 days).

Effects of Immunosuppression on Islet Homografts

Further confirmation of the immunological etiology of the recurrence of diabetes in homograft recipients was forthcoming when immunosuppression was found to prolong the normoglycemic period. Seven DA recipients of ACI islets were treated with 1 cc of horse antirat serum daily for five days prior to transplantation. This extended the functional islet survival group from the control MST of 8.1 to 30.5 days. Two rats in this group were normoglycemic for more than 100 days.

However, when AgB incompatibility applied (Fischer → ACI), immunosuppression was much less effective (MST was 1.8 days in eight recipients despite ALS [1 cc] daily starting five days prior to transplant and continuing thereafter until rejection)

Survival of Islet Homografts Compared with Skin or Vascularized Whole Organs (Table 2)

To determine the relative position of islets in the spectrum of immunological requirements for success, skin and whole organ heart transplants were done in the same rat strains. In an AgB incompatible combination (Fischer → ACI), the islet survival failed to exceed five days whether or not immunosuppression (1 cc of ALS daily starting five days before transplant) was used. An identical ALS protocol extended skin homograft survival from 7.2 to 18.4 days and heart survival from 8.4 to more than 50 days.

As mentioned above, when AgB compatible ACI donors were used, diabetic DA recipients of islet transplants remained normoglycemic for a median of 8.1 days, and ALS extended this normoglycemic period to 30.5 days and for as long as 150 days in two of seven animals. ACI skin homografts, on the other hand, had a normal MST of 12.0 days on DA hosts, and immunosuppression was even more effective in increasing this than in the case of islet

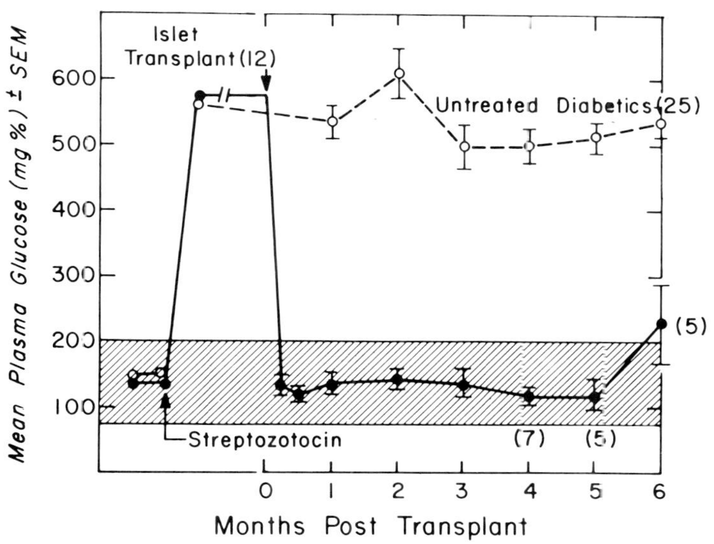

FIG. 1. Plasma glucose after isologous islet transplantation. Plasma glucose values in 25 untreated diabetic rats (broken line) are compared with those seen in 12 previously diabetic recipients of pancreatic islet isografts (solid line). Eight currently remain normoglycemic at 2, 2, 3, 3, 4, 4, 10, and 11 months after treatment.

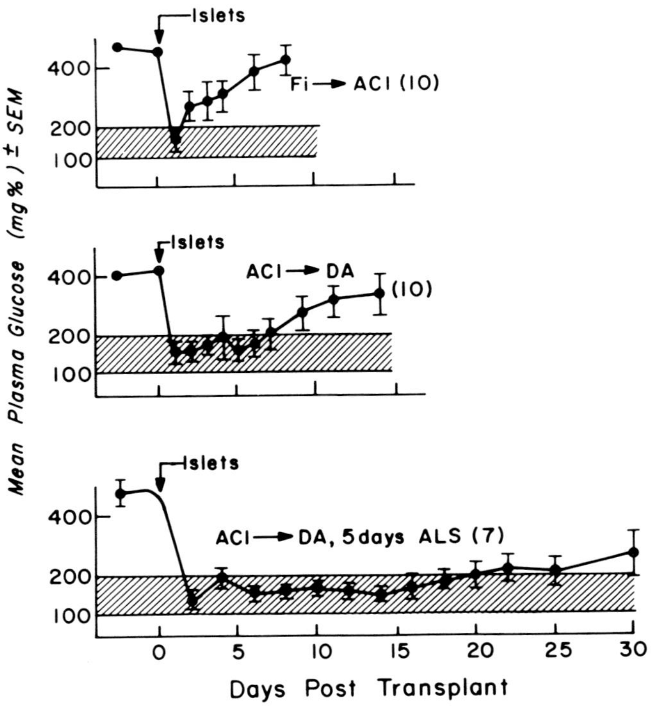

FIG. 2. Plasma glucose after homologous islet transplantation. Duration of normoglycemia after islet homografts in diabetic rats depends on histocompatibility. Fischer islets function only a few days in AgB incompatible ACI hosts although some of these animals received ALS. ACI islets function longer in AgB compatible DA rats especially if ALS is given.

transplants (more than 50 days by five days of pretreatment with ALS). All five ACI auxiliary heart homografts continued to beat for more than 100 days in DA hosts without benefit of any immunosuppression.[3]

TABLE 2. *Functional Survival of Pancreatic Islet Grafts Compared With That of Skin and Heart Transplants*

Donor → recipient	Type of graft	No. of animals with successful grafts (total no. treated)	Median survival time (days) ± 95% confidence limits (S.D.)
ACI → ACI	Islets	12 (16)	>120
ACI → DA	Islets	10 (18)	8.1 ± 1.17 (1.3)
	Skin	10	12.0 ± 6.8 (1.0)
	Heart	5	>100
ACI → DA (5 days of ALS therapy)	Islets	7 (14)	30.5 ± 19.9 (2.37)
	Skin	6	>50
Fischer → ACI	Islets	4 (8)	<3
	Skin	8	7.2 ± 1.01 (1.03)
	Heart	5	8.4 ± 0.72 (1.10)
Fischer → ACI (ALS, 1 c.c., daily starting 5 days pre-transplant)	Islets	8	1.8 ± 0.91 (1.50)
	Skin	10	18.0 ± 1.4 (1.07)
	Heart	5	>100
Fischer → Lewis	Skin (normal hosts)	10	10.0 ± 0.8 (1.15)
	Skin (hosts pretreated with Fischer islets)	6	<7

Glucose Tolerance and Plasma Insulin

Immunoreactive insulin levels were determined on plasma obtained from unfasted normal, diabetic, and normoglycemic islet-treated animals. The values in microunits per cubic centimeter were 34 6 ± 3.69 (S.D., 7.39) for five normal animals; 24.5 ± 3.67 (S.D., 11.02) for ten diabetics; and 49.8 ± 10.1 (S.D., 41.8) for 18 islet recipients. The difference between the unmodified diabetic rat and the islet-treated rats was statistically significant ($p = < 0.05$). Despite the normal random plasma insulin levels, the response to a challenge with intravenous glucose (1 mg per gram of body weight) was abnormal in the islet recipients. Glucose tolerance curves were somewhat flat and insulin levels rose slowly as compared to the immediate response seen in normal rats. Some islet-treated animals did eventually demonstrate a twofold increase in their plasma insulin about two hours after the glucose infusion.

Discussion

The desirability of attempting clinical pancreatic transplantation depends on several factors, some of which can be studied in animals: (1) whether the procedure is technically feasible and safe; (2) whether it is permanently effective in controlling hyperglycemia and other metabolic consequences of diabetes; (3) how readily rejection can be controlled; and (4) whether long-term vascular complications are more likely to be avoided by pancreatic replacement than with insulin therapy.

Whole organ pancreatic transplantation has proved dangerous,[1] but improvements in technique, such as avoidance of a duodenal conduit[7] may be expected to minimize complications. Still, the injection of a tiny volume of a pure islet preparation would unquestionably be safer and more convenient for the patient. On the other hand, the ease in administering this type of transplant would be achieved at the expense of a tedious technical effort in preparing the islet inoculum as well as in a substantial loss of islet tissue from each donor pancreas. Islets from six pancreata would probably be necessary to achieve normoglycemia. We hope that technical refinements may overcome this problem, since only 200 of a probable total of about 15,000 islets[8] are currently being isolated from each rat pancreas. It is somewhat surprising that only 1,200 (8 percent of the number in the intact pancreas) are needed to overcome diabetes.

Whole organ pancreatic transplantation has been shown to achieve long-term normoglycemia in diabetic rats,[11] dogs,[6] and humans.[12] It is, however, not a foregone conclusion that isolated pancreatic islets, outside their usual milieu and deprived of a normal blood supply, would function efficiently. Some tissues are at a disadvantage when taken out of a normal dermal-epithelial relationship.[4] However, Ballinger and Lacy[2] demonstrated that the diabetic state could be dramatically improved by isolated islet transplantation, with polyuria and glycosuria being diminished and weight gain restored. The present experiments confirm these findings and also demonstrate that normoglycemia can be achieved in 75 percent of diabetic rats by intraperitoneal isologous islet injections and that normal plasma glucose levels may last for as long as 11 months. Whether these transplanted animals achieve fully normal islet function remains in doubt. Although plasma immunoreactive serum insulin levels were in a normal range in our "cured diabetics," these rats had abnormal glucose tolerance curves, and the insulin response to an intravenous glucose challenge was sluggish. Another suggestion that our animals remained abnormal was the currence of hyperglycemia in three of them after normal plasma glucose had been maintained for five to six months after islet transplantation. In an earlier series of transplants[16] in which a smaller islet dose was given, apparent cures sometimes lasted for only one to two months. We speculate that this indicates that the islet mass transplanted was often barely adequate to achieve normal glucose levels and that, eventually, overworked intraperitoneal islets became exhausted and ceased functioning, a situation akin to that theorized in adult onset diabetes. It is also possible, however, that some other mechanism was responsible for the late failures such as an autoimmune attack on the islets, the cell surfaces of which were no longer embedded in and protected by their usual pancreatic envelope.

Since endocrine tissue may be antigenically poor,[5] it has been thought by some that isolated islets were unlikely to provoke an immune response. That islets have appeared spared in rejected pancreas[12] might also indicate that they are a privileged tissue which is less than normally vulnerable to rejection. Our experiments indicate that transplanted islets evoke an immune state characterized by subsequent accelerated rejection of donor strain skin grafts. The present islet preparation is somewhat contaminated by acinar tissue which could contribute to the antigenic load but even if this were avoided by differential centrifugation or picking out individual islets, it seems doubtful that contaminating passenger leukocytes could be excluded from an islet preparation. As few as 50,000 such cells will evoke an immune response.[19]

That islets of Langerhans are themselves vulnerable to rejection is evident from this report. Normoglycemia persisted for a median of only 1.8 days in diabetic rats receiving islets from homologous donors differing at the major (AgB) locus. It is in fact difficult to invoke an immune mechanism to explain such acute destruction. A period of voluntary starvation which sometimes followed islet injections and the passive release of insulin from damaged islets are alternative explanations for the transient normoglycemia in these animals. A two- to threefold increase in plasma immunoreactive insulin in several of these animals 24 hours after islet transplantation may indicate either passive or active hormone release. The results of treating diabetic DA rats with islets from ACI donors were more revealing, leaving no doubt that, although homografted islets will function, they are as subject to the laws of transplantation biology as are other tissues. These strains are identical at the AgB locus but, since they differ by antigens determined at multiple minor loci, acutely reject exchanged skin grafts (MST, 12.0 days). Functional islet survival time with this combination was 8.1 days. By means of a brief period (five days) of ALS prior to islet transplantation, normoglycemia of up to 150 days (MST, 30.5) was achieved.

Although these results with minimal immunosuppression seem rather favorable, they should be examined in the light of results of skin and whole organ grafting in identical genetic settings. In the AgB *compatible* (ACI → DA) combination, 1 cc of ALS daily extended skin survival to more than 50 days while no immunosuppression was required to achieve auxiliary heart transplant survival of 100 days. It should be remembered that the rat is somewhat anomalous in his response to whole organ grafts and the ease with which their survival may be prolonged, perhaps because of the phenomenon of enhancement.[21] However, it appears that when compared to skin, a particularly exacting type of graft in its immunologic requirements for success, the pancreatic islet does not compare favorably. Perhaps the disruption inherent in the isolation process exposes the islets to the same immunologic forces which make dissociated tumor or lymphoid cell transplants more susceptible to damage by humoral mechanisms than skin or other fixed tissue grafts.

Although we have shown that transplanted isologous islets of Langerhans will allow diabetic rats to remain normoglycemic for many months, their behavior depends on classical histocompatibility requirements and homografts are at least as vulnerable to rejection as skin or whole organ transplants.

ACKNOWLEDGMENTS

We thank Dr. W. K. Silvers for helpful criticism of the manuscript, Drs. A. I. Winegrad and R. E. Billingham for advice, Dr. D. T. Rowlands for review of the histology, and Dr. J. R. Hansell for making it possible to obtain immunoreactive insulins. George Sawchuck, Brigitte Koeberlein, and Pat Weigand provided expert technical assistance.

REFERENCES

1. ACS/NIH Organ Transplant Registry: Second scientific report, J.A.M.A. 1972;221:1486.
2. Ballinger WF, and Lacy PE. Transplantation of intact pancreatic islets in rats, Surgery 1972;72:175.
3. Barker CF, and Billingham RE. Comparison of the fates of AgB locus compatible homografts of skin and hearts in inbred rats, Nature 1970;225:851.
4. Billingham RE, and Silvers WK. Studies on the conservation of epidermal specificities of skin and certain mucosas in adult animals, J. Exp. Med. 1967;125:429.
5. Billingham RE, and Silvers WK. The immunobiology of transplantation, Englewood Cliffs, N.J., 1971, Prentice-Hall, Inc., p. 82.
6. Bergan JJ, Hoehn JG, Porter N, and Dry L. Total pancreatic allografts in pancreatectomized dogs, Arch. Surg. 1965;90:521.
7. Gold M, Whittaker JR, Vieth FJ, and Gliedman ML. Evaluation of ureteral drainage for pancreatic exocrine secretion, Surg. Forum. 1972;23:375.
8. Haist RE, and Pugh EJ. Volume measurement of the islets of Langerhans and the effects of age and fasting. Am. J. Physiol. 1948;152:36.

9. Junod A, Lambert AE, Stauffacher W, and Renold AE. Diabetogenic action of streptozotocin: Relationship of dose to metabolic response. J. Clin. Invest. 1969;48:2129.
10. Lacy PE, and Kostianovsky M. Method for the isolation of intact islets of Langerhans from the rat pancreas. Diabetes 1967;16:35.
11. Lee S, Chandler JG, Krubel R, Nakaji NT, Rosen H, and Orloff MJ. Relief of diabetes mellitus by heterotopic transplantation of the whole pancreas in inbred rats. Surg. Forum 1971;22:75.
12. Lillehei RC, Simmons RL, Najarian JS, Weil R, Uchida H, Ruiz JC, Kjellstrand CV, and Goetz FC. Pancreatico-duodenal allotransplantation, experimental and clinical experience, Ann. Surg. 1970;172:405.
13. Litchfield JT, Jr. A method for rapid graphic solution of time and percent effect curves. J. Pharmacol. Exp. Ther. 1949;97:399.
14. Moskalewski S. Studies on the culture and transplantation of isolated islets of Langerhans in the guinea pig. Proc. K. Ned. Akad. Wet. (Biol. Med.) 1969;72:157.
15. Ono K, Lindsey ES, and Creech O, Jr. Transplanted rat heart: Local graft irradiation. Transplantation 1969;7:176.
16. Reckard CR, and Barker CF. Transplantation of isolated pancreatic islets across strong and weak histocompatibility barriers. Transplant. Proc. 1973;5:761.
17. Reemtsma K. Experimental islet cell grafting: A transplantation model, Transplant. Proc. 1970;2:513.
18. Siperstein MD. The relationship of carbohydrate derangement to the microangiopathy of diabetes, in Cerasi E, and Luft R, editors: Pathogenesis of diabetes mellitus, New York, 1970, Wilegand and Sons, pp. 81–96.
19. Steinmuller D, and Weiner LJ. Evocation and persistence of transplantation immunity in rats. Transplantation 1963;1:97.
20. Strautz RL. Studies of hereditary-obese mice (OBOB) after implantation of pancreatic islets in Millipore filter capsules. Diabetologia 1970;6:306.
21. Stuart FP, Saitoh T, Fitch FW, and Spargo BH. Immunologic enhancement of renal allografts in the rat. Surgery 1968;64:17.

Curriculum Vitae & Bibliography

Name Jonathan Evans Rhoads

Place of Birth Philadelphia, Pennsylvania

Date of Birth May 9, 1907

Office Address 3400 Spruce Street, Philadelphia, Pennsylvania 19104

Home Address 131 West Walnut Lane, Philadelphia, Pennsylvania 19144

Parents Edward G. Rhoads and Margaret (Ely) Paxson Rhoads

Married Teresa Folin Rhoads

Children Margaret Rhoads Kendon, Jonathan Evans, Jr., George Grant, Edward Otto Folin, Philip Garrett, and Charles James

Education
Germantown Friends School, Philadelphia, Pennsylvania 1913–1921

Westtown School, Westtown, Pennsylvania 1921–1924

B.A. Haverford College, Haverford, Pennsylvania 1928

M.D. Johns Hopkins University School of Medicine, Baltimore, Maryland 1932

D.Sc.Med. University of Pennsylvania, Graduate School of Medicine, Philadelphia, Pennsylvania 1940

Honorary Degrees
LL.D. University of Pennsylvania, Philadelphia, Pennsylvania 1960

D.Sc. Haverford College, Haverford, Pennsylvania 1962

D.Sc. Swarthmore College, Swarthmore, Pennsylvania 1969

M.A. University of Pennsylvania, Philadelphia, Pennsylvania 1971

D.Sc. The Medical College of Pennsylvania, Philadelphia, Pennsylvania 1974

D.Sc. Hahnemann Medical College, Philadelphia, Pennsylvania 1978

D.Sc. Duke University, Durham, North Carolina 1979

D.Litt. Jefferson University, Philadelphia, Pennsylvania 1979

D.Sc. Georgetown University School of Medicine, Washington, D.C. 1981

D.Sc. Medical College of Ohio at Toledo, 1985

Licensure Pennsylvania 1934

Specialty Certification The American Board of Surgery 1940

Internship Hospital of the University of Pennsylvania, Philadelphia, Pennsylvania 1932–1934

Residency

Assistant Chief Resident Physician, Hospital of the University of Pennsylvania, 1934

Fellow in General Surgery, Hospital of the University of Pennsylvania, 1934–1939

Assistant Instructor in Surgery, University of Pennsylvania School of Medicine, 1934–1935

Instructor in Surgery, University of Pennsylvania School of Medicine, 1935–1939

Hospital and University Positions Held

Associate in Surgery, University of Pennsylvania School of Medicine, 1939–1947
Assistant Surgeon, Pennsylvania Hospital, Philadelphia, 1939–1946
Associate in Surgery, University of Pennsylvania Graduate School of Medicine, 1940–1945
Assistant Surgeon, Hospital of the University of Pennsylvania, 1940–1946
Acting Chief, Surgical Service B, Hospital of the University of Pennsylvania, 1942–1946
Assistant Surgeon, Children's Hospital of Philadelphia, 1942–1947
Acting Director, Harrison Department of Surgical Research, University of Pennsylvania School of Medicine, 1944–1945
Assistant Professor of Surgery, University of Pennsylvania Graduate School of Medicine, 1945–1950
Assistant Professor of Surgery, University of Pennsylvania School of Medicine, 1946–1947
Chief, Surgical Division II, Hospital of the University of Pennsylvania, 1946–1956
Special Consultant, Friends Hospital, Philadelphia, 1947–1949
Associate Professor of Surgery, University of Pennsylvania School of Medicine, 1947–1949
Professor of Surgery, University of Pennsylvania School of Medicine, 1949–1951
J. William White Professor of Surgical Research, University of Pennsylvania School of Medicine, 1949–1951
Professor of Surgery and Surgical Research, University of Pennsylvania School of Medicine, 1951–1957
Assistant Director, Harrison Department of Surgical Research, University of Pennsylvania School of Medicine, 1946–1959
Professor of Surgery, University of Pennsylvania School of Medicine, 1957–1959
Assistant Chief, Department of Surgery, Hospital of the University of Pennsylvania, 1956–1959
Provost, University of Pennsylvania, 1956–1959
Professor of Surgery, University of Pennsylvania Graduate School of Medicine, 1950–1964
John Rhea Barton Professor of Surgery and Chairman, Department of Surgery, University of Pennsylvania School of Medicine, 1959–1972
Director of the Harrison Department of Surgical Research, University of Pennsylvania School of Medicine, 1959–1972
Chairman of the Department of Surgery, Hospital of the University of Pennsylvania, 1959–1972
Director, Department of Surgery, Pennsylvania Hospital, Philadelphia, 1972–1974

Current Hospital and University Positions

Professor of Surgery, University of Pennsylvania School of Medicine, 1972–
Surgical Staff, Hospital of the University of Pennsylvania, 1939–
Consultant, Department of Surgery, Germantown Hospital and Medical Center, 1958–
Senior Surgeon, Visiting Staff, 1948–1972; Consultant in Surgery, Children's Hospital of Philadelphia, 1972–
Consultant in Surgery, Veterans Administration Hospital, Philadelphia, 1953–
Consulting Surgeon, The Pennsylvania Hospital, Philadelphia, 1974–
Provost Emeritus, University of Pennsylvania, 1977–

Editorial Positions

Annals of Surgery, Editorial Board, 1947, Chairman, 1971–1973

Cancer, Journal of the American Cancer Society, Editor, 1972

Journal of Surgical Research, Founding Member and Editorial Board, 1960–1971

Oncology Times, Editorial Board, 1979–

Transactions and Studies of The College of Physicians of Philadelphia, Editorial Committee, 1979–

The Journal of Clinical Surgery, Senior Editorial Advisory Board, 1981–

The Classics of Surgery, Leslie B. Adams, Jr., M.A., J.D., LLD., Publisher, Editorial Advisory Board, 1982–

Honorary Fellowships and Memberships

Alpha Omega Alpha
American Society of Nutritional Support Services
Association of Surgeons of India, Fellow
Buffalo Surgical Society, Fellow
Chicago Surgical Society, Fellow
Deutsches Gesellschaft fur Chirurgie, Corresponding Member
Greater Philadelphia First Foundation, Celebration of Excellence Honorary Committee Member, May 1987
The Halsted Society
Hollandsche Maatchappij der Wetenschappen, Fellow
International Federation of Surgical Colleges, Honorary President, 1987
James Ewing Society
Die Kollege van Geneeskunde van Suid-Afrika, Fellow
National Foundation for Ileitis and Colitis, Philadelphia Chapter
Osler Library at McGill University, Curator (*ex officio*), 1952–1954
Phi Beta Kappa
Phi Beta Kappa Associates
Philomathean Society
Polish Association of Surgeons, Fellow
Royal College of Physicians and Surgeons of Canada, Fellow
Royal College of Surgeons of Edinburgh, Fellow
Royal College of Surgeons of England, Fellow
The Royal Society of Arts, Benjamin Franklin Fellow
H. William Scott, Jr. Society
Society of Graduate Surgeons, Los Angeles County Hospital
Society of Sigma XI
Southeastern Surgical Congress, Fellow
Sphinx Senior Society

Government Service

National Research Council
Member representing the American Surgical Association, 1959–1962
Member at Large, 1962–1965
Member, Executive Committee of the Division of Medical Sciences, 1961–1965
Former member, Advisory Committee on Scientist to Scientist Communication in the Biomedical Field
Former member and Chairman of the Committee on Trauma
Former member of the Committee on Shock
Former member of the Medical Fellowship Board

United States Department of Health, Education and Welfare, Food and Drug Administration, Chairman, Surgical Drugs Advisory Committee, 1971–1974

United States Public Health Service
Special Consultant, Surgery Study Section, 1956–1960
Member of the General Clinical Research Center Committee, Division of Research Grants, 1961–1963

Consultant to the Division of General Medical Sciences, 1962–1965
Member of the National Advisory General Medical Sciences Council, National Institutes of Health, 1963–1967
National Cancer Advisory Board, 1972–1979; Chairman, 1972–1979

United States Senate Panel of Consultants on the Conquest of Cancer 1970

Veterans Administration
Consultant to the Bureau of State Services, Cancer Control Program, Department of Medicine and Surgery, 1963
Selections Committee, 1964–1970

Honors and Awards
American Cancer Society Award for Distinguished Service to Cancer Control, 1957
Award of Merit, General Alumni Society of the University of Pennsylvania, 1960
Humanitarian Award, the Kain Moses Group for Cancer Research, Philadelphia Division, American Cancer Society, 1963
Strittmatter Award, Philadelphia County Medical Society, 1968
American Medical Association Joseph Goldberger Award in Clinical Nutrition (co-recipient with Dr. Stanley J. Dudrick), 1970
Citation from the Association for Academic Surgery, 1971
Mount Scopus Citation of Honor, American Friends of the Hebrew University, Philadelphia Physicians' Division, 1972
Dr. Roswell Park Medal for Eminent Service to Profession and to Humanity, Buffalo Surgical Society, 1973
Orville C. King Teaching Award of the Pennsylvania Hospital, 1973
American Cancer Society National Award, 1973
Modern Medicine Award for Distinguished Achievement, 1974
James Ewing Lecturer Award of the James Ewing Society, 1974
Distinguished Service Award of the Pennsylvania Medical Society, 1975
Papanicolaou Award for Distinguished Service, Papanicolaou Cancer Research Institute, 1977
The Philadelphia Award for 1976
Physician of the Year Award, National Foundation for Ileitis and Colitis (Philadelphia Chapter), 1977
Distinguished Service Award, The American Surgical Association, 1979
Distinguished Service Award, The American Trauma Society, 1979
Prix de la Société Internationale de Chirurgie, 1979
American Medical Association Dr. Rodman E. and Thomas G. Sheen Award for 1979 for Scientific Accomplishment, 1980
National Cancer Institute Medal, 50th Anniversary of the National Coalition for Cancer Research, 1987
The Surgeon General's Medallion, 1987
The Swanberg Award, American Medical Writers Association, 1987
Distinguished Service Award, College of Physicians of Philadelphia 1987
Medal of the Surgeon General of the United States, 1988
Benjamin Franklin Medal of The American Philosophical Society, 1988

Membership in Academies and Professional Societies
American Academy of Arts and Sciences, Member of Council, 1977–1981
American Association for the Advancement of Science, Council Delegate of Electorate N, 1982–1985 Secretary Section N 1985
American Association for Cancer Research
American Association for the Surgery of Trauma
American Association of University Professors
American Geriatrics Society
American Heart Association
American Institute of Biological Sciences
American Institute of Nutrition

American Medical Association
American Medical Writers Association
American Philosophical Society, Secretary, 1963–1966; President, 1977–1984, Executive Committee, Chairman 250th Anniversary Celebration,
American Physiological Society
American Public Health Association
American Society for Parenteral and Enteral Nutrition, Board of Advisors
American Society of Contemporary Medicine and Surgery
American Surgical Association, President, 1972–1973; Council, 1972–1976
Association for Academic Surgery, Executive Council, 1971
Association for the Advancement of Medical Instrumentation
Association of American Medical Colleges, Executive Council, 1967–1972; Council of Academic Societies, Chairman, 1968–1969; Administrative Board, 1969–1972; Distinguished Service Member, 1974–
Association of Community Cancer Centers
Association of Governing Boards of Colleges and Universities
College of Physicians of Philadelphia, Chairman, Library Committee, 1952–1954; President, 1958–1960; ex-Presidential Councilor, 1960; Censor, 1965–1975; Steering Committee of Francis Clark Wood Institute, 1982–; Council; Committee on Planning and Development; Editorial Committee; Board Member, 1987–; Ad Hoc Committee on Interdisciplinary Colloquia,
Collegium Internationale Chirurgiae Digestivae
Council of Medical Specialty Societies, Chairman, 1968–1969
Digestive Disease Foundation
Federation of American Societies for Experimental Biology
Fellows in American Studies
Gerontological Society
Hawthorne Surgical Society
International Federation of Surgical Colleges, Executive Council, 1969–; Vice President, 1972–1978; President, 1978–1981, Honorary Pres., 1987–
International Society of Blood Transfusion
International Surgical Group, President, 1958–1959
Johns Hopkins Medical and Surgical Association
Medical Club
Medical Club of Philadelphia
Medical Society for the Study of Education
John Morgan Society
New York Academy of Sciences (Life Member)
Pan-American Medical Association
Pan-Pacific Surgical Association, Vice President, 1974–1977
Pennsylvania Association of Blood Banks
Pennsylvania Medical Society
Pennsylvania Public Health Association
Pennsylvania Society for Advancing Medical Research
Philadelphia Academy of Surgery, Recorder, 1950–1954; Chairman, Committee on Scientific Business, 1955–1959; Council Member at Large, 1960–1961; First Vice President, 1962–1963; President, 1964–1966
Philadelphia County Medical Society, President, 1970; Investment Committee, Chrm. 1987–8. Past Presidents' Council; Deans' Committee
Philadelphia Medico-Legal Institute
Physiological Society of Philadelphia
Ravdin-Rhoads Surgical Society
Royal Society for the Promotion of Health
Royal Society of Medicine
Société Internationale de Chirurgie
Society for Academic Achievement
Society for Health and Human Values
Society of Clinical Surgery, President, 1958–1960

Society of Surgical Chairman, President, 1966–1968
Society of University Surgeons
Southern Surgical Association
Surgeons Travel Club, President, 1975–1976
Surgical Infection Society, Founding Member; Chairman, Education Committee, Pres. 1985–6.
Allen O. Whipple Surgical Society
Wistar Association, Executive Committee, 1971–1973
World Medical Association
Worcester Foundation for Experimental Biology

Miscellaneous

Adult Education Council of Philadelphia
American Council for the United Nations University, 1977–
Council of Biology Editors
Citizens Crime Commission of Philadelphia
Franklin Institute
Germantown Friends School, School Committee and Chairman, Finance Committee, Treasurer.
Johns Hopkins University Philadelphia Alumni Association
Life Insurance Medical Research Fund, Advisory Council, 1961–1965
Papanicolaou Cancer Research Institute, Scientific Advisory Committee, 1971–1976
Pennsylvania Citizens Association
The Pennsylvania Society
Philadelphia Athenenaeum
Philadelphia Commission on AIDS, Member, 1987–
Philadelphia Medical Political Action Committee
Philadelphia Orchestra Association
Philadelphia Society for the Preservation of Landmarks
Milford D. Schulz Lectureship Committee
Science and Art Club of Germantown
Sunday Breakfast Club
University of Miami School of Medicine, Visiting Committee, 1969–1973
University of Pennsylvania Twenty-Five Year Club, Chairman, 1984
University of Texas System Cancer Center, Consultant to the Director of Scientific Affairs, 1973–1976
Widows and Single Women's Society of Philadelphia, Advisory Board, 1973–
William Penn Statue Restoration Fund, Co-Chairman, Philadelphia Yearly Meeting of Friends, 1987

Board Memberships

Advisory Committee on the John Scott Award for the Board of Directors of City Trusts, Philadelphia, 1975–
American Board of Surgery, Representative of the American Surgical Association, 1963–1969; Senior Member, 1969–
The American Cancer Society, Director at Large, 1965–1969; Executive Committee, 1967–1971; Medical and Scientific Committee, Chairman, 1967–1968; Vice President and President-elect, 1968–1969; President, 1969–1970; Past Officer Director, 1971–1977; Honorary Life Member, 1977–; Board of Directors, Philadelphia Division, 1951–; President; Philadelphia Division, 1955–1956; Honorary Life Member, 1978–
American College of Surgeons, Governor, 1954–1961; Board of Regents, 1961–1970; Vice Chairman, Board of Regents 1965–1967; Chairman, Board of Regents, 1967–1969; President-elect, 1970–1971; President, 1971–1972; Advisory Council to the Board of Regents, 1972–
American Trauma Society, Founding Member, Board of Directors, Executive Committee, Finance Committee, Chairman, 1987–8
Associated Universities, Board of Trustees, 1961–1963
Board of Public Education of the City of Philadelphia, December 1965–January 1971

Bryn Mawr College, Board of Trustees, 1960–1979; Board of Directors, 1969–1979; Trustee Emeritus, 1979–

Fox Chase Cancer Center, Board of Directors, 1975–

Friends Hospital, Board of Managers, 1952–; Finance Committee, 1978–

General Motors Cancer Research Foundation, Chairman of Awards Assembly, 1978–; Board of Trustees, 1978–

Haverford College, Board of Managers of the Corporation, 1947–; President of the Corporation, 1963–1977; Chairman of the Board of Managers, 1963–1972; Finance Committee, 1968–

Independence Hall Association, Board of Directors, 1980–1987; Council of Advisors, 1987–

The Institute for Medical Research, Board of Trustees, 1957–; Vice President for Scientific Affairs, 1964–76

InTerAx, Board of Directors, 1973–1975

Benjamin and Mary Siddons Measey Foundation, Board of Directors, 1971–; Chairman, 1978–

Pennwalt Corporation, Board of Directors, 1966–1977

Philadelphia Health Management Corporation, Board of Directors, 1973–1981

Philadelphia Professional Standards Review Organization, Board of Directors, 1974–1981; Executive Committee, 1974–1981; President, 1974–1981

Philadelphia Yearly Meeting, Society of Friends, Representative Meeting, 1973–; Chairman, Bequests Committee, 1980–

Provident Mutual Life Insurance Company, Board of Directors, 1956–1977

The Quadrangle, Board of Directors, 1981–

J. E. Rhoads and Sons, Board of Directors, 1976–

Society for Surgery of the Alimentary Tract, President, 1967–1968; Board of Trustees, 1968–1970

Westtown School, Executive Committee; Finance and Budget Committees; Committee in Charge of Westtown School; Capital Campaign Steering Committee, 1980; National Chairman, Third Century Fund, 1981–1985.

Pennsylvania Hospital, Honorary Member, Board of Managers

Club Memberships

Cosmos Club

Faculty Club of the University of Pennsylvania

Haverford Club of Philadelphia

Peale Club

Penn Club

Philadelphia Art Alliance

Philadelphia Club

Rittenhouse Club

Union League of Philadelphia

Visiting Professorships and Lectureships

Surgeon-in-Chief pro tem—Rhode Island Hospital, Providence, R.I., 1957

Visiting Professor of Surgery—University of Manitoba, Winnepeg, Canada, 1958

Visiting Lecturer—Ogden Surgical Society, Ogden, Utah, 1960

Visiting Lecturer—Reno Surgical Society, Reno, Nevada, 1960

Visiting Professor of Surgery—Hartford Hospital, Hartford, Conn., 1960

Visiting Professor of Surgery—Marquette University, Milwaukee, Wisconsin, 1963

Visiting Professor—University of Illinois, Abraham Lincoln School of Medicine, Chicago, Ill., 1973

Visiting Lecturer—Roswell Park Memorial Institute, Buffalo, N.Y., 1973

Visiting Lecturer—Milwaukee Surgical Society, Milwaukee, Wisconsin, 1973

Visiting Professor of Surgery—Allegheny General Hospital, Pittsburgh, Pa., 1973

Visiting Professor of Surgery—Vanderbilt University (Barney Brooks Lecture), Nashville, Tenn., 1973
Visiting Professor of Surgery—Downstate Medical Center, Brooklyn, N.Y., 1973
Address to the Royal College of Surgeons of Edinburgh, Edinburgh, Scotland, 1973
Visiting Lecturer—Washington Hospital Center, Washington, D.C., 1974
Visiting Lecturer—Rutgers Medical School, Piscataway, N.J., 1974
Visiting Lecturer—Maui Memorial Hospital, Wailuku, Maui, Hawaii, 1974
James Ewing Lecturer—Maui, Hawaii, 1974
Visiting Lecturer—Bryn Mawr Hospital (Third Annual Dr. Alan Parker Memorial Lecture), Bryn Mawr, Pa., 1974
Visiting Professor—University of Mississippi Medical Center (AOA Lecture), Jackson, Mississippi, 1974
Visiting Lecturer—Southwestern Michigan Surgical Society, Kalamazoo, Mich., 1974
President d'honneur—Congres International de Nutrition Parenterale, Montpellier, France, 1974
Visiting Professor of Surgery—Norfolk General Hospital and Eastern Virginia Medical School, Norfolk, Va., 1974
Alumni Day Lecturer—California Institute of Technology, Pasadena, Ca., 1975
Visiting Professor of Surgery—State University of New York at Stony Brook, Stony Brook, N.Y., 1975
Visiting Professor of Surgery—University of Texas Medical School at Houston, 1975
Visiting Professor of Surgery—Hospital for Joint Diseases and Medical Center, New York, 1976
Visiting Professor of Surgery—Medical Center of Western Massachusetts, Springfield, Mass., 1976
Visiting Professor—Einstein College of Medicine of Yeshiva University, Bronx, N.Y., 1977
Visiting Lecturer—Massachusetts General Hospital, Boston, Mass., 1978
Visiting Professor—Duke University, Durham, N.C., 1979
Visiting Lecturer—American Cancer Society, California Division (John W. Cline Memorial Lecture), Sacramento, Ca., 1979
Visiting Lecturer—Clinical Oncological Society of Australia, Sydney, Australia, 1979
Visiting Lecturer—The Cancer Institute (Peter McCallum Lecture), Melbourne, Australia, 1979
Visiting Professor—Ohio State University Department of Surgery, Columbus, Ohio, 1980
Visiting Lecturer—College of Medicine & Dentistry of New Jersey, Newark, N.J., 1981
Visiting Lecturer—North Ridge General Hospital Symposium, Ft. Lauderdale, Fla., 1982
Roswell Park Memorial Lecture, Buffalo, New York, 1982
Visiting Professor of Surgery—University of South Florida, Tampa, Fla., 1982
Visiting Professor of Surgery—AOA Lecture, Temple University, Philadelphia, 1982
Visiting Professor of Surgery—University of Iowa, Iowa City, Iowa, 1982
Third Sonneborn Memorial Lecture, Jeanes Hospital & Fox Chase Cancer Center, 1982
Visiting Professor of Surgery—Temple University Hospital, 1982
Samuel Harvey Lecture, Yale University, 1983
Visiting Professor—Rutgers Medical School, Camden, N.J., 1983
Althouse Lecture, Hershey Medical Center, Hershey, Pa., 1983
Visiting Professor—Guthrie Clinic, Sayre, Pa., 1984
Visiting Professor at Stony Brook, New York, 1984
Visiting Professor—University of Illinois Medical School, Rockford, Ill., 1984
Longmire Lecture, Los Angeles, California, 1984
Shumacker Lecture, Indiana Chapter ACS, 1985
William H. Muller Visiting Professor—University of Medicine, Gainesville, Fla., 1988

Bibliography

1. Ravdin, I. S. and Rhoads, J. E. Certain Problems Illustrating the Importance of a Knowledge of Biochemistry by the Surgeon. *Surg Clin North Am* 15:85–100, 1935.
2. Rhoads, J. E. and Mecray, P. M., Jr. Recurrence in Mixed Tumors of the Soft Palate. *Am J Med Sci* 193:389–394, 1937.
3. Rhoads, J. E., Hottenstein, H. F. and Hudson, I. F. The Decline in the Strength of Catgut after Exposure to Living Tissues. *Arch Surg* 34:377–397, 1937.

4. Ravdin, I. S. and Rhoads, J. E. Regional Ileitis and Fibroplastic Appendicitis. *Ann Surg* 106:394–406, 1937.
5. Rhoads, J. E. and Terrell, A. W. Ovarian Fibroma with Ascites and Hydrothorax (Meigs' Syndrome). *JAMA* 109:1684–1687, 1937.
6. Rhoads, J. E. The Use of Zinc Peroxide in Microaerophilic Infections. *Surgery* 2:937–942, 1937.
7. Thompson, W. D., Ravdin, I. S., Rhoads, J. E. and Frank, I. L. Use of Lyophile Plasma in Correction of Hypoproteinemia and Prevention of Wound Disruption. *Arch Surg* 36:509–518, 1938.
8. Ravdin, I. S., Rhoads, J. E., Frazier, W. D. and Ulin, A. W. The Effect of Recent Advances in Biliary Physiology on the Mortality following Operation for Common Duct Obstruction. *Surgery* 3:805–814, 1938.
9. Rhoads, J. E. and Stein, E. Splenectomy and Ligation of Gastric Coronary Vessels. *Am J Dis Children* 56:119–125, 1938.
10. Rhoads, J. E. Peritoneal Lavage in the Treatment of Renal Insufficiency. *Am J Med Sci* 196:642–647, 1938.
11. Rhoads, J. E. and Panzer, L. M. The Prothrombin Time of "Bank Blood". *JAMA* 112:309–310, 1939.
12. Rhoads, J. E., Stengel, A., Jr., Riegel, C., Cajori, F. A. and Frazier, W. D. The Absorption of Protein Split Products from Chronic Isolated Colon Loops. *Am J Physiol* 125:707–712, 1939.
13. Rhoads, J. E. The Relation of Vitamin K to the Hemorrhagic Tendency in Obstructive Jaundice, with a Report of Cerophyl as a Source of Vitamin K. *Surgery* 5:794–808, 1939.
14. Rhoads, J. E. The Management of Regional Ileitis and Certain Other Ulcerative Lesions of the Intestines. *Pa Med J* 42:1050–1953, 1939.
15. Warren, R. and Rhoads, J. E. The Hepatic Origin of the Plasma-prothrombin Observations after Total Hepatectomy in the Dog. *Am J Med Sci* 198:193–197, 1939.
16. Lockwood, J. S. and Rhoads, J. E. The Use of Sulfanilamide in the Treatment of Peritonitis. *Surg Clin North Am* 19:1457–1464, 1939.
17. Ravdin, I. S., Rhoads, J. E. and Lockwood, J. S. The Use of Sulfanilamide in the Treatment of Peritonitis Associated with Appendicitis. *Ann Surg* 111:53–63, 1940.
18. Rhoads, J. E. and Fliegelman, M. T. The Use of 2-Methyl-1, 4-Naphthoquinone (A Synthetic Vitamin K Substitute) in the Treatment of Prothrombin Deficiency in Patients. *JAMA* 114:400–401, 1940.
19. Rhoads, J. E. The Treatment of Prothrombin Deficiencies with Vitamin K. *New Int Clin* 1:209–220, 1940.
20. Rhoads, J. E. and Ravdin, I. S. The Control of Hemorrhage in Patients Operated on for Obstructive Jaundice. *Rev Gastroenterol* 7:169–176, 1940.
21. Ravdin, I. S., Lockwood, J. S. and Rhoads, J. E. The Use of Sulfanilamide in the Treatment of Peritonitis of Appendiceal Origin. *Pa Med J* 43:1100, 1940.
22. Wolff, W. A., Elkinton, J. R. and Rhoads, J. E. Liver Damage and Dextrose Tolerance in Severe Burns. *Ann Surg* 112:158–160, 1940.
23. Rhoads, J. E. Physiologic Factors Regulating the Level of the Plasma Prothrombin. *Ann Surg* 112:568–574, 1940.
24. Rhoads, J. E., Wolff, W. A. and Lee, W. E. The Use of Adrenal Cortical Extract in the Treatment of Traumatic Shock of Burns. *Ann Surg* 113:955–968, 1941.
25. Fliegelman, M. T., Panzer, L. M. and Rhoads, J. E. The Effect of Colloidal Aluminum Hydroxide on Certain Aspects of Blood Coagulation. *Surgery* 10:387–390, 1941.
26. Rhoads, J. E. and Fitz-Hugh, T., Jr. Idiopathic Hyproprothrombinemia—An Apparently Unrecorded Condition. *Am J Med Sci* 202:662–670, 1941.
27. Rhoads, J. E., Warren, R. and Panzer, L. M. Experimental Hypoprothrombinemia. *Am J Med Sci* 202:847–861, 1941.
28. Rhoads, J. E. and Norris, R. F. Effect of Vitamin K Therapy on Plasma Prothrombin Level of Patients without Prothrombin Deficiency. *Bull Ayer Clin Lab*, Pennsylvania Hospital 3:359–363, 1941.
29. Rhoads, J. E. and Kasinskas, W. The Influence of Hypoproteinemia on the Formation of Callus in Experimental Fracture. *Surgery* 11:38–44, 1942.
30. Rhoads, J. E., Fliegelman, M. T. and Panzer, L. M. The Mechanism of Delayed Wound Healing in the Presence of Hypoproteinemia. *JAMA* 118:21–25, 1942.
31. Rhoads, J. E. and Lee, W. E. The Advantages of Combining Local Infiltration Anesthesia with Controlled Fractional Spinal Anesthesia in Substandard Surgical Risks. *Ann Surg* 115:156–158, 1942.
32. Rhoads, J. E., Wolff, W. A., Saltonstall, H. and Lee, W. E. The Use of Plasma in the Treatment of Shock Due to Burns. *Clinics* 1:37–42, 1942.
33. Lee, W. E., Wolff, W. A., Saltonstall, H. and Rhoads, J. E. Recent Trends in the Therapy of Burns. *Ann Surg* 115:1131–1139, 1942.
34. Rhoads, J. E. The Advantages and Dangers of Blood and Plasma Banks. *Hospitals* 16:80, 1942.
35. Rhoads, J. E., Wolff, W. A. and Lee, W. E. The Use of Sulfonamides in the Local Treatment of Burns. *Pa Med J* 46:13–16, 1942.
36. Wolff, W. A., Rhoads, J. E. and Lee, W. E. Recent Developments in the Treatment of Severe Third Degree Burns. *Nebr State Med J* 27:369–374, 1942.
37. Ravdin, I. S., Lockwood, J. S. and Rhoads, J. E. The Results of Sulfonamide Prophylaxis in the Surgery of the Large Bowel. *Surg Clin North Am* 22:1585–1591, 1942.
38. Ravdin, I. S., Thorogood, E., Riegel, C., Peters, R. and Rhoads, J. E. The Prevention of Liver Damage and the Facilitation of Repair in the Liver by Diet. *JAMA* 121:322–324, 1943.
39. Rhoads, J. E. Progress and Conservatism in Anesthesia. *Jackson Co Med Bull* Feb 27, 1943.

40. Maris, E. P., McGuinness, A. C., Lee, H. R., Rhoads, J. E. and Lee, W. E. The Pre- and Post-operative Use of Metal Tipped Gastroduodenal Tube as an Aid in the Surgical Treatment of Duodenal Obstruction in the Newborn. *Ann Surg* 117:348, 1943.
41. Rhoads, J. E. Problems of Fluid Balance in the Traumatized Patient. *Ann Intern Med* 18:988–990, 1943.
42. Ravdin, I. S., Royster, H. P., Riegel, C. and Rhoads, J. E. Surgical Care of Patients with Gastric Cancer before and after Operation. *Arch Surg* 46:871–878, 1943
43. Rhoads, J. E., Riegel, C., Koop, C. E. and Ravdin, I. S. The Problem of Nutrition in Patients with Gastric Lesions Requiring Surgery. *Western J Surg Gynec Obstet* 51:229–233, 1943.
44. Rhoads, J. E., Walker, J. and Panzer, L. Control of Blood Coagulability with Coumarin and Other Drugs. *Northwest Med* 42:182–185, 1943.
45. Zintel, H. A., Rhoads, J. E. and Ravdin, I. S. The Use of Intravenous Ammonium Chloride in the Treatment of Alkalosis. *Surgery* 14:728–741, 1943.
46. Rhoads, J. E., Wolff, W. A., Saltonstall, H. and Lee, W. E. Further Experiences with Adrenal Cortical Extract in the Treatment of Burn Shock. *Ann Surg* 118:932–987, 1943.
47. Horn, R. C., Jr. and Rhoads, J. E. Regional Enteritis Involving Meckel's Diverticulum: Perforation of the Diverticulum and Fistula Formation. *Ann Surg* 119:274–278, 1944.
48. Walker, J. and Rhoads, J. E. Effect of Dicumarol on Susceptibility to Action of Heparin. *Surgery* 15:859–865, 1944.
49. Ravdin, I. S., McNamee, H. G., Kamholz, J. H. and Rhoads, J. E. Effect of Hypoproteinemia on Susceptibility to Shock Resulting from Hemorrhage. *Arch Surg* 48:491–492, 1944.
50. Lee, W. E. and Rhoads, J. E. The Present Status of the Tannic Acid Method in the Treatment of Burns. *JAMA* 125:610–612, 1944.
51. Zintel, H. A., Riegel, C., Peters, R., Rhoads, J. E. and Ravdin, I. S. Intravenous Administration of Dextrose in the Treatment of Patients with Disease of the Biliary Tract. *Arch Surg* 49:238–240, 1944.
52. Rhoads, J. E. and Ravdin, I. S. The Influence of Sulfonamides on Postoperative Complications. *Ann Surg* 120:463–467, 1944. *Trans Am Surg Assoc* 62:463, 1944.
53. Rhoads, J. E. Symposium on Recent Advances in Surgery. *Surg Clin North Am* 24:1281–1289, 1944.
54. Saltonstall, H., Walker, J., Jr., Rhoads, J. E. and Lee, W. E. The Influence of Local Treatment of Burns on Liver Function. *Ann Surg* 121:291–300, 1945.
55. Rhoads, J. E. Some Newer Aspects of the Treatment of Burns. *Clinics* 3:1618–1622, 1945.
56. Riegel, C., Rhoads, J. E., Koop, C. E., Grigger, R. P., Bullitt, L. and Barrus, D. Dietary Requirements for Nitrogen Equilibrium in the Period Immediately Following Certain Major Surgical Operations. *Am J Med Sci* 210:133–134, 1945.
57. Riegel, C., Koop, C. E., Grigger, R. P., Rhoads, J. E. and Bullitt, L. The Protein Requirements of Surgical Patients during the Postoperative Period. *Surg Clin North Am* 25:1096–1105, 1945.
58. Zintel, H. A., Flippin, H. F., Nichols, A. C., Wiley, M. M. and Rhoads, J. E. Studies on Streptomycin in Man. 1. Absorption, Distribution, Excretion and Toxicity. *Am J Med Sci* 210:421–430, 1945.
59. Rhoads, J. E. The Peritoneum. Chapter 76 in Bockus, H. L., *Gastroenterology*. Philadelphia, W. B. Saunders Company, 1945, pp. 902–925.
60. Rhoads, J. E. The Mesentery and Omentum. Chapter 77 in Bockus, H. L., *Gastroenterology*. Philadelphia, W. B. Saunders Company, 1945, pp. 926–946.
61. Rhoads, J. E. The Skin and Subjacent Tissues: Wounds. Chapter 5 in *Davis-Christopher Textbook of Surgery*, 4th Edition. Philadelphia, W. B. Saunders Company, 1945, pp. 98–112.
62. Walker, J., Jr., Saltonstall, H., Rhoads, J. E. and Lee, W. E. Toxemia Syndrome after Burns: Biochemical and Pathologic Observations and Studies. *Arch Surg* 52:177–186, 1946.
63. Chandy, J. and Rhoads, J. E. Experimental Studies on the Mechanism of the Formation of Intraperitoneal Adhesions. *Fed Proc* 5:218, 1946.
64. Koop, C. E., Drew, J. H., Riegel, C. and Rhoads, J. E. Studies on Nutrition. The Effect of Preoperative Force-feeding on Surgical Patients. *Am J Med Sci* 211:752, 1946. *Ann Surg* 124:1165–1176, 1946.
65. Rhoads, J. E. The Pathologic Physiology of Hyperthyroidism. *Surg Clin North Am* 26:1454–1461, 1946.
66. Riegel, C., Koop, C. E., Drew, J., Stevens, L. W. and Rhoads, J. E. The Nutritional Requirements for Nitrogen Balance in Surgical Patients during the Early Postoperative Period. *J Clin Invest* 26:18–23, 1947.
67. Zintel, H. A., Wiley, M., Nichols, A. and Rhoads, J. E. The Use of Streptomycin in Surgical Patients. *Surgery* 21:175–183, 1947.
68. Horn, R. C., Jr., Welty, R. F., Brooks, F. P., Rhoads, J. E. and Pendergrass, E. P. Carcinoma of the Thyroid. *Ann Surg* 126:140–155, 1947.
69. Harris, T. N., Rhoads, J. E. and Stokes, J., Jr. A Study of the Role of the Thymus and Spleen in the Formation of Antibodies in the Rabbit. *J Immunol* 58:27–32, 1948.
70. Kirby, C. K. and Rhoads, J. E. The Present Status of the Treatment of Thrombosis and Embolism in Surgical Patients. *Pa Med J* 51:638–641, 1948.
71. Rhoads, J. E., Pipes, R. L. and Randall, J. P. A Simultaneous Abdominal and Perineal Approach in Operations for Imperforate Anus with Atresia of the Rectum and Rectosigmoid. *Ann Surg* 127:552–556, 1948.
72. Rhoads, J. E. Recent Advances in Pre- and Postoperative Care. *Pa Med J* 52:207–209, 1948.
73. Rhoads, J. E. Wounds. Chapter 17 in *Davis-Christopher Textbook of Surgery*, 5th Edition. Philadelphia, W. B. Saunders Company, 1949, pp. 689–702.

74. Rhoads, J. E. The Use of Antibiotics in Surgery. *Southwestern Med* May 1949, pp. 88–92.
75. Rhoads, J. E. Surgical Therapy in Ulcerative Colitis. *Rev Gastroenterol* 16:480–486, 1949.
76. Sawyer, P. N., Rhoads, J. E. and Panzer, R. An Evaluation of Electrogastrography in the Diagnosis of Gastric Cancer. *Surgery* 26:479–487, 1949.
77. Machella, T. E., Rhoads, J. E. and Hobler, R. E. Gastric Hyperchlorhydria with Three Primary Jejunal Ulcers and Hypoproteinemia. *Gastroenterol* 13:357–366, 1949.
78. Rhoads, J. E. The Place of Research in a Surgical Training Program (Editorial). *Ann Surg* 130:855–856, 1949.
79. Rhoads, J. E. The Surgical Physiology of the Gastrointestinal Tract. *Surg Clin North Am* 29:1764–1774, 1949.
80. Rhoads, J. E., Howard, J. M. and Moss, N. H. Clinical Experiences with Surgical Lesions of the Pancreas. *Surg Clin North Am* 29:1801–1816, 1949.
81. Rhoads, J. E. and Zintel, H. A. The Use of Antibiotics in Surgery. Reprinted from *Adv Surg* 1:221–268, 1949.
82. Rhoads, J. E. Indications for and Results of Surgical Procedures in Pronounced Portal Hypertension. Reprinted from Bockus, H. L., *Postgraduate Gastroenterology.* Philadelphia, W. B. Saunders Company, 1950, pp. 1–7.
83. Rhoads, J. E. Nutritional Requirements for the Surgical Patient. *Conn State Med J* 14:189–195, 1950.
84. Howard, J. M., Moss, N. H. and Rhoads, J. E. Hyperinsulinism and Islet Cell Tumors of the Pancreas. *Surg Gynec Obstet* 90:417–455, 1950.
85. Rhoads, J. E. Symposium on the Diagnosis and Management of Benign and Malignant Lesions of the Stomach: Surgical Aspects. *Del State Med J* 22:98–106, 1950.
86. Thomas, J., Jackson, G., Portnoff, C., Chandy, J. and Rhoads, J. E. Further Experiments on Influence of Hyaluronidase on Formation of Intraperitoneal Adhesions in the Rat. *Proc Soc Exp Biol Med* 74:497–498, 1950.
87. Thomas, J. W. and Rhoads, J. E. Adhesions Resulting from Removal of Serosa from an Area of Bowel: Failure of "Oversewing" to Lower Incidence in the Rat and the Guinea Pig. *Arch Surg* 61:565–567, 1950.
88. Rhoads, J. E. The Use and Abuse of the Miller-Abbott Tube (Editorial). *Surg Gynec Obstet* 92:244–246, 1951.
89. Rhoads, J. E. and Darrow, R. P. Acute Appendicitis and Its Complications. *Pa Med J* 54:435–439, 1951.
90. Rhoads, J. E., Liboro, O., Fox, S., Gyorgy, P. and Machella, T. E. Observations on the *in vivo* Action of a New Lipotropic Fraction of the Pancreas. *Am J Med Sci* 221:595, 1951.
91. Rhoads, J. E. Surgical Considerations in Management of Thromboembolic Disease. *Phila Med* 46:1496–1497, 1951.
92. Rhoads, J. E., Liboro, O., Fox, S., Gyorgy, P. and Machella, T. E. *In vivo* Action of a New Lipotropic Fraction of the Pancreas. *Am J Physiol* 166:436–440, 1951.
93. Rhoads, J. E. A Career in Surgery (Editorial). *Ann Surg* 134:782, 1951.
94. Rhoads, J. E. The Diagnosis and Management of Carcinoma of the Stomach. *Surg Clin North Am* 31:1705–1711, 1951.
95. Maxwell, D. B., Horn, R. C., Jr. and Rhoads, J. E. Cysts of the Parathyroid: Report of Three Cases Clinically Simulating Nodular Goiter. *Arch Surg* 64:208–213, 1952.
96. Rhoads, J. E., Zintel, H. A. and Horn, R. C., Jr. Masculinovoblastoma or Masculinizing Adrenal Rest Tumor of Ovary: Report of a Case. *JAMA* 148:551–552, 1952.
97. Rhoads, J. E. Malignancy of the Colon and Rectum. *VA Tech Bull*, Series TB 10-82, 1952, pp. 1–13.
98. Rhoads, J. E. and Kirby, C. K. The Use of Anticoagulants in Thromboembolic Disease. *Advances in Medicine and Surgery.* Philadelphia, W. B. Saunders Company, 1952, pp. 217–226.
99. Rose, E. K., Enterline, H. T., Rhoads, J. E. and Rose, E. Adrenal Cortical Hyperfunction in Childhood: Report of a Case with Adrenocortical Hyperplasia and Testicular Adrenal Rests. *Pediatrics* 9:475–484, 1952.
100. Rhoads, J. E. Protein Nutrition in Surgical Patients. *Surg Gynec Obstet* 94:417–427, 1952.
101. Rhoads, J. E. Protein Nutrition in Surgical Patients. *Fed Proc* 11:659–665, 1952.
102. Rhoads, J. E. The Current Status of Plasma Volume Expanders. *Southwestern Med* 33:326–332, 1952.
103. Rhoads, J. E. Various Plasma Expanders in Man. *Ann NY Acad Sci* 55:522–525, 1952.
104. Rhoads, J. E. Studies on the Formation of Peritoneal Adhesions (Annual Address, 1948. *Trans Phila Acad Surg 1943–1950* 28:76–89, 1952.
105. Rhoads, J. E. The Management of Burns with Special Reference to Rehabilitation. *Phys Ther Rev* 33:509–513, 1952.
106. Hagan, W. H. and Rhoads, J. E. Inguinal and Femoral Hernias: A Follow-up Study. *Surg Gynec Obstet* 96:226–232, 1953.
107. Thomas, J. W., Lehr, H. B. and Rhoads, J. E. Clinical Experience with Fluid Gelatin. *Surgical Forum.* Philadelphia, W. B. Saunders Company, 1953, pp. 154–157.
108. Rosenthal, O., Stainback, W. C., Rhoads, J. E. and Engelberg, J. The Utilization of Invert Sugar and Glucose following Intravenous Administration of Postoperative Patients. *Surgical Forum.* Philadelphia, W. B. Saunders Company, 1952, pp. 585–589.
109. Rhoads, J. E. Mass Treatment of Burns. *Pa Med J* 56:191–194, 1953.
110. Blakemore, W. S., Dumke, P. R. and Rhoads, J. E. Gangrene Following Intra-arterial Transfusion: Report of Two Cases. *JAMA* 151:988–989, 1953.

111. Ravdin, I. S., Walker, J. M. and Rhoads, J. E. Blood Volume Maintenance and Regulation. *Ann Rev Physiol* 15:165–194, 1953.
112. Rhoads, J. E. Supranormal Dietary Requirements of Acutely Ill Patients. *J Am Diet Assoc* 29:897–903, 1953.
113. Zintel, H. A., Enterline, H. T. and Rhoads, J. E. Benign Cystadenoma of Pancreas: Report of Four Treated Cases, One by Whipple Type of Resection. *Surgery* 35:612–620, 1954.
114. Dyson, W. L., Hodes, P. J. and Rhoads, J. E. Late Results in the Surgical Treatment of Regional Enteritis. *Pa Med J* 57:433–438, 1954.
115. Pitts, F. W. and Rhoads, J. E. Studies of a Drain of a Non-reactive Plastic Teflon. *Surgical Forum.* Philadelphia, W. B. Saunders Company, 1955, pp. 828–830.
116. Scott, S. M., Bevilacqua, J. E., Lehr, H. B., Vars, H. M., Rosenthal, O. and Rhoads, J. E. Clinical Experimental Studies of Fat Emulsions for Intravenous Use. *Trans Southern Surg Assoc* 66:5–7, 1954.
117. Rhoads, J. E. The Transfer of Surgical Experience (Editorial). *Ann Surg* 141:283–284, 1955.
118. Rhoads, J. E. Extensive Superficial Burns. *Pa Med J* 58:391–394, 1955.
119. Kirby, C. K., Senior, J. R., Howard, J. M. and Rhoads, J. E. Death Due to Delayed Hemorrhage in Acute Pancreatitis. *Surg Gynec Obstet* 100:458–462, 1955.
120. Rhoads, J. E., Senior, J. R., Kirby, C. K. and Rhoads, D. V. Surgery of the Pancreas. *Miss Doctor* 33:55–58, 1955.
121. Rhoads, J. E. and Koop, C. E. The Surgical Management of Imperforate Anus. *Surg Clin North Am* 35:1251–1257, 1955.
122. Rhoads, J. E. and Alexander, C. E. Nutritional Problems of Surgical Patients. *Ann NY Acad Sci* 63:268–275, 1955.
123. Rhoads, J. E., Vaun, W. S., Perkins, W. M., Ben, M. and Vars, H. M. Shock. *Surg Clin North Am* 35:1585–1595, 1955.
124. Rhoads, J. E. The Surgical Management of Pancreatic Tumors. *West J Surg Obstet Gynec* 64:62–69, 1956.
125. Rhoads, J. E., Roberts, B. and Helwig, J., Jr. The Metabolic Response to Trauma. *Ann Rev Med* 7:141–156, 1956.
126. Rhoads, J. E., Allen, J. G., Harkins, H. N. and Moyer, C. A. Surgical Philosophy. Chapter 1 in Allen, J. G., Harkins, H. N., Moyer, C. A. and Rhoads, J. E. *Surgery: Principles and Practice.* Philadelphia, J. B. Lippincott Company, 1957, pp. 1–5.
127. Rhoads, J. E. Fluid and Electrolytes. Chapter 5 in Allen, J. G., Harkins, H. N., Moyer, C. A. and Rhoads, J. E. *Surgery: Principles and Practice.* Philadelphia, J. B. Lippincott Company, 1957, pp. 65–79.
128. Rhoads, J. E. Nutrition. Chapter 6 in Allen, J. G., Harkins, H. N., Moyer, C. A. and Rhoads, J. E. *Surgery: Principles and Practice.* Philadelphia, J. B. Lippincott Company, 1957, pp. 80–96.
129. Moyer, C. A. and Rhoads, J. E. Neoplastic Disease—General Considerations. Chapter 10 in Allen, J. G., Harkins, H. N., Moyer, C. A. and Rhoads, J. E. *Surgery: Principles and Practice.* Philadelphia, J. B. Lippincott Company, 1957, pp. 163–174.
130. Moyer, C. A. and Rhoads, J. E. Skin and Subcutaneous Tissues. Chapter 24 in Allen, J. G., Harkins, H. N., Moyer, C. A. and Rhoads, J. E. *Surgery: Principles and Practice.* Philadelphia, J. B. Lippincott Company, 1957, pp. 485–500.
131. Rhoads, J. E. Liver, Gallbladder and Bile Passages. Chapter 30 in Allen, J. G., Harkins, H. N., Moyer, C. A. and Rhoads, J. E. *Surgery: Principles and Practice.* Philadelphia, J. B. Lippincott Company, 1957, pp. 687–714.
132. Rhoads, J. E. Pancreas. Chapter 31 in Allen, J. G., Harkins, H. N., Moyer, C. A. and Rhoads, J. E. *Surgery: Principles and Practice.* Philadelphia, J. B. Lippincott Company, 1957, pp. 715–740.
133. Rhoads, J. E. Trends in Medical Education. *Arch Phys Med Rehabil* 38:587–591, 1957.
134. Rhoads, J. E., Zintel, H. A. and Helwig, J., Jr. Results of Operations of the Whipple Type in Pancreaticoduodenal Carcinoma. *Ann Surg* 146:661–668, 1957.
135. Rhoads, J. E. Development of Preventive Surgery in the Field of Cancer *Ann Surg* 146:782–789, 1957.
136. Rhoads, J. E. Surgical Management of Ulcerative Colitis. *Med Clin North Am* 41:6:1667–1671, 1957.
137. Lehr, H. B., Rosenthal, O., Rawnsley, H. M., Rhoads, J. E. and Sen, M. B. Clinical Experience with Intravenous Fat Emulsions. *Metabolism* 6:6(2):666–672, 1957.
138. Rhoads, J. E. Common Operations—Refinements in a Technique. Introduction. *Surg Clin North Am* 37:1523, 1957.
139. Zintel, H. A., Rhoads, J. E. and Helwig, J., Jr. Surgical Treatment of Carcinoma of the Pancreas. *J Am Geriat Soc* 6(2):143–146, 1958.
140. Rhoads, J. E. Inaugural Remarks. *Trans Stud Coll Physicians Phila* 25:191, 1958.
141. Rhoads, J. E. and Best, R. J. Surgery in the Therapy of Thyroid Disease. *Curr Med Pract* 2:373–379, 1958.
142. Rhoads, J. E. and Orloff, M. J. Pancreatitis. Chapter in Conn, Howard F., Ed., *Current Therapy.* Philadelphia, W. B. Saunders Company, 1959, pp. 226–231.
143. Lyday, J. E., Markarian, M. and Rhoads, J. E. Perforated Duodenal Ulcer in a 2,100 Gram Female Infant, with Survival. *Am J Surg* 97:346, 1959.
144. Rhoads, J. E. President's Address. *Trans Stud Coll Physicians Phila* 26:167–170, 1959.
145. Rhoads, J. E. and Patterson, L. T. Experiences in Treatment of Surgical Lesions of the Pancreas. *Manitoba Med Rev* 39:665, 1959.

146. Zintel, H. A., Rhoads, J. E. and Helwig, J., Jr. Results of Subtotal Pancreatectomy in the Treatment of Carcinoma of the Pancreas. *Western J Surg Obstet Gynec* 67:293, 1959.
147. Rhoads, J. E., Zintel, H. A. and Helwig, J., Jr. An Evaluation of Palliative and Curative Operations in the Treatment of Pancreatoduodenal Carcinomas. *Acta Int Union against Cancer* 16:1397–1401, 1960.
148. Moss, N. H. and Rhoads, J. E. Hyperinsulinism and Islet Cell Tumors of the Pancreas. Chapter 21 in Howard, J. M. and Jordan, G. L., Eds. *Surgical Diseases of the Pancreas.* Philadelphia, J. B. Lippincott Company, 1960, pp. 321–441.
149. Rhoads, J. E. The Increasing Value of Medical Care. *Trans Stud Coll Physicians Phila* 27:147–149, 1960.
150. Rhoads, J. E. Nutrition in Surgery (Symposium: Nutrition; Current Advances with Clinical Applications). *Mod Med* August 1, 1960, pp. 116–123.
151. Rhoads, J. E. Treatment of Pancreatoduodenal Carcinoma by Radical Duodenopancreatectomy, in Mulholland, J. H., Ellison, E. H., and Friesen, S. R., Eds. *Current Surgical Management,* 2nd Edition. Philadelphia, W. B. Saunders Company, 1960, pp. 85–91.
152. Machella, T. E. and Rhoads, J. E. Complications of Gastrointestinal Intubation. Chapter 37 in Artz, C. P. and Hardy, J. D., *Complications of Surgery and Their Management.* Philadelphia, W. B. Saunders Company, 1960, pp. 662–638.
153. Rhoads, J. E. Cancer. *The Encyclopedia Americana,* c. 1961.
154. Rhoads, J. E. Annual Report of the President. *Trans Coll Physicians Phila* 28:149–153, 1961.
155. Grimson, K. S., Moyer, C. A. and Rhoads, J. E. The Dog in Medical Research. *US Public Health Serv Pub No. 312.* Washington, U.S. Government Printing Office, 1961, pp. 1–15.
156. Rhoads, J. E., Allen, J. G., Harkins, H. N. and Moyer, C. A. Surgical Philosophy. Chapter 1 in Harkins, H. N., Moyer, C. A., Rhoads, J. E. and Allen, J. G. *Surgery: Principles and Practice,* 2nd Edition. Philadelphia, J. B. Lippincott Company, 1961, pp 1–5.
157. Rhoads, J. E. Fluid and Electrolytes. Chapter 5 in Harkins, H. N., Moyer, C. A., Rhoads, J. E. and Allen, J. G. *Surgery: Principles and Practice,* 2nd Edition. Philadelphia, J. B. Lippincott Company, 1961, pp 71–85.
158. Rhoads, J. E. Nutrition. Chapter 6 in Harkins, H. N., Moyer, C. A., Rhoads, J. E. and Allen, J. G. *Surgery: Principles and Practice,* 2nd Edition. Philadelphia, J. B. Lippincott Company, 1961, pp 86–103.
159. Moyer, C. A. and Rhoads, J. E. Neoplastic Disease—General Considerations. Chapter 10 in Harkins, H. N., Moyer, C. A., Rhoads, J. E. and Allen, J. G. *Surgery: Principles and Practice,* 2nd Edition. Philadelphia, J. B. Lippincott Company, 1961, pp 172–184.
160. Rhoads, J. E. Liver, Gallbladder and Bile Passages. Chapter 30 in Harkins, H. N., Moyer, C. A., Rhoads, J. E. and Allen, J. G. *Surgery: Principles and Practice,* 2nd Edition. Philadelphia, J. B. Lippincott Company, 1961, pp. 721–754.
161. Rhoads, J. E. Pancreas. Chapter 31 in Harkins, H. N., Moyer, C. A., Rhoads, J. E. and Allen, J. G. *Surgery: Principles and Practice,* 2nd Edition. Philadelphia, J. B. Lippincott Company, 1961, pp. 755–782.
162. Rhoads, J. E. Influences of Voluntary and Governmental Health Agencies in Formulating the Task of our Medical Schools. *J Med Educ* (Part II) 36:171–177, 1961.
163. Rhoads, J. E. Summation of Conference on Shock. *Fed Proc* (Part III) 20:235–237, 1961.
164. Rhoads, J. E. Diuretics as an Adjuvant in Disposing of Extra Water as a Vehicle in Parenteral Hyperalimentation (Abstract). *Fed Proc* 21:389, 1962.
165. Lehr, H. B., Rhoads, J. E., Rosenthal, O. and Blakemore, W. S. The Use of Intravenous Fat Emulsions in Surgical Patients. *JAMA* 181:745–749, 1962.
166. Miller, L. D., Mackie, J. A. and Rhoads, J. E. The Pathophysiology and Management of Intestinal Obstruction. *Surg Clin North Am* 42:1285–1307, 1962.
167. Rhoads, J. E. Foreword to a Symposium on Methods of Improving Morbidity and Mortality Rates in Standard Operations. *Surg Clin North Am* 42:1385–1386, 1962.
168. Rhoads, J. E. The Impact of the Natural Sciences upon Natural Selection. In Morris, Clarence, Ed. *Trends in Modern American Society.* (The Benjamin Franklin Lectures of the University of Pennsylvania, 7th Series). Philadelphia, The University of Pennsylvania Press, 1962, pp. 83–99.
169. Rhoads, J. E. and Howard, J. M. *The Chemistry of Trauma.* Springfield, Illinois, Charles C Thomas Company, 1963.
170. Rhoads, J. E. Fluid and Electrolyte Disturbances Associated with Surgery—General Considerations. *Am J Cardiol* 13:639, 1963.
171. Rhoads, J. E. The Acute Abdomen. *Chicago Med* 66:23:959–962, 1963.
172. Rhoads, J. E. Academic Medicine and the Seven Stages of Man. *Tex Rep Biol Med* 21:476–479, 1963.
173. Rhoads, J. E. Physiologic Approach to the Evaluation of Bleeding Problems. *Ann NY Acad Sci* 115:113–115, 1964.
174. Rhoads, J. E. Postoperative Wound Infection (Editorial). *Ann Surg* 160:332, 1964.
175. Rhoads, J. E. and Miller, L. D. Foreword to a Festschrift for Dr. Isidor Schwaner Ravdin. *Surgery* 56:604–608, 1964.
176. Dudrick, S. J., Lehr, H. B., Senior, J. R. and Rhoads, J. E. Nutritional Care of the Surgical Patient. *Med Clin North Am* 48:1253–1269, 1964.
177. Rhoads, J. E. and Mackie, J. A. Sliding Inguinal Hernia (Special Comment). In Chapter 6 in Nyhus, L. M. and Harkins, H. N., Eds. *Hernia.* Philadelphia, J. B. Lippincott Company, 1964, pp. 148–149.
178. Rhoads, J. E. Charles Franklin Mitchell, 1875–1962. *Trans Am Surg Assoc* 81:432–434, 1964.

179. Rhoads, J. E. The Peritoneum. Chapter 81 in Bockus, H. L., *Gastroenterology*, 2nd Edition, Volume II. Philadelphia, W. B. Saunders Company, 1964, pp. 1125–1135.
180. Rhoads, J. E. The Mesentery and Omentum. Chapter 84 in Bockus, H. L, *Gastroenterology*, 2nd Edition, Volume II Philadelphia, W. B. Saunders Company, 1964, pp. 1166–1184.
181. Rhoads, J. E., Rawnsley, H. M., Vars, H. M., Crichlow, R. W., Nelson, H. M., Spagna, P. M., Dudrick, S. J. and Rhoads, J. E., Jr. The Use of Diuretics as an Adjunct in Parenteral Hyperalimentation for Surgical Patients with Prolonged Disability of Gastrointestinal Tract. *Bull Int Soc Surg* 24:59–70, 1965.
182. Dudrick, S. J., Lehr, H. B., Senior, J. R. and Rhoads, J. E. Evaluation of Nutritional Care of Surgical Patients (Abstract) *Med Digest* 11:35, 1965.
183. Rhoads, J. E. and Mackie, J. A. The Colon. Chapter 27 in Nealon, T. F., Jr., *Management of the Patient with Cancer*. Philadelphia, W. B. Saunders Company, 1965, pp. 657–673.
184. Rhoads, J. E. and Schwegman, C. W. One-stage Combined Abdominoperineal Resection of the Rectum (Miles) Performed by Two Surgical Teams. *Surgery* 58:600–606, 1965.
185. Rhoads, J. E. Educational Preparation for the Medical Curriculum. *Pahlavi U Mag*, 1965.
186. Rhoads, J. E. Shock. Chapter 5 in Committee on Trauma of the American College of Surgeons. *The Management of Soft Tissue Injuries and Fractures*. Philadelphia, W. B. Saunders Company, 1965, pp. 27–43.
187. Rhoads, J. E. Introduction to the Philip Syng Physick Paper. *Medical Affairs*. The University of Pennsylvania, September 1965, p. 60.
188. Rhoads, J. E. Remarks on the Occasion of the Bicentennial of the School of Medicine of the University of Pennsylvania. *Ann Surg* 162:327–328, 1965.
189. Rhoads, J. E. Chronic Pancreatitis: Signs and Symptoms. *Bull Int Soc Surg* 24:594–619, 1965.
190. Rhoads, J. E., Allen, J. G., Harkins, H. N. and Moyer, C. A. Surgical Philosophy. Chapter 1 in Moyer, C. A., Rhoads, J. E., Allen, J. B. and Harkins, H. N. *Surgery: Principles and Practice*, 3rd Edition. Philadelphia, J. B. Lippincott Company, 1965, pp. 1–6.
191. Moyer, C. A. and Rhoads, J. E. Fluid and Electrolytes. Chapter 5 in Moyer, C. A., Rhoads, J. E., Allen, J. G. and Harkins, H. N. *Surgery: Principles and Practice*, 3rd Edition. Philadelphia, J. B. Lippincott Company, 1965, pp. 78–104.
192. Rhoads, J. E. Nutrition. Chapter 6 in Moyer, C. A., Rhoads, J. E., Allen, J. G. and Harkins, H. N. *Surgery: Principles and Practice*, 3rd Edition. Philadelphia, J. B. Lippincott Company, 1965, pp. 105–123.
193. Moyer, C. A. and Rhoads, J. E. Neoplastic Disease—General Considerations. Chapter 10 in Moyer, C. A., Rhoads, J. E., Allen, J. G. and Harkins, H. N. *Surgery: Principles and Practice*, 3rd Edition. Philadelphia, J. B. Lippincott Company, 1965, pp. 204–217.
194. Moyer, C. A. and Rhoads, J. E. Skin and Subcutaneous Tissues. Chapter 24 in Moyer, C. A., Rhoads, J. E., Allen, J. G. and Harkins, H. N. *Surgery: Principles and Practice*, 3rd Edition. Philadelphia, J. B. Lippincott Company, 1965, pp. 603–620.
195. Rhoads, J. E. Liver, Gallbladder and Bile Passages. Chapter 30 in Moyer, C. A., Rhoads, J. E., Allen, J. G. and Harkins, H. N. *Surgery: Principles and Practice*, 3rd Edition. Philadelphia, J. B. Lippincott Company, 1965, pp. 820–855.
196. Rhoads, J. E. Pancreas. Chapter 31 in Moyer, C. A., Rhoads, J. E. Allen, J G. and Harkins, H. N. *Surgery: Principles and Practice*, 3rd Edition. Philadelphia, J. B. Lippincott Company, 1965, pp. 856–884.
197. Rhoads, J. E. Diagnosis and Treatment of Cancer of the Rectum. *Fifth National Cancer Conference Proceedings*. Philadelphia, J. B. Lippincott Company, 1965, pp. 621–626.
198. Rhoads, J. E., Mackie, J. A. and Schwegman, C. W. Cancer of the Rectum. *NY State J Med* 65:3056–3059, 1965.
199. Rhoads, J. E. and Dudrick, S. J. Hypovolemic Shock—Current Clinical Concepts of Diagnosis and Management. *Postgrad Med* 39:3–10, 1966.
200. Dudrick, S. J., Vars, H. M., Rawnsley, H. M. and Rhoads, J. E. Total Intravenous Feeding and Growth in Puppies (Abstract). *Fed Proc* 25:481, 1966.
201. Rhoads, J. E., Dudrick, S. J. and Miller, L. D. Colectomy for Cancer: Technique and Pitfalls. *Surg Clin North Am* 46:1163–1177, 1966.
202. Rhoads, J. E. Surgical Treatment of Malignant Lesions of the Colon and Rectum. Chapter 18 in Blakemore, W. S. and Ravdin, I. S. Eds. *Current Perspectives in Cancer Therapy*. New York, Hoeber Medical Division of Harper & Row, Inc., 1966, pp. 144–151.
203. Rhoads, J. E., Mackie, J. A. and Curreri, P. W. Gallbladder and Bile Ducts. Chapter 25 in Ulin, A. W. and Gollub, S. S., *Surgical Bleeding*. New York, McGraw-Hill Book Company, 1966, pp. 171–178.
204. Park, C. D., Mackie, J. A. and Rhoads, J. E. Pancreaticogastrostomy. *Am J Surg* 113:85–90, 1967.
205. Rhoads, J. E. The Shift from Solo Physician to Organized Group Practice. *New Physician* 16:2, 1967.
206. Rhoads, J. E. Shock: Preoperative, Operative, Postoperative. Chapter 8 in Hawthorne, H. R. et al., Eds. *Acute Abdomen and Emergent Lesions of the Gastrointestinal Tract*. Springfield, Illinois, Charles C Thomas Company, 1967, pp. 96–103.
207. Rhoads, J. E. Surgical Treatment of Carcinoma of the Pancreas. Chapter 16 in Blakemore, W. S. and Ferguson, L. K. *Current Perspectives in Gastroenterology*. New York, Hoeber Medical Division of Harper & Row, 1967, pp. 144–149.
208. Rhoads, J. E. The Relationship of the Council of Academic Societies to the Association of American Medical Colleges (Editorial). *Arch Environ Health* 15:273–274, 1967.

209. Dudrick, S. J., Vars, H. M. and Rhoads, J. E. Growth of Puppies Receiving All Nutritional Requirements by Vein. *Fortschr Parent Ernährung*, pp. 1–4, 1967.
210. Berkowitz, H. D., Bovee, K., Miller, L. D., Itskovitz, H. D. and Rhoads, J. E. Renal Function and Intrarenal Blood Distribution in the Isolated Kidney (Abstract). *Fed Proc* 27:630, 1968.
211. Dudrick, S. J., Wilmore, D. W., Vars, H. M. and Rhoads, J. E. Long-term Total Parenteral Nutrition with Growth, Development, and Positive Nitrogen Balance. *Surgery* 64:134, 1968.
212. Dudrick, S. J., Wilmore, D. W., Vars, H. M. and Rhoads, J. E. Long Term Total I.V. Feeding Will Maintain Growth (Abstract). *Mod Med* 36:134–142, 1968.
213. Wilmore, D. W., Dudrick, S. J., Vars, H. M. and Rhoads, J. E. Long-term Intravenous Hyperalimentation (Abstract). *Fed Proc* 27:486, 1968.
214. Rhoads, J. E. Francis Clark Grant, 1891–1967. *Trans Am Surg Assoc* 86:477–479, 1968.
215. Dudrick, S. J., Wilmore, D. W., Steiger, E. and Rhoads, J. E. Reversal of Uremia and Body Wasting with Intravenous Essential Amino Acids (Abstract). *Fed Proc* 28:808, 1968.
216. Steiger, E., Wilmore, D. W., Dudrick, S. J. and Rhoads, J. E. Total Intravenous Nutrition in the Management of Inflammatory Disease of the Intestinal Tract (Abstract). *Fed Proc* 28:808, 1968.
217. Rhoads, J. E., Dudrick, S. J. and Miller, L. D. Colectomy for Cancer: Technic and Pitfalls (Abstract). *Year Book of Cancer*, 1967–1968 Series. Chicago, Year Book Medical Publishers, Inc., c1968, pp. 167–168.
218. Rhoads, J. E. Approaches to an Artificial Gastrointestinal Tract. *Am J Surg* 117:3–10, 1969.
219. Dudrick, S. J., Wilmore, D. W., Vars, H. M. and Rhoads, J. E. Can Intravenous Feeding as the Sole Means of Nutrition Support Growth in the Child and Restore Weight Loss in an Adult?—An Affirmative Answer. *Ann Surg* 169:974–984, 1969.
220. Tsou, K. C., Vucicevic, Z. M., Miller, E. E., Scheie, H. G. and Rhoads, J. E. A Cytochemical Approach to Ruby Laser Microsurgery: Preliminary Study in Tissue Culture and Rabbit Eye. *Surg Forum* 20:487–488, 1969.
221. Pitman, G. H. and Rhoads, J. E. Osteitis Deformans (Paget's Disease of Bone) Complicating Hypoparathyroidism. *Ann Surg* 170:286–291, 1969.
222. Reber, H. A., Wolf, C. J. and Rhoads, J. E. Permeability Characteristics of the Main Pancreatic Duct (Abstract). *Fed Proc* 28:274, 1969.
223. Rhoads, J. E. Detection and Diagnosis of Carcinoma of the Breast. *Cancer* 24:1182, 1969.
224. Steiger, E., Dudrick, S. J., Daly, J. M., Wilmore, D. W., Vars, H. M. and Rhoads, J. E. Growth and Development of Puppies Nourished Intravenously with Crystalline Amino Acids as the Sole Source of Dietary Nitrogen (Abstract). *Fed Proc* 29:2, 1970.
225. Dudrick, S. J., Long, J. M., Steiger, E. and Rhoads, J. E. Intravenous Hyperalimentation. *Med Clin North Am* 54:577–589, 1970.
226. Rhoads, J. E. Current Techniques in Surgical Management of Cancer of the Colon and Rectum. *Sixth National Cancer Conference Proceedings*. Philadelphia, J. B. Lippincott Company, 1970, pp. 455–458.
227. Rhoads, J. E., Allen, J. G., Harkins, H. N. and Moyer, C. A. Surgical Philosophy. Chapter 1 in Rhoads, J. E., Allen, J. G., Harkins, H. N. and Moyer, C. A. *Surgery: Principles and Practice*, 4th Edition. Philadelphia, J. B. Lippincott Company, 1970, pp. 1–7.
228. Moyer, C. A. and Rhoads, J. E. Fluid and Electrolytes. Chapter 5 in Rhoads, J. E., Allen, J. G., Harkins, H. N. and Moyer, C. A. *Surgery: Principles and Practice*, 4th Edition. Philadelphia, J. B. Lippincott Company, 1970, pp. 75–100.
229. Rhoads, J. E. Nutrition. Chapter 6 in Rhoads, J. E., Allen, J. G., Harkins, H. N. and Moyer, C. A. *Surgery: Principles and Practice*, 4th Edition. Philadelphia, J. B. Lippincott Company, 1970, pp. 101–120.
230. Harkins, H. N. and Rhoads, J. E. Shock. Chapter 7 in Rhoads, J. E., Allen, J. G., Harkins, H. N. and Moyer, C. A. *Surgery: Principles and Practice*, 4th Edition. Philadelphia, J. B. Lippincott Company, 1970, pp. 121–148.
231. Moyer, C. A. and Rhoads, J. E. Neoplastic Disease—General Considerations. Chapter 10 in Rhoads, J. E., Allen, J. G., Harkins, H. N. and Moyer, C. A. *Surgery: Principles and Practice*, 4th Edition. Philadelphia, J. B. Lippincott Company, 1970, pp. 209–223.
232. Moyer, C. A. and Rhoads, J. E. Skin and Subcutaneous Tissues. Chapter 26 in Rhoads, J. E., Allen, J. G., Harkins, H. N. and Moyer, C. A. *Surgery: Principles and Practice*, 4th Edition. Philadelphia, J. B. Lippincott Company, 1970, pp. 649–667.
233. Rhoads, J. E. Liver, Gallbladder and Bile Passages. Chapter 32 in Rhoads, J. E., Allen, J. G., Harkins, H. N. and Moyer, C. A. *Surgery: Principles and Practice*, 4th Edition. Philadelphia, J. B. Lippincott Company, 1970, pp. 880–915.
234. Rhoads, J. E. Pancreas. Chapter 33 in Rhoads, J. E., Allen, J. G., Harkins, H. N. and Moyer, C. A. *Surgery: Principles and Practice*, 4th Edition. Philadelphia, J. B. Lippincott Company, 1970, pp. 916–946.
235. Dudrick, S. J., Wilmore, D. W., Steiger, E., Vars, H. M. and Rhoads, J. E. Intravenous Essential Amino Acids and Hypertonic Glucose in the Treatment of Renal Failure. In Berg, G., Ed. *Advances in Parenteral Nutrition*. Stuttgart, Georg Thieme Verlag, 1970, pp. 152–165.
236. Rhoads, J. E. Introduction: Proceedings of an International Symposium. In Meng, H. C. and Law, D. H., Eds. *Parenteral Nutrition*. Springfield, Charles C Thomas, 1970, pp. 8–12.
237. Dudrick, S. J., Steiger, E., Long, J. M. and Rhoads, J. E. Role of Parenteral Hyperalimentation in Management of Multiple Catastrophic Complications. *Surg Clin North Am* 50:1031–1038, 1970.

238. Dudrick, S. J., Steiger, E., Long, J. M. and Rhoads, J. E. The Use of Carbohydrates and Proteolysates for Long-term Parenteral Feeding. Chapter 4 in Fox, C. L., Jr. and Nahas, G. G. *Body Fluid Replacement in the Surgical Patient.* New York, Columbia University Press, 1970, pp. 301–313.
239. Dudrick, S. J. and Rhoads, J. E. New Horizons for Intravenous Feeding. *JAMA* 215:939–949, 1971.
240. Rhoads, J. E. Surgical Societies: The Role of the American College of Surgeons in the Continuing Education of the Surgeon. Chapter 2 in Barker, H. G., Ed. *The Continuing Education of the Surgeon (Transactions of the 12th Annual Meeting of the Allen O. Whipple Surgical Society).* Springfield, Charles C Thomas, 1971, pp. 22–32.
241. Ruberg, R. L., Dudrick, S. J., Long, J. M., Allen, T. R., Steiger, E. and Rhoads, J. E. Pre- and Postoperative Nutrition Using Crystalline Amino Acids as the Sole Source of Nitrogen (Abstract). *Fed Proc* 30:2, 1971.
242. Rhoads, J. E. Surgical Treatment of Precancerous Lesions of the Rectum and Colon. *Chirurg Gastroenterol* 5:229–230, 1971.
243. Rhoads, J. E. Management of Colon and Rectal Cancer, and Polyps. *Cancer* 28:144, 1971.
244. Saik, R. P., Walz, C. A. and Rhoads, J. E. Evaluation of a Bacitracin-Neomycin Surgical Skin Preparation. *Am J Surg* 121:557–560, 1971.
245. Rhoads, J. E. Preparation of Surgeons for Academic Responsibilities at Home and Abroad. *J Royal Coll Surg Edinburgh* 16:225–229, 1971.
246. Dudrick, S. J. and Rhoads, J. E. Intravenous Hyperalimentation. Chapter 30 in Hardy, J. D., Ed. *Critical Surgical Illness.* Philadelphia, W. B. Saunders Company, 1971, pp. 654–665.
247. Rhoads, J. E. The Horizons and the Clouds in Surgery. *Ann Royal Coll Surg England* 49:212–214, 1971.
248. Rhoads, J. E. Special Problems of Fluids in Septic Shock. Chapter 19 in Hershey, S. J., DelGuercio, L. R. M., McConn, R., Eds. *Septic Shock in Man.* Boston, Little Brown and Company, 1971, pp. 265–269.
249. Dudrick, S. J., Long, J., Steiger, E. and Rhoads, J. E. Technique of Long-term Parenteral Nutrition. In Lang, K., Fekl W. and Berg, G. *Balanced Nutrition and Therapy.* Stuttgart, Georg Thieme Verlag, 1971, pp. 138–150.
250. Rhoads, J. E. National Health Policies for Improving the Care of the Surgical Patient. *Bull Am Coll Surg* 56:7–10, 1971.
251. Rhoads, J. E. Alimentary and Metabolic Life Support Techniques: Long-term Parenteral Alimentary Support. *Transplantation Proc* 3:1503–1507, 1971.
252. Rhoads, J. E. Does the Present Status of Cancer Research Warrant the Funding Proposed? *Cincinnati J Med* 53:23–27, 1972.
253. MacFadyen, B. V., Dudrick, S. J., Maynard, A. T., Law, D. and Rhoads, J. E. Triglyceride and Free Fatty Acid Clearances in Patients Receiving Complete Parenteral Hyperalimentation with 10% Soybean Oil Emulsion (Abstract). *Fed Proc* 31:716, 1972.
254. Dudrick, S. J. and Rhoads, J. E. Total Intravenous Feeding. *Sci Am* 226:73–80, 1972.
255. Rhoads, J. E. The Role of the Surgeon in Health Maintenance Organizations. *Trans Southern Surg Assoc* 83:152–158, 1971. *Ann Surg* 175:752–758, 1972.
256. Dudrick, S. J. and Rhoads, J. E. Metabolism in Surgical Patients: Protein, Carbohydrate and Fat Utilization by Oral and Parenteral Routes. Chapter 7 in *Davis-Christopher Textbook of Surgery,* 10th Edition. Philadelphia, W. B. Saunders Company, 1972, pp. 147–174.
257. Rhoads, J. E. The Contribution of the Surgeon to Preclinical Sciences. *Langenbecks Archiv fur Chirurgie.* Berlin, Springer-Verlag, 1972, pp. 561–562.
258. Rhoads, J. E. National Health Policies. *Med Affairs* (University of Pennsylvania) Winter 1972, pp. 3–7.
259. Dudrick, S. J., Steiger, E., Long, J. M., Ruberg, R. L., Allen, T. R., Vars, H. M. and Rhoads, J. E. Chapter: General Principles and Technique of Administration in Complete Parenteral Nutrition. *Intravenous Hyperalimentation* G. F. Cowan, Jr. and W. L. Scheetz, Eds. Philadelphia, Lea and Febiger, 1972, pp. 222–233.
260. Dudrick, S. J., Steiger, E., Long, J. M., Ruberg, R. L., Allen, T. R., Vars, H. M. and Rhoads, J. E. Introduction. In Cowan, G. F., Jr. and Scheetz, W. L., Eds. *Intravenous Hyperalimentation.* Philadelphia, Lea and Febiger, 1972, pp. 3–14.
261. Rhoads, J. E. In Memoriam: I. S. Ravdin, M. D., 1894–1972. *Phila Med* 68:848, 1972.
262. Rhoads, J. E. In Memoriam: John H. Gibbon, Jr., M. D. 1903–1973. *Phila Med* 69:216–217, 1973.
263. Rhoads, J. E. Joseph Stokes, Jr. (1896–1972). *Year Book, American Philosophical Society 1972.* Philadelphia, George H. Buchanan Company, 1973, pp. 239–244.
264. Rhoads, J. E. and Dudrick, S. J. Weight Gain, Growth, and Development Induced in Man by the Intravenous Administration of Pure Chemicals. *Proc Am Philosophical Soc* 117:152–161, 1973.
265. Rhoads, J. E. Memoir of John W. Bransfield, 1888–1973. *Trans Stud Coll Physicians Phila* 41:37, 1973.
266. Rhoads, J. E. Writing for the Readers. *Med Communications* 2:3–6, 1973.
267. Rhoads, J. E. Memoir of Samuel Emlen Stokes, 1894–1973. *Trans Stud Coll Physicians Phila* 41:148–149, 1973.
268. Rhoads, J. E. The Quality of Surgical Scholarship. *Ann Surg* 178:227–231, 1973.
269. MacFadyan, B. V., Jr., Dudrick, S. J., Tagudar, E. P., Maynard, A. T., Law, D. K. and Rhoads, J. E. Triglyceride and Free Fatty Acid Clearances in Patients Receiving Complete Parenteral Nutrition Using a Ten per cent Soybean Oil Emulsion. *Surg Gynec Obstet* 137:813–815, 1973.
270. Rhoads, J. E. and Rhoads, G. G. Preventive Cancer Surgery. Chapter 13 in Raven, R. W., Ed.

Modern Trends in Oncology—1. Part Two: Clinical Progress. London, Butterworths, 1973, pp. 281–293.

271. Rhoads, J. E. Address to New Diplomates of the Royal College of Surgeons of Edinburgh. *J Royal Coll Surg Edinburgh* 18:380–383, 1973.
272. Rhoads, J. E. Memoir of John Heysham Gibbon, Jr., 1903–1973. *Trans Stud Coll Physicians Phila* 41:194–197, 1974.
273. Johnson, J. and Rhoads, J. E. Memoir: I. S. Ravdin, 1894–1972. *Trans Am Surg Assoc* 91:69–72, 1973.
274. Rhoads, J. E. Memoir: I. S. Ravdin, 1894–1972. *Trans Southern Surg Assoc* 84:350–352, 1973.
275. Rhoads, J. E. Fission and Fusion in the Field of Surgery. *Laryngoscope* 84:1741–1747, 1974.
276. Rhoads, J. E. A Clinician's View of the Cancer Problem. *Cancer* 35:705–709, 1975.
277. Mackie, J. A., Rhoads, J. E. and Park, C. D. Pancreaticogastrostomy: A Further Evaluation. *Ann Surg* 181:541–545, 1975. *Trans Southern Surg Assoc* 86:55–59, 1975.
278. Rhoads, J. E. Introduction: The History of Intravenous Nutrition. In Committee on Pre- and Postoperative Care of the American College of Surgeons *Manual of Surgical Nutrition.* Philadelphia, W. B. Saunders Company, 1975, pp. 1–9.
279. Rhoads, J. E. The Control of Large Bowel Cancer: Present Status and Its Challenges. *Cancer* 36:2314–2318, 1975.
280. Mackie, J. A. and Rhoads, J. E. Pancreaticogastrostomy following Radical Pancreaticoduodenal Resection. *Bull Soc Int Chir* 34:303–304, 1975.
281. Rhoads, J. E. Preliminary Remarks for the Symposium on New Approaches in the Study of Neoplasia. *Proc Am Philosophical Soc* 120:67–68, 1976.
282. Rhoads, J. E. Surgery for the Tricentennial. In *Philadelphia: A Medical Panorama of 200 Years, 1776–1976.* Philadelphia, Philadelphia County Medical Society, 1976, pp. 104–106.
283. Rhoads, J. E. and Mackie, J. A. The Colon. Chapter 26 in Nealon, T. F., Jr., *Management of the Patient with Cancer.* 2nd Edition. Philadelphia, W. B. Saunders Company, 1976, pp. 524–541.
284. Rhoads, J. E. Foreword. In Committee on Control of Surgical Infections of the Committee on Pre- and Postoperative Care of the American College of Surgeons. *Manual on Control of Infection in Surgical Patients.* Philadelphia, J. B. Lippincott Company, 1976, pp. v–vi.
285. Rhoads, J. E. History and Bases of Parenteral Nutrition. *Proceedings of the International Congress of Parenteral Nutrition.* Montpellier, University de Montpellier, 1976, pp. 13–16.
286. Rhoads, J. E. and Rhoads, J. E., Jr. The Peritoneum. Chapter 147 in Bockus, H. L., Ed. *Gastroenterology,* 3rd Edition, Vol. 4. Philadelphia, W. B. Saunders Company, 1976, pp. 33–47.
287. Rhoads, J. E. Nutrition: The General Principles of Nutrition. Chapter 11 in Hardy, James D., Ed. *Rhoads Textbook of Surgery: Principles and Practice,* 5th Edition, Vol. 1. Philadelphia, J. B. Lippincott Company, 1977, pp. 149–156.
288. Dudrick, S. J. and Rhoads, J. E. Metabolism in Surgical Patients: Protein, Carbohydrate and Fat Utilization by Oral and Parenteral Routes. *Davis-Christopher Textbook of Surgery,* 11th Edition. Philadelphia, W. B. Saunders Company, 1977, pp. 150–171.
289. Tsou, K. C., Lo, K. W., Rhoads, J. E. and Mackie, J. A. An Electroncytochemical Study of 5'-Nucleotide Phosphodiesterase in Hepatoma, Cirrhosis and Hepatitis. In Chapter 3 Nieburgs, H. E., Ed., *Prevention and Detection of Cancer,* Part I, Vol. 1. New York, Marcel Dekker, Inc., 1977, pp. 331–342.
290. Rhoads, J. E. Some Advances in Clinical Practice. *Yale J Biol Med* 50:245–251, 1977.
291. Rhoads, J. E. The Long-Range Goals of the National Cancer Plan. *Cancer* 40:2572–2575, 1977.
292. Mackie, J. A. and Rhoads, J. E. The Restoration of Pancreatic Flow by Pancreaticogastrostomy following Whipple Resection. *Chir Gastroenterol* 11:347–352, 1977.
293. Rhoads, J. E. Charles Harrison Frazier, M.D., 1870–1936. *Surg Neurol* 7:5:254, 1977.
294. Rhoads, J. E. Loren C. Eiseley (1907–1977). *The American Philosophical Society Year Book, 1978.* Philadelphia, George H. Buchanan Company, 1978, pp. 73–77.
295. Rhoads, J. E. Memoir of Robert C. Horn, Jr. (1913–1976). *Trans Stud Coll Physicians Phila* 45(5):292–293, 1978.
296. Rhoads, J. E. Memoir of J. Montgomery Deaver, 1901–1978. *Trans Stud Coll Physicians Phila* 1(1):75–77, 1979.
297. Rhoads, J. E. and Paskin, D. L. Patients Made Operable by Intravenous Hyperalimentation. *JPEN* 3:5:372–373, 1979.
298. Rhoads, J. E. and Paskin, D. L. Certain Surgical Patients Made Operable by Intravenous Hyperalimentation. *Acta Chir Scand Suppl* 1979, pp. 226–227.
299. Rhoads, J. E. The Impact of Nutrition on Infection. *Surg Clin North Am* 60:1:41–47, 1980.
300. Rhoads, J. E. Memoir of Lessing J. Rosenwald, 1891–1979. *Trans Stud Coll Physicians Phila* 5(2):71–73, 1980.
301. Rhoads, J. E. Past and Future Role of the Organ Site Programs. *Cancer* 45:6:1090–1092, 1980.
302. Rhoads, J. E. The Right to Die and the Chance to Live. *J Med Ethics* 6:53–54, 1980.
303. Rhoads, J. E. Development of Surgical Nutrition at the University of Pennsylvania. *JPEN* 4(5):464–466, 1980.
304. Rhoads, J. E. Memoir of William Thomas Fitts, Jr., 1915–1980. *Trans Stud Coll Physicians Phila* 5(2):319–321, 1980.
305. Rhoads, J. E. J. Montgomery Deaver, 1901–1978. *Trans Am Surg Assoc* 98:60–62, 1980.
306. Rhoads, J. E. Thoughts about Cancer Research from a Surgical Viewpoint. In Fortner, J. G. and Rhoads, J. E., Eds. *Accomplishments in Cancer Research 1980.* Philadelphia, J. B. Lippincott Company, 1980, pp. 159–167.

307. Rhoads, J. E., Vars, H. M. and Dudrick, S. J. The Development of Intravenous Hyperalimentation. Chapter in Mullen, J. L. et al. *Surgical Nutrition and Metabolism.* Surgical Clinics of North America, Philadelphia, W. B. Saunders and Company, 1981, pp. 429–435.

308. Dudrick, S. J. and Rhoads, J. E. Metabolism in Surgical Patients: Protein, Carbohydrate and Fat Utilization by Oral and Parenteral Routes. *Davis-Christopher Textbook of Surgery,* 12th Edition. Philadelphia, W. B. Saunders Company, 1981, pp. 144–171.

309. Rhoads, J. E. The Evolution of Intravenous Hyperalimentation. *World J Surg* 6:144–148, 1982.

310. Rhoads, J. E. History of the Founding of the Society of Surgical Chairmen. *Trans Stud Coll Physicians Phila* 5(4):87–97, 1982.

311. Rhoads, J. E. Memoir of George Washington Corner, 1889–1981. *Trans Stud Coll Physicians Phila* 5(4):162–165, 1982.

312. Rhoads, J. E. Prize Selection Process. Fortner, J. G. and Rhoads, J. E., Eds., *Accomplishments in Cancer Research 1981.* J. B. Lippincott Co. 1982, p. 6.

313. Rhoads, J. E. Foreword to Alexander-Williams, J. and Irving, M. *Intestinal Fistulas.* John Wright & Sons Ltd., Bristol, 1982.

314. Rhoads, J. E. Foreword in Silberman, H. and Eisenberg, D. *Parenteral and Enteral Nutrition for the Hospitalized Patient.* Appleton-Century-Crofts, 1982.

315. Chang, A. E. and Rhoads, J. E. Malignant Duodenocolic Fistulas: A Case Report and Reivew of the Literature, *J Surg Onc* 21:33–36, 1982.

316. Rhoads, J. E. Academic Pitfalls in America—1907–1982. *J Surg Onc* 21:74–80, 1982.

317. Rhoads, J. E. Memoir of Herbert Reid Hawthorne, 1894–1981 *Trans Am Surg Assoc* 100:90–92, 1982.

318. Rhoads, J. E. *Preface* for Rombeau, J. L. and Caldwell, M. D., Eds. *Clinical Nutrition: Enteral and Tube Feeding,* Vol. I. W. B. Saunders Co. 1982.

319. Rhoads, J. E. *Foreword,* Cook, John, Ed. *Collected Papers of the International Federation of Surgical Colleges.* 1982.

320. Rhoads, J. E. The Prize Selection Process. Fortner, J. G. and Rhoads, J. E.. Eds, *Accomplishments in Cancer Research 1982.* J. B. Lippincott Co., 1983, pp. 9–10.

321. Caroline, D. F., Creteur, V., Kressel, H. Y. and Rhoads, J. E. Verification of Superficial Biopsy Sites by Barium Enema. *Am J Roentgenology* 140:945–946, 1983.

322. Rhoads, J. E. Chapter in The History and Development of Nutritional Assessment of the Hospitalized Patient, in *Nutritional Assessment.* Wright, R. A., Ed., Butterworth, 1983.

323. Rhoads, J. E. *Editorial,* Preventive Surgery, *Oncology,* 1983.

324. Rhoads, J. E. Contribution to the Memorial Issue, *Cancer Detection and Prevention,* 1983.

325. Rhoads, J. E. Contracoastal Views of the Surgery of the Pancreas. *Surgical Rounds* 7(10):66–74, Oct. 1984.

326. Rhoads, J. E. *Book Review, Principles of Surgery—4th Edition,* Schwartz, S. I., Shires, G. T., Spencer, F. C., and Storer, E. H. McGraw Hill Book Co., 1984.

327. Rhoads, J. E. *Review, Conservative Management of Breast Cancer: New Surgical and Radiotherapeutic Techniques,* Harris, J. R., Hellman, S., Silen, W. J. B. Lippincott Co, 1983. (For the *New Eng J of Med,* 1984)

328. Rhoads, J. E. Greetings to the Symposium of Parenteral and Enteral Nutrition, Japan, November 16–17, 1983, *Parenteral and Enteral Hyperalimentation,* Ogoshi, S. and Okada, A., Eds. Elsevier Science Publishing Co. Inc., 1984.

329. Rhoads, J. E. Gastrointestinal Surgery: Then and Now. *Am J Surg* Vol 149: 15–22, Jan 1985.

330. Rhoads, J. E. William A. Altemeier, M. D.: Surgeon & Bacteriologist. *Arch Surg* Vol 120:13–16, Jan 1985.

331. Rhoads, J. E. *Overview,* Long-Term Total Parenteral Nutrition with Growth Development and Positive Nitrogen Balance, Dudrick, S. J., Wilmore, D. W., Vars, H. M. and Rhoads, J. E. *Contemporary Nutrition,* July/Aug 1985.

332. Rhoads, J. E. *Overview, Surgical Treatment of Digestive Disease,* Moody, F., Skinner, D., et al, Eds. Year Book Publishers, Oct 1985.

333. Rhoads, J. E. *Overview, Nutritional and Metabolic Support of Hospitalized Patients,* Bernard, M. A., Jacobs, D. O., Rombeau, J. W. B. Saunders Co., 1985.

334. Rhoads, J. E., Mackie, J. A. Chapter on The Colon, *Management of the Patient with Cancer,* 3rd Edition, Nealon Jr., T. F., Ed. W. B. Saunders Co, 1985.

335. Rhoads, J. E. Memoir: Luther L. Terry, 1911–1985. *Trans Stud Coll Physicians Phila.,* 7(4):91–93, 1985.

336. Rhoads, J. E. *Foreword and Chapter, Clinical Nutrition: Total Parenteral Nutrition,* Vol. II, Rombeau, J. L. and Caldwell, M. D., Eds. W. B. Saunders Co., 1986.

337. Rhoads, J. E. Memoir: Maurice B. Visscher. American Philosophical Society, 1986.

338. Rhoads, J. E. *Preface, Current Aspects of Total Parenteral Nutrition,* Okada, A. (in press).

339. Rhoads, J. E. The History of Surgery of the Pancreas, *Surgical Diseases of the Pancreas,* Howard J. M., Jordan, Jr., G. L. and Reber, H. A., Eds. Lea and Ferbiger, pp. 3–10, 1987.

340. Rhoads, J. E. Introductory *Statement, Nutrition and Cancer: Etiology and Therapy,* Michael M. Meguid, Guest Ed., Surg. Cl of N.A., W. B. Saunders Co.

341. Rhoads, J. E. *Foreword, Atlas of Nutritional Support Techniques,* Rombeau, J. L., Caldwell, M. D., et al Eds. (in press).

342. Rhoads, J. E. Memoir—Julian Johnson, M. D. *Transactions and Studies, The College of Physicians of Philadelphia* (in press).

343. Rhoads, J. E. Memoir—Julian Johnson, M. D. *Transactions of the American Surgical Association* (in press).